Ethnopharmacological Investigation of Indian Spices

Neha Mishra
Sam Higginbottom University of Agriculture, Technology, and Sciences, India

A volume in the Advances in Medical Diagnosis, Treatment, and Care (AMDTC) Book Series

IGI Global
DISSEMINATOR OF KNOWLEDGE

Published in the United States of America by
IGI Global
Medical Information Science Reference (an imprint of IGI Global)
701 E. Chocolate Avenue
Hershey PA, USA 17033
Tel: 717-533-8845
Fax: 717-533-8661
E-mail: cust@igi-global.com
Web site: http://www.igi-global.com

Library of Congress Cataloging-in-Publication Data

Names: Mishra, Neha, 1984- editor.
Title: Ethnopharmacological investigation of Indian spices / Neha Mishra, editor.
Description: Hershey, PA : Medical Information Science Reference, [2020] | Includes bibliographical references and index. | Summary: “”This book explores the biosynthesis, phytochemistry, and pharmacology of Indian spices”--Provided by publisher.
Identifiers: LCCN 2019040958 (print) | LCCN 2019040959 (ebook) | ISBN 9781799825241 (hardcover) | ISBN 9781799825258 (ebook)
Subjects: MESH: Spices | Ethnopharmacology--methods | Plant, Medicinal--chemistry | India
Classification: LCC SB305 (print) | LCC SB305 (ebook) | NLM QV 752 | DDC 641.3/383--dc23
LC record available at https://lccn.loc.gov/2019040958
LC ebook record available at https://lccn.loc.gov/2019040959

This book is published in the IGI Global book series Advances in Medical Diagnosis, Treatment, and Care (AMDTC) (ISSN: 2475-6628; eISSN: 2475-6636)

British Cataloguing in Publication Data
A Cataloguing in Publication record for this book is available from the British Library.

For electronic access to this publication, please contact: eresources@igi-global.com.

Advances in Medical Diagnosis, Treatment, and Care (AMDTC) Book Series

ISSN:2475-6628
EISSN:2475-6636

Mission

Advancements in medicine have prolonged the life expectancy of individuals all over the world. Once life-threatening conditions have become significantly easier to treat and even cure in many cases. Continued research in the medical field will further improve the quality of life, longevity, and wellbeing of individuals.

The **Advances in Medical Diagnosis, Treatment, and Care (AMDTC)** book series seeks to highlight publications on innovative treatment methodologies, diagnosis tools and techniques, and best practices for patient care. Comprised of comprehensive resources aimed to assist professionals in the medical field apply the latest innovations in the identification and management of medical conditions as well as patient care and interaction, the books within the AMDTC series are relevant to the research and practical needs of medical practitioners, researchers, students, and hospital administrators.

Coverage

- Disease Prevention
- Diagnostic Medicine
- Cancer Treatment
- Disease Management
- Internal Medicine
- Patient Interaction
- Alternative Medicine
- Medical Procedures
- Medical Testing
- Patient-Centered Care

IGI Global is currently accepting manuscripts for publication within this series. To submit a proposal for a volume in this series, please contact our Acquisition Editors at Acquisitions@igi-global.com or visit: http://www.igi-global.com/publish/.

The Advances in Medical Diagnosis, Treatment, and Care (AMDTC) Book Series (ISSN 2475-6628) is published by IGI Global, 701 E. Chocolate Avenue, Hershey, PA 17033-1240, USA, www.igi-global.com. This series is composed of titles available for purchase individually; each title is edited to be contextually exclusive from any other title within the series. For pricing and ordering information please visit http://www.igi-global.com/book-series/advances-medical-diagnosis-treatment-care/129618. Postmaster: Send all address changes to above address.

Titles in this Series

For a list of additional titles in this series, please visit: www.igi-global.com/book-series/advances-medical-diagnosis-treatment-care/129618

Ethnomedicinal Plant Use and Practice in Traditional Medicine
Akash (Gurukul Kangri University, India) Navneet (Gurukul Kangri University, India) and B.S. Bhandari (Garhwal University, India)
Medical Information Science Reference • © 2020 • 300pp • H/C (ISBN: 9781799813200) • US $295.00

Interdisciplinary Approaches to Altering Neurodevelopmental Disorders
Tanu Wadhera (Dr. B. R. Ambedkar National Institute of Technology, Jalandhar, India) and Deepti Kakkar (Dr. B. R. Ambedkar National Institute of Technology, Jalandhar, India)
Medical Information Science Reference • © 2020 • 300pp • H/C (ISBN: 9781799830696) • US $295.00

Advanced Pharmacological Uses of Medicinal Plants and Natural Products
Ajeet Singh (National Dairy Research Institute, India) Padam Singh (Vaccine and Infectious Disease Research Centre, Translational Health Science and Technology Institute, India) and Navneet Bithel (Gurukul Kangri University, India)
Medical Information Science Reference • © 2020 • 540pp • H/C (ISBN: 9781799820949) • US $425.00

Quality Control of Cellular Protein in Neurodegenerative Disorders
Md. Sahab Uddin (Southeast University, Bangladesh) and Ghulam Md. Ashraf (King Abdulaziz University, Saudi Arabia)
Medical Information Science Reference • © 2020 • 515pp • H/C (ISBN: 9781799813170) • US $295.00

Multidimensional Perspectives and Global Analysis of Universal Health Coverage
Yeter Demir Uslu (Istanbul Medipol University, Turkey) Hasan Dinçer (Istanbul Medipol University, Turkey) and Serhat Yüksel (İstanbul Medipol University, Turkey)
Medical Information Science Reference • © 2020 • 499pp • H/C (ISBN: 9781799823292) • US $265.00

Examining Biological Foundations of Human Behavior
Barre Vijaya Prasad (Dharwad Institute of Mental Health and Neurosciences, India)
Medical Information Science Reference • © 2020 • 266pp • H/C (ISBN: 9781799828600) • US $285.00

Handbook of Research on Medical Interpreting
Izabel E.T. de V. Souza (Osaka University, Japan) and Effrossyni (Effie) Fragkou (National and Kapodistrian University of Athens, Greece)
Medical Information Science Reference • © 2020 • 511pp • H/C (ISBN: 9781522593089) • US $345.00

IGI Global
DISSEMINATOR OF KNOWLEDGE

701 East Chocolate Avenue, Hershey, PA 17033, USA
Tel: 717-533-8845 x100 • Fax: 717-533-8661
E-Mail: cust@igi-global.com • www.igi-global.com

Table of Contents

Detailed Table of Contents

Spices take an important place in common man's everyday life mainly because of their flavor, taste, and medicinal values. Spice usage grew with the increased use of processed products. India is the largest producer of spices in the world. Growth in Indian spices and spice product exports clearly show that Indian spices and spice products have a great demand in international markets. India is the land of spices and could exploit the fast-growing nutraceutical sector with its high intrinsic quality spices. The scope of spices like turmeric, ginger, fenugreek, garlic, and red pepper in the nutraceutical industry with their possible role in the control and prevention of important health disorders are examined. The demand for nutraceutical products has gone up as more people are turning to natural products for treating lifestyle diseases. This review deals with the history and origin of spices and their potential uses as well as future prospects in treatment of various diseases in a natural way.

Plants, principally spices and herbs, have been given much more attention because they are considered important for flavoring and coloring foods and their use as condiments. Herbs and spices have been used for generations by humans as food and also to treat ailments since they are full of medicinal and antioxidant properties and contain bioactive compounds like tannins, alkaloids, phenolics, flavonoids, polyphenols, and vitamins, which help in healing diseases. Spices and herbs contain biomolecules that play a crucial role in healthcare and fitness levels. Spices and herbs have been considered as esoteric food adjuncts as they play numerous roles like being coloring agents, flavoring agents, preservatives, food additives, and having uses in the medicinal and pharmaceutical industries.

The term "spices" has been derived from the word "species," which was connected to the group of exotic foods in medieval times. Spices and herbs have a long history of culinary use, medicinal properties, and as additives and thus have a distinct place in Ayurveda. Exhibiting the merits of spices by scientific methods still remains a challenge. This review investigates the anti-diabetic properties in preventing and managing diabetics and associated complications with commonly used spices. The bioactive compounds in these spices are additionally discussed. The major aim and object of the present work is to investigate the customary therapeutic usage of basic Indian spices and to corelate their observed pharmacological activities with the presence of explicit bioactive compounds present for the treatment or counteractive action of diabetes. This includes the basic underlying mechanism of their blood glucose lowering property including exploratory experimental evidence from proposed animal and human trials.

Myristica fragrans or nutmeg is a ground spice of the family Myristicaceae. Its tree has dark leaves mainly cultivated in Grenada, Malaysia, and Kerala. It is majorly a source of two spices derived from its fruit: nutmeg (jaiphal) from its seed and mace (javitri) from the covering of seed. The important bioactive constituents present in nutmeg include macelignan, carvacrol, myristicin, β-caryophyllene, β-pinene, α-pinene, p-cymene, and eugenol. Low doses of nutmeg do not cause any side effects whereas after consuming 5g toxic overdose occurs, and central nervous system (CNS) effects were induced after consuming 1 to 2 mg/kg b.wt. of nutmeg. Various therapeutic or medicinal applications were shown by nutmeg such as antioxidant, antimicrobial, aphrodisiac, anticancer, hepatoprotective, anti-inflammatory, antidepressant, and cardioprotective activity. This review chapter focuses on ethnobotany, phytochemistry, acceptable daily intake, and different pharmacological actions of this medicinal plant.

Ginger (Zingiber officinale) has been traditionally employed in south East Asia as well as India and China for treatment of nausea, asthma, fever, vomiting, cough, constipation, pain, arthritis, inflammation, etc. This chapter discusses the phytochemical composition and pharmacological studies of ginger extracts, ginger essential oil (GEO), and active bioactive constituents. The essential oil of fresh and dry ginger was ranged between 0.2% - 2.62% and 0.72% - 4.17% respectively. The bioactive constituent zingiberene, β-sesquiphellandrene, curcumene, β-bisabolene, β-farnesene, camphene, and gingerol and shogal are the major constituents in ginger extracts. These compounds are chief bioactive substances responsible for pharmacological activities such antioxidant, antidiabetic, anticancer, anticoagulant, antiradiation, anti-inflammatory, gastrointestinal, antimicrobial, cardiovascular, anti-obesity, and weight loss effects. Future research needs to investigate the suitable duration, maximum dosage of ginger, concerns of overdosage, and its side effects in animal models and humans.

Saffron spice also known as Crocus sativus (Saffron crocus) belongs to the family of iridaceae. Many studies have proved its potential role in disease eradication. It has been reported to possess the attributes of a sedative, an anti-asthma, an emmenagogue, an expectorant, and an adaptogenic agent. Crocin, crocetin, and safranal are the most important biochemically active ingredients that were found in different parts of the plants in varying proportions like the peels, fruits, seeds, and rind of Crocus sativus. The in vitro and in vivo studies showed that saffron has got its therapeutic implication in health management via anti-oxidant, anti-microbial, hepatoprotective, and anti-tumour activity. This review attempts to reveal the potential pharmacological properties of Crocus sativus. It also draws attention towards the use of herbs and spices in various ailments without facing the harmful side effects of chemically derived medicine.

Illicium verum, as a spice and pharmaceutical treatment of many harmful diseases, has been widely used in most Asian countries. The Ministry of Health of the People's Republic of China considered it as both food and medicine due to its non-toxicity towards human health. In the present study, the review focuses mainly on food and medical applications of I. verum. The fruits are commonly used as an ingredient of the traditional "five-spice" powder of Chinese cooking, and the essential oil of I. verum can be used as flavoring. The extraction from I. verum has carminative, stomachic, stimulant, and diuretic properties, and is used as a pharmaceutical supplement. Shikimic acid extracted from I. verum is one of the main ingredients in the antiviral drug Tamiflu, which is used to fight avian influenza. It has also been reported to possess antimicrobial and antioxidative properties as well as significant anticancer potential. This review presents a detailed compilation of the literature on phytochemicals and pharmacological properties of Illicium verum.

The plant science that studies the historical and current uses of plants is called ethnobotany. Spices and herbs have since medieval times been categorized as having medicinal properties. India is a land of spices, and several spices have been grown in the country. Buchanania lanzan Spreng, commonly known as char,

and modifier gastric stimulant. It has a valuable influence on digestion and also has the capability to modify food texture. In modern food technology, it is used as a food stabilizer, adhesive, and emulsifying agent due its fiber, protein, and gum content. Recent pharmocological exploration of the seed extract of this plant discovered anticancer properties. Although it has many potential effects, there are some side effects as well; therefore, there is a greater need to study the pharmacological and toxicological effects of fenugreek to examine its clinical efficacy and safety.

Mamta Sahu, Department of Agricultural Biochemistry, Chandra Shekhar Azad University of Agriculture and Technology, Kanpur, India
Suman Devi, Department of Agricultural Biochemistry, Chandra Shekhar Azad University of Agriculture and Technology, Kanpur, India
Pragya Mishra, Department of Agricultural Biochemistry, Chandra Shekhar Azad University of Agriculture and Technology, Kanpur, India
Ena Gupta, Department of Home Science, University of Allahabad, India

Brassica juncea, known as Indian mustard, has been used for centuries for its nutritional and medicinal values. L. brassica is a genus of plants in the mustard family, Brassicaceae. The members of the genus are informally known as cruciferous vegetables, cabbages, or mustard plants. Among the different varieties of mustard, the three principals are Brassica hirta or Alba (yellow-white), B. nigra (black), and B. juncea (brown). In Asian countries, India ranks first in mustard production, and mustard is the primary cooking oil used. In folkloric medicine, different parts of the plants are obtained to treat a wide variety of human aliments. Mustard seed is good source of protein, fibre, minerals, vitamins, antioxidants, and phytonutrients. The plant has several health benefits acting as antimicrobial, antibacterial, anti-diabetic, antimalarial, etc. The present study aims to discuss the up to date information regarding the botany, traditional uses, phytochemistry, and pharmacological applications of mustard seed and its essential oil.

Mazia Ahmed, Center of Food Technology, University of Allahabad, India
Urvashi Srivastava, Center of Food Technology, University of Allahabad, India
Chitra Gupta, Center of Food Technology, University of Allahabad, India

Turmeric (Curcuma longa) is a rhizomatous crop found in tropical regions and belongs to the family Zingiberaceae. It was used in the form of a spice, flavoring substance, coloring agent, and as a therapeutic agent for the treatment of several human ailments for centuries. Turmeric, along with its extracts, has a very broad and diverse field of application. It is an exclusive and versatile naturally occurring plant product having properties of not only a spice but also food colorant, medicine or drug, and cosmetics. In ethnic delicacies, turmeric is a commonly used flavoring ingredient. It is also a popularly used natural food color. It exhibits several biological activities such as having antioxidant, anti-inflammatory, anticarcinogenic, antimutagenic, antimicrobial, antiviral, and antiparasitic properties. It is well known as a skincare product and a healthy food ingredient. It is found to have the capability to prevent or retard a wide range of ailments.

Preface

A spice is a seed (cumin), root (ginger), bark(cinnamon), bud (clove), flower, stigma(saffron) or other plant substance primarily used for flavoring, coloring or preserving food. The word *spice* derived from the old French word *espice*, which means *epice*, and from the Latin root *spec* means species which signifies the groups of exotic foodstuffs. The spices have been used in South Asia and the Middle East as far back as 2000 BCE. India is known as home of medicinal herbs and spices as no country in the world grows as many varieties of spices as India. It is the world's largest exporter of spices and more than 70% of drug is derived from medicinal plants.

Around the world, spices are commonly used for its characteristic flavor, aroma and color in culinary art. Plant secretes secondary metabolites in small amount to attract pollens, to adopt environmental stress or to protect itself from invaders such as microorganism, insect and predators. These secondary metabolites are used commercially as biologically active compounds as model compounds for drug synthesis by the pharmaceutical industries. Extensive studies are going on around the word for isolation and characterization of bioactive compounds, owing to its biological activities Medicinal properties of spices have being used to treat diverse human ailments since prehistoric times. In traditional medicine such as Ayurveda, Unani, the medicinal properties of spices have been practices for decades but only very few have been studied chemically and pharmacologically for their potential medicinal value. Researchers are turning towards natural medicinal plants from synthetic compounds as they are more safe and cheaper. Several synthetic antibiotics have resulted in the emergence of multiple drug resistant bacteria and it has created alarming clinical situations in the treatment of infections. Previous studies reported that along with medicinal properties spices also enhances the absorption and utilization of other therapeutic substance.

Natural flora offers great possibilities for the discovery of new compounds with important medicinal applications for treatment of diverse diseases. The aim and objective of the current work was to explore the traditional therapeutic usage of common Indian spices and to correlate their observed pharmacological actions with the presence of specific chemical compounds in them. Some of the common medicinal plants that are used as spices in India are Jeerak, Haldi, Lanka, Dhania, Palandu, Rason, Methi, Adrakh, Elaichi, Tejapatra, Daruchini, Jaiphal, Kababchini, Marich, Lavang, Sarson, Ajwoin, Saunf, and Heeng. The specific plant parts contain active compounds present provide traditional therapeutic uses and pharmacological properties of the important Indian spices have been reviewed.

ABOUT THE BOOK

The book provides systematic and comprehensive collection of available information on the biosynthesis, phytochemistry, and pharmacology of Indian spices which help to design new drug. Spices are rich in biologically active metabolites which governs its nutritional, therapeutic and functional properties. The aim of the book to explore the facts related to the phytochemistry and biosythetic pathway of active constituents of Indian spices. In addition, this describes its ethanomedicinal importance, appropriate dosages and side effects. This book compiles the recent discoveries in related field which help to design new therapeutic drugs and possible utility in food Industry.

This book is written for the academicians, graduate, post graduate students, professionals and researchers working in the field of public nutrition, food technology, hotel management and pharmaceutical. Moreover, the book will provide insights and serve as a valuable resource of information to other allied botanical and alternative healthcare science students as well as researchers and industrialists working in the field of pharmaceutical, biochemistry, biotechnology, food and nutrition.

This book is written in systematic and lucid manner to explain the concepts. The book is written in a simple and systematic format by covering all the important topics suited to the students and researchers of Food and Nutrition/ Health Science and pharmacy. Enough tables and figures are incorporated in the text that simplify the difficult concept and to review the previous studies in easiest and quickest way. This book provides the structural approach to learning in a simple, uniform and systematic format.

ORGANIZATION OF THE BOOK

Under theses constraints this book consist of 18 chapters that covers the major aspects regarding traditional use, phytochemical compounds and their therapeutic activity. A brief description of each of the chapters follows:

Chapter 1 enlightened the history and origin of spices in India. Author discussed common practices and importance of these spices in Indian tradition. The spices and other medicinal plants have been the basis of traditional medicine system such as Ayurveda, Unani and Sindh for centuries. The spices are high in secondary metabolites that exhibit wide range of biological activities that could use for diverse human aliments. Since they are safe, author summarized the role of spices in modern medicine and in food process industry.

Chapter 2 reviews the role of spices beyond flavoring and coloring agents. From ancient eras, plant principally spices and herbs have been given much more attention for flavoring and coloring in foods and their use as condiments. They contain array of bioactive compounds like tannins, alkaloid, phenolic, flavonoid, polyphenols and vitamins which help in healing diseases. Authors have discussed the importance of bioactive compounds which apart from their primary role as organoleptic enhancers in culinary, also have diverse medicinal action like laxative, carminative, diuretic, anti-tumourigenic, antioxidative, anticarcinogenic, anti-inflamatory and cholesterol lowering activities. Medicinal plants are the most recent alternatives of medicines because they posses no side effects to our body as well as they are cheaper to afford by the maximum population.

Chapter 3 emphasized the anti-diabetic properties of spices and their role in preventing diabetes and associated complications. Authors enlisted the observed pharmacological activities with the explicit bioactive compounds present in them for the treatment and management of diabetes. Their basic underlying mechanism for the blood glucose lowering property is also discussed. Utilization of anti-diabetic drugs has been limited by their pharmacokinetic properties, auxiliary failures and potential side effects. Therefore, spice therapies have emerged as an effective way in the management of diabetes.

Chapter 4 focuses on ethanobotany, phytochemistry, acceptable daily intake and different pharmacological actions of Nutmeg. Nutmeg is considered as an importance spice all over the world and is used to enhance the taste and aromatic flavor of the food. It is a unique culinary ingredient frequently used in bakery foods, confections, puddings, meats, sausages, sauces, vegetables and beverages. Various therapeutic or medicinal applications were shown by nutmeg such as antioxidant, antimicrobial, aphrodisiac, anticancer, hepatoprotective, anti-inflammatory, antidepressant and cardioprotective activity.

Chapters 5 discusses the phytochemical composition and pharmacological studies of ginger extracts, ginger essential oil (GEO) and bioactive constituents. The bioactive constituent zingiberene, β-sesquiphellandrene, curcumene, β-bisabolene, β-farnesene, camphene, and gingerol and shogal are the major constituents in ginger extracts and responsible for pharmacological activities. Author enlisted the studies extensively investigated for discover the therapeutic potential of ginger extracts, GEO and its bioactive compounds such as α-zingiberene, gingerol and shogaol in humans and animal models. Gingerol is the key pungent constituent, is a major bioactive compounds accumulated in rhizome of fresh ginger and used for chemoprevention of cancer.

Chapter 6 summarizes the pharmacological activities of saffron the most expensive spice, also known as red gold. *C. sativus* (saffron) is an important herb of medicinal importance grown extensively and cultivated for economic and nutritional purpose. Saffron has wide applications in different fields of pharmaceutics and global food industry. Traditionally, saffron is dense in bioactive constituents especially safranal, crocin and crocetin, which is reported to posses therapeutic applications in fighting multiple diseases like diabetes, cancer, renal, cardiovascular and retinal complications. It is considered as a promising candidate with potentials for designing new drugs.

Chapter 7 presents a detailed compilation of the literature on phytochemicals and pharmacological properties of *Illicium verum.* Commonly *Illicium verum* is known as star anise or star aniseed or Chinese star anise It is a spice that very similar to anise in flavor, obtained from the star-shaped pericarp of the plant. The star anise is a major source of chemical compound, such as shikimic acid, a primary precursor in the pharmacological synthesis of anti influenza drugs namely Oseltamivir (Tamiflu).There is a growing demand for star anise as a source of shikimic acid for the manufacture of anti-viral drugs widely used in the treatment and prophylaxis of avian flu (commonly bird flu).

Chapter 8 discusses the cultivation, uses, chemical constituents, and therapeutic activities of *Buchanania lanzan Spreng* as well emphasis on the need and importance of pharmacognostic study of *Buchanania lanzan Spreng*. It is an integral and indispensable part of the traditional system of medicine practiced worldwide because of their economical viability, easy accessibility and century's old experience. As natures gift, these are considered to be biocompatible, environment friendly, non-toxic, much cheaper and quite freely available in comparison to synthetic substances.

Chapter 9 focuses on the pharmacological as well as traditional properties of bay leaves. *Laurus nobilis* commonly known as bay leaves, belong to Lauraceae family. It is a native spice of India and grown in Himalaya's range at altitude of 900 to 2500 meters. The dried leaves are used extensively in cooking as naturally occurring essential oil is used to enhance the flavor. Around the world concern, this medicinal plant have received attraction due to its antimicrobial, antifungal and antioxidant activity.

Chapter 10 reviews the ethanomedicinal importance, phytochemistry and wide spectrum of pharmacological and therapeutic applications of Cinnamon. It has been used as a folk medicine for the treatment of array of human aliments. Therapeutic properties of cinnamon are due to presence of bioactive constituents such *p*-coumaric, cinnamaldehyde, cinnamic acid and eugenol. Cinnamaldehyde and eugenol is the major active constituent responsible of its characteristic flavor, aroma and therapeutic properties. Pharmacological studies found that it could be a promising candidate with potentials for designing new drugs.

Chapter 11 elucidates the nutritional and pharmacological properties of Fenugreek. It is one of the oldest traditional medicinal plants, cultivated in the Indian subcontinent, parts of west Asia, Middle East, North Africa, United Kingdom, Russia, Mediterranean Europe, Australia, US and Canada. Since prehistoric time it is consumed as preservatives, as traditional medicine and flavouring agent. Authors have emphasized the biologically active compounds which exhibit specific pharmacological effects and also the need to study the pharmacological and toxicological effects of fenugreek to examine their clinical efficacy and safety.

Chapter 12 described the therapeutic potential of mustard, the world's third most important spice after salt and pepper. *Brassica juncea is* known as Indian mustard whose different parts are obtained to treat diverse human aliments and culinary purposes for century. Author have discussed the botany, traditional uses, phytochemistry and pharmacological applications of mustard seed and essential oil.

Chapter 13 reviews one of the most extensively used spice "Turmeric" for its strong flavor and vibrant color throughout the world. It is the member of the Zingiberaceae family. Since prehistoric time, turmeric is used in the Ayurvedic system of medicines with a number of biological applications. These biological activities make it a good candidate for development of pharmaceuticals, nutraceuticals, or food ingredients with functional properties. The active ingredient present in turmeric is Curcumin which is found to have a broad range of remedial or therapeutic effects and also has been used as an ingredient in preparing medicinal oils, creams/ointments and poultice in the Indian system of medicine as a stomachic, carminative, stimulant or tonic, vermicide, blood purifier, and an antiseptic.

Chapter 14 highlights the cultural and historical information about coriander. The author reviewed exhaustively the photochemical constituents of seed, leaf and fruit and therapeutic potential of coriander has explained well.

Chapter 15 aims to discuss the botany, traditional uses, medicinal and industrial applications of coriander extracts and essential oil. Coriander (*Coriandrum sativum L)* is an annual herb which belongs to the family Apiaceae (Umbelliferae) and commonally known as dhanya. Its different portion stem, leaves and fruits all are edible and have a distinct pleasant flavor and odor. Since century there parts majorly leaves and ripe seeds are used in folk medicine in addition to use for culinary purposes.

Chapter 16 discussed the role of Nano biotechnology for enhancing the antimicrobial activity of spices. Nanoformulation of spices and its active constituents is emerging as a novel technique to enhance solubility and targeted delivery to increase bioavailability. Antimicrobial activity of spices is well known and proved. Authors have described the different methods for nanoformulates of spices have different medicinal property like antimicrobial, anti-inflammatory, antioxidant, anticancer property.

Chapter 17 presents a concise approach for pest-crop- pathogen management system of coriander crop. Coriander is one of the first spices to be used by mankind but highly susceptible for various diseases, which is responsible for crop loss for small and marginal farmers every year. Authors overviewed the better cultivation technology to prevent the plants from pests and pathogen, and listed the preventive measures required. They also discussed the various controlling strategies must be followed by the farmers for enhancing the soil fertility.

Chapter 18 presents Chili as a popular and unique spice that is known for its burning sensation and hot, punget flabor. Chili is commercially important and has a large genetic diversity. The authors give a description of the crop in respect to its origin, distribution, description, standard crop husbandry, protection, management, and biotic stresses.

The authors are grateful to our professional colleagues and friends for their encouragements and valuable suggestions. I would like to give sincere thanks to publisher for bringing out this book timely. Authors are also thankful to their husband and family for their encouragement and pleasant support.

We shall welcome the constructive suggestions of readers for improvement of the book.

Acknowledgment

In compiling the book, I have extensively referred a vast number of standard books, journals, proceedings of seminars and conferences and workshop manuals.

I express my deep sense of indebtedness to the students, learned colleagues and scientist for providing the necessary stimulus for writing this book. I am equally grateful to the reviewer of the manuscript of this book who made extremely valuable suggestions and has thus contributed in enhancing the standard of the book. During the commencement of the book, I have taken the assistance of my expert friends in the field whom I wish to recognize with the appreciation although I cannot name them individually. I have given credit for the sources and I thank them all very much.

A special acknowledgement is owed to my husband Dr. Saurabh Mishra for initiating to bring this book and for constant encouragement in this endeavor. I extended my special thanks to my teachers, colleagues and several individuals who play significant role in the project.

Finally, I thank all my family members and chapter contributors who cooperated me at various stages by encouraging the work without which it would not have been possible to honor the deadlines.

I shall feel ample rewarded if the book proves helpful in the development of genuine research studies. I look forward to suggestions from all readers especially from experienced researchers and scholar for further improving the subject content as well as the presentation of this book. It is hoped that the book shall provide guidelines to all interest in research studies of one sort or the other.

Chapter 1
Historical and Future Perspective of Indian Spices

Priyanka Singh
Centre of Food Technology, University of Allahabad, India

ABSTRACT

Spices take an important place in common man's everyday life mainly because of their flavor, taste, and medicinal values. Spice usage grew with the increased use of processed products. India is the largest producer of spices in the world. Growth in Indian spices and spice product exports clearly show that Indian spices and spice products have a great demand in international markets. India is the land of spices and could exploit the fast-growing nutraceutical sector with its high intrinsic quality spices. The scope of spices like turmeric, ginger, fenugreek, garlic, and red pepper in the nutraceutical industry with their possible role in the control and prevention of important health disorders are examined. The demand for nutraceutical products has gone up as more people are turning to natural products for treating lifestyle diseases. This review deals with the history and origin of spices and their potential uses as well as future prospects in treatment of various diseases in a natural way.

HISTORY AND ORIGIN OF SPICES IN INDIA

Spices can be derived from different parts of the plant. Cloves are the buds, cinnamon is the bark, ginger from the roots, peppercorns from the berries, cumin as the aromatic seeds, and saffron being the stigma of a flower. Various aromatic seeds used as spices are actually collected from plants after finishing the flowering stage. For example, coriander leaves are referred to as an herb, having their seeds(dried) used as a spice. The stem and roots of coriander, used in cooking, and onions, garlic, and the bulbs of fennel, are classified as herbs as these parts of their plants are often used fresh and applied in a similar way in cooking.

In India, Ayurveda for traditional medicine came into existence more than 5000 years ago in the Himalayas, and the knowledge was transmitted orally until it was written down in the Vedas by around 1500 BCE, but it flourished in the 7th century. Ayurveda mainly focuses on prevention from diseases and promotion for health through the importance of diet (Govindrajan et al,2005). Health Effects such

DOI: 10.4018/978-1-7998-2524-1.ch001

as the use of turmeric for jaundice, heart protection through basil, the mace in stomach infections, cinnamon in stimulating circulation, and ginger as the universal medicine, chiefly for relieving nausea and indigestion. These are some of the examples of Ayurvedic use of herbs and spices. Most of these spices are utilized in Indian cooking to impart flavor and significant quantities are consumed in a regular meal. It has also been reported that such spices can supply appreciable quantities of nutrients as well, such as iron. India produces 75 varieties of spices of the 109 listed by ISO, and is also the world's largest producer of spices (Thatte et al, 1986).

THE HEALTH BENEFITS OF SPICES

Although herbs and spices are not often consumed in large quantities, and even small doses of them can be a powerful source of anti-inflammatories, nutrients, antioxidants agents, cancer-fighting constituents, minerals, vitamins, and more.

Cinnamon

Cinnamon has the property of lowering blood sugar levels and has a potential anti-diabetic effect. It is a very popular spice, which is found in all sorts of recipes and baked goods. Cinnamaldehyde, the prime constituent of cinnamon, is responsible for it's medicinal properties. Cinnamon has high antioxidant activity, which helps fight inflammation and has also been shown to reduce cholesterol and triglycerides in blood serum. But the most important activity of cinnamon is its action on blood sugar levels. Cinnamon has several mechanisms to lower blood sugar, including slowing down the breakdown of carbs in the digestive tract and increasing insulin sensitivity. Studies have revealed that cinnamon can reduce fasting blood sugars by a significant amount, ie. 10-29% in diabetic patients. The effective dose of cinnamon to have beneficial effects is typically 0.5-2 teaspoons of cinnamon per day or 1-6 grams.

Turmeric

Turmeric contains curcumin, a substance with powerful anti-inflammatory effects. Although it contains various compounds with medicinal properties, the most important of them is curcumin. Curcumin is a significant potential antioxidant, which helps in fighting with oxidative damage and also boosting the body's own antioxidant enzymes. Oxidative damage is believed to be one of the key mechanisms behind aging and many diseases; hence, it very important to reduce these kinds of reactions in the body. Curcumin is also strongly anti-inflammatory, as it matches the effectiveness of many anti-inflammatory drugs. Many studies have also suggested that it can improve brain functioning, fight against Alzheimer's, subside the risk of heart disease and cancer, and relieve arthritis to a large extent.

Fenugreek

Fenugreek plays a vital role in improving blood sugar control. In ancient times fenugreek was commonly used in Ayurveda, chiefly to enhance libido and masculinity. Although, studies are inconclusive for its effects on testosterone levels. Fenugreek does seem to have beneficial effects on blood sugar. It posses the plant protein 4-hydroxyisoleucine, which is useful in improving the function of the hormone insulin.

Several studies have concluded that at least 1 gram of fenugreek extract per day could be a potential agent for lowering blood sugar levels, particularly in diabetics.

Ginger

Ginger is another versatile spice that is easy to use. Fresh ginger and ground ginger are both beneficial. It's commonly known as a powerful remedy for a stomachache, but its benefits extend far beyond that. It is anti-inflammatory and soothing for an upset stomach, which is often a root cause of inflammation. Ginger can decrease markers of inflammation, such as C- reactive protein. Ginger can also prevent stomach ulcers and menstrual cramps. It could also be a relief from nausea and diarrhea. Ginger tea is used for relieving flu symptoms. Raw ginger is relatively high in minerals like potassium, manganese, copper, niacin, magnesium, phosphorus, and iron. Ginger can be used as a raw root, which provides the most bioavailable source of minerals; hence, it's easier to get a substantial amount of vitamins from it compared to other spices. We can get a high amount of vitamin B6 and vitamin C from the ginger. This may be the reason for its great potential in enhancing immunity. It is also a great prebiotic food for gut health.

Chili

Chili derived from pepper contains even more vitamin C than an orange does. They contain up to seven times the amount of vitamin C of an orange. Chilli also contains vitamin A and vitamin E. It has a tremendous immune-boosting action. The capsaicin found in the spices derived from the pepper is particularly beneficial in inhibiting the neuropeptides related to inflammatory processes that take place in the body, and it may also subside the pain in individuals having symptoms of sensory nerve fiber disorders (psoriasis, arthritis, etc.). Capsaicin can also reduce congestion and stuffy nose.

Cumin

Cumin aids in digestion problems. One of its main compounds, thymol, helps in the production of bile, stomach acid, and digestive enzymes, which can improve the efficiency of digestion, naturally, treat hemorrhoids, and reduce the complications of gas. It is also a good source of antioxidants due to the presence of vitamin E, which is also good for healthy, glowing skin. Cumin is also an anti-congestive, antiviral, and antibacterial agent. It's also pretty high in vitamin C, so like many spices on my list today, it can be a powerful immune booster.

FUTURE PERSPECTIVE OF SPICES

Spices, the predominant flavoring, coloring, and aromatic agents in foods and beverages, are now gaining importance for their diversified uses. **Curcumin**, the coloring pigment present in turmeric, **capsaicin**, the pungent principle in red pepper, **allicin**, the active principle in garlic, **gingerol**, the pungent principle in ginger, and **saponin**, the fiber present in fenugreek are all immensely valuable in health care with their multiple physiological effects. In the present scenario, the anti-diabetic, anti-hyper cholesterolemic, anti-carcinogenic, and anti-inflammatory effects of spices have paramount importance, as the key health issues of mankind nowadays are diabetes, cardiovascular diseases, arthritis, and cancer. These metabolic diseases and age-related degenerative disorders are closely associated with oxidative processes in the body (Jacob et al., 2003). Spices or their active principles could be used as possible ameliorative or preventive agents for these health disorders as spices are a source of antioxidants to combat oxidation, which requires further attention. Immediate studies should focus on validating the antioxidant capacity of spices after harvest, as well as testing their effects on markers of oxidation. Extensive studies on animal models carried out indicate that spices could be consumed at higher dietary levels without any adverse effects on growth, organ weights, and food efficiency ratio and blood constituents (Liu et al., 2003). With time, we can expect to see a greater body of scientific evidence supporting the benefits of spices in the overall maintenance of health and protection from disease.

REFERENCES

Liu, R. H. (2003). Health benefits of fruit and vegetables are from additive and synergistic combinations of phytochemicals. *The American Journal of Clinical Nutrition, 78*(3), 517S–520S. doi:10.1093/ajcn/78.3.517S PMID:12936943

Thatte, U. M., & Dahanukar, S. A. (1986). Ayurveda and contemporary scientific thought. *Trends in Pharmacological Sciences, 7*, 247–251. doi:10.1016/0165-6147(86)90336-6

ADDITIONAL READING

Govindarajan, R., Vijayakumar, M., & Pushpangadan, P. (2005). Antioxidant approach to disease management and the role of 'Rasayana' herbs of Ayurveda. *Journal of Ethnopharmacology, 99*(2), 165–178. doi:10.1016/j.jep.2005.02.035 PMID:15894123

Jacobs, D. R. Jr, & Steffen, L. M. (2003). Nutrients, foods, and dietary patterns as expo-sures in research: A framework for food synergy. *The American Journal of Clinical Nutrition, 78*(3), 508S–513S. doi:10.1093/ajcn/78.3.508S PMID:12936941

Tapsell, L. C., Hemphill, I., Cobiac, L., Patch, C. S., Sullivan, D. R., Fenech, M., ... Inge, K. E. (2006, August 21). *Health benefits of herbs and spices: the past, the present, the future*. Retrieved from https://www.ncbi.nlm.nih.gov/pubmed/17022438

Chapter 2
Role of Spices Beyond a Flavouring Agent:
The Antioxidant and Medicinal Properties

Anuradha Patel
University of Allahabad, India

Sanjesh Tiwari
https://orcid.org/0000-0002-1335-0267
University of Allahabad, India

Neeraj Pandey
University of Allahabad, India

Divya Gupta
University of Allahabad, India

Sheo Mohan Prasad
University of Allahabad, India

ABSTRACT

Plants, principally spices and herbs, have been given much more attention because they are considered important for flavoring and coloring foods and their use as condiments. Herbs and spices have been used for generations by humans as food and also to treat ailments since they are full of medicinal and antioxidant properties and contain bioactive compounds like tannins, alkaloids, phenolics, flavonoids, polyphenols, and vitamins, which help in healing diseases. Spices and herbs contain biomolecules that play a crucial role in healthcare and fitness levels. Spices and herbs have been considered as esoteric food adjuncts as they play numerous roles like being coloring agents, flavoring agents, preservatives, food additives, and having uses in the medicinal and pharmaceutical industries.

DOI: 10.4018/978-1-7998-2524-1.ch002

INTRODUCTION

Since ancient eras, spices and herbs have been known to play a vital role in the lifestyle of human beings. Herbs, as well as spices, are seasonings derived from plants and used for different purposes. The terms 'herbs' and 'spices' are two sides of the same coin, or often used interchangeably, but they are defined sparsely. Herbs store flavor components in their leaves, whereas spices store in their seeds, bark, and root. A spice may be any part of the plant such as bud (clove), bark (cinnamon), root (ginger), aromatic seed (cumin), and flower stigma (saffron) of a plant. Among the whole world, India is rich in herbs and spices and has been recognized as a country for spices and traditional medicine; that is having a wide range of physiological and pharmacological properties. Being a biodiversity-rich country, in India, there is extensive use of spices and herbs. It was observed that the consumption of these food additives is found to be doubled between 1970 and 2005, and among them, the use of garlic has increased more than six-fold (USDA ERS, 2011).

Spices are esoteric food adjuncts that have been known for thousands of years which enhance the sensory quality of food. The quantity and variety consumed in tropical countries is particularly extensive. These spices impart uniquely characteristic flavors, aromas, or piquancy and colors to foods. Apart from their role in flavoring, spices often are used for preservation, medicinally, pharmaceutically, and for health maintenance purposes (Opara and Chohan, 2014).

Besides being ornamental in food quality and aiding as a source of basic nutritional requirements, spices are beneficial for therapeutic diseases (Lobo et al., 2010). They have several bioactive compounds that behave as antioxidants and have antimicrobial, pharmaceutical, and nutritional properties. The bioactive molecules, including secondary metabolites secreted by plants, possess a distinct pharmacological property and are also involved in defense against stress (Newman and Cragg, 2012). This plant constituent is known to function against repellents and pathogens called allelochemicals, and several active compounds like flavanols, tocopherols, geraniolthymol, carvacrol, and benzoic acid which are major antibacterial and antifungal compounds. (Adeyemi, 2011). Currently, studies focused enormously on the medicinal and nutritional properties of spices. They are a potential source of bioactive compounds such as polyphenols, antioxidants, and essential oils, and antimicrobial chemicals that can deal with the current situation of stress, depression, hormonal imbalance, and metabolic disorders that are common issues in today's lifestyle. A bioactive molecule like polyphenols from ginger (*Zingiber offcinale*) and turmeric (*Curcuma longa* L.) both display anti-inflammatory, anti-cancerous, and radical scavenging properties (Scalbert and Williamson, 2000). Antioxidants from turmeric, curcumin, clove, eugenol, and red pepper capsaicin control oxidative stress in cells due to their antioxidant properties and they scavenge the oxygen radicals in aerobic metabolism that interferes with signal transduction pathways (Rubió*et al.*, 2013; Srinivasan, 2014). These metabolites play a constructive role in treating chronic disorders such as cancer, diabetes, and diseases associated with respiratory and cardiovascular problems (Kaefer and Milner, 2011). Here this chapter deals with the role of spices in flavoring, nutritional, medicinal, and pharmacological aspects. Their potential role in traditional systems of medicine for combating chronic diseases is also discussed.

Traditional Uses of Spices

Traditionally, spices are a part of our diet and have been almost requisite in the culinary art of flavoring foods since ancient times. Spices, whether in fragmented or pounded form, are aromatic vegetable substances whose significant function is in seasoning rather than nutrition in food. For many generations, humans have used herbs and spices in food to treat various ailments. Bio-molecules involved in the plants play a vital role in health recovery and promotion (Sachan et al., 2018). In history, different parts have served numerous roles, such as coloring agents, flavoring agents, preservatives, food additives, and as medicine. In Ayurveda, spices and herbs have distinctive functions like carminative properties, cold & cough relief, diuretic action, and cardiac stimulation. Traditionally, *Elettaria Cardamomum* has a protective gastrointestinal property and is also used against urinary and kidney disorders. It's oil has an anti-inflammatory and antibacterial property (Zuhair et al., 1996). Traditionally, infections related to urinary, digestive, and respiratory problems were diagnosed by *Coriandrum Sativum* through stimulant action (Gilani et al., 2007). In medicines, *Foenum-graecum* is used as an aphrodisiac property, demulcent action, astringent carminative, diuretic, emollient, expectorant, emmenagogue, lactogogue, restorative, and a tonic (Acharya et al., 2008). In Ayurvedic and Siddha medicine, sinus problems are reduced by the juice of garlic, and most importantly, its rhizome is used to overcome gastrointestinal disorders, vomiting and motion sickness (Agarwal et al., 2001). In Unani medicine, the dried bulb of *Zingiber officinale* is adopted to treat ulcers, fever, and colic pains as well as to aid in abortion and menstruation problems in females. As a traditional remedy in Sidha medicine, various disorders like rheumatism, body aches (Ammon and Wahl., 1991) skin disease, diarrhea (Bernard et al., 1982), hepatic, urinary, dental and arthritis diseases were all treated by *Curcuma longa* and *Trachyspermum ammi* (Sachan et al., 2016; Khajehdehi, 2012; Zuhair et al., 1996; Gilani et al., 2007).). In Nigeria, plant parts of *P. guineense*have have folkloric and ethnomedical uses (Ekanemet al., 2010). This plant is also used for the preparation of soaps for post-parturient women due to its pungent smell and flavoring essence (Chiwenduet al., 2016). The important uses of this plant are from the seeds which are suggested to women after giving birth to flush out the placenta, and other remnants of the womb, by enhancing the contraction of the uterine lining (Ekanemet al., 2010). It is also used as an anti-asthmatic agent (Sofowora, 1982). Leaves are found to be effective in regulating the female menstrual cycle, and infertility, but also with the consumption of their fruits and roots is a remedy treatment for sexually transmitted diseases (Iwu, 2014). Spices and herbs also play a role in the preservation of foods and preventing the spoilage of food due to antimicrobial and antioxidant properties. All spices have a wide variety of bio-functions and their additive and synergistic actions that protect the human body are very well known to have a holistic approach, which is discussed in further headings.

BIOACTIVE MOLECULES IN SPICES AND ITS FUNCTION

In India, spices have been traditionally used for several years to improve the taste of food and to aid in various diseases. Spices improve the characteristics of food, and the bioactive molecules are the key flavoring agent that impart characteristics of aroma, fragrance, and taste in food and they are also vital for health care (Gunasekar et al., 2012). The bioactive molecule comprises polyphenols, antioxidants, essential oils, and several active compounds such as thymol, carvacrol, flavanols, tocopherols, geraniol, and benzoic acid along with other antibacterial and antifungal compounds (Jiang et al., 2019). Spices are also an important source for natural antioxidants; antioxidants are the largest group of the bioactive compound which includes flavonoids, phenolic compounds, sulfur-containing compounds, tannins, alkaloids, phenolic diterpenes, and vitamins (McCormick, 2017). Spices like turmeric (*Curcuma longa*), ginger (*Zingiber officinalis*), garlic (*Alliumsativum*), clove (*Syzygium aromaticum*), black cumin (*Nigella sativum*), red pepper (*Capsicum annuum*) and black pepper (*Piper nigrum*) contain several natural antioxidant biomolecules. The polyphenols from Cinnamon (*Cinnamomumverum*), Cloves (*Syzygium aromaticum*), Coriander seed (*CoriandrumsativumL.*) Ginger (*Zingiber officinale*), Nutmeg (*Myristicafragans*), and Turmeric (*Curcuma longa* L.) are widely known for their antioxidant properties; however, they exert other biological effects (anti-inflammatory, anti-cancer and neuroprotective) also. Culinary herbs and spices have also been shown to possess these properties. Essential oil also plays a prominent role like turmeric oil, a constituent of the turmeric (Curcuma longa) rhizome which showed a decrease in inflammatory swelling and acted as an anti-inflammatory and an anti-arthritic (Chandra & Gupta 1972). Macelignan extracted from Nutmeg (Myristicafragrans) protects microglial cells (Jin et al., 2005). The essential oil from Oregano is high in antioxidant and antimicrobial property, which mainly contains terpenoids, mainly the monoterpenoid phenols of thymol and carvacrol. Primarily phenolics and terpenoids have been identified from various species of turmeric, including twenty-two diarylheptanoids and diarylpentanoids, and eight phenylpropenes as well as other phenolics (Li *et al.*, 2011). From those compounds curcuminoids (mostly curcumin) and essential oils (monoterpenes) are the major bioactive constituents showing different bioactivities. Volatile oil in *Nigela Sativa* contains active basic components such as thymoquinone, dithymoquinone and thymohydroquinone (Gullu&Gulcan, 2013; Kaya *et al.*, 2003). Thymoquinone, which is one of the most important bioactive components of *N. sativa* exists as a volatile oil (Yuncu*et al.*, 2013). Antimicrobials are also derived from plant sources that are phytochemicals, which are important for the proper functioning of the plant. These antimicrobial compounds helped the plants as a defense mechanism to protect them from plant pathogens and other predators. The major bioactive compounds in spices and their role is displayed in Table 1 and 2.

FUNCTIONS OF BIOACTIVE MOLECULES OF SPICES

Besides the important role of spices and herbs in food, and the cosmetics and perfume industry, coloring and flavoring agents have also been used in pharmaceutical industries and play a direct role in human health in the form of various medicines in their raw as well as extracted form. They have been used for generations by humans as food and in the treatment of various diseases and ailments due to these bioactive compounds (Sachan et al., 2018).

Table 1. List of bioactive compounds in some spices and their role

1.	*Capsicum annuum*	•Capsaicinoids (0.2-2%) •Capsaicin (50-70%) •Capsacinoids and Dihydrocapasaicin (20–25%)	•Red pepper capsaicin has antioxidant potential in mitigating oxidative stress •Suppress obesity-induced •Beneficial effects on the cardiovascular system •Defend against heart diseases •Lowers the blood glucose level and maintain healthy function of insulin •Increases production of body heat / regulate (thermogenesis) •Increases basic metabolic rate •Beneficial effect on gut microbiota •Possess antibacterial activity	Anandakumar et al., 2008 Spiller et al., 2008 Chaiyata et al., 2003 Chaiyasit et al., 2009 Janssens et al., 2014 Karlsson et al., 2013
2.	*Cinnamomum verum*	•Essential oils like Cinnamaldehyde, Cinnamic, cinnamate (60–80%) •Eugenol (leaf oil; 10%), and polyphenols (4–10%)	•Possess antibacterial and antifungal activity •Majorly attack the pathogens associated with respiratory and gastrointestinal tract •Beneficial against typhoid and diarrhea •Regulate anti and pro-inflammatory gene responses •Lowers blood sugar level •Act as hepato protectant, protect liver •Possesss neuro-protective property	Fabio et al., 2007 Rosti and Gastaldi (2005) Cao et al., 2008 Preuus et al., 2006
3.	*Zingiber officinale*	•Gingerol •Shogaols •Paradols •Zingerone	•Effective for decreasing nausea and vomiting •Possess free radicle scavenging property •Possess anti-inflammatory and antioxidant response •Has anticlotting activity •Reduces joint swelling •Also reduces body mass index •Reduces ageing	Smith et al., 2004 Grzanna et al.,2004
4.	*Piper nigrum*	•Piperine5 to 9%, •Various alkaloid such as alkamides, piptigrine, wisanine, and dipiperamide	•Possess anti-inflammatory, anti-allergic and antioxidative responses •Piperine protect against oxidative damage •Quenches free radicle and reactive oxygen species •Immunomodulator •Accelerate digestive process by stimulating secretion of digestive enzymes •Maintain body weight •Enhances absorption of nutrient and drugs •Also it is an anti- depressant	Delecroix et al., 2017 Kim et al., 2009 Matsuda et al., 2008 Li et al., 2007
5.	*Curcuma longa*	•Curcuminoids including curcumin (diferuloylmethane), de-methoxy curcumin, bis de-methoxy curcumin, and tetra-hydro curcumin.	•Possess anti-inflammatory and antioxidative effect •Protective effect on cardiac function and vascular health •Reduces the cholesterol •Boost hepatic system •Reduces joint swelling and improves muscle health •Control blood sugar level •Manages body weight •Reduces proliferation of cancerous cell thus preventing cancer	Ahmed and Gilani, (2009) Kuptniratsaiku et al., 2009 Kim et al., 2009 Wang et al., 2009
6.	*Trigonella foenum-graecum*	•Steroidal saponins like diosgenin and trigogenin •Flavonoids. and alkaloids like gentianine and trigonelline.	•Lipid lowering activity •Regulate blood glucose metabolism •Improves liver health •Sexual fitness •Balances androgen deficiency •Improve mental alertness and reduces mood swings	Rao et al., 2015 Rao et al., 2016 Maheshwari et al., 2017
7.	*Allium sativum*	•Allicin, ajoene, and other organosulfur constituents such as S-allyl-L-cysteine (SAC).	•Anti-inflammatory responses •Promote cardiovascular health •Lowers blood cholesterol •Lowers blood pressure •Lowers blood glucose level and help in curing diabetes •Promote brain health •Immune-modulatory activity	Gupta et al., 2009 Gupta and Rao (2007) Jiang (2019)
8.	Syzygium aromaticum	•Eugenol the main bioactive compound of clove •Phenolic acid like caffeic, ferulic, elagic and salicylic acids.	•Possess antioxidant activity •Antimicrobial activity •Anticandidal property •Antinociceptive •Antiviral activity	Shaan et al., 2005 Pérez-Jiménez et al., 2010
9.	Mentha piperita	•Limonene •Menthol •Eriodictyol, •Hesperitin, •Apigenin, •Luteolin	•cure indigestion issues •increase bile secretion •easy digestion •maintains cholesterol level	Blumenthal 1998
10.	Rosamarium officinalis	•Carnasol, carnosic acid, cineole, geraniol, α-pinene, •β-carotene, apigenin, limonene, naringin, luteolin •caffeic acid, rosmarinic acid, rosmanol, •vanillic acid	•Neurologically protective in nature •Memory enhancer •Prevents ageing •Macular degeneration •Anti- cancerous •Aid digestion	Derwich, et al. 2011
11.	Crocus Sativus	•Crocetin, crocin, β-carotene, safranal, all trans retinoic acid	•Anti-tumor activity •Skin healer •Immunity booster •Wound healing •Anti-inflammatory	Garcia-Olmo et al., 1999
12.	Nigella sativa	•Thymoquinone •Dithymoquinone	•Decrease membrane damage •Increased antioxidant •Enzymatic reaction	Abdulazeez et al., 2015
13.	*Cinnamomum*	•Cinnamaldehyde	•Anti-microbial activity against Listeria monocytogenes, Staphylococcus aureus and Salmonella enterica	Shan et al., 2009

Table 2. List of bioactive compounds in some spices and their corresponding role with their structure (taken and modified)

Sr.no.	Phytochemical	Structure	Target	References
1.	Capsaicinoid	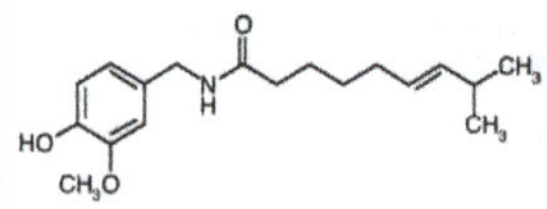	• Interact neuropeptide- and activate a "vanilloid" receptor • Opens channel, mediate influx of Ca^{2+} and Na^{+}, depolarization of the neuron, and releases neuropeptides.	Szallasi and Blumberg, 1990 Martling, 1987
2.	Cinnamaldehyde	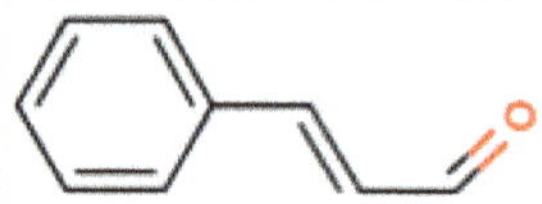	• Enhance insulin resistance, and glucose transporter-4 in 3T3-L1 adipocytes.	Jakhetia et al., 2010
3.	Eugenol	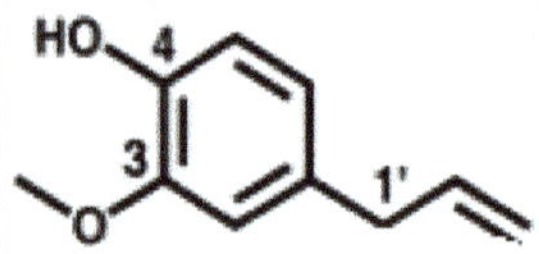	• interacts with the Ca^{2+} channel cyclooxygenese, and opens chloride ion channel	Yasushi et. al. 2016
4.	Gingerol	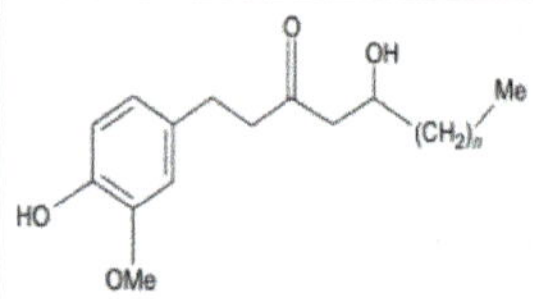	• inhibited the expression of IL-6 and reduced production of PGE2 • Inhibit expression and production of inflammatory factors IL-1β, TNF-α, IL-6, IL-10, iNOS, • Interfere with the NO production	Bang et al. (2009) Umar et al., 2013; Li et al., 2015
5.	Piperine	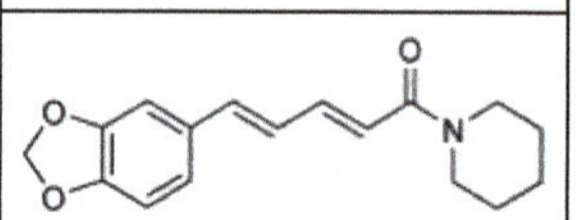		
6.	Allicine	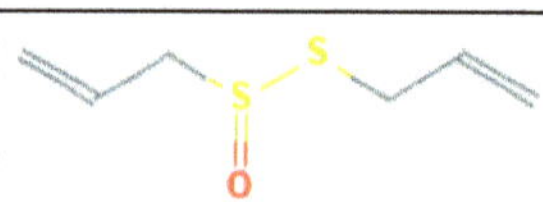	• Inhibit T-cell migration • Inhibit T-cell polarization and T-cell adhesion to fibronectin.	Sela et al. (2004)
7.	Limonene	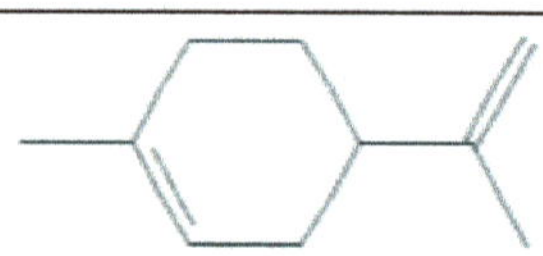	• Inhibition of GTP-binding proteins	Li et al., 2015
8.	Menthol	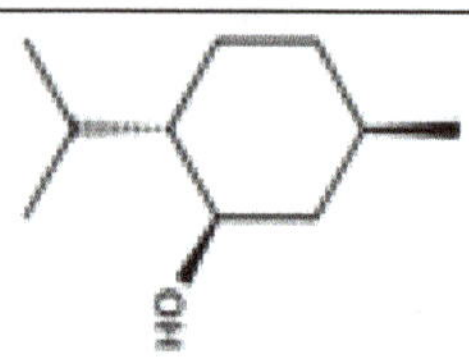	• Menthol exerts a wide range of TRPM8-independent effects, generally at somewhat higher concentrations than those that adequately activate TRPM8.	Rory Mitchell et al.
9.	Eriodictyol	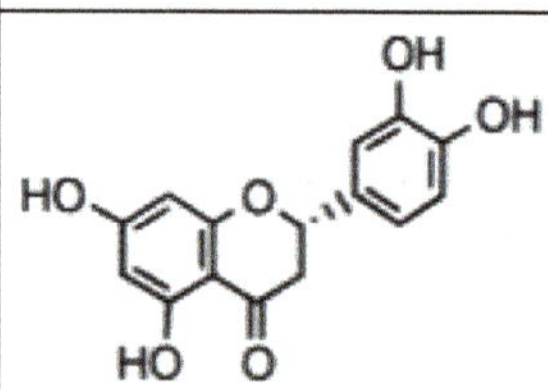	• It reduces oxidative stress- induced cell death through modulating Heme Oxygenase-1 Expression	Lee et al., 2015
10.	Hesperetin	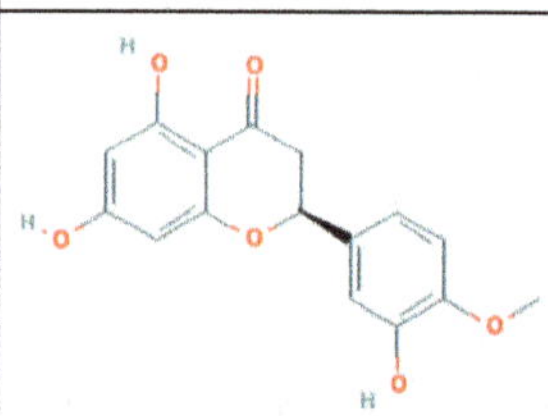	• Hesperetin inhibits the activity of acyl-coenzyme • It reduces microsomal triglyceride transfer protein (MTP) activity. • Antioxidant • Possess anti-inflammatory, anti-allergic • Enhances anti- carcinogenic property	Kara et al., 2014

continued on following page

Table 2. Continued

Sr.no.	Phytochemical	Structure	Target	References
11.	Apigenin	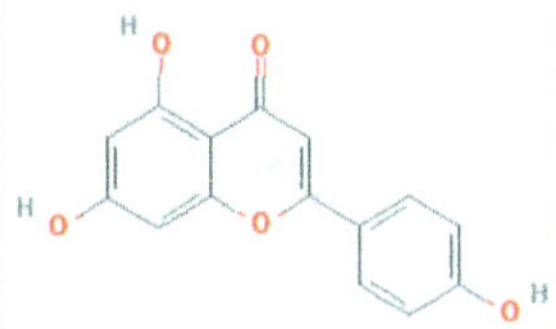	• Apoptotic. Anti-inflammatory and function as antioxidant • Check cell cycle by arresting G1/S and G2/M phase by CDKs	Salehi et al., 2019
12.	Luteolin	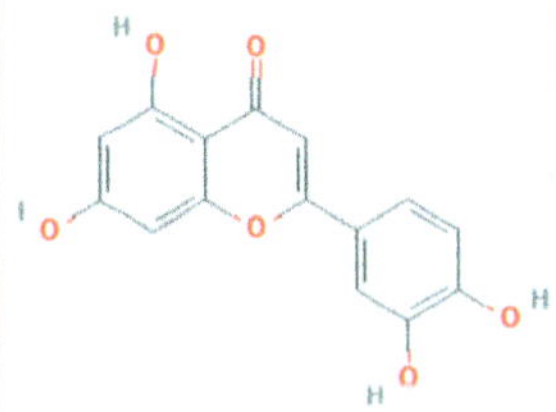	• kinase activity inhibition, apoptosis induction, suppression of the secretion of matrix metalloproteinases and of tumor invasive behavior	Kandaswami et al., 2005
13.	Carnosol	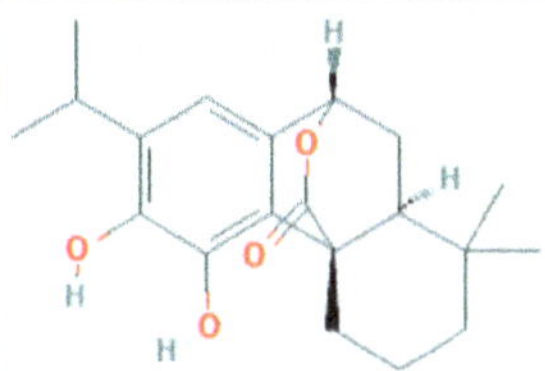	• scavenging free radicals induced by CCl_4, consequently avoiding the propagation of lipid peroxides.[223]	ErikaRamos-Tovar (2019)
14	Vanillic acid	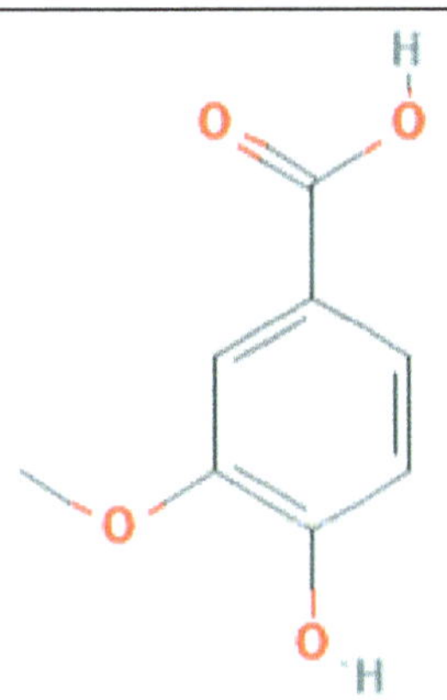	• It specifically inhibits 5'nucleotidase activity.	ErikaRamos-Tovar (2019)
15	Thymoquinone	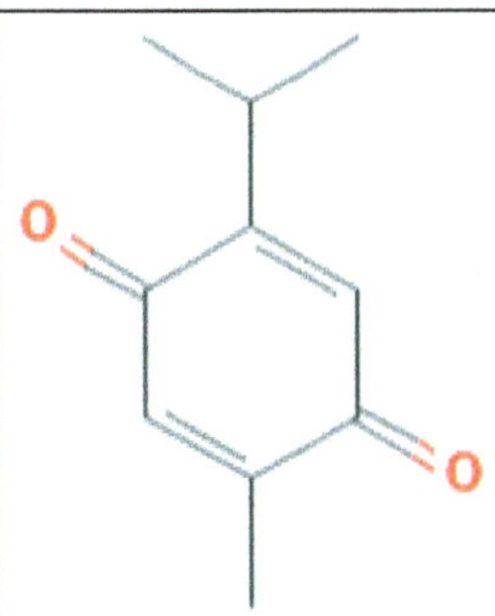	• Inhibits constitutive and TNF-α-mediated activation of NF-κB in • And reduced the transport of NF-κB from the cytosol to the nucleus • Affecting the metabolic process	Cheh et al., 2009 J.P.Dzoyem

Table 3. List of a few spices, their part as a source and their role in curing diseases

S.no	Plant name	Common name	Plant belongs to family	Plant part	uses	References
1.	*Syzygium aromaticum*	Cloves	Myrtaceae	Buds of the flower	Used in seasoning food and rich in antioxidants. Regulates bone health and blood sugar, improvse liver and reduces stomach problems. Clove oil is used for curing tooth-ache and sore gums and also in coughs and colds.	Ghadermazi et al., 2017 Duke et al., 2003
2.	*Elettaria cadamomum Amomum subulatum*	Cardamom	Zingiberaceae	Dried fruits and seed	Flavoring agent that possesses antioxidant and diuretic properties, anti-inflammatory, anti-cancerous compounds and for treating chronic ailments.	Jafri et al., 2001 Duke et al., 2003
3.	*Coriandrum sativum*	Coriander	Umbelliferae	Leaves and seed	Used for the treatment of stomach disorders loss of appetite, bowl spasm and diarrhea as well as reduces bacterial infection.	Dhanapakiam et al., 2008
4.	*Ferula-assa-foetida*	Asafoetida	Umbelliferae	Leaves Gum resin and starch from the roots	A medicinal herb used for seasoning food and medicinally helpful in curing whooping cough and acts mainly on the treatment of stomach disorders and strengthens the gastro-intenstinal tract	Basu et al., 2008
5.	*Laurus nobilis*	Bay leaf	Lauraceae	Leaves	Used as a flavoring agent And possesses medicinal properties. Its oil has antifungal and antibacterial properties.	Alam et al., 2009
6.	*Cinnamommum verum*	Cinnamon	Lauraceae	Bark and berry fruits	It has powerful medicinal properties, loaded with antioxidant and anti-inflammatory responses, reduces the risk of heart diseases, lowers blood sugar and has an anti diabetic property.	Kim et al., 2007 Roussel et al., 2009
7.	*Cuminum cyminum*	Cumin	Apiaceae	Seed	A rich source of iron and promotes digestion, reduces sugar level and blood cholesterol, promotes fat loss and possesses a narcotic property.	Zheng et al., 2001
8.	*Murraya Koenigii*	Curry leaves	Rutaceae	Leaves	Leaves are rich source of carbohydrate, fiber, calcium, phosphorous, iron, magnesium, zinc, multi vitamins and flavonoids, used in curing Anemic condition against diabetes and indigestion and in treating skin ailment.	Irfan and Ali (2016)
9.	*Allium Sativum*	Garlic	Amaryllidaceae	Leaves	Used in food flavoring and possesses potent medicinal properties, and is known to combat cold and cough and sickness, reduces blood pressure and lowers cholesterol.	Butt et al., 2009 Ban et al., 2009
10.	*Trigonella foenum-graceum*	Fenugreek	Fabaceace	Seeds	Balances cholesterol, reduces fat and appetite and maintains liver and stomach, also reduces fiver and muscular pain.	Srichamroen et al., 2008 Narender et al., 2006
11.	*Zingiber officinale*	Ginger	Zingiberaceae	Rhizome or root stem	Contains gingerol that possess medicinal property, act as anti-inflamatory and used in reducing muscular pain and soreness	Stoilova et al., 2007
12.	*Myristica fragrans*	Nutmeg	***Myristicaceae***	Seed	Full of medicinal property and used in treating cancer and kidney diseases and in treating insomnia	Blumenthal (1998)
13.	*Brassica juncea Brassica nupus Brassica hitra*	Mustard	***Brassicaceae***	Leaves and seed	Used in flavouring and seasoning curry, oil is used on large scale. Rich in nutrient selenium, high anti-inflammatory effect, reduces the asthma attacks and lowers the blood pressure and against rheumatoid arthritis	Yoo et al., 2001
14.	*Pipper nigrum*	Pepper	Piperaceae	Dried fruits	The pungency and heating property, help in metabolism and digestion of food, also clear congestion in respiratory system	Kapoor et al.,2009 Kim et al., 2007
15.	*Crocus sativus*	Saffron	Iridaceace	Stigma and sometime petals	Powerful antioxidant, treat depressive symptoms, anti-cancerous property, reduces appetite and maintenance of weight loss, act as aphrodisiac.Used in asthma, cough, sore throat, whooping cough and loosen phlegm.	Abdullaev (2002)
16.	*Curcuma longa*	Turmeric	Zingiberaceae	Roots	Bioactive compound curcumin, control heart disease, Alzheimers and cancer, anti-inflamatory against arthristis and full of antioxidants, also heals depression	Srivastava and Mehta (2009) Fang et al., 2009
17.	*Illicium verum*	Star anise	Schisandraceae	Fruits	The oil is rich source of thymol, terpinol and anethole used in treatment of cough and cold, thr flu. Improves digestion, cramps and reduces nausea, decoction also reduces bloating and obesity	Abhishek et al., 2009

continued on following page

Table 3. Continued

S.no	Plant name	Common name	Plant belongs to family	Plant part	uses	References
18.	*Piper guineense*	Uziza/kale	Piperaceae	Dried fruits	Useful in treating intestinal disorders, cough, bronchitis and rheumatism. And also for the treatment of infertility in women and low sperm count in men	Asfaw. (2019)
19.	*Rosmarinus officinale*	Rosemary	Lamiaceae	Leaves	It helps in alleviating muscle pain, boosts memory, boosts the immune and circulatory system and promotes hair growth. Cures digestion problem, heartburn and loss of appetite.	McCaffrey et al., 2009 Machado et al., 2009
20.	*Capsicum annuum*	Paprika	Capsiceae	Fruits	Helps in healing wound, for treatment of skin problem, improve digestion, prevent hair loss, induces sleep, reduces the risk of heart attacks, anti-inflammatory properties	Kawabata et al., 2006 Snitker et al., 2009
21.	*Trachyspermum ammi*	Ajowan	Apiaceae	Leaves an seed-like fruit	Instantaneous relief from acidity and indigestion and treatment for common cold, cures tooth ache, prevents graying if hair, possess skin cleansing property	Gilani et al., 2007
22.	*Sesamum indicum*	Sesame	Pedaliaceae	Seed	Good source of fiber, lowers the cholesterol level, maintain low blood pressure, anti- inflammatory, goof source of vitamins, aid blood formation, reduces ageing	Park et al., 2010
23.	*Nigella sativa*	Fennel	Apiaceae	Seed	Possess carminative, diaphoretic, digestive, diuretic, emmenagogue, excitant, laxative, expectorant, antipyretic, antihelminthic, resolvent, stimulant, sudorific, parasiticide, stomachic, property	Sachan et al., 2016

It has been reported that the bioactive constituents of culinary spices and herbs are responsible for their biological activities such as anti-tumourigenic, antioxidative, anticarcinogenic, anti-inflammatory and cholesterol-lowering activities. Furthermore, they have aphrodisiac properties that affect cognition and mood (Tapsell et al., 2006; Srinivasan et al., 2005; Neveu et al., 2010; Craig, 1999). These properties have been actively practiced in therapeutic, clinical and preclinical trials for the investigation of new treatments and diseases. In a recent study, it was assessed that people enjoy consuming spices to improve their health and reduce the risk of mortality due to cancer, heart, ischemic and respiratory diseases (Lv et al., 2015). It was concluded in one of the observational studies, that the application of spices declines salt preferences, its daily intake, and blood pressure by modifying neural processing and behavioral intervention of salt taste in the brain (Li et al., 2017). Many spices especially turmeric (curcumin), clove (eugenol) and capsicum (red and green pepper) are antioxidant-rich, they scavenge the reactive oxygen radicles by enhancing the antioxidant properties through signal transduction pathways and lessening oxidative stress (Rubióet al., 2013; Srinivasan, 2014

The phytochemistry behind these spices and herbs has bioactive compounds in their different parts, such as alkaloids, flavonoids, tannins, saponins, terpenes, resins, and phenols which imparts medicinal and nutritive properties (Okoye and Ebeledike, 2013). Alkaloid contains heterocyclic nitrogen exhibit anti-arrhythmic, anti-hypertensive, anti-cancer, anti-malarial properties, and also proves to be powerful analgesics as a CNS stimulant (Heikens*et al.*, 1995; Ashok and Upadhyaya, 2012). Saponins have been reported to exhibit antimalarial effects (Besong*et al.*, 2016). Flavonoids and phenols possess antiallergic, anti-inflammatory, antitumor, antiplatelet and antioxidant properties (Pal and Verma, 2013). The presence of minerals such as calcium in spices and herbs have been reported to help in supporting the maintenance of teeth and bones (Omotayo*et al.*, 2013). Vitamins such as A, C, E and traces of B1, B2, B3 in spices point out antioxidant properties, especially Vitamin E. The right quantity of Vitamin C has a protective and healing role towards the formation of teeth and healthy gums (Ogbunugaforet al., 2011). Iweala et al.(2015) found the anticancerous activity against the human myeloid leukemia (HL-60) cell line and hepatocellular carcinoma (SMMC-7721), human breast adenocarcinoma (MFC-7), human lung carcinoma (A-549) and colon cancer (SW-480) in the extract of dichloromethane leaf and hexane extract of the leaves and seeds. Some of the Indian spices such as pepper, turmeric, chilli, coriander, cumin and fennel are major importers from Germany, US, the UAE, China and Malaysia. These spices are listed to aid digestion, drop the temperature of the body, enhances the rate of sweat. Most importantly, they are the source excellent carminative, antioxidant, antiseptic, and stimulant properties, as suggested by Jiang (2019) The health benefits of spices are discussed in Table 3.

ANTIOXIDANT PROPERTIES OF SPICES

Reactive oxygen species (ROS) at higher concentrations subsequently damage the macromolecules like DNA, lipids, and proteins. Every organism exhibits an array of antioxidant machinery that includes enzymatic as well as non-enzymatic antioxidant systems to cope with these damaging effects (Singh et al., 2016). Spices and herbs serve as an immense source of these antioxidants systems, and other metabolites actively participate in neutralizing the free radicals (Bi et al., 2017). They consist of secondary metabolities includeing flavonoids, phenolics, sulfur-containing compounds, tannins, alkaloids, and vitamins that protect membrane lipids against oxidative stress (Brewer, 2011). Among antioxidants, typically flavonoids and phenolics are abundant in spices and herbs that possess antioxidant properties. Aromatic herbs are good sources of flavonoids that are glycosylated derivatives, and the antioxidant activity of phenolic compounds is mainly due to their redox properties such as quenching and neutralizing free radicals. In general, flavonoids have higher antioxidant activities against proxy-radicals than do phenolic acids due to the presence of multiple hydroxyl groups. There are a number of herbs such as *Syzygium aromaticum* (clove), *Anethum graveolens* (dill), *Carum carvi* (Persian fennel), *Coriandrum sativum* (coriander), *Rosmarium officinalis* (rosemary), *Origanum vulgare* (oregano) and *Ocimum basilicum* (basil), that are a good source of flavonoids. They have the polyphenolic group, improve health, and increase the tolerance against various physiological and biochemical disorders. A part of flavanoids, phenolics behaves as antioxidant, antiviral and anticancer and anti-inflammatory activities due to inherent biochemical and pharmacological properties present in *Capsaicin* (chilly), *Curcuma longa* (turmeric), *Piper Nigrum* (black pepper), *Zingiber officinale* (ginger). These metabolites actively up-regulate the cell signaling pathway and increase the health benefits, an example is rosemarinic acid which is an active metabolite dominant in *Rosmarium Officinalis* (rosemary), *Laurus nobilis* (bay leaf), *Origanum vulgare* (Oregano) and *Curcuma longa* (turmeric). It is a conjugate acid with antioxidant and anti-inflammatory properties and also mediates various physiological effects. In turmeric oil, the major component is curcuminoid that inhibits trypsin and hyaluronidase activity, arachidonic acid metabolism, cyclooxygenase (COX), lipoxygenase, and cytokines resulting in the stabilization of the lysosomal membrane. It also increased oxidative phosphorylation and behaved as a strong O_2 radical scavenging activity associated with decreasing inflammatory swelling, acting as a boon in arthritis (Mae et al. 2007), decreasing the levels of total serum, triglyceride and free fatty acid (FFA), and increasing the level of high-density lipoprotein. Besides this, *Myristica fragrans* (nutmeg) has macelignan that actively reduces the ROS generation in neuronal hippocampal cells, as well as regulating the COX-2 expression in primary microglial cells (Jin et al. 2005). It also has anti-inflammatory activity due to suppression of mitogen-activated protein kinases (MAPKs) associated with the degradation of inhibitory–kappa B and stimulation of microglial cells (Ma et al. 2009). Damage in membrane lipids significantly reduces the intake of spices like oregano, ginger, and cloves that are rich in antioxidants that are extensively used in cooking processes (Li et al. 2006). Similarly, *Trigonella foenum-graecum* has a biological compound that has an antioxidant property named galactomannans (GAL) which reduces appetite and body weight. A compound named 2- methoxycinnamaldehyde extracted from *Cinnamomum verum* has antioxidant and anti-inflammatory properties that protect myocardial injury and cure inflammatory disorders (Hwa et al., 2012). The polyphenols in cocoa (*Cocoa bean*) and cinnamon play an important role in treating cardiovascular diseases by regulating enzymes that convert angiotensin. Angiotensin is considered as a central component of the renin- angiotensin system (RAS) that controls the level of sugar in blood (Persson et al., 2011) and also glucose metabolism activity (Anderson et al., 2004). Fenugreek seeds take active participation in glycaemic control hence improving a decreasing resistance to insulin (Vijayakumar and Bhat 2008). Besides this, extracts of turmeric also decreased the blood glucose level in type-II diabetes and activated the differentiation of human adipocyte. The compounds that are responsible for this are curcumin, demethoxy-curcumin, bis-demethoxy-curcumin (BDMC), and arturmerone (Minpei et al. 2005). During the process of weight maintenance, the compound capsaicin that is present in chilies regulate fat oxidation (Lejeune et al. 2003). Due to the scavenging of nitric oxide, curcumin accelerated gastric ulcer healing. Extracts made from sweet basil, thyme, cardamom, cinnamon, mustard, and clove have antimicrobial activity and control the infections induced by *Staphylococcus aureus, Escherichia coli, Salmonella typhimurium, Pseudomonas aeruginosa* and *Candida albicans* (Hussien et al. 2011). Besides this, plants such as lemon balm, rosemary, sage, and thyme also have antimicrobial properties against *Bacillus cereus, E. coli, Listeria monocytogenes* and *P. aeruginosa* (Gutierrez et al. 2008). Major antimicrobial compounds are β-pinene, cineole, limonene, linalool and geranylacetate which mediate a protective role against these pathogens (Chen et al. 2008; Sandasi et al. 2008). Antifungal and antibacterial properties are rich in oregano, savory, and thyme due to the occurrence of terpenes, carvacrol, p-cymene, and thymol (Bendahou et al. 2008).

Synthetic antioxidants such as butylated hydroxyanisole (BHA)/ butylated hydroxytoluene (BHT) extracted from the oil of rosemary extract also function in a similar way to natural antioxidants (Broek van der 2004). The free radical scavenging activity of black pepper (*Piper nigrum* L.) could be a potential source of natural antioxidants that are also reactive nitrogen species (RNS), and superoxide radicals generated via xanthine/xanthine oxidase system (Singh et al. 2008). Compound β-tocopherols extracted from pine bark extract (*Pinus sylvestris* L.) and grape seed extract (*Vitis vinifera* L.) also have antioxidant activity. It actively decreased the lipid peroxidation more than curcumins or synthetic antioxidant BHT (Toda et al. 1985; Majeed 1995; Sreejayan and Rao 1994). Due to having a similar structure to phenolics, the compounds curcuminoids, curcumins, demethoxycurcumin and BDMC have strong antioxidant properties by neutralizing the free radicals and by interacting with oxidative chemical chain reactions which prevented the harmful outcome by quenching the available oxygen and making it less available for oxidative reactions.

THERAPEUTIC PROPERTIES OF SPICES

With progressive findings over spices, apart from their primary role as organoleptic enhancers in culinary instances, they have a useful role in health care. Several herbs and shrubs are currently being investigated for their potential health benefits (Ogbunugafor et al., 2017). Spices not only enhance the flavor, aroma and color of food and beverages, but they may also protect against the development of acute, chronic and non-communicable diseases and help people maintain health (Jiang, 2019). Spices impart a protective role against ongoing cardiovascular and neurodegenerative diseases, type 2 diabetes mellitus and cancer (Iriti et al., 2010). Medicines extracted from spices and herbs are categorized under herbal medicine and are best described in Chinese and Indian (*Ayurvedic*) systems of medicine and their role were reviewed by Mahindru (1982). The following sections briefly discuss important human health disorders and their cure by spices.

Respiratory Diseases

Diseases associated with the respiratory system or lungs are either caused by toxic micro-organisms present in the environment or the presence of various toxic chemicals. The microbes generally attack organisms that have low nutritional values or weak immunological responses. Common respiratory disorders include the respiratory flu, tonsillitis, bronchitis, pneumonia, influenza, and pneumonia that results in a cold and cough, fever, headache, throat irritation, ears or muscle aches, and tiredness (Shah et al., 2015). A lot of work has been done to describe the role of medicinal plants to treat respiratory disorders and they are found to be more active instead of allopathic medicines (Coon and Ernst, 2004; Hetzman et al., 2005; Jari et al., 2007). Among spices, cardamom is widely used in India and used to treat throat troubles, congestion of the lungs, asthma, and pulmonary tuberculosis induced by infections present in the teeth and gums. With cold and cough, cardamom mixed with neem leaf is used to prepare nasal preparation and secrete out the mucous present in the mouth and will also relieve sore throats (Duke et al., 2003). Coriander is considered as a major spice excesscively used in Asia, North Africa, and India that is used to treat different respiratory disorders as well as used to treat anxiety and insomnia, sore throat, nosebleeds, and a cough (Gilani et al., 2007). Ginger is also used to treat respiratory disorders, including bronchitis (Benavides et al., 2007). Besides this, in the study of Shah et al. (2015), there are a number of plants that are commonly used to treat respiratory disorders. Plants such as *Abiespindrow, Achyranthesaspera, Achilleamellefolium, Adiantum, Camellia sinensis,* and *Curcuma longa* were used to treat cold, cough, chest infections, influenza, mucus problems, soothing of the throat, and to treat phlegm.

Gastrointestinal Diseases

Digestive disorders collectively studied under functional abdominal pain disorders (FAPDs) result from visceral hypersensitivity, gut dysbiosis, motility abnormalities, abnormal gastrointestinal reactivity to physiological (e.g., dietary) or noxious stimuli (toxin) or psychological stress (Beinvogl et al., 2018). Digestive disorders cause sleep problems, comorbid somatic pains, depression, and anxiety all resulting in an overall decreased quality of life (Varni et al., 2015). To treat digestive disorders, first improve food intake and include a large amount of fibers in diet, minerals, and nutrition and exclude lactose and gluten for patients (Portincasa et al., 2017). A lot of spices and herbs are implemented to treat gastrointestinal diseases. Among them, ulcer diseases of the stomach are treated by the use of capsaicin which is regarded as having gastro-protective agents (Mozsik et al., 2005). The mechanism behind the healing of ulcers is that capsaicin stimulates the secretion of alkali and mucus secretion while inhibiting the acid release from the pancreas which results in the prevention of ulcers (Satyanarayana, 2003). The contractility and motility of the human esophagus is maintained by consuming red pepper sauce (which is high in capsaicin). Many spices and herbs possess anti-microbial activity and inhibit the *Helicobacter pylori* and other bacteria and fungi (Lai and Roy, 2004). Furthermore, an herb named *Menthaepiperitae (a* source of peppermint oil), relaxes the smooth muscle tissue by blocking the Ca^{2+} channels (Grigoleit et al., 2005), and also relaxes the esophagus by helping to diffuse oesophageal spasms (Pimentel et al., 2001). The overall efficiency of the digestive system was accelerated by enhancing the secretion of gastric and bile acids *via* consuming black pepper and reducing food transit time (Srinivasan, 2007). Digestive enzymes such as amylase, lipase, trypsin and chymotrypsin were up-regulated when piperine was consumed with the diet (Patel and Srinivasan, 2004). Similarly, peptic ulcers were also treated *via* consuming curcumin (500 mg/day) which also improves dyspepsia symptoms (Khonche et al., 2016) in the human by having an anti-helicobacter regimen. In China and India, consumption of cardamom was significantly used to treat various digestive disorders including stomach ache disorders, constipation problems, and dysentery in children. It is also an effective herbal medicine to treat bladder problems when cardamom pods are mixed with mastic and milk. In a study of Yuki et al. (2015), a mixture of extracts of three medicinal plants such as *Zingiberis rhizome, Ginseng radix* and *Zanthoxylifructus* was found very effective in chronic constipation and bloating as well as improving bacterial growth in the small intestine. In brief, natural herbal medicines (spices and herbs) play a very important role in treating many gastrointestinal and pain disorders; their use is abdominal pains, especially in pediatrics remains unclear. This would help increase therapeutic options and tailor treatments for patients with functional gastrointestinal pain symptoms.

Liver Disease

Curcumin is also effective in treating steatohepatitis (Rahmani et al., 2016) and improves the BMI, total cholesterol, LDL-C, triglycerides, liver enzymes, and uric acid when compared with the placebo group. Ling (2012) elucidates the role of turmeric oil in the prevention of liver damage. The fat content of liver was reduced up-to 78.9% as compared to patients with non-alcoholic fatty liver disease via the application of curcumin.

Cancer

Across the world a major death-causing disease is cancer (one of the major and common diseases among human beings). In 2012, approximately 8.2 million deaths were reported due to cancer, and 14 million new cases of cancer were reported (Arends, 2010; WHO, 2016). Treatment of cancer is done by various methods, and among them surgery, radiotherapy and chemotherapy are major treatment processes. However, these treatment techniques are found to be effective for localized and small tumors as well as inducing certain side effects. Hence, to minimize the side effects induced by chemotherapy, there is a need to use herbal medicines that include spices and herbs which have low side effects and also treat chemotherapy-induced indigestion, nausea, vomiting, and metallic taste (Giacosa et al., 2015; Ijpma et al., 2015).

Spices and herbs were reported to act as anticancer drugs. Furthermore, the study revealed that phlegm-eliminating herbs have an array of chemical compounds with antitumor effects i.e. provokes apoptosis, inhibits invasion, and metastasis as well as reducing the effects of chemotherapeutic drugs. In tumor cells, the basic apoptosis process is distorted, and the cell survives, and for apoptosis, a major role is played by caspase and arrests of the cell cycle and anticancer drugs target the apoptosis process (Debatin, 1999). In traditional Chinese medicine (TCM), one of the most important anti-cancer herbs is *Citrus reticulata*. It reported to induce apoptosis and have significant effects on several tumor cell lines includes gastric cancer (Kim et al., 2005; Lee et al., 2012b), colorectal cancer (Zhengetal., 2002), and lung cancer cells (Xiao et al.,2009) (Silalahi, 2002; Ariasand Ramon-Laca, 2005). Active ingredients of this herb are flavonoids that increased the level of Ca^{2+} and activating Ca dependent apoptotic proteases and increased apoptosis (Qiu et al., 2010). Further, *Platycodongrandiflorus* is also used to induce apoptosis in SKOV-3 human ovarian tumor cells (Hu et al., 2010), MCF-7 human breast tumor cells (Yu and Kim, 2010) and U-937 human leukemia cells (Shin et al., 2009).

Spices such as turmeric (*Curcuma longa*) have an array of anti-cancer compounds including curcumin terpenoids and alkaloids. These compounds suppressed the activation of NF-κB, that down-regulates TNF-α induced NF-κB activation, blocks IκBα degradation, cytokine-induced NF-κB DNA binding activity, IKK activity in HT-29, RelA nuclear translocation, IκB serine 32 phosphorylation, Caco-2, and EC-6 cells (Mughal et al., 2019). It also reduced the level of IL-8 and LPS-mediated TLR2 mRNA induction on mouse splenic macrophages in human monocytes and gingival fibroblasts through suppressing NF-κB activation (Kato et al., 2004). Further, eugenol is a major compound present in clove (*Eugenia caryophyllata*) which down-regulates the H-ras, c-Myc, and Bcl2 expression along with up-regulates the Bax, p53 and the active caspase-3 expression in the skin lesions of rats (Kaur et al., 2010) and protects against DNA damage. Similarly, basil (*Ocimum sanctum*) has a large number of anti-cancer compounds that suppress the cell proliferation, migration of tumor cells, and promotes apoptosis. Besides this, it also suppresses the induction of apoptosis and down-regulates the anti-apoptotic proteins (Bcl-2 and Bcl-xL) (Kothari et al., 2004). Several other spices such as bay leaf (*Cinnamomumtamala*), black cumin seed (*Nigella sativa*), cardamom (*Elettariacardamomum*), cinnamon (*Cinnamomum cassia*), coriander (*Coriandrumsativum*), fennel(*Foeniculumvulgare*), saffron (*Crocus sativus*) and garlic (*Allium sativa*) also have a vast variety of anti-cancer compounds with a low level of health risks.

Cardiovascular Disease

A major death-causing disease is heart disease (cardio-vascular disease). It is very common due to a change in the lifestyle of human beings or excessive consumption of fast foods or fat-containing foods which significantly increase the level of cholesterol in the heart (Jiang et al., 2017). Besides allopathic treatments, the use of herbal medicine in treating heart diseases is well documented by several workers (Ghayur et al., 2005; Tanwar et al., 2010; Lee et al., 2015; Guldiken et al., 2018). Major spices that are extensively used to lower cardiovascular diseases are focussed on the use of garlic, ginger, turmeric, onions, and tulsi. Garlic (*Allium sativa*) is used as a common spice all over the world that has phenolics as it's major compounds as well as allicin, S-allyl cysteine, and alliin (sulfur-containing). These compounds have anti-thrombotic, anti-atherogenic, anti-lipidemic, anti-hypertensive, and anti-glycemic effects (Schwingshackl et al., 2016). The garlic extract also significantly works on blood pressure and lowers the risk associated with a change in blood pressure and reduces hypertension (Ried et al., 2016). Further, curcumin extracted from turmeric gives a yellow color and is frequently used in Asian cooking (Prasad et al., 2014). It plays an important role in enhancing the cardiac function as it stabilized the cytoskeleton structure, which in turn is attributed to the Hsp27 expression along with a reinforced antioxidant defense system (Tanwar et al., 2010). Some other active compounds such as gingerol and shogaol extracted from ginger lower blood pressure and act as vasodilators and a cardio-suppressant (Ghayur et al., 2005). In one of the studies, it was reported that ginkgo significantly inhibits the angiotensin-converting enzyme and modulates the endothelial NO release in animal models (Mansour et al., 2011). Overall, in brief, both *in vivo* and clinical study results suggested that herbs and spice-containing diets have been recommended for heart health. The secondary metabolites such as digoxin and digitoxin extracted from *Digitalis lanata* and *Digitalis purpurea;*; reserpine extracted from *Rauwolfia serpentine* and acetylsalicylic acid (aspirin) extracted from willow bark, have medicinal properties to cure cardio-vascular disease and psychosis (Hussain et al., 2004; Slim et al., 2011).

Other

Furthermore, green tea (Camellia sinensis), which is rich in flavonoids (mainly catechins) is used to enhance mental alertness as well as reduce cholesterol levels, control diabetes, and also prevent cardio-vascular events (Stangl et al., 2006). Besides these, the gymnosperm named *Ginkgo biloba leaves* is a rich source of ginkgolides, bilobalides, and flavonoids that are used to treat asthma, bronchitis, fatigue, and tinnitus as well as to boost memory and cure dementia and coronary heart disease.

CONCLUSION

Spices are potentially endowed with several bioactive molecules, thus performing various bio-functions, and these synergistic effects protect that human body. Conventionally, spices are part of the diet, regulating physiological and biochemical processes. Apart from their role in flavoring, spices are used for preservation, medicinal, pharmaceutical, and health maintenance purposes. They are rich sources of micronutrients, such as iron, magnesium, calcium, and many others, and are essential elements to a diet. Theseh spices display anti-inflammatory, anti-cancerous, and radical scavenging properties and have antioxidants that control oxidative stress in cells. These metabolites from spices and herbs play a constructive role in treating chronic disorders such as cancer, diabetes, and diseases associated with respiratory and cardiovascular problems. Thus, spices play a potential role in flavoring, nutritional, medicinal and pharmacological aspects, and in traditional systems of medicine by combatting chronic diseases.

REFERENCES

Acharya, S. N., Thomas, J. E., & Basu, S. K. (2008). Fenugreek, an alternative crop for semiarid regions of North America. *Crop Science*, *48*(3), 841–853. doi:10.2135/cropsci2007.09.0519

Adeyemi, M. M. H. (2011). A review of secondary metabolites from plant materials for post-harvesting. *IJPAS*, *6*, 94–102.

Ahmed, T., & Gilani, A. H. (2009). Inhibitory effect of curcuminoids on acetylcholinesterase activity and attenuation of scopolamine-induced amnesia have medicinal use of turmeric in Alzheimer's disease. *Pharmacology, Biochemistry, and Behavior, 91*(4), 554–559. doi:10.1016/j.pbb.2008.09.010 PMID:18930076

Alam, K., Goher, Z., & Anderson, R. A. (2009). Bay leaves improves glucose and lipid profile of people with type 2 diabetes. *Journal of Clinical Biochemistry and Nutrition, 44*(1), 52–56. doi:10.3164/jcbn.08-188 PMID:19177188

Ammon, H. P., & Wahl, M. A. (1991). Pharmacology of Curcuma longa. *Planta Medica, 57*(01), 1–7. doi:10.1055-2006-960004 PMID:2062949

Anandakumar, P., Kamaraj, S., Jagan, S., Ramakrishnan, G., Vinodjkumar, R., & Devaki, T. (2008). Capsaicin modulates pulmonary antioxidant defense system during benzo(a)pyrene-induced lung cancer in swiss albino mice. *Phytotherapy Research, 22*(4), 529–533. doi:10.1002/ptr.2393 PMID:18338764

Anderson, R. A., Broadhurst, C. L., Polansky, M. M., Schmidt, W. F., Khan, A., Flanagan, V. P., ... Graves, D. J. (2004). Isolation and characterization of polyphenol type-A polymers from cinnamon with insulin-like biological activity. *Journal of Agricultural and Food Chemistry, 52*(1), 65–70. doi:10.1021/jf034916b PMID:14709014

Arends, J. (2010). Metabolism in cancer patients. *Anticancer Research, 30*, 1863–1868. PMID:20592393

Arias, B. A., & Ramon-Laca, L. (2005). Pharmacological properties of citrus and their ancient and medieval uses in the Mediterranean region. *Journal of Ethnopharmacology, 97*(1), 89–95. doi:10.1016/j.jep.2004.10.019 PMID:15652281

Asfaw, D., (2019) Review on Use of Bioactive Compounds in Some Spices in Food Preservation. *Food Sci and Quality Manag., 87.*

Ashok, P. K., & Upadhyaya, K. (2012). Tannins are asrigent. *Journal of Pharmacognosy and Phytochemistry, 1*, 45–50.

Ban, J. O., Oh, J. H., Kim, T. M., Kim, D. J., Jeong, J. S., Han, S. B., & Hong, J. T. (2009). Anti-inflammatory and arthritic effects of thiacremonone, a novel sulfur compound isolated from garlic via inhibition of NF-κB. *Arthritis Research & Therapy, 11*(5), R145. doi:10.1186/ar2819 PMID:19788760

Basu, S. K., Acharya, S. N., & Thomas, J. E. (2008). Application of phosphate fertilizer and harvest management for important fenugreek (Trigonellafoenum-graecumL.) seed and forage yield in a dark brown soil zone of Canada. *KMITL Sci Tech J, 8*(1), 1–7.

Beinvogl, B., Burch, E., Snyder, J., Schechter, N., Hale, A., Okazaki, Y., ... Nurko, S. (2018). Multidisciplinary treatment of pediatric functional gastrointestinal disorders results in improved pain and functioning. *Clinical Gastroenterology and Hepatology.*

Benavides, G. A., Squadrito, G. L., Mills, R. W., Patel, H. D., Isbell, T. S., Patel, R. P., ... Kraus, D. W. (2007). Hydrogen sulfide mediates the vasoactivity of garlic. *Proceedings of the National Academy of Sciences of the United States of America, 104*(46), 17977–17982. doi:10.1073/pnas.0705710104 PMID:17951430

Bendahou, M., Muselli, A., Grignon-Dubois, M., Benyoucef, M., Desjobert, J. M., Bernardini, A. F., & Costa, J. (2008). Antimicrobial activity and chemical composition of OriganumglandulosumDesf. Essential oil and extract obtained by microwave extraction. Comparison with hydro distillation. *Food Chemistry, 106*(1), 132–139. doi:10.1016/j.foodchem.2007.05.050

Bernard, G. T., Esteban, P., & Christopher, J. S. (1982). Turmerones: Isolation from turmeric and their structure determination. *Chemical Communications, 6*, 363.

Besong, E. E., Balogun, M. E., Djobissie, S. F. A., Mbamalu, O. S., & Obimma, J. N. (2016). A review of *Piper guineense*(African Black Pepper). *Inter J of Pharm and Pharma Res, 6*, 368–384.

Bi, X., Lim, J., & Henry, C. J. (2017). Spices in the management of diabetes mellitus. *Food Chemistry, 217*, 281–293. doi:10.1016/j.foodchem.2016.08.111 PMID:27664636

Blumenthal, M. (1998). *The complete German Commission E monographs: therapeutic guide to herbal medicines*. Austin, TX: American Botanical Council.

Brewer, M.S. (2011) Natural Antioxidants: Sources, Compounds, Mechanisms of Action, and Potential Applications. *Inst food technol, 10*, 221-247.

Broek, H., Robbins, K., & Randall, J. (2004). Rosemary extract: Taking freshness back to basics. In: Fats and oils-their role in food and health. In *Proceedings of the biennial conference*. Australian Section of the American Oil Chemists Society.

Butt, M. S., Sultan, M. T., Butt, M. S., & Iqbal, J. (2009). Garlic: Nature's Protection Against Physiological Threats. *Critical Reviews in Food Science and Nutrition, 49*(6), 538–551. doi:10.1080/10408390802145344 PMID:19484634

Cao, H., Urban, J. F. Jr, & Anderson, R. A. (2008). Cinnamon Polyphenol Extract Affects Immune Responses by Regulating Anti- and Proinflammatory and Glucose Transporter Gene Expression in Mouse Macrophages. *The Journal of Nutrition, 138*(5), 833–840. doi:10.1093/jn/138.5.833 PMID:18424588

Chaiyasit, K., Khovidhunkit, W., & Wittayalertpanya, S. (2009). Relationships between Free Radical Scavenging and Antioxidant Activity in Foods. *Journal of the Medical Association of Thailand, 92*, 108–113. PMID:19260251

Chandra, D., & Gupta, S. S. (1972). Anti-inflammatory and antiarthritic activity of volatile oil of Curcuma longa. *The Indian Journal of Medical Research, 60*, 138–142. PMID:5029117

Chen, N., Chang, C. C., Ng, C. C., Wang, C. Y., Shyu, Y. T., & Chang, T. I. (2008). Antioxidant and antimicrobial activity of Zingiberaceae plants in Taiwan. *Plant Foods for Human Nutrition (Dordrecht, Netherlands), 63*(1), 15–20. doi:10.100711130-007-0063-7 PMID:18157743

Chiwendu, S., Ejike, E. N., Ejeke, B. U., Oti, W., & Uwachukwu, I. (2016). Phytochemical properties of Uziza leave (*Piper guineesnse*). *J of Pure and App Chem, 3*, 12–15.

Craig, W. J. (1999). Health-promoting properties of common herbs. *The American Journal of Clinical Nutrition, 70*(3), 491–499. doi:10.1093/ajcn/70.3.491s PMID:10479221

Debatin, K. M. (1999). Activation of apoptosis pathways by anticancer drugs. *Advances in Experimental Medicine and Biology, 457*, 237–244. doi:10.1007/978-1-4615-4811-9_25 PMID:10500798

Delecroix, B., Abaïdia, A. E., Leduc, C., Dawson, B., & Dupont, G. (2017). Article. *Journal of Sports Science & Medicine, 16*, 147–153. PMID:28344463

Derwich, E., Benziane, Z., & Chabir, R. (2011). *Aromatic and medicinal plants of Morocco: Chemical composition of essential oils of Rosmarinus officinalis and Juniperus Phoenicea*. Academic Press.

Dhanapakiam, P., & Joseph, J., Mini, Ramaswamy, V. K. M., Moorthi, & Senthil Kumar, A. (2008). The cholesterol lowering property of coriander seeds (Coriandrumsativum): Mechanism of action. *Journal of Environmental Biology, 29*(1), 53–56. PMID:18831331

Duke, J. A., Bogenschutz-Godwin, M. J., deCellier, J., & Duke, P. K. (2003). Elettaria cardamomum Maton (Zingiberaceae) Cardamon, Malabar or Mysore cardamon. CRC Handbook of Medicinal Spices, 120-138.

Duke, J. A., Bogenschutz-Godwin, M. J., deCellier, J., & Duke, P. K. (2003). *Syzygiumaromaticum(L.) Merr.and L. M. Perry (Myrtaceae) Clavos, Clove, Clovetree. In CRC Handbook of Medicinal Spices* (p. 281). Washington, DC: CRC Press.

Dzoyem, J. P., McGaw, L.J., Kuete, V., & Bakowsky, U. (2017). *Medicinal Spices and Vegetables from Africa*. Academic Press.

Ekanem, A. P., Udoh, V. F., & Oku, E. E. (2010). Effects of ethanol extract of *Piper guineense* seeds (Schum and Thonn) on the conception of mice (MuaMusculus). *African Journal of Pharmacy and Pharmacology, 4*, 362–367.

Fabio, A., Cermelli, C., Fabio, G., Nicoletti, P., & Quaglio, P. (2007). Screening of the antibacterial effects of a variety of essential oils on microorganisms responsible for respiratory infections. *Phytotherapy Research, 21*(4), 374–377. doi:10.1002/ptr.1968 PMID:17326042

Fang, X. D., Yang, F., Zhu, L., Shen, Y. L., Wang, L. L., & Cheng, Y. Y. (2009). Curcumin ameliorates high glucose-induced acute vascular endothelial dysfunction in rat thoracic aorta. *Clinical and Experimental Pharmacology & Physiology, 36*(12), 1177–1182. doi:10.1111/j.1440-1681.2009.05210.x PMID:19473193

Garcia-Olmo, D. C., Riese, H. H., Escribano, J., Ontanon, J., Fernandez, J. A., Atienzar, M., & Garcia-Olmo, D. (1999). Effects of long-term treatment of colon adenocarcinoma with crocin, a carotenoid from saffron (Crocussativus L.): An experimental study in the rat. *Nutrition and Cancer, 35*(2), 120–126. doi:10.1207/S15327914NC352_4 PMID:10693164

Ghadermazi, R., Keramat, J., & Goli, S. A. H. (2017). Antioxidant activity of clove (Eugenia caryophyllataThunb), oregano (Oringanumvulgare L) and sage (Salvia officinalis L) essential oils in various modelsystems. *International Food Research Journal, 24*(4), 1628–1635.

Ghayur, M. N., Gilani, A. H., Afridi, M. B., & Houghton, P. J. (2005). Cardiovascular effects of ginger aqueous extract and its phenolic constituents are mediated through multiple pathways. *Vascular Pharmaco, 43*(4), 234-241.

Giacosa, A., Morazzoni, P., Bombardelli, E., Riva, A., Bianchi, P. G., & Rondanelli, M. (2015). Can nausea and vomiting be treated with ginger extract? *European Review for Medical and Pharmacological Sciences*, *19*, 1291–1296. PMID:25912592

Gilani, A. H., Bashir, S., & Khan, A. U. (2007). Pharmacological basis for the use of *Borago officinalis* in gastrointestinal, respiratory and cardiovascular disorders. *Journal of Ethnopharmacology*, *114*(3), 393–399. doi:10.1016/j.jep.2007.08.032 PMID:17900837

Grigoleit, H. G., & Grigoleit, P. (2005). Gastrointestinal clinical pharmacology of peppermint oil. *Phytomedicine*, *12*(8), 607–611. doi:10.1016/j.phymed.2004.10.006 PMID:16121522

Grzanna, R., Phan, P., Polotsky, A., Lindmark, L., & Fondoza, C. G. (2004). Ginger Extract Inhibits β-Amyloid Peptide–Induced Cytokine and Chemokine Expression in Cultured THP-1 Monocytes. *Journal of Alternative and Complementary Medicine (New York, N.Y.)*, *10*(6), 1009–1013. doi:10.1089/acm.2004.10.1009 PMID:15673995

Guldiken, B., Özkan, G., Catalkaya, G., Ceylan, F.D., Yalçınkaya, İ. E., & Capanoglu, E. (2018). Phytochemicals of herbs and spices: Health versus toxicological effects. *Food and Chemical Toxicology*. doi:10.1016/j.fct.2018.05.050 PMID:29802945

Gunasekar, M., Geemon, K., & Mariwala, S. J. (2012). Health benefits of bioactive molecules from spices and aromatic plants. *JOSAC21*, 87–101.

Gupta, A., Gupta, R., & Lal, B. (2001). Effect of Trigonellafoenum-graecum (fenugreek) seeds on glycemic control and insulin resistance in type-2 diabetes mellitus: A double blind placebo controlled study. *J Assoc Physi Ind*, *49*, 1057–1061. PMID:11868855

Gupta, V. B., Indi, S. S., & Rao, K. S. (2009). Garlic extract exhibits antiamyloidogenic activity on amyloid-beta fibrillogenesis: Relevance to Alzheimer's disease. *Phytotherapy Research*, *23*(1), 111–115. doi:10.1002/ptr.2574 PMID:18844255

Gupta, V. B., & Rao, K. S. (2007). Anti-amyloidogenic activity of S-allyl-L-cysteine and its activity to destabilize Alzheimer's beta-amyloid fibrils in vitro. *Neuroscience Letters*, *429*, 75–80.

Shan, B., Cai, Y. Z., Sun, M., & Corke, H. (2005). Antioxidant capacity of 26 spice extracts and characterization of their phenolic constituents. *Journal of Agricultural and Food Chemistry*, *53*(20), 7749–7759.

Gutierrez, J., Barry-Ryan, C., & Bourke, P. (2008). The antimicrobial efficacy of plant essential oil combinations and interactions with food ingredients. *International Journal of Food Microbiology*, *124*(1), 91–97. doi:10.1016/j.ijfoodmicro.2008.02.028 PMID:18378032

Gutierrez, J., Barry-Ryan, C., & Bourke, P. (2009). Antimicrobial activity of plant essential oils using food model media: Efficacy, synergistic potential and interactions with food components. *Food Microbiology*, *26*(2), 142–150. doi:10.1016/j.fm.2008.10.008 PMID:19171255

Heikens, H., Fliers, E., Endert, E., Acknermans, M., & van Montfrans, G. (1995). Linquorice-induced hypertension—A new understanding of an old disease. *Journal of Medicinal Chemistry*, *5*, 230–234.

Heitzman, M. E., Neto, C. C., Winiarz, E., Vaisberg, A. J., & Hammond, G. B. (2005). Ethnobotany, phytochemistry and pharmacology of Uncaria (Rubiaceae). *Phytochemistry*, *66*(1), 5–29. doi:10.1016/j.phytochem.2004.10.022 PMID:15649507

Hu, Q., Pan, R., Wang, L., Peng, B., Tang, J., & Liu, X. (2010). Platycodongrandiflorum induces apoptosis in SKOV3 human ovarian cancer cells through mitochondrial-dependent pathway. *The American Journal of Chinese Medicine*, *38*(02), 373–386. doi:10.1142/S0192415X10007919 PMID:20387232

Hussain, F., Sher, H., & Ibrar, M. (2004). Ethnobotanical profile of some plants of District Swat, Pakistan. *Pak J Pl Sci*, *10*, 85–104.

Hussain, Z., Swindle, J., & Hauptman, P. J. (2006). Digoxin useand digoxin toxicity in the post-DIG trial era. *Journal of Cardiac Failure*, *12*(5), 343–346. doi:10.1016/j.cardfail.2006.02.005 PMID:16762795

Hussien, J., Teshale, C., & Mohammed, J. (2011). Assessment of the antimicrobial effects of some Ethiopian aromatic spice and herb hydrosols. *International Journal of Pharmacology*, *7*(5), 635–640. doi:10.3923/ijp.2011.635.640

Hwa, J. S., Jin, Y. C., Lee, Y. S., Ko, Y. S., Kim, Y. M., Shi, L. Y., ... Chang, K. C. (2012). 2- Methoxycinnamaldehyde from Cinnamomum cassia reduces rat myocardial ischemia and reperfusion injury in vivo due to HO-1 induction. *Journal of Ethnopharmacology*, *139*(2), 605–615. doi:10.1016/j.jep.2011.12.001 PMID:22179023

IJpma, I., Renken, R. J., Ter Horst, G. J., & Reyners, A. K. (2015). Metallic taste in cancer patients treated withchemotherapy. *Cancer Treatment Reviews*, *41*(2), 179–186. doi:10.1016/j.ctrv.2014.11.006 PMID:25499998

Irfan, U., & Ali, S. (2016). The antibacterial effect of curry leaves (*Murraya Koenigii*). *Euro J. Pharma. and Medi Resea.*

Iriti, M., Vitalini, S., Fico, G., & Faoro, F. (2010). Neuroprotective Herbs and Foods from Different Traditional Medicines and Diets. *Molecules (Basel, Switzerland)*, *15*(5), 3517–3555. doi:10.3390/molecules15053517 PMID:20657497

Iweala, E. E. J., Liu, F. F., Cheng, R. R., Li, Y., Ononhinmin, C. A., & Zhand, Y. J. (2015). Anticancer and free radical scavenging acivity of some Nigerian food plants *in vitro*. *International Journal of Cancer Research*, *11*(1), 41–51. doi:10.3923/ijcr.2015.41.51

Iwu, M. M. (2014). *Handbook of African medicinal plants*. Boca Raton, FL: Francis & Taylorn Group. doi:10.1201/b16292

Jafri, M. A., Farah, Javed, K., & Singh, S. (2001). Evaluation of the gastric antiulcerogenic effect of large cardamom (fruits of AmomumsubulatumRoxb). *Journal of Ethnopharmacology*, *75*(2-3), 89–94. doi:10.1016/S0378-8741(00)00398-6 PMID:11297839

Janssens, P. L., Hursel, R., & Westerterp-Plantenga, M. S. (2014). Capsaicin increases sensation of fullness in energy balance, and decreases desire to eat after dinner in negative energy balance. *Appetite*, *77*, 44–49. doi:10.1016/j.appet.2014.02.018 PMID:24630935

Jari, Ä. (2007). An ethnobotanical study on the usage of wild medicinal herbs from Kopaonik Mountain (Central Serbia). *Journal of Ethnopharmacology, 111*(1), 160–175. doi:10.1016/j.jep.2006.11.007 PMID:17145148

Jiang, S., Han, J., Li, T., Xin, Z., Ma, Z., Di, W., & Wang, D. (2017). 880 Curcumin as a potential protective compound against cardiac diseases. *Pharmacological Research, 119*, 373–383. doi:10.1016/j.phrs.2017.03.001 PMID:28274852

Jiang, T. A. (2019). Health Benefits of Culinary Herbs and Spices. *Journal of AOAC International, 102*(2), 395–411. doi:10.5740/jaoacint.18-0418 PMID:30651162

Jiang, Y., Wu, N., Fu, Y. J., Wang, W., Luo, M., Zhao, C. J., ... Liu, X. L. (2011). Chemical composition and antimicrobial activity of the essential oil of rosemary. *Environmental Toxicology and Pharmacology, 32*(1), 63–68. doi:10.1016/j.etap.2011.03.011 PMID:21787731

Jin, D. Q., Lim, C. S., Hwang, J. K., Ha, I., & Han, J. S. (2005). Anti-oxidant and anti-inflammatory activities of macelignan in murine hippocampal cell line and primary culture of rat microglial cells. *Biochemical and Biophysical Research Communications, 331*(4), 1264–1269. doi:10.1016/j.bbrc.2005.04.036 PMID:15883012

Kaefer, C. M., & Milner, J. A. (2011). Herbs and Spices in Cancer Prevention and Treatment. In Source Herbal Medicine: Biomolecular and Clinical Aspects (2nd ed.). CRC Press/Taylor & Francis. doi:10.1201/b10787-18

Kandaswami, C., Lee, L. T., Lee, P. P., Hwang, J. J., Ke, F. C., Huang, Y. T., & Lee, M. T. (2005) The antitumor activities of flavonoids. In Vivo, 19(5), 895-909.

Kapoor, I. P., Singh, B., Singh, G., De-Heuluan, C. S., De Lampasona, M. P., & Catalan, C. A. N. (2009). Chemistry and in Vitro Antioxidant Activity of Volatile Oil and Oleoresins of Black Pepper (*Piper nigrum*). *Journal of Agricultural and Food Chemistry, 57*(12), 5358–5364. doi:10.1021/jf900642x PMID:19456163

Kara, S., Gencer, B., Karaca, T., Tufan, H., Arikan, S., Ersan, I., … Volkan, H. (2019). *Protective Effect of Hesperetin and Naringenin against Apoptosis in Ischemia/Reperfusion-Induced Retinal Injury in Rats*. Academic Press.

Karlsson, F. H., Tremaroli, V., Nookaew, I., Bergström, G., Behre, C. J., Fagerberg, B., ... Bäckhed, F. (2013). Gut metagenome in European women with normal, impaired and diabetic glucose control. *Nature, 498*(7452), 99–103. doi:10.1038/nature12198 PMID:23719380

Kato, S., Yuzawa, Y., Tsuboi, N., Maruyama, S., Morita, Y., Matsuguchi, T., & Matsuo, S. (2004). Endotoxin-induced chemokine expression in murine peritoneal mesothelial cells: The role of toll-like receptor 4. *Journal of the American Society of Nephrology, 5*, 1289–1299. PMID:15100369

Kaur, G., Athar, M., & Alam, M. S. (2010). Eugenol precludes cutaneous chemical carcinogenesis in mouse by preventing oxidative stress and inflammation and by inducing apoptosis. *Molecular Carcinogenesis, 49*(3), 290–301. PMID:20043298

Kawabata, F., Inoue, N., Yazawa, S., Kawada, T., Inoue, K., & Fushiki, T. (2006). Effects of CH-19 Sweet, a Non-Pungent Cultivar of Red Pepper, in Decreasing the Body Weight and Suppressing Body Fat Accumulation by Sympathetic Nerve Activation in Humans. *Bioscience, Biotechnology, and Biochemistry*, *70*(12), 2824–2835. doi:10.1271/bbb.60206 PMID:17151481

Khajehdehi, P. (2012). Turmeric: Reemerging of a neglected Asian traditional remedy. *Journal of Nephropathology*, *1*(1), 17–22. doi:10.5812/jnp.5 PMID:24475382

Khan, A., Safdar, M., Ali Khan, M. M., Khattak, K. N., & Anderson, R. A. (2003). Cinnamon improves glucose and lipids of people with type-2 diabetes. *Diabetes Care*, *26*(12), 3215–3218. doi:10.2337/diacare.26.12.3215 PMID:14633804

Khonche, A., Biglaria, O., Panahi, Y., Valizadegan, G., Soflaei, S. S., Ghamarchehreh, M. E., ... Sahebkar, A. (2016). Adjunctive Therapy with Curcumin for Peptic Ulcer: A Randomized Controlled Trial. *Drug Research (Stuttgart)*, *66*(08), 444–448. doi:10.1055-0042-109394 PMID:27351245

Kim, D. H., Kim, C. H., Kim, M. S., Kim, J. Y., Chung, J. H., Lee, J. W., ... Chung, H. Y. (2007). Suppression of age-related inflammatory NF-κB activation by cinnamaldehyde. *Biogerontology*, *8*(5), 545–554. doi:10.100710522-007-9098-2 PMID:17486422

Kim, M. J., Park, H. J., Hong, M. S., Kim, M. S., Leem, K. H., Kim, J. B., ... Kim, H. K. (2005). Citrus Reticulatablanco induces apoptosis in human gastric cancer cells SNU-668. *Nutrition and Cancer*, *51*(1), 78–82. doi:10.120715327914nc5101_11 PMID:15749633

Kim, S. H., & Lee, Y. C. (2009). Piperine inhibits eosinophil infiltration and airway hyperresponsiveness by suppressing T cell activity and Th2 cytokine production in the ovalbumin-induced asthma model. *The Journal of Pharmacy and Pharmacology*, *61*(3), 353–359. doi:10.1211/jpp.61.03.0010 PMID:19222908

Kim, T., Davis, J., Zhang, A. J., He, X., & Matthews, S. T. (2009). Curcumin activates AMPK and suppresses gluconeogenic gene expression in hepatoma cells. *Biochemical and Biophysical Research Communications*, *388*(2), 377–382. doi:10.1016/j.bbrc.2009.08.018 PMID:19665995

Kothari, S. K., Bhattacharya, A. K., & Ramesh, S. (2004). Essential oil yield and quality of methyl eugenol rich Ocimumtenuiflorum L. f. (syn. O. sanctum L.) grown in South India as influenced by method of harvest. *Journal of Chromatography. A*, *1054*(1-2), 67–72. doi:10.1016/j.chroma.2004.03.019 PMID:15553132

Lai, P. K., & Roy, J. (2004). Antimicrobial and Chemopreventive Properties of Herbs and Spices. *Current Medicinal Chemistry*, *11*(11), 1451–1460. doi:10.2174/0929867043365107 PMID:15180577

Lee, D.H., Park, K.I., Park, H.S., Kang, S.R., Nagappan, A., Kim, J.A., … Kim, G.S. (2012b). Flavonoids isolated from Korea Citrus aurantium L. induce G2/M phase arrest and apoptosis in human gastric cancer AGS Cells. *Evid.-Based Complement.Altern Med: eCAM*, 515901.

Lee, K. H., Abas, F., Alitheen, M., Banu, N., Shaari, K., Lajis, N. H., & Syahida, A. (2015). Chemopreventive effects of a curcuminlike diarylpentanoid [2,6-bis (2, 5-dimethoxybenzylidene) cyclohexanone] in cellular targetsof rheumatoid arthritis in vitro. *International Journal of Rheumatic Diseases*, *18*(6), 616–627. doi:10.1111/1756-185X.12341 PMID:24832356

Lejeune, M. P., Kovacs, E. M., & Westerterp-Plantenga, M. S. (2003). Effect of capsaicin on substrate oxidation and weight maintenance after modest body-weight loss in human subjects. *British Journal of Nutrition*, *90*(3), 651–659. doi:10.1079/BJN2003938 PMID:13129472

Li, Q., Cui, Y., Jin, R., Lang, H., Yu, H., Sun, F., ... Zhu, Z. (2017). Enjoyment of Spicy Flavor Enhances Central Salty-Taste Perception and Reduces Salt Intake and Blood Pressure. *Hypertension*, *70*(6), 1291–1299. doi:10.1161/HYPERTENSIONAHA.117.09950 PMID:29089370

Li, S., Wan, C., Wang, M., Li, W., Matsumoto, K., & Tang, Y. (n.d.). *Antidepressant like effects of piperine in chronic mild stress treated mice and its possible mechanisms*. Academic Press.

Li, T. Y., Brennan, A. M., Wedick, N. M., Petersen, J. M., Stonehouse, O. W., Jerling, J. C., ... White, Z. (2006). Anti-oxidant rich spice added to hamburger meat during cooking results in reduced meat, plasma, and urine malondialdehyde concentrations. *The American Journal of Clinical Nutrition*, *84*, 95–135.

Ling, J., Wei, B., Lv, G., Ji, H., & Li, S. (2012). Antihyperlipidaemic and antioxidant effects of turmeric oil in hyperlipidaemic rats. *Food Chemistry*, *130*(2), 229–235. doi:10.1016/j.foodchem.2011.07.039

Lobo, V., Patil, A., Phatak, A., & Chandra, N. (2010). Free radicals, antioxidants and functional foods: Impact on human health. *Pharmacognosy Reviews*, *4*(8), 118–126. doi:10.4103/0973-7847.70902 PMID:22228951

Ma, J., Hwang, Y. K., Cho, W. H., Han, S. H., Hwang, J. K., & Han, J. S. (2009). Macelignan attenuates activations of mitogen-activated protein kinases and nuclear factor kappa B induced by lipopolysaccharide in microglial cells. *Biological & Pharmaceutical Bulletin*, *32*(6), 1085–1090. doi:10.1248/bpb.32.1085 PMID:19483320

Machado, D. G., Bettio, L. E., Cunha, M. P., Capra, J. C., Dalmarco, J. B., Pizzolatti, M. G., & Rodrigues, A. L. S. (2009). Antidepressant-like effect of the extract of Rosmarinus officinalis in mice: Involvement of the monoaminergic system. *Progress in Neuro-Psychopharmacology & Biological Psychiatry*, *33*(4), 642–650. doi:10.1016/j.pnpbp.2009.03.004 PMID:19286446

Mae, T., Nishiyama, T., Kishida, H., Takagaki, R., & Yamamoto, M. (2007). *Agent for preventing/ameliorating life style related diseases containing turmeric essential oil component*. European Patent Application, Intl Nat Pub No. WO 2005/115366, EP1752144A1, 1–12. Spices and aromatic plants–health benefits 100.

Maheshwari, A., Verma, N., Swaroop, A., Bagchi, M., Preuss, H. G., Tiwari, K., & Bagchi, D. (2017). Efficacy of Furosap™, a novel *Trigonella foenum-graecum* seed extract, in Enhancing Testosterone Level and Improving Sperm Profile in Male Volunteers. *International Journal of Medical Sciences*, *14*(1), 58–66. doi:10.7150/ijms.17256 PMID:28138310

Mahindru, S. N. (1982). *Spices in Indian Life*. New Delhi: Sultanchand and Sons.

Majeed, M. (1995). *Curcuminoids: Antioxidant Phytonutrient*. NutriScience Publishers Inc.

Mansour, S. M., Bahgat, A. K., El-Khatib, A. S., & Khayyal, M. T. (2011). Ginkgo biloba extract (EGb 761) normalizes hypertensionin 2K, 1C hypertensive rats: Role ofantioxidant mechanisms, ACE inhibiting activityand improvement of endothelial dysfunction. *Phytomedicine*, *18*(8-9), 641–647. doi:10.1016/j.phymed.2011.01.014 PMID:21353510

Matsuda, D., Ohte, S., Ohshiro, T., Jiang, W., Rudel, L., Hong, B., ... Tomoda, H. (2008). Ectomycorrhizal fungal community of naturally regenerated *Pinus thunbergii* seedlings in a coastal pine forest. *Biological & Pharmaceutical Bulletin*, *31*, 1063–1066. doi:10.1248/bpb.31.1063 PMID:18520030

McCaffrey, R., Thomas, D. J., & Kinzelman, A. O. (2009). The effects of lavender and rosemary essential oils on test-taking anxiety among graduate nursing students. *Holistic Nursing Practice*, *23*(2), 88–93. doi:10.1097/HNP.0b013e3181a110aa PMID:19258850

McCormick. (2017). *The History of Spices*. Available online: https://www.mccormickscienceinstitute.com/resources/history-of-spices

Minpei, K., Yoshihiro, M., Tozo, N., Tatsumasa, M., Hideyuki, K., Misuzu, T., ... Mikio, K. (2005). Hypoglycemic effects of turmeric (Curcuma longa L.) rhizomes on genetically diabetic KK-Ay mice. *Biological & Pharmaceutical Bulletin*, *28*(5), 937–939. doi:10.1248/bpb.28.937 PMID:15863912

Mitchell, R., & Fleetwood-Walker, S. (2015). *TRP Channels As Therapeutic Targets*. Academic Press.

Mughal, M. H. (2019). Spices; a mechanistic anticancer treatise. *J Nutr Food Technol.*, *2*(1), 14–19. doi:10.30881/jnfrt.00016

Narender, T., Puri, A., Shweta, A., Khaliq, T., Saxena, R., Bhatia, G., & Chandra, R. (2006). 4-hydroxyisoleucine an unusual amino acid as antidyslipidemic and antihyperglycemic agent. *Bioorganic & Medicinal Chemistry Letters*, *16*(2), 293–296. doi:10.1016/j.bmcl.2005.10.003 PMID:16246556

Neveu, V., Perez-Jiménez, J., Vos, F., Crespy, V., & du Chaffaut, L. (2010). *Database*. doi:/bap024 doi:10.1093/database

Newman, D. J., & Cragg, G. M. (2012). Natural Products as Sources of New Drugs over the 30 Years from 1981 to 2010. *Journal of Natural Products*, *75*(3), 311–335. doi:10.1021/np200906s PMID:22316239

Ogbunugafor, H. A. (2011). Physico-chemical and antioxidant properties of *Moringaoleifera*seed oil. *Pakistan Journal of Nutrition*, *10*(5), 409–414. doi:10.3923/pjn.2011.409.414

Ogbunugafor, H. A., Ugochukwu, C. J., & Kyrian-Ogbonna, A. E. (2017). The role of spices in nutrition and health: a review of three popular spices used in Southern Nigeria. *J Food QualSaf*, *1*, 171–185.

Okoye, E. I., & Ebeledike, A. O. O. (2013). *Phytochemical constituents of Piperguineense(Uziza) and their health implications on some microorganisms*. Academic Press.

Omotayo, O. A., Adepoju, O., Thomas, K., & Oluremi, O. (2013). Evaluation of micronutrient potentials of seven commonly consumed indigenous spices from Nigeria. *American Journal of Food and Nutrition*, *3*(3), 122–126. doi:10.5251/ajfn.2013.3.3.122.126

Opara, E. I., & Chohan, M. (2014). Culinary Herbs and Spices: Their Bioactive Properties the Contribution of Polyphenols and the Challenges in Deducing Their True Health Benefits. *International Journal of Molecular Sciences*, *15*(10), 19183–19202. doi:10.3390/ijms151019183 PMID:25340982

Pal, D., & Verma, P. (2013). Flavonoids: A powerful and abundant source of antioxidants. *Interl J of Pharm and Pharmaceu Sci*, *5*, 97–106.

Park, S. H., Ryu, S. N., Bu, Y., Kim, H., Simon, J. E., & Kim, K. S. (2010). Antioxidant components as potential neuroprotective agent in sesame (Sesamumindicum L.) food rev. *Int.*, *26*, 103–121.

Pérez-Jiménez, J., Neveu, V., Vos, F., & Scalbert, A. (2010). Identification of the 100 richest dietary sources of polyphenols: An application of the phenol-explorer database. *European Journal of Clinical Nutrition*, *64*(3), 112–120. doi:10.1038/ejcn.2010.221 PMID:21045839

Persson, I. A., Persson, K., Hägg, S., & Andersson, R. G. (2011). Effects of cocoa extract and dark chocolate on angiotensin-converting enzyme and nitric oxide in human endothelial cells and healthy volunteersanutrigenomics perspective. *Journal of Cardiovascular Pharmacology*, *57*(1), 44–50. doi:10.1097/FJC.0b013e3181fe62e3 PMID:20966764

Pimentel, M., Bonorris, G. G., Chow, E. J., & Lin, H. C. (2001). Peppermint oil improves the manometric findings in diffuse esophageal spasm. *Journal of Clinical Gastroenterology*, *33*(1), 27–31. doi:10.1097/00004836-200107000-00007 PMID:11418786

Platel, K., & Srinivasan, K. (2004). Article. *The Indian Journal of Medical Research*, *119*, 167–179. PMID:15218978

Portincasa, P., Bonfrate, L., de Bari, O., Lembo, A., & Ballou, S. (2017). Irritable bowel syndrome and diet. *Gastroenterology Report*, *5*(1), 11–19. doi:10.1093/gastro/gow047 PMID:28110300

Prasad, S., Gupta, S. C., Tyagi, A. K., & Aggarwal, B. B. (2014). Curcumin, acomponent of golden spice: From bedside to bench and back. *Biotechnology Advances*, *32*(6), 1053–1064. doi:10.1016/j.biotechadv.2014.04.004 PMID:24793420

Preuss, H. G., Echard, B., Polansky, M. M., & Anderson, R. (2006). Whole Cinnamon and Aqueous Extracts Ameliorate Sucrose-Induced Blood Pressure Elevations in Spontaneously Hypertensive Rats. *Journal of the American College of Nutrition*, *25*(2), 144–150. doi:10.1080/07315724.2006.10719525 PMID:16582031

Qiu, P., Dong, P., Guan, H., Li, S., Ho, C. T., Pan, M. H., ... Xiao, H. (2010). Inhibitory effects of 5-hydroxy polymethoxyflavones on colon cancer cells. *Molecular Nutrition & Food Research*, *54*(S2), S244–S252. doi:10.1002/mnfr.200900605 PMID:20397199

Rahmani, S., Asgary, S., Askar, G., Keshvari, M., Hataminpour, M., Feizi, A., & Sahebkar, A. (2016). Treatment of Non-alcoholic Fatty Liver Disease with Curcumin: A Randomized Placebo-controlled Trial. *Phytotherapy Research*, *30*(9), 1540–1548. doi:10.1002/ptr.5659 PMID:27270872

Ramos-Tovar, E. (2019). Dietary Interventions in Liver Disease. *Foods, Nutrients, and Dietary Supplements*, 101-121.

Rao, A., Steels, E., Beccaria, G., Inder, W. J., & Vitetta, L. (2015). Influence of a Specialized Trigonella foenum-graecum Seed Extract (Libifem), on Testosterone, Estradiol and Sexual Function in Healthy Menstruating Women, a Randomised Placebo Controlled Study. *Phytotherapy Research, 29*(8), 1123–1130. doi:10.1002/ptr.5355 PMID:25914334

Rao, A., Steels, E., Inder, W. J., Abraham, S., & Vitetta, L. (2016). Testofen, a specialised Trigonella foenum-graecum seed extract reduces age-related symptoms of androgen decrease, increases testosterone levels and improves sexual function in healthy aging males in a double-blind randomised clinical study. *The Aging Male, 19*(2), 134–142. doi:10.3109/13685538.2015.1135323 PMID:26791805

Ried, K., Travica, N., & Sali, A. (2016). The effect of aged garlic extract on bloodpressure and other cardiovascular risk factors in uncontrolled hypertensives: The AGE at Heart trial. *Integrated Blood Pressure Control, 9*, 9. doi:10.2147/IBPC.S93335 PMID:26869811

Rosti, L., & Gastaldi, G. (2005). Chronic Salmonellosis and Cinnamon. *Pediatrics, 116*(4), 1057. doi:10.1542/peds.2005-1521 PMID:16199729

Roussel, A. M., Hininger, I., Benaraba, R., Ziegenfuss, T. N., & Anderson, R. A. (2009). Antioxidant Effects of a Cinnamon Extract in People with Impaired Fasting Glucose That Are Overweight or Obese. *Journal of the American College of Nutrition, 28*(1), 16–21. doi:10.1080/07315724.2009.10719756 PMID:19571155

Rubió, L., Motilva, M. J., & Romero, M. P. (2013). Recent advances in biologically active compounds in herbs and spices: A review of the most effective antioxidant and anti-inflammatory active principles. *Critical Reviews in Food Science and Nutrition, 53*(9), 943–953. doi:10.1080/10408398.2011.574802 PMID:23768186

Sachan, A.K., Rao, C.V., & Sachan, N.K. (2016). Ethnobotanicalsurvey of indigenous medicines practiced in Chambal valley of Uttar Pradesh. *Bharatiya Vaigyanik Evam Audyogik Anusandhan Patrika, 23*(2), 132-135.

Sachan, A. K., Das, D. R., & Kumar, M. (2016). Carum carvi- An important medicinal plant. *Journal of Chemical and Pharmaceutical Research, 8*, 529–533.

Sachan, A. K. R., Kumar, S., Kumari, K., & Singh, D. (2018). Medicinal uses of spices used in our traditional culture world wide. *JMPS, 6*, 116–122.

Sachan, P. L., Singh, M., Patel, M. L., & Sachan, R. A. (2018). Study on cervical cancer screening using pap smear test and clinical correlation. *Asia-Pacific Journal of Oncology Nursing, 5*(3), 337–341. doi:10.4103/apjon.apjon_15_18 PMID:29963597

Sandasi, M., Leonard, C. M., & Viljoen, A. M. (2008). The effect of five common essential oil components on Listeria monocytogenes biofilms. *Food Control, 19*(11), 1070–1075. doi:10.1016/j.foodcont.2007.11.006

Satyanarayana, M. N. (2006). Capsaicin and Gastric Ulcers. *Critical Reviews in Food Science and Nutrition, 46*(4), 275–328. doi:10.1080/1040-830491379236 PMID:16621751

Schwingshackl, L., Missbach, B., & Hoffmann, G. (2016). An umbrella review of garlic intake and risk of cardiovascular disease. *Phytomedicine*, *23*(11), 1127–1133. doi:10.1016/j.phymed.2015.10.015 PMID:26656227

Shah, G. M., Hussain, M., & Abbasi, A. M. (2015). *Medicinal Plants Used to Treat Respiratory Tract Illness in Kaghan Valley*. Himalayan Region-Pakistan.

Shin, D. Y., Kim, G. Y., Li, W., Choi, B. T., Kim, N. D., Kang, H. S., & Choi, Y. H. (2009). Implication of intracellular ROS formation, caspase-3 activation and Egr-1 induction in platycodon D-induced apoptosis of U937 human leukemia cells. *Biomedicine and Pharmacotherapy*, *63*(2), 86–94. doi:10.1016/j.biopha.2008.08.001 PMID:18804340

Silalahi, J. (2002). Anticancer and health protective properties of citrus fruit components. *Asia Pacific Journal of Clinical Nutrition*, *11*(1), 79–84. doi:10.1046/j.1440-6047.2002.00271.x PMID:11890643

Singh, R., Singh, N., Saini, B. S., & Rao, H. S. (2008). In vitro antioxidant activity of pet ether extract of black pepper. *International Journal of Pharmacology*, *40*, 147–151. PMID:20040947

Singh, R., Singh, S., Parihar, P., Mishra, R. K., Tripathi, D. K., Singh, V. P., ... Prasad, S. M. (2016). Reactive Oxygen Species (ROS): Beneficial Companions of Plants' Developmental Processes. *Front Plant Sci*, *7*, 1299. doi:10.3389/fpls.2016.01299 PMID:27729914

Slim, H. B., Black, H. R., & Thompson, P. D. (2011). Older bloodpressure medications-do they still have a place? *The American Journal of Cardiology*, *108*(2), 308–316. doi:10.1016/j.amjcard.2011.03.041 PMID:21550576

Smith, C., Crowther, C., Willson, K., Hotham, N., & McMillian, V. (2004). A randomized controlled trial of ginger to treat nausea and vomiting in pregnancy. *Obstetrics and Gynecology*, *103*(4), 639–645. doi:10.1097/01.AOG.0000118307.19798.ec PMID:15051552

Snitker, S., Fujishima, Y., Shen, H., Ott, S., Pi-Sunyer, X., Furuhata, Y., ... Takahashi, M. (2009). Effects of novel capsinoid treatment on fatness and energy metabolism in humans: Possible pharmacogenetic implications. *The American Journal of Clinical Nutrition*, *89*(1), 45–50. doi:10.3945/ajcn.2008.26561 PMID:19056576

Sofowora, A. (1982). *Medicinal plant and traditional medicine in Africa*. New York: John Wiley and Sons.

Soureshjan, E. H., & Heidari, M. (2014). In vitro variation in antibacterial activity plant extracts on Glaucium elegansand saffron (Crocus sativus). *Bangladesh Journal of Pharmacology*, *9*, 275–278.

Spiller, F., Alves, M. K., Vieira, S. M., Carvalho, T. A., Leite, C. E., Lunardelli, A., ... de Oliviera, J. R. (2008). Anti-inflammatory effects of red pepper (Capsicum baccatum) on carrageenan- and antigen-induced inflammation. *The Journal of Pharmacy and Pharmacology*, *60*, 473–478.

Chaiyata, P., Puttadechakum, S., & Komindr, S. (2003). Bioactives from spices and herbs. *Journal of the Medical Association of Thailand*, *86*, 854–860.

Sreejayan, N., & Rao, M. N. A. (1994). Curcuminoids as potent inhibitors of lipid peroxidation. *The Journal of Pharmacy and Pharmacology*, *46*(12), 1013–1016. doi:10.1111/j.2042-7158.1994.tb03258.x PMID:7714712

Srichamroen, A., Field, C. J., Thomson, A. B., & Basu, T. K. (2008). The Modifying Effects of Galactomannan from Canadian-Grown Fenugreek (*Trigonella foenum-graecum L.*) on the Glycemic and Lipidemic Status in Rats. *Journal of Clinical Biochemistry and Nutrition*, *43*(3), 167–174. doi:10.3164/jcbn.2008060 PMID:19015751

Srinivasan, K. (2005). Role of Spices Beyond Food Flavoring: Nutraceuticals with Multiple Health Effects. *Food Reviews International*, *21*(2), 167–188. doi:10.1081/FRI-200051872

Srinivasan, K. (2007). Black Pepper and its Pungent Principle-Piperine: A Review of Diverse Physiological Effects. *Critical Reviews in Food Science and Nutrition*, *47*(8), 735–748. doi:10.1080/10408390601062054 PMID:17987447

Srinivasan, K. (2014). Antioxidant potential of spices and their active constituents. *Critical Reviews in Food Science and Nutrition*, *54*(3), 352–372. doi:10.1080/10408398.2011.585525 PMID:24188307

Srivastava, G., & Mehta, J. L. (2009). Currying the Heart: Curcumin and Cardioprotection. *Journal of Cardiovascular Pharmacology and Therapeutics*, *14*(1), 22–27. doi:10.1177/1074248408329608 PMID:19153099

Stangl, V., Lorenz, M., & Stangl, K. (2006). The role of tea and tea flavonoids in cardiovascular health. *Molecular Nutrition & Food Research*, *50*(2), 218–228. doi:10.1002/mnfr.200500118 PMID:16404706

Stoilova, I., Krastanv, A., Stoyanova, A., Denev, P., & Gargova, S. (2007). Antioxidant activity of a ginger extract (Zingiber officinale). *Food Chemistry*, *102*(3), 764–770. doi:10.1016/j.foodchem.2006.06.023

Tanwar, V., Sachdeva, J., Golechha, M., Kumari, S., & Arya, D. S. (2010). Curcumin protects rat myocardium against isoproterenol-induced ischemic injury: Attenuation of ventricular dysfunction through increased expression of hsp27alongwith strengthening antioxidant defense system. *Journal of Cardiovascular Pharmacology*, *55*(4), 377–384. doi:10.1097/FJC.0b013e3181d3da01 PMID:20125031

Tapsell, L. C., Hemphill, I., Cobiac, L., Patch, C. S., Sullivan, D. R., Fenech, M., ... Inge, K. (2006). Health benefits of herbs and spices: The past, the present, the future. *The Medical Journal of Australia*, *185*(S4), S1–S24. doi:10.5694/j.1326-5377.2006.tb00548.x PMID:17022438

Toda, S., Miyase, T., & Arich, H. (1985). Natural Antioxidants. III. Antioxidative components isolated from rhizomes of Curcuma longa L. *Chemical & Pharmaceutical Bulletin*, *33*(4), 1725–1728. doi:10.1248/cpb.33.1725 PMID:4042250

USDA/ERS. (2011). Food availability (Per Capita) Data System. *United States Department of Agriculture Economic Research Service*. Available at: http://www.ers.usda.gov/Data/ FoodConsumption/

Varni, J. W., Bendo, C. B., Nurko, S., Shulman, R. J., Self, M. M., Franciosi, J. P., ... Pohl, J. F. (2015). Pediatric Quality of Life Inventory (PedsQL) Gastrointestinal Symptoms Module Testing Study Consortium Health-related quality of life in pediatric patients with functional and organic gastrointestinal diseases. *The Journal of Pediatrics*, *166*(1), 85–90. doi:10.1016/j.jpeds.2014.08.022 PMID:25241177

Vijayakumar, M. V., & Bhat, M. K. (2008). Hypoglycemic effect of a novel dialysed feungreek seeds extract is sustainable and is mediated, in part, by the activation of hepatic enzymes. *Phytotherapy Research*, *22*(4), 500–505. doi:10.1002/ptr.2351 PMID:18338783

Wang, S. L., Li, Y., Wen, Y., Chen, Y. F., Na, L. X., Li, S. T., & Sun, C. H. (2009). Curcumin, a potential inhibitor of up-regulation of TNF-alpha and IL-6 induced by palmitate in 3T3-L1 adipocytes through NF-kappaB and JNK pathway. *Biomedical and Environmental Sciences*, *22*(1), 32–39. doi:10.1016/S0895-3988(09)60019-2 PMID:19462685

Xiao, H., Yang, C. S., Li, S., Jin, H., Ho, C. T., & Patel, T. (2009). Monodemethylatedpolymethoxyflavones from sweet orange (Citrus sinensis) peel inhibit growth of human lung cancer cells by apoptosis. *Molecular Nutrition & Food Research*, *53*(3), 398–406. doi:10.1002/mnfr.200800057 PMID:19065586

Yoo, M. J., Kim, Y. S., & Shin, D. H. (2006). Antibacterial effects of natural essential oils from ginger and mustard against Vibrio species inoculated on sliced raw flatfish. *Food Science and Biotechnology*, *15*, 462–465.

Yu, J. S., & Kim, A. K. (2010). Platycodin D induces apoptosis in MCF-7 human breast cancer cells. *Journal of Medicinal Food*, *13*(2), 298–305. doi:10.1089/jmf.2009.1226 PMID:20412017

Yuki, M., Komazawa, Y., Kobayashi, Y., Kusunoki, M., Takahashi, Y., Nakashima, S., ... Kinoshita, Y. (2015). Effects of Daikenchuto on abdominal bloating accompanied by chronic constipation:A prospective, single-center randomized open trial. *Current Therapeutic Research, Clinical and Experimental*, *77*, 58–62. doi:10.1016/j.curtheres.2015.04.002 PMID:27069528

Zheng, G., Kenney, P. M., & Lam, L. K. (1992). Myristicin: A potential cancer chemopreventive agent from parsley leaf oil. *Journal of Agricultural and Food Chemistry*, *40*(1), 107–110. doi:10.1021/jf00013a020

Zheng, Q., Hirose, Y., Yoshimi, N., Murakami, A., Koshimizu, K., Ohigashi, H., ... Mori, H. (2002). Further investigation of the modifying effect of various chemopreventive agents on apoptosis and cell proliferation in human colon cancer cells. *Journal of Cancer Research and Clinical Oncology*, *128*(10), 539–546. doi:10.1007/00432-002-0373-y PMID:12384797

Zheng, W., & Wang, S. Y. (2001). Antioxidant activity and phenolic compounds in selected herbs. *Journal of Agricultural and Food Chemistry*, *49*(11), 5165–5170. doi:10.1021/jf010697n PMID:11714298

ADDITIONAL READING

Abdullah, I. H., Farooq, A., Poonam, S. N., Satyajit, D. S., John, E. M., Juluri, R. R., & Anisha, M. (2011). Antibacterial activity of some Lamiaceae essential oils using resazurin as an indicator of cell growth. LWT - Food. *Sciences et Techniques (Paris)*, *44*, 1199–1206.

Abishek, I., Panchal, S., Poudyal, H., & Brown, L. (2009). Potential health benefits of Indian spices in the symptons of metabolic syndrome: A review. *Indian Journal of Biochemistry & Biophysics*, *46*, 461–481.

Agrawal, M., Walia, S., Dhingra, S., & Khambay, B. P. S. (2001). Insect growth inhibition antifeedant and antifungal activity of compounds isolated derived from *Zingiber officinale* Roscoe, ginger rhizome. *Pest Management Science*, *57*(3), 289–300. doi:10.1002/ps.263 PMID:11455660

Al-Zuhair, H., el-Sayeh, B., Ameen, H. A., & Al-Shoora, H. (1996). Pharmacological studies of cardamom oil in animals. *Pharmacological Research*, *34*(1-2), 79–82. doi:10.1006/phrs.1996.0067 PMID:8981560

Bakkali, F., Averbeck, S., Averbeck, D., & Idaomar, M. (2008). Biological effects of essential oils - A review. *Food and Chemical Toxicology*, *46*(2), 446–475. doi:10.1016/j.fct.2007.09.106 PMID:17996351

Chacon, P. A., Buffo, R. A., & Holley, R. A. (2006). Inhibitory effects of microencapsulated allylisothiocyanate (AIT) against Escherichia coli O157:H7 in refrigerated, nitrogen packed and finely chopped beef. *International Journal of Food Microbiology*, *107*(3), 231–237. doi:10.1016/j.ijfoodmicro.2005.08.030 PMID:16266766

Coon, J. T., & Ernst, E. (2004). Andrographispaniculata in the treatment of upper respiratory tract infections: A systematic review of safety and efficacy. *Planta Medica*, *70*(4), 293–298. doi:10.1055-2004-818938 PMID:15095142

Delaquis, P. J., Stanich, K., Girard, B., & Mazza, G. (2002). Antimicrobial activity of individual and mixed fractions of dill, cilantro, coriander, and eucalyptus essential oils. *International Journal of Food Microbiology*, *74*(1-2), 101–109. doi:10.1016/S0168-1605(01)00734-6 PMID:11929164

Erturk, O. (2006). Antibacterial and antifungal activity of ethanolic extracts from eleven spice plants. *Biologia*, *61*(3), 275–278. doi:10.247811756-006-0050-8

Ghanbari, H., Saghravanian, N., & Zakery, M. (2008). Histological evaluation of Curcuma longa ghee formulation and hyaluronic acid on gingival healing in dog. *Journal of Ethnopharmacology*, *120*(3), 335–341. doi:10.1016/j.jep.2008.09.011 PMID:18929638

Güllü, E. B., & Gülcan, A. (2013). Timokinon: Nigella sativa' nınBiyoaktifKomponenti. *Kocatepe Vet J*, *6*, 51–61.

Gulluce, F., Sahin, F., Sokmen, M., Ozer, H., Daferera, D., Sokmen, A., ... Ozkan, H. (2007). Antimicrobial and antioxidant properties of the essential oils and methanol extract from Menthalongifolia L. ssp. *Longifolia. Food Chem.*, *103*(4), 1449–1456. doi:10.1016/j.foodchem.2006.10.061

Haeri, M. R., Izaddoost, M., Ardekani, M. R., Nobar, M. R., & White, K. N. (2008). The effect of fenugreeek 4-hydroxyisoleucine on liver function biomarkers and glucose in diabetic and fructose-fed rats. *Phototh Res*, *23*(1), 61–64. doi:10.1002/ptr.2557

Hayouni, E. A., Chraief, I., Abedrabba, M., Bouix, M., Leveau, J. Y., Mohammed, H., & Hamdi, M. (2008). Tunisian Salvia officinalis L. and Schinusmolle L. essential oils: Their chemical compositions and their preservative effects against Salmonella inoculated in minced beef meat. *International Journal of Food Microbiology*, *125*(3), 242–251. doi:10.1016/j.ijfoodmicro.2008.04.005 PMID:18511141

Kuptniratsaikul, V., Thanakhumtorn, S., Chinswangwantanakul, P., Wattanamongkonsil, L., & Thamlikitkul, V. (2009). Efficacy and safety of Curcuma domestica extracts in patients with knee osteoarthritis. *Journal of Alternative and Complementary Medicine (New York, N.Y.)*, *15*(8), 891–897. doi:10.1089/acm.2008.0186 PMID:19678780

Mahattanadul, S., Nakamura, T., Panichayupakaranant, P., Phdoongsombut, N., Tungsinmunkong, K., & Bouking, P. (2009). Comparative anti-ulcer effect of bisdemethoxycurcumin and curcumin in a gastric ulcer model system. *Phytom*, *16*(4), 342–351. doi:10.1016/j.phymed.2008.12.005 PMID:19188055

Mózsik, G., Szolcsányi, J., & Rácz, I. (2005). Involvement of serum retinoids and Leiden mutation in patients with esophageal, gastric, liver, pancreatic, and colorectal cancers in Hungary. *World Journal of Gastroenterology*, *11*(48), 5180–5184. doi:10.3748/wjg.v11.i48.7646 PMID:16127749

Santos, F. S., Guadalupe, M., & Novales, M. (2012). Essential oils from aromatic herbs as antimicrobial agents. *Current Opinion in Biotechnology*, *23*(2), 136–141. doi:10.1016/j.copbio.2011.08.005 PMID:21903378

Shahidi, F., Pegg, R. B., & Saleemi, Z. O. (2007). Stabilization of meat lipids with ground spices. *Journal of Food Lipids*, *2*(3), 145–153. doi:10.1111/j.1745-4522.1995.tb00038.x

Sharma, R. D., Raghuram, T. C., & Rao, N. S. (1990). Effect of fenugreek seeds on blood glucose and serum lipids in type I diabetes. *European Journal of Clinical Nutrition*, *44*, 301–306. PMID:2194788

Tajkarimi, M. M., Ibrahim, S. A., & Cliver, D. O. (2010). Antimicrobial herb and spice compounds in food. *Food Control*, *21*(9), 1199–1218. doi:10.1016/j.foodcont.2010.02.003

Tallon, M. J. (2008). Spicing up health with capsaicin. *Nat Foods Merchand*, *28*, 38–40.

Tripathi, R. M., Gupta, S. S., & Chandra, D. (1973). Antitrypsin and antihyaluronidase activity of volatile oil of Curcuma longa (Haldi). *International Journal of Pharmacology*, *5*, 260–261.

Weerakkody, N. S., Caffin, N., Lambert, L. K., Turner, M. S., & Dykes, G. A. (2011). Synergistic antimicrobial activity of galangal (Alpiniagalanga), rosemary (Rosmarinusofficinalis) and lemon iron bark (Eucalyptus staigerana) extracts. *Journal of the Science of Food and Agriculture*, *91*(3), 461–468. doi:10.1002/jsfa.4206 PMID:21218479

Chapter 3
Spices:
Pharmacological and Anti-Diabetic Activities

Nisha
Central University of Rajasthan, India

Deepika
University of Rajasthan, India

ABSTRACT

The term "spices" has been derived from the word "species," which was connected to the group of exotic foods in medieval times. Spices and herbs have a long history of culinary use, medicinal properties, and as additives and thus have a distinct place in Ayurveda. Exhibiting the merits of spices by scientific methods still remains a challenge. This review investigates the anti-diabetic properties in preventing and managing diabetics and associated complications with commonly used spices. The bioactive compounds in these spices are additionally discussed. The major aim and object of the present work is to investigate the customary therapeutic usage of basic Indian spices and to corelate their observed pharmacological activities with the presence of explicit bioactive compounds present for the treatment or counteractive action of diabetes. This includes the basic underlying mechanism of their blood glucose lowering property including exploratory experimental evidence from proposed animal and human trials.

INTRODUCTION

The term "spices" has been derived from the word "species," which was connected to the group of exotic foods since medieval times. These aromatically rich, home-grown, herbal food stuff has been utilized for ages to enhance food flavors and nourishments. Spices and herbs might be characterized as a group of obscure sustenance, subordinates that have been used to intensify the organoleptic qualities of foods. Generally, if a plant leaf is used in minor quantities during cooking, it might be alluded to be a culinary herb, and if some other piece of the plant is regularly dried and used, then it is known as a spice. Different parts of the plant may be used as a spice such as the buds (cloves), bark (cinnamon),

DOI: 10.4018/978-1-7998-2524-1.ch003

roots (ginger), berries (peppercorns), fragrant seeds (cumin), and even the stigma of a flower (saffron). Ayurveda, the traditional medicinal system of India that has been developed over 5000 years prior, in the Himalayas and the learning being transmitted orally until it was recorded in Sanskrit verse — the Vedas — around 1500 BC. Ayurveda centers around ailment, counteractive action and wellbeing promotion, with an accentuation on the diet and eating pattern. Herbs and spices are used not only as additives or an aromatically flavoring substance but also as a pharmaceutical agent owing to its medicinal properties for a long time and thus have a distinct place in Ayurveda. In India, these herbs and spices are used in reasonable amounts in meal preparation, and significant quantities have been observed to be consumed in a single meal. It has been reported that such herbs and spices can supply good amounts of nutrients to the body. In the ninth century, the Emperor Charlemagne is cited as saying, "a herb is a companion of doctors and the praise of cooks", recommending the dual role of herbs and spices for food flavouring and health benefits, though the theory of health benefits has been established, but the mechanism is yet to be postulated. Keeping in mind the age-old history of utilization of herbs and spices, with strong roles in social legacy, in the valuation for sustenance and its connection to wellbeing, they might be viewed as one of the first-ever recorded functional food or foods with nutraceutical properties. Exhibiting the merits of spices by scientific methods still remains a challenge, especially when contrasted and compared with pharmaceutical agents. Pharmaceuticals are little atomic weight mixes expended in a purified and concentrated form. Food is generally eaten in mixes with other stuffs, in moderately huge, unmeasured amounts, under profoundly mingled conditions. The real challenge lies not in demonstrating whether herbs and spices have medicinal benefits but lies in characterizing these benefits and developing the techniques to define them by scientific methods. The manner by which foods are today examined isn't constrained to ideas of averting clinical deficiencies and maintaining homeostasis, but rather includes a growing recognition of the way in which food components actively interact with the body to support health and prevent abnormality and overt disease. Setting up this job would include distinguishing novel bioactive mixes to help recognize target benefits with a proposed system of activity. The role of nutrition in the appropriate functionality of the immune system is well established since ancient times (Saeed *et al.*, 2016).

This review investigates the anti-diabetic properties in preventing and management diabetics and associated complications by commonly used spices, for example, cinnamon, fenugreek, garlic, onion, cloves, ginger, turmeric, curry leaves, and cumin. There are different ways to deal with the treatment and prevention of diabetes as well as secondary related complications. Nonetheless, the determination of spices may rely upon a few components, which incorporates the stage of diabetes and types of comorbidities that the patients may be suffering from. The bioactive compounds in these spices are additionally discussed. The major aim and object of the present work is to investigate the customary therapeutic usage of basic Indian spices and to co-relate their observed pharmacological activities with the explicit bioactive compounds present in them for the treatment or counteractive action of morbid disorder *i.e;* diabetes, including their basic underlying mechanism for the blood glucose-lowering property including the exploratory, experimental evidences from proposed animal and human trials.

Diabetics Mellitus

Diabetes Mellitus - a silent ailment, is currently perceived as the fastest growing threat to public health, in practically all the nations of the world. According to the WHO fact sheet, around 422 million people are suffering from this disease, of which 69.2 million are Indians (WHO, 2016). It is the third most non-

Figure 1.Sources of blood glucose and normal routes of its control

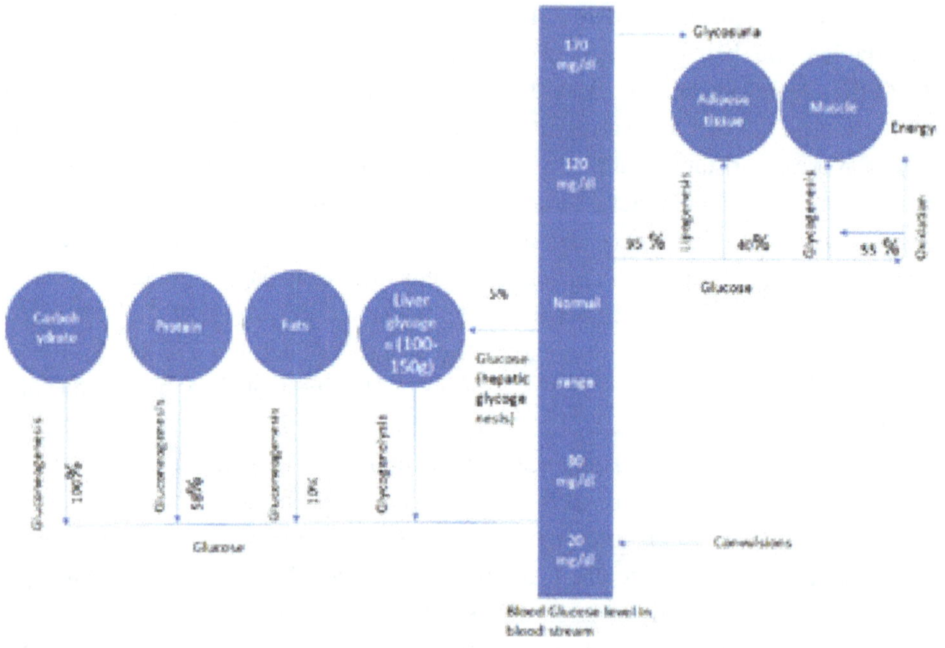

communicable disease, first being hypertension in terms of public health nutrition. Diabetes (Type 2) is described not by absolute insulin inadequacy but by its resistance and relativity instead. It is a more typical type of diabetes affecting around 90 percent of the diabetic populace. Diabetes Mellitus can develop because of the resistance from the receptor cells or elevated production of endogenous glucose by the liver (ADA, 2006) and is clinically portrayed by hyperglycemia, which may result in the glycation of body proteins and cause severe complexities. These complexities are classified into intense metabolic and systemic complications. Hyperglycemia is a condition, which results due to the insufficiency of insulin or it is due to the incapability of the insulin produced *i.e*; fault in the structure of produced insulin. Such an insufficiency leads to an elevation of the glucose concentration in the blood, which may harm the body's metabolism, specifically the veins and nerves prompting oxidative stress inside the body (Ayodhya *et. al.,* 2010). For a better understanding of the disease, it is important to have knowledge of the various biochemical pathways involved in the maintenance of normal blood glucose level (Figure 1).

Managing diabetes with no side effects is yet a challenge to the medicinal community. Several drugs such as biguanides, metformin, sulfonylurea, and thiazolidinediones are generally used these days in diabetes mellitus. The utilization of these medications is limited by their pharmacokinetic properties, auxiliary failures, and potential side effects.

Mechanism of Glucose Homeostasis

Diabetes mellitus is a metabolic dysregulation of normal glucose metabolism and is generally accompanied by long-term complications, which are characteristic of the disease. The complications of diabetes mellitus include retinopathy, nephropathy, and neuropathy. Patients, both IDDM and NIDDM, are sensitive and susceptible to develop these complications, if they are suffering from this disease from a long period and if the disease is not under strict control. Spices have been known for their cancer, preventing action and anti-diabetic properties. Figure 2 elucidates the possible key sites for the action by the various bioactive compounds present in different spices. Carbohydrate enters the body in complex form and is broken down to glucose before its absorption can take place in blood. The bioactive compounds from several spices act as a mild inhibitor to α amylase, thereby preventing the digestion and absorption of carbohydrates. At the same time few bioactive components from spices acts as a strong inhibitor to α glucosidase present in the small intestine which breaks down disaccharides to its simplest forms (monosaccharides).

Figure 2. Entry of glucose in blood & its control via bioactive compounds present in spices

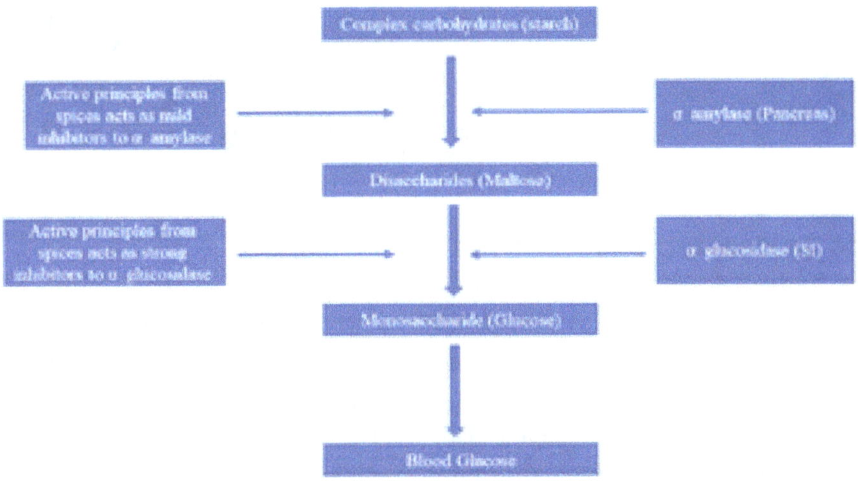

Spice polyphenols apart from its action on the above-stated enzymes, has also found to affect various other organs like small intestine, liver, pancreas and muscle. It is beneficial in bringing about glucose homeostasis either by decreasing the glucose uptake as in small intestine by inhibiting α amylase, α glucosidase and SGLT 1 or by increasing the uptake of glucose by the liver *via* increase in glycogenesis and glycolysis or decrease in gluconeogenesis. In muscle cells, spices activate the AMP kinase and increase GLUT 2 and GLUT 4; therefore, increasing glucose uptake. Some of the bioactive compounds present in the spices have been reported to protect the β cells of Langerhans from oxidative damage, thereby increasing insulin production and secretion (Figure 3).

Figure 3. Action of bioactive compounds in spices on various organs during carbohydrate metabolism

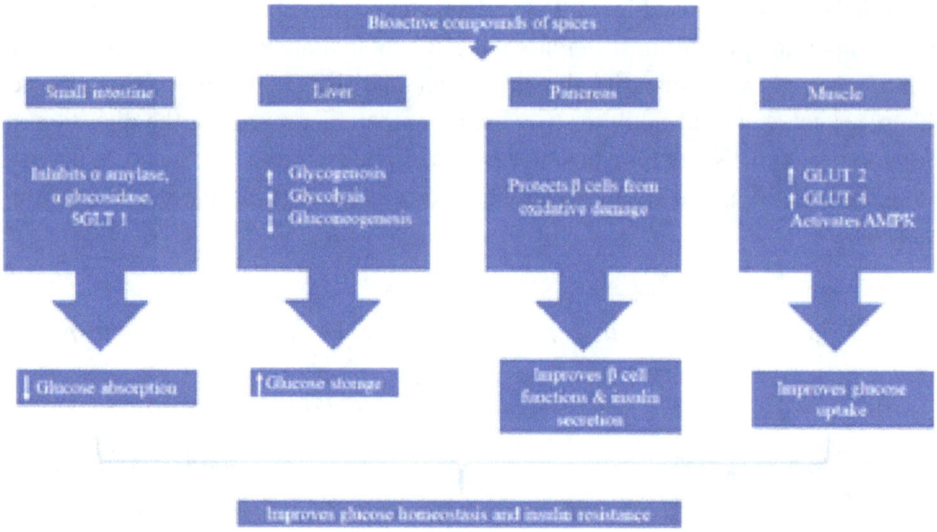

Anti-diabetic Spices and Their Dosage

Several *in vitro, in vivo* and human trials, have established the fact that some of the common spices like cinnamon, fenugreek, garlic, onion, turmeric, cumin *etc.* possess anti-diabetic properties. In the case of some spices, this fact has been established even through human trials. When there is a conjunction of these hypoglycemic spices along with the antidiabetic drugs, they have shown to demonstrate a better therapeutic activity and have even resulted in lowering the dosage of the medicine. Researches have established an effective dosage, of these spices *i.e.,* about 25-50g fenugreek seeds, 5-/6 cloves garlic, 50 g (1 bulb) onion and 1 g turmeric powder if consumed daily by diabetics, is observed to be quite supportive and effective in the management and prevention of long/term morbidities and complications. This anti-diabetic activity of the spices is generally mediated through either of the below listed methods or by a combination of them. Spices may

(i) Increase the secretion of insulin by the pancreas,
(ii) Hinder in uptake glucose by the body and
(iii) The bio-active compounds present in spices may demonstrate insulin-sparing action (Table I).

Such amounts of these spices can be easily expended in our daily routine, with the exception of spices that carry strong odor (garlic). Incorporation of these spices at levels a lot higher than the normal, by various segments of the population, may really be practically possible depending on the culinary inclinations. Indeed, even among those segments of populace where the use of spices may not be high, utilization of portions of these could be practically possible.

Cinnamon

Cinnamon is mainly used owing to its aromatic qualities in foods, perfumes and medicinal industries. Around 250 species have been recognized and they have been scattered all around the world. The two commonly found species are *cinnamomum cassia,* which is mainly sold as cinnamon in US, whereas *Cinnamomum zeylanicum* commonly known as Ceylon cinnamon, which is also called sweet cinnamon or true cinnamon is found in India, Srilanka, and parts of Asia (Rao and Gan, 2014). The major constituents of cinnamon are cinnamaldehyde, cinnamate, cinnamic acid, and numerous essential oils (Singh *et. al.,* 2007). Procyanidins, tannins, mucilage and coumarin is also present in cinnamon (Yeh et al., 2013). The most important constituent of the cinnamon bark oil, i.e., cinnamaldehyde (trans-cinnamaldehyde) and eugenol, is found in the leaf oil (Sangal, 2011). Owing to the presence of these bioactive compounds cinnamon is antimicrobial, antifungal, antioxidant, anti-inflammatory, antiemetic, insecticidal, antimycotic and anti-cancerous. Since the past 20 years, cinnamon has been investigated as a potentially valuable treatment for diabetes mellitus.

Researchers have reported that cinnamon powder lowers fasting blood sugar level, glycosylated hemoglobin, intestinal glycosidase activity among diabetes patients (*i.e.,* type 2) with uncontrolled sugar level, it also increases serum insulin levels, HDL cholesterol, serum glutathione and superoxide dismutase (Shahib *et. al.,* 2016; Kim *et al.,* 2006; Kumar *et. al.,*2013; Anderson *et. al.,*2016; Al-Yasiry *et. al.,* 2014; Governa *et. al.,*2018)

Several scientists have tried to identify the potential mechanism of action of cinnamon in the body that is helpful in diabetes mellitus type 2. Cinnamon has a hypoglycemic action as it stimulates the insulin receptors, activates and regulates the enzymes that regulate carbohydrate metabolism such as glycolysis, gluconeogenesis, stimulates the uptake of glucose by cells, increases glucose transporter 4 receptor synthesis, stimulates insulin secretion, increases glucagon-like peptide 1 (GLP-1), delays the gastric emptying time, inhibits the activity of α glucosidase, and also increases GLUT 4 expression and stimulates phosphorylation of insulin receptor beta subunits on adipocytes and others (Medagama, 2015 and Adisakwattana *et. al.,* 2011).

Fenugreek

Fenugreek, botanically known as *Trigonellafoenum graecum,* belongs to the family *Fabaceae.* The major compounds present in the fenugreek seeds are galactomanans, 4-hydroxyisoleucine, a pseudo alkaloid trigonelline, steroids like sitosterol, steroidal saponins like trigogenin and gitogenin. Other than these, linolenic and linoleic acid, g-lactone, sotolone (major component that is responsible of the distinct odour), trigocoumarin, diosgenin, trigomethylo coumarin, mucilage and fiber are also found (Grover, *et. al.,* 2002). Fenugreek possess several health beneficial properties such as demulcent, emollient, carminative, tonic, astringent, diuretic, emmenagogue, restorative, vermifugal, expectorant, and aphrodisiac. The pharmacological properties of fenugreek are owing to the presence of nitrogen containing compound, polyphenolic compounds, steroids, flavonoids like luteolin, apigenin, isovitexin, quercetin, vitexin, orientin, amino acids, and volatile constituents (Raju, *et. al.,* 2004). In germinated, sprouted or powder form fenugreek seeds displays anti-diabetic properties (Broca, *et. al.,* 2004). Hannan *et. al.,* (2003) documented the hypo-cholesterolemic, glycemic, insulemic properties of fenugreek. Devi and co-workers (2003) reported that fenugreek had an effect on the carbohydrate metabolic enzymes and also had an effect on thyroxine-initiated hyperglycaemia. According to Coon and Earnest (2003) fenugreek

Table 1. Mode of antidiabetic action of spices

Name of spice	Major bioactive compounds	Trials	Possible action	Effect	Toxicity	Reference
Cinnamon	Cinnamaldehyde Cinnamate Cinnamic acid	*In vivo* studies Human trials (T2DM subjects)	Reduced phosphorylation of the insulin receptors; Delaying gastric emptying Enhance the activity of insulin	Reduced postprandial blood glucose, Hypolipidemic Antioxidant, Potentiate insulin action	Potential effects may be overcome using aqueous extracts of cinnamon	Cusi *et. al.*, (2000), Khan *et. al.*, (2003), Cao *et. al.*, (2008), Hlebowicz *et. al.*, (2007), Qin *et. al.*, (2010) Subhash Babu, *et. al;* (2007) Lu *et. al.*, (2011)
Fenugreek	Galactomanans 4-hydroxyisoleucine Trigonelline Steroids Linoleic and linolenic acid Diosgenin Trigocoumarin Trigomethylo Coumarin	Human trials (T2DM subjects)	Delay of gastric emptying Suppressing release of gastric inhibitory peptides and insulinotropic hormones Fibre and gums act as a direct hindrance in the absorption of glucose Acts synergistically with 4-hydroxy isoleucine to increase insulin secretion Suppress the action of gluconeogenic enzymes Stimulates the action of enzymes involved glycolysis	Reduced fasting blood sugar Improved glucose tolerance	Lack of toxic effect at proposed/used levels	Yeh *et. al.*, (2003), Srinivasan (2005)
Garlic (*A. sativum*)	Allicin	*In vivo* studies Human studies (T2DM)	Allicin (di(2-propenyl) disulfide) helps in the production of insulin within the body Reacts with endogenous thiol-containing molecules thus spraining insulin from -SH inactivation	Decreases serum cholesterol Reduces LDL Improves LDL/HDL ratio Increases HDL Also shows an effect on elevated triglyceride levels		Liu *et. al.*, 2006 Ashraf *et. al.*, 2011
Onion (*A. cepa*)	Allyl propyl di sulfide Thiopropanal s-oxide Phosphoric acid	*In vitro* studies *In vivo* studies	Insulin sparing action by this sulfur compound (spares insulin from _/ SH inactivation by reacting with endogenous thiol containing molecules) Inhibits α glucosidase activity	Hypoglycemic Increases glucose uptake by cells		Jain and Vyas, 1974
Clove	Oleanolic acid Dehydrodieugenol Dehydrodieugenol B	*In vivo* studies	Delays digestion of carbohydrates, Protects the liver from damage, Improves lipid proðle & maintains membrane integrity, Suppresses oxidative stress Inhibits α amylase and α glucosidase	Hypoglycemic, Hepatoprotective, Hypolipidemic		Oboh *et. al.*, 2015 Ngubane *et. al.*, 2011 Prasad *et. al.*, 2005 Atawodi *et.al.*, 2011
Curry leaves	Oxalic acid Vitamin A Koenigin, Bicyclomahanimbicine Cyclomahanimbine Murrayastine Coumarine Koenidine Pypayafolinecarbazole	*In vitro* studies	Antioxidant, Pancreatic β cells regeneration	Hypolipidemia Hypoglycemia		Gupta & Watal, 2005 Xie *et. al.*, 2006 Arulselvan *et. al.*, 2014
Ginger	Terpenes Oleoresin	*In vivo* studies	Improves secretion or reduces the uptake of glucose by the body Lowers the LDL and VLDL profile Possess antioxidant activity	Anti hyperglycemic Hypolipidemic		Islam and Choi, 2008 Goyal and Kadnur, 2006
Turmeric (*C. longa*)	Curcuminoids α -turmeron β-turmeron Curlon Zingiberen	*In vivo* studies	Increases insulin secretion Hypolipidemic Antioxidative properties helps in amelioration of kidney lesion	Hypoglycemic		Ferreira *et. al.*, 2006 Aggarwal *et. al.*, 2005 Eshrat and Hussain, 2002 Nishizono *et. al.*, 2000
Cumin (*C. cyminum*)	Cuminaldehyde Cuminic alcohol	*In vivo* studies Human trials (T2DM)	Flavonoids act synergistically with insulin demonstrating anti-hyperglycaemic and hypoglycemic activity Potential antioxidant Hepatoprotective	Hypoglycemic Reduces LDL, VLDL & cholesterol		(Karnick, 1991 Willatgamuwa *et. al.*, 1998
Coriander (*C. sativum*	Linalool α- pinene γ- terpine Geranylacetate Camphor	*In vivo* studies	Stimulates insulin secretion Hypolipidemic Inhibition of α glucosidase Hypoglycemic	Reduces LDL, VLDL & cholesterol Increases HDL Reduces blood glucose uptake Regenerating pancreatic β cell		Dhanapakiam *et. al.*, 2008 Sogara, 2014 Abderrahmane *et.al.*, 2011, Aligita *et. al.*, 2018

seed have been accounted to decrease blood sugar levels and so it has been used as an oral insulin substitute. The fiber and galactomannan present in the fenugreek seeds possess antidiabetic and the blood cholesterol lowering properties (Rathi, *et. al.,* 2002). The amino acid n-hydroxyisoleucine is related to the insulinotropic and anti-diabetic properties, which directly stimulates the β cells for delaying gastric emptying and inhibiting glucose transport (Tahiliani and Kar, 2003).

Garlic

Garlic botanically known as *Allium Sativum Linn*, is a good source of sulphur containing compounds, if cells are damaged, allicin (diallyl disulphide oxide) is produced enzymatically from alliin (S-2-propeny-L-cysteine sulfoxide). In pharmacological or therapeutic terms, it possesses anti-asthmatic, antiseptic, antithelmentic, anticholesterolemic, diaphoretic, expectorant, stimulant, febrifuge, tonic and vasodilator pharmacological properties. Total serum cholesterol is decreased by 10-12% by consuming a dose of about 10mg of allin or by garlic supplementation. Garlic affects the LDL/HDL ratio more profoundly than the cholesterol; it increases HDL and lowers LDL cholesterol. Garlic has also been found to have moderate action on the elevated triglycerides. Several animal studies have shown that garlic possesses antioxidant and blood sugar lowering properties (Lee *et al.,* 2009; Al-Qattan *et al.,* 2008; Eidi *et al.,* 2006; Jeloder *et al.,* 2005, Banerjee *et al.,* 2003).

Devaki and associates (1992) observed that garlic oil led to an increase in insulin levels in diabetic rats. Kasuga *et al.,*(1999) found it to be effective in preventing adrenal hypertrophy, elevated of corticosterone, and blood glucose levels. Sheela and co-workers (1995) reported that S-allyl cysteine sulfoxide (alliin), possessed a comparable efficacy to the standard antidiabetic agents like glibenclamide and insulin in controlling hyperglycemia in diabetic animals.

Onion

Onion is botanically known as *Allium cepalinn.* Allyl propyl disulphide, thiopropanal s-oxide and phosphoric acid are the main chemical constituents present in it. Based on to these bioactive compounds, onion is observed to be antimicrobial, diuretic, expectorant, stimulant and lachrymatory pharmacological properties. Jain and Vyas (1974) reported that onion extracts possessed hypoglycemic properties and reduced blood glucose concentration in diabetic rabbits by increasing glucose uptake by the cells. It was also found to decrease fasting plasma glucose and HbA1c (Kang *et al.*, 2010).

Cloves

Clove is the bud of an evergreen flowering plant belonging to the family of *Myrtaceae.* It is commonly used in Asia, Africa, and other parts of the world. Apart from its distinct position in the culinary world, its oil holds an important place in the pharmacological world. Kuroda and co workers (2005) identified and reported that oleanolic acid, dehydrodieugenol and dehydrodieugenol B are the main components of clove oil. Several therapeutic effects like antifungal, antibacterial, antiphlogistic, analgesic, antivomiting, antispasmodic, anticarminative, antiseptic, kidney reinforcement and insecticidal activities have been reported. Traditionally clove is used as a ñavoring and antimicrobial agent in food.

Several researches reported that clove exhibited anti-hyperglycemic activity in diabetic rats by attenuation of the activities of glycogenic enzymes with concomitant increases of hepatic and muscle glycogen concentrations (Ngubane *et. al.,* 2011). Prasad *et. al.* (2005) reported the insulin-like actions of clove bud extract in hepatocytes and hepatoma cells by reducing phosphoenolpyruvate carboxykinase and glucose 6-phosphatase gene expression. Clove has also been reported to prevent disease related to oxidative stress such as diabetics, CVD and cancer (Atawodi *et.al.*, 2011). The inhibition of α amylase, α glucosidase, lipid peroxidation and radicle scavenging activities by the essential oils present in clove are the possible mechanisms for control and prevention of type 2 diabetics (Oboh, *et. al.,*2015).

Curry Leaves

In India, curry leaves are widely and regularly used. In preclinical investigations, the aqueous extracts demonstrated its hypoglycemic property. Curry leaves are frequently utilized as a culinary flavor because of its sweet-smelling nature. It is a rich source of organically dynamic carbazole alkaloids and has pharmacological activities like, anti-cancer, antioxidant, hepatoprotective, and anti- tumourous. The bioactive constituents, includes oxalic acid, vitamin A, koenigin, bicyclomahanimbicine, cyclomahanimbine, murrayastine, coumarine, koenidine and pypayafolinecarbazole.

The curry leaves concentrate has been accounted to lower blood cholesterol and blood glucose levels in diabetic creatures (Gupta and Watal, 2005; Xie *et. al.,* 2006). Curry leaves are a good source of numerous minerals and trace elements, which are significant for maintaining normoglycemia, by actuating of pancreatic β-cells. Arulselvan and associates (2014) proposed that curry leaves might be helpful for the administration of DM. Clinical research is subsequently expected to further affirm the genuine adequacy of curry leaves in the administration of DM.

Ginger

Botanically known as *Zingiber officinale* and is well known in India as the spice. It has been found to possess antinociceptive, anti-inflammatory, aromatic, carminative, spasmolytic, antipyretic, analgesic, hypotensive, antitussive and absorbent pharmacological properties. The lipid-lowering and antioxidant potential of ethanolic extract of ginger was evaluated in streptozotcin (STZ) induced diabetes in rats. In diabetic rats ethanolic extract of *zingiber officinale* (200mg/kg) fed orally for 20 days produced the significant anti-hyperglycaemic effect. Goyal and Kadnur, (2006) observed that methanolic and ethanolic extracts of ginger at 250 mg per kg helps in the improvement of insulin sensitivity. The mechanisms underlying these actions are associated with the inhibition of key enzymes controlling carbohydrate metabolism and increased insulin release/sensitivity, resulting in enhanced glucose uptake in peripheral adipose and skeletal muscle tissues (Islam and Choi, 2008;Yiming, *et. al.,* 2012)

Turmeric

Turmeric belongs to *Zingiberaceae,* family botanically it is *curcumalonga.* Turmeric is one of the oldest spices that has been used since ages. It is a food preservative, a colorant, a drug, and a cosmetic. The major constituent present in turmeric is called curcuminoids, it is a combination of mono and bisedemethoxy derivatives. Minor amounts of resins and oils are also present, these include α-turmeron, β-turmeron, curlon, zingiberen. Ayurveda has used it since long for the treatment of diabetes as it reduces blood glucose, potentiates insulin activity more than three folds and increases glucose metabolism. Ferreira and co-workers (2006) portrayed that the extracts of turmeric lowered blood glucose level in experimentally induced- diabetic rats. Aggrawal *et. al.,* (2005) observed that curcumin lowered blood glucose and glycosylated heamoglobin levels significantly in an alloxan-induced diabetic rat model. Nishizono *et. al.,* (2000) documented that several animals studies proved that curcumin could overcome insulin resistance and can delay cataract incidence in diabetic patients. Shishu (2011) reported that in the present-day curcumin is used in polyherbal formulations *viz.* Diabecon.

Cumin

Cumin (*Cuminum cyminum*) belongs to the family *Apiaceae,* it is native to the Mediterranean region of India. It has a strong, distinct flavor, which is owing to the essential oil content. The major aromatic compounds present in cumin seeds are cuminaldehyde and cuminic alcohol. Substituted pyrazines, 2methoxy-3-sec-butylpyrazine, 2-methoxy-3ethylpyrazineand 2-ethoxy-3-isopropylpyrazine are the compounds formed in roasted cumin. Other components include γ-terpinene, safranal, p-cymene, and β-pinene (Li and Jiang, 2004). The essential oils found in the cumin possess high antioxidant activity, as well as the non-volatile extracts, also possess free radical inhibition properties. Cumin has been documented and validated to possess health beneficial properties, mainly diabetes, hypertension, dyslipidemia, inflammatory diseases, respiratory disorders, and cancer. It also possesses immune-stimulatory, hepatoprotective, gastroprotective, neuroprotective, and nephroprotective activities.

Karnick (1991) documented that cumin seeds possessed antidiabetic properties after conducting trials on humans. Researcher also reported that cumin improved fasting and postprandial blood sugar levels and helped in alleviating diabetes-related metabolic abnormalities in STZ-diabetic rats (Willatgamuwa *et. al.,* 1998). Cumin seed powder (2 g/kg) lowered the blood glucose levels in hyperglycaemic rabbits when given orally as indicated by the reduction in hyperglycaemia and glucosuria (Jain *et al.,* 1994). It also alleviated other metabolic alterations (Willatgamuwa *et al.,* 1998). Cuminaldehyde and cuminol (25 μg/ml) demonstrated 3.34- and 3.85-fold increased secretion of insulin, respectively portraying their insulinotropic activities. The insulinotropic action of both components was observed to be glucose-dependent and was owing to the increase in intracellular Ca^{2+} concentration and closure of ATP-sensitive K (K^+ -ATP) channel. The potentiality of cumin seeds to protect β-cell was also noted (Al-Snafi, 2016).

Coriander Seeds

Coriander (*Coriandrum sativum L.*), comes from the *Umbelliferae* family and is one of the highly reputed ayurvedic medicinal plants. Almost all the parts of the plant are edible, but mainly, the seed and leaves are used. Czygan and associates (2001) reported that traditionally, the seeds are used for the treatment of cold, thrush, gastric inflammatory, dizziness, nausea, and irregular menstruation. The main constituents of coriander are linalool, essential oils, and fatty oil. Aligita and associates (2018) conducted *in vitro* and *in vivo* studies and reported that the ethanolic extract of coriander (*Coriandrum sativum L.*) leaves had the antidiabetic activity at a dose of 400 mg/kg body weight by improving and regenerating the β cell in the pancreas and inhibiting the α-glucosidase enzyme in the small intestine.

Dhanapakiam *et al.,* (2008) and Duke (2002) documented that the ethanolic extract of coriander seeds lowered blood glucose levels in diabetic animals. The researcher also documented that coriander has a significant hypolipidemic action and reduced LDL, VLDL levels in experimental animals, and increased HDL level. Eguale and co-workers (2007) showed that the methanolic extract of coriander leaves portrayed antidiabetic activity in alloxan-induced animals.

CONCLUSION

A balanced diet prepared well with spices is likely to make life not only more "spicy" but more healthy also. Spices and herbs are supplementary dietary stuff used widely in Indian foods as coloring agent, flavoring agent, and preservatives from thousands of years. Spices possess various types of phytochemicals and thus portray variety of pharmacological actions and physiological actions including the digestive stimulatory, anti-inflammatory, antioxidant, anti-diabetic, hypolipidemic, anti-mutagenic. Some of the common spices such as cinnamon, garlic, curry leaves, cumin turmeric, *etc.* have been established to possess anti-diabetic properties based on several *in vitro* and *in vivo* studies. The anti-diabetic potency of some spices is also evident in human trials. Still, the research over spices is having a wide span of exploration and probability to evaluate spice therapy as a substitute and complementary in various lifestyle-related disorders.

REFERENCES

Abderrahmane, A., Soumia, Z., Zafar, H., & Badiaam, I. L. (2011). Hypoglycemic and hypolipidemic effects of *Coriandrum sativum* L. in *Merionesshawi* rats. *Journal of Ethnopharmacology, 137*(1), 652–661. doi:10.1016/j.jep.2011.06.019 PMID:21718774

Adisakwattana, S., Lerdsuwankij, O., Poputtachai, U., Minipun, A., & Suparpprom, C. (2011). Inhibitory activity of cinnamon bark species and their combination effect with acarbose against intestinal α-glucosidase and pancreatic α-amylase. *Plant Foods for Human Nutrition (Dordrecht, Netherlands), 66*(2), 143–148. doi:10.100711130-011-0226-4 PMID:21538147

Aggarwal, B. B., Kumar, A., & Aggarwal, M. S. (2005). Curcumin derived from turmeric (Curcuma longa): a spice for all seasons. In P. D. Debases Bagchi & H. G. Preuss (Eds.), *Phytochemicals in Cancer Chemoprevention* (pp. 349–387). New York: CRC Press.

Al-Qattan, K., Thomson, M. and Ali, M., (2008). Garlic (Allium sativum) and ginger (Zingiberofficinale) attenuate structural nephropathy progression in streptozotocin-induced diabetic rats. *Eur E J Clin NutrMetab, 3*, e62-e71.

Al-Snafi, A. E. (2016). The pharmacological activities of Cuminumcyminum - A review. *IOSR Journal of Pharmacy., 6*(6), 46–65.

Al-Yasiry, K., Kathum, W., & Al-Ganimi, Y. (2014). Evaluation of antidiabetic effect of cinnamon in patients with diabetes mellitus type Ii in Kerbala City. *Journal ofNatural Sciences Research, 4*(4), 43–45.

Aligita, W., Susilawati, E., Sukmawati, I.K., Holidayanti, L. & Riswanti, J. (2018). Article. *The Indonesian Biomedical Journal, 10*(2), 165. DOI: 20 doi:10.18585/inabj.v10i2.405

Anderson, R. A., Zhan, Z., Luo, R., Guo, X., Guo, Q., Zhou, J., ... Stoecker, B. A. (2016). Cinnamon extract lowers glucose, insulin and cholesterol in people with elevated serum glucose. *Journal of Traditional and Complementary Medicine, 6*(4), 332–336. doi:10.1016/j.jtcme.2015.03.005 PMID:27774415

Arulselvan, P., Ghofar, H. A. A., Karthivashan, G., Halim, M. F. A., Ghafar, M. S. A., & Fakurazi, S. (2014). Antidiabetic therapeutics from natural source: A systematic review. *Biomedicine & Preventive Nutrition*, *4*(4), 607–617. doi:10.1016/j.bionut.2014.07.009

Ashraf, R., Aamir, K., Shaikh, R. A., & Ahmed, T. (2005). Effects of garlic on dyslipidemia in patients with type 2 diabetes mellitus. *Journal of Ayub Medical College*, *17*(3), 60–64. PMID:16320801

Atawodi, S. E., Atawodi, J. C., Idakwo, G. A., Pfundstein, B., Haubner, R., & Wurtel, G. (2011). Spiegelhalder & Owen, R.W. (2011). *Journal of Medicinal Food*, *12*(6), 1316. doi:10.1089/jmf.2008.0211 PMID:20041787

Ayodhya, S., Kusum, S., & Anjali, S. (2010). Hypoglycaemic activity of different extracts of various herbal plants. *International Journal of Research in Ayurveda and Pharmacy*, *1*(1), 212–224.

Banerjee, S. K., Mukherjee, P. K., & Maulik, S. K. (2003). Garlic as an antioxidant: The good, the bad and the ugly. *Phytotherapy Research*, *17*(2), 97–106. doi:10.1002/ptr.1281 PMID:12601669

Bi, X., Lim, J., & Henry, C. J. (2017). Spices in the management of diabetes mellitus. *Food Chemistry*, *217*, 281–293. doi:10.1016/j.foodchem.2016.08.111 PMID:27664636

Broca, C., Breil, V., Cruciani-Guglielmacci, C., Manteghetti, M., Rouault, C., Derouet, M., ... Taouis, M. (2004). The insulinotrophic agent 1D1101(4-hydroxyisoleucine) activates insulin signaling in rat. *American Journal of Physiology. Endocrinology and Metabolism*, *287*(3), E463–E471. doi:10.1152/ajpendo.00163.2003 PMID:15082420

Cao, J., Liu, Y., Jia, L., Jiang, L. P., Geng, C. Y., Yao, X. F., ... Zhong, L. F. (2008). Curcumin attenuates acrylamide-induced cytotoxicity and genotoxicity in HepG2 cells by ROS scavenging. *Journal of Agricultural and Food Chemistry*, *56*(24), 12059–12063. doi:10.1021/jf8026827 PMID:19012407

Coon, J. S. T., & Ernst, E. (2003). Herbs for serum cholesterol reduction: A systematic view. *The Journal of Family Practice*, *52*, 468–478. PMID:12791229

Cusi, K., & DeFronzo, R. (2000). Recombinant human insulin-like growth factor I treatment for 1 week improves metabolic control in type 2 diabetes by ameliorating hepatic and muscle insulin resistance. *The Journal of Clinical Endocrinology and Metabolism*, *85*, 3077–3084. PMID:10999789

Czygan, F. C. D., Frohne, C., Holtzel, A., Nagell, & Pfander, H. J. (2001). Norman Grainger Bisset and max Wichtl. Herbal Drugs and Phytopharmaceuticals. In A Handbook for practices on a scientific basics with reference to German commission and Monographs (2nd ed.). Medpharm Scientific Publishers.

Devaki, T., Venmahdi, S., & Govindaraju, P. (1992). Alterations in protein metabolism in ethanol-ingested rats treated with garlic. *Medical Science Research*, *20*, 725–727.

Devi, B. A., Kamalakkannan, N., & Prince, P. S. (2003). Supplementation of fenugreek leaves to diabetic rats-Effect on carbohydrate metabolic enzymes in diabetic liver and kidney. *Phytotherapy Research*, *17*(10), 1231–1233. doi:10.1002/ptr.1357 PMID:14669264

Dhanapakiam, P., Mini Joseph, J., Ramaswamy, V. K., Moorthi, M., & Senthil Kumar, A. (2008). The cholesterol lowering property of coriander seeds (Coriandrum sativum): Mechanism of action. *Journal of Environmental Biology*, *29*(1), 53–56. PMID:18831331

Duke, J. A. (2002). *Handbook of Medicinal Herbs* (2nd ed.). Boca Raton, FL: CRC Press LLC. doi:10.1201/9781420040463

Eguale, T., Tilahun, G., Debella, A., Feleke, A., & Makonnen, E. (2007). In vitro and in vivo anthelmintic activity of crude extracts of Coriandrum sativum against Haemonchuscontortus. *Journal of Ethnopharmacology*, *110*(3), 428–433. doi:10.1016/j.jep.2006.10.003 PMID:17113738

Eidi, A., Eidi, M., & Esmaeili, E. (2006). Antidiabetic effect of garlic (Allium sativum L.) in normal and streptozotocin-induced diabetic rats. *Phytomedicine*, *13*(9-10), 624–629. doi:10.1016/j.phymed.2005.09.010 PMID:17085291

Eshrat, H., & Hussain, M. A. (2002). Hypoglycemic, hypolipidemic and antioxidant properties of combination of curcumin from Curcuma longa Linn. and partially purified product from Abromaaugusta Linn. in streptozotocin induced diabetes. *Indian Journal of Clinical Biochemistry*, *17*(2), 33–43. doi:10.1007/BF02867969 PMID:23105348

Ferreira, E. B., Neves, F. E. A., da Costa, M. E. D., do Prado, W. A., Ferri, L. A., & … . (2006). Comparative effects of Stevia rebaudiana leaves and stevioside on glycaemia and hepatic gluconeogenesis. *Planta Medica*, *72*(08), 691–696. doi:10.1055-2006-931586 PMID:16732523

Governa, P., Baini, G., Borgonetti, V., Cettolin, G., Giachetti, D., Magnano, A. R., ... Biagi, M. (2018). Phytotherapy in the management of diabetes: A review. *Molecules (Basel, Switzerland)*, *23*(1), 1–22. doi:10.3390/molecules23010105 PMID:29300317

Goyal, R. K., & Kadnur, S. V. (2006). Beneðcial effects of *Zingiber officinale* on gold thioglucose induced obesity. *Fitoterapia*, *77*(3), 160–163. doi:10.1016/j.fitote.2006.01.005 PMID:16513292

Grover, J. K., Rathi, S. S., & Vats, V. (2002). Amelioration of experimental diabetic neuropathy and gastropathy in rats following oral administration of plant (Eugenia jambolana, Mucunapruriens and Tinosporacordifolia) extracts. *Indian Journal of Experimental Biology*, *40*, 273–276. PMID:12635695

Gupta, R. K., & Watal, G. (2005). Hypoglycemic effects of Murrayakoenigii on normal and alloxan-diabetic rabbits. *Journal of Ethnopharmacology*, *97*(2), 247–251. doi:10.1016/j.jep.2004.11.006 PMID:15707761

Hannan, J. M., Rokeya, B., Faruque, O., Nahar, N., Mosihuzzaman, M., Azad Khan, A. K., & Ali, L. (2003). Effect of soluble dietary fibre fraction of Trigonellafoenum-graecum on glycemic, insulenimic, lipidemic and platelet aggregation status of Type II diabetic model rats. *Journal of Ethnopharmacology*, *88*(1), 73–77. doi:10.1016/S0378-8741(03)00190-9 PMID:12902054

Hlebowicz, J., Wickenberg, J., & Ingemansson, S. L. (2007). Effects of Curcuma longa (turmeric) on postprandial plasma glucose and insulin in healthy subjects. *Nutrition Journal*, *9*, 43. PMID:20937162

Huang, E. S., Shook, M., Jin, L., Chin, M. H., & Meltzer, D. O.ADA. (2006). The impact of patient preferences on the cost-effectiveness of intensive glucose control in older patients with new-onset diabetes. *Diabetes Care*, *29*(2), 259–264. doi:10.2337/diacare.29.02.06.dc05-1443 PMID:16443870

Islam, M. S., & Choi, H. (2008). Comparative effects of dietary ginger (Zingiberofficinale) and garlic (Allium sativum) investigated in a type2 diabetes model of rats. *Journal of Medicinal Food*, *11*(1), 152–159. doi:10.1089/jmf.2007.634 PMID:18361751

Jain, R. C., & Vyas, C. R. (1974). Hypoglycemic action of onion on rabbits. *British Medical Journal*, *2*(5921), 730. doi:10.1136/bmj.2.5921.730-b PMID:4852817

Jain, S. C., Purohit, M., & Jain, R. (1992). Pharmacological evaluation of Cuminumcyminum. *Fitoterapia*, *63*(4), 291–294.

Jelodar, G. A., Maleki, M., Motadayen, M. H., & Sirus, S. (2005). Effect of fenugreek, onion and garlic on blood glucose and histopathology of pancreas of alloxan induced diabetic rats. *Indian Journal of Medical Sciences*, *59*(2), 64–69. doi:10.4103/0019-5359.13905 PMID:15738612

Kang, J. H., Tsuyoshi, G., Han, I. S., Kawada, T., Kim, Y. M., & Yu, R. (2010). Dietary capsaicin reduces obesity induced insulin resistance and hepatic steatosis in obese mice fed a high fat diet. *Obesity (Silver Spring, Md.)*, *18*(4), 780–787. doi:10.1038/oby.2009.301 PMID:19798065

Karnick, C. R. (1991). A clinical trial of a composite herbal drug in the treatment of diabetes mellitus. *Aryavaidyan.*, *5*, 36–46.

Kasuga, S., Ushijima, M., Morihara, N., Itakura, Y., & Nakata, Y. (1999). Effect of aged garlic extract (AGE) on hyperglycemia induced by immobilization stress in mice. *Nippon Yakurigaku Zasshi*, *114*(3), 191–197. doi:10.1254/fpj.114.191 PMID:10553583

Khan, A., Safdar, M., Ali Khan, M.M., Khattak, K.N. & Anderson, R.A. (2003). Cinnamon improves glucose and lipids of people with type 2. *Diabetics Care, 26*, 3215-3218.

Kim, S. H., Hyun, S. H., & Choung, S. Y. (2006). Anti-diabetic effect of cinnamon extract on blood glucose in db/db mice. *Journal of Ethnopharmacology*, *104*(1-2), 119–123. doi:10.1016/j.jep.2005.08.059 PMID:16213119

Kumar, S., & Mukkadan, J. (2013). Anti diabetic effect of oral administration of cinnamon in Wistar Albino Rats. *Bali Medical Journal*, *2*(3), 97–99.

Kuroda, M., Mimaki, Y., Nishiyama, T., Mae, T., Kishida, H., Tsukagawa, M., & Kitahara, M. (2005). Hypoglycemic effects of turmeric (Curcuma longa L. rhizomes) on genetically diabetic KK-Ay mice. *Biological & Pharmaceutical Bulletin*, *28*(5), 937–939. doi:10.1248/bpb.28.937 PMID:15863912

Lee, Y. M., Gweon, O. C., Seo, Y. J., Im, J., Kang, M. J., Kim, M. J., & Kim, J. I. (2009). Antioxidant effect of garlic and aged black garlic in animal model of type 2 diabetes mellitus. *Nutrition Research and Practice*, *3*(2), 156–161. doi:10.4162/nrp.2009.3.2.156 PMID:20016716

Li, R., & Jiang, Z. (2004). Chemical composition of the essential oil of Cuminumcyminum L. from China. *Flavour and Fragrance Journal*, *19*(4), 311–313. doi:10.1002/ffj.1302

Liu, C. T., Wong, P. L., Lii, C. K., Hse, H., & Sheen, L. Y. (2006). Antidiabetic effect of garlic oil but not diallyl disulfide in rats with streptozotocin-induced diabetes. *Food and Chemical Toxicology*, *44*(8), 1377–1384. doi:10.1016/j.fct.2005.07.013 PMID:16690190

Lu, X., Rasco, B. A., Jabal, J. M. F., Aston, D. E., Lin, M., & Kondel, M. E. (2011). Investigating antibacterial effects of garlic (*Allium sativum*) concentrate and garlic-derived organosulfur compounds on *Campylobacter jejuni* by using fourier transform infrared spectroscopy, raman spectroscopy, and electron microscopy. *Applied and Environmental Microbiology, 77*(15), 5257–5269. doi:10.1128/AEM.02845-10 PMID:21642409

Medagama, B. (2015). The glycaemic outcomes of Cinnamon, a review of the experimental evidence and clinical trials. *Nutrition Journal, 14*(108), 2015. doi:10.118612937-015-0098-9 PMID:26475130

Ngubane, P. S., Masola, B., & Musabayane, C. T. (2011). The effects of Syzygiumaromaticum-derived oleanolic acid on glycogenic enzymes in streptozotocin-induced diabetic rats. *Renal Failure, 33*(4), 434–439. doi:10.3109/0886022X.2011.568147 PMID:21529273

Nishizono, S., Hayami, T., Ikeda, I., & Imaizumi, K. (2000). Protection against diabetogenic effect of feeding tert-butylhydroxyquinone to rats prior to the administration of streptozotocin. *Bioscience, Biotechnology, and Biochemistry, 64*(6), 1153–1158. doi:10.1271/bbb.64.1153 PMID:10923784

Oboh, G., Agunloye, O. M., Adefegha, S. A., Akinyemi, A. J., & Ademiluyi, A. O. (2015). Caffeic and chlorogenic acids inhibit key enzymes linked to type 2 diabetes (in vitro): A comparative study. *Journal of Basic and Clinical Physiology and Pharmacology, 26*(2), 165–170. doi:10.1515/jbcpp-2013-0141 PMID:24825096

Prasad, R. C., Herzog, B., Boone, B., Sims, L., & Waltner-Law, M. (2005). An extract of Syzygiumaromaticum represses genes encoding hepatic gluconeogenic enzymes. *Journal of Ethnopharmacology, 96*(1-2), 295–301. doi:10.1016/j.jep.2004.09.024 PMID:15588682

Qin, B., Polansky, M. M., Sato, Y., Adeli, K., & Anderson, R. A. (2010). Cinnamon extract inhibits the postprandial overproduction of apolipoprotein B48-containing lipoproteins in fructose-fed animals. *The Journal of Nutritional Biochemistry, 20*(11), 901–908. doi:10.1016/j.jnutbio.2008.08.005 PMID:18993048

Raju, J., Patlolla, J. M., Swamy, M. V., & Rao, C. V. (2004). Diosgenin, a steroid saponin of *Trigonellafoenum graecum* (Fenugreek), inhibits azoxymethane-induced aberrant crypt foci formation in F344 rats and induces apoptosis in HT-29 human colon cancer cells. *Cancer Epidemiology, Biomarkers & Prevention, 13*, 1392–1398. PMID:15298963

Rao, P. V., & Gan, S. H. (2014). Cinnamon: A multifaceted medicinal plant. *Evidence-Based Complementary and Alternative Medicine*. PMID:24817901

Rathi, S. S., Grover, J. K., Vats, V., & Biswas, N. R. (2002). Prevention of experimental diabetic cataract by Indian Ayurvedic plant extracts. *Phytotherapy Research, 16*(8), 774–777. doi:10.1002/ptr.1064 PMID:12458487

Saeed, F., Nadeem, M., Ahmad, R. S., Nadeem, M. T., Arshad, M. S., & Ullah, A. (2016). Studying the impact of nutritional immunology underlying the modulation of immune responses by nutritional compounds – A review. *Food and Agricultural Immunology, 27*(2), 205–229. doi:10.1080/09540105.2015.1079600

Sahib, S. (2016). Anti-diabetic and antioxidant effect of cinnamon in poorly controlled type-2 diabetic Iraqi patients: A randomized, placebocontrolled clinical trial. *Journal of Intercultural Ethnopharmacology*, *5*(2), 108–113. doi:10.5455/jice.20160217044511 PMID:27104030

Sangal, A. (2011). Role of cinnamon as beneficial antidiabetic food adjunct: A review. *Advances in Applied Science Research*, *2*(4), 440450.

Sheela, C. G., Kumud, K., & Augusti, K. T. (1995). Antidiabetic effect of onion and garlic sulfoxide amino acids in rats. *Planta Medica*, *61*(04), 356–357. doi:10.1055-2006-958099 PMID:7480182

Shishu, N. A. (2011). A Review of Recent Investigations on Medicinal Herbs Possessing Anti-Diabetic Properties. *Journal of Nutritional Disorders & Therapy*, *1*(102), 2.

Singh, G., Maurya, S., & Catalan, C. A. (2007). A comparison of chemical, antioxidant and antimicrobial studies of cinnamon leaf and bark volatile oils, oleoresins and their constituents. *Food and Chemical Toxicology*, *45*(9), 1650–1661. doi:10.1016/j.fct.2007.02.031 PMID:17408833

Sogara, P. P. U. (2014). Pengaruh ekstrak etanol buah ketumbar (coriandrum sativum l.) Terhadap penurunan kadar gula darah tikus putih yang diinduksi aloksan. *Pharmacon, 3*(3).

Srinivasan, K. (2005). Spices as influencers of body metabolism: An overview of three decades of research. *Food Research International*, *38*(1), 77–86. doi:10.1016/j.foodres.2004.09.001

Subash Babu, P., Prabuseenivasan, S., & Ignacimuthu, S. (2007). Cinnamaldehyde--a potential antidiabetic agent. *Phytomedicine*, *14*(1), 15–22. doi:10.1016/j.phymed.2006.11.005 PMID:17140783

Tahiliani, P., & Kar, A. (2003). Mitigation of thyroxine induced hyperglycaemia by two plant extracts. *Phytotherapy Research*, *17*(3), 294–296. doi:10.1002/ptr.1121 PMID:12672166

Willatgamuva, S. A., Platel, K., Sarawathi, G., & Srinivasan, K. (1998). Antidiabetic influence of dietary cumin seeds (Cuminumcyminum) in streptozotocin induced diabetic rats. *Nutrition Research (New York, N.Y.)*, *18*(1), 131–142. doi:10.1016/S0271-5317(97)00207-8

Williams, S. R. (1973). *Nutrition and diet therapy*. Jones & Bartlett Publishers.

World Health Organization. (2016). *Global report on diabetes*. World Health Organization.

Xie, J. T., Chang, W. T., Wang, C. Z., Mehendale, S. R., Li, J., Ambihaipahar, R., & Yuan, C. S. (2006). Curry leaf (MurrayakoenigiiSpreng.) reduces blood cholesterol and glucose levels in ob/ob mice. *The American Journal of Chinese Medicine*, *34*(02), 279–284. doi:10.1142/S0192415X06003825 PMID:16552838

Yeh, G. Y., Eisenberg, D. M., Kaptchuk, T. M., & Phillips, R. S. (2003). Systematic review of herbs and dietary supplements for glycemic control in diabetes. *Diabetes Care*, *26*(4), 1277–1294. doi:10.2337/diacare.26.4.1277 PMID:12663610

Yeh, H. F., Luo, C. Y., Lin, C. Y., Cheng, S. S., Hsu, Y. R., & Chang, S. T. (2013). Methods for thermal stability enhancement of leaf essential oils and their main constituents from indigenous cinnamon (*Cinnamomumosmophloeum*). *Journal of Agricultural and Food Chemistry*, *61*(26), 6293–6298. doi:10.1021/jf401536y PMID:23738884

Yiming, Li., Tran, V. H., Duke, C. C., & Roufogalis, B. D. (2012). Preventive and protective properties of Zingiberofficinale (ginger) in diabetes mellitus, diabetic complications, and associated lipid and other metabolic disorders: A brief review. *Evidence-Based Complementary and Alternative Medicine*.

Chapter 4
Elucidating the Phytochemical and Pharmacological Potential of *Myristica fragrans* (Nutmeg)

Ena Gupta
Department of Home Science, University of Allahabad, India

ABSTRACT

Myristica fragrans or nutmeg is a ground spice of the family Myristicaceae. Its tree has dark leaves mainly cultivated in Grenada, Malaysia, and Kerala. It is majorly a source of two spices derived from its fruit: nutmeg (jaiphal) from its seed and mace (javitri) from the covering of seed. The important bioactive constituents present in nutmeg include macelignan, carvacrol, myristicin, β-caryophyllene, β-pinene, α-pinene, p-cymene, and eugenol. Low doses of nutmeg do not cause any side effects whereas after consuming 5g toxic overdose occurs, and central nervous system (CNS) effects were induced after consuming 1 to 2 mg/kg b.wt. of nutmeg. Various therapeutic or medicinal applications were shown by nutmeg such as antioxidant, antimicrobial, aphrodisiac, anticancer, hepatoprotective, anti-inflammatory, antidepressant, and cardioprotective activity. This review chapter focuses on ethnobotany, phytochemistry, acceptable daily intake, and different pharmacological actions of this medicinal plant.

INTRODUCTION

The term 'Myristica' was derived from Greek term 'Myron', meaning a sweet liquid cleansed from the plant (Everett, 1981). "Myristica" is a genus having nine species and few are most commonly found in India, such as *Myristica fragrans*, *Myristica malabarica*, and *Myristica beddomeii*. The common name of *Myristica fragrans* is known as nutmeg, which belongs to Myristicaceae family. The two important condiments mainly recognized for their production are nutmeg and mace. (Krishnamoorthy and Rema 2001). The seed present inside the fruit is nutmeg, and the delicate red coating on the kernel is mace (Pal et al., 2011), as shown in figure 1. It is the native of East Indonesia, formally known as 'spice islands'. Later, it is broadly distributed in India, North Australia, Srilanka, Pacific islands, and South East Asia.

DOI: 10.4018/978-1-7998-2524-1.ch004

In India, nutmeg is chiefly cultivated in southern parts, mostly in Tamil Nadu. It is a medium-sized, evergreen aromatic tree, usually growing to about 5 to13 m high, even up to 25m.

Figure 1. Diagram of different parts of ground spice Myristica fragrans or nutmeg

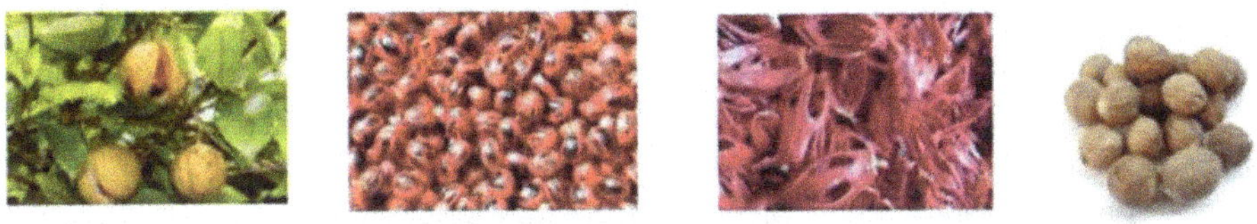

Nutmeg tree | **Seeds wrapped with mace** | **Mace** | **Nutmeg seeds**

Nutmeg is considered as an important spice all over the world and is used to enhance the taste and aromatic flavor of the food. It is a unique culinary ingredient frequently used in bakery foods, confections, puddings, meats, sausages, sauces, vegetables, and beverages.

Nutmeg is utilized as a folklore medicine since the middle ages in the treatment of many health issues like stomachic, appetite stimulant, diarrhea, and controlling flatulence (**Min et al., 2011**).

Studies report that essential oil obtained from nutmeg cures paralysis, infectious skin diseases, and rheumatism. The plant is also used for anti-inflammatory, analgesic, sedative, hypnotic, and antimicrobial actions (**Kokate et al., 2010; Chelladurai et al., 2017**).

An array of compounds have been identified in nutmeg through phytochemical analysis such as phenolics, flavonoids, carotenoids, alkaloids, lignins, and terpenoids, which are mainly responsible for their therapeutic and pharmacological applications (**Saxena and Patil, 2012**). The nutmeg is a bitter aromatic astringent, and chemical analysis showed the presence of volatile and non-volatile compounds that give the characteristic pleasant fragrance and aroma. The aim of this review article is to sum up the pharmacological/biological activities of nutmeg and its bioactive constituents with possible therapeutic applications.

Taxonomical Classification (Forrester, 2005)

Kingdom: Plantae
Division: Magnoliophyta
Class: Magnoliopsida
Subclass: Magnoliidae
Order: Magnoliales
Genus: *Myristica Gronov*
Family: Myristicaceae
Species: *Myristica fragrans*

Botanical Description

Table 1. Macroscopic Study

Macroscopic Study	
Tall	Grows to nearly 5 to 13 m
Leaf	Alternately arranged dark green leaves, 9.5-22 x 3.7-10 cm, elliptic, tip pointed, glossy and hairless
Flowers	Flowers unisexual, urn-shaped and lightly creamy, smooth, chubby, and tumble-shaped.
Fruit	single seed, typically with a ruminate endosperm, covered to various degrees by a fatty white-reddish aril
Bark	greenish-black, smooth, blaze reddish

Ethnobotany

Myristica fragrans (Nutmeg) is a dark-leaved fruits bearing green tree, cultivated for majorly two spices from its fruit: a single seed nutmeg and its bright red aril or seed covering called mace. Primarily it is used as a flavoring agent in cooking and in the preparation of many sweet snacks known as 'pala gulu' or 'pala manis'. Oils obtained from nutmeg are used for flavoring food products and in curing the number of problems like diarrhea, headaches, flu and stomach aches. Studies reports that nutmeg and mace boosts the immune system, maintain healthy blood vessels and nerve cells, prevent headaches and eye problems. Phytosterols present in nutmeg slow down cancer cell reproduction in the large intestine and protects against colon cancer by reducing inflammation. Therefore, nutmeg shows different nutritional effects for maintaining good health.

Phytochemistry

The primary metabolites such as fixed oils, pigments, starch, and protein are the main constituents of nutmeg (more than 70% of nutmeg kernel's weight). Plants can synthesize secondary metabolites to protect themselves against adverse conditions. These compounds are highly varied in chemical composition and also exhibit beneficial effects on human diseases. Nutmeg is an important medicinal plant with characteristic pleasant flagrance and bitter taste due to the presence of diverse volatile and non-volatile compounds. The most commonly identified compounds include volatile substances, terpenoids, phenolics, lignin compounds, proteins, mucilage, starch, fiber and vitamin A, C and E (Naikodi et al., 2011; El-Alfy et al., 2009).

The seeds also contain 25% - 30% fixed oils (myristic, stearic, palmitic, oleic, linoleic, and lauric acids) and 10% of essential oil. The major chemical constitutes are terpene hydrocarbons (α-pinenes, camphene, p-cymene, sabinene, β-phellandrene, γ-terpinene, limonene, myrcene (60% to 90%), terpene derivatives (linalool, geraniol, terpineol-5% to 15%) and phenylpropanes (myristicin, elemicin, safrole-2% to 20%) (Qiu et al., 2004; Yang et al., 2008). Thirty-seven numbers of compounds were identified in the essential oil, including elemicin, camphene, eugenol, isoeuglenol, isoelemicin, methoxyeugenol and elimicin (Piaru et al., 2012; Wahab et al., 2009). In another study by Gupta (2013) identified 32 different compounds (99.49% of the total extract) in acetone extract of nutmeg seed such as sabinene (28.61%), b-pinene (10.26%), apinene (9.72%) terpinen-4-ol (5.80%), myristicin (4.30%), limonene (3.76%), cterpinene (3.71%), (Z)-p-menth-2-en-1-ol (3.21%), isoeugenol (2.72%), elemicin (2.67%), (E)-p-menth-2-en-1-ol (2.15%), myrcene (2.14%), a-phellandrene (1.84%),p-cymene (1.81%), terpinolene (1.63%) and linalool (1.12%). Myristicin is a principle that constitutes of nutmeg, which is responsible for most of its pharmacological effects. Besides, the seeds contain saponins, polyphenols, tannins, epicatechin, triterpenic sapogenins, and fats (**Latha et al., 2005**). Some important bioactive constituents in nutmeg seed oil are shown in figure 2.

Figure 2. The structures of some important constituents of nutmeg seed oil:β-Caryophyllene, safrole, β –Phellandrene, eugenol and isoeugenol
(source Gupta and Rajpurohit, 2011)

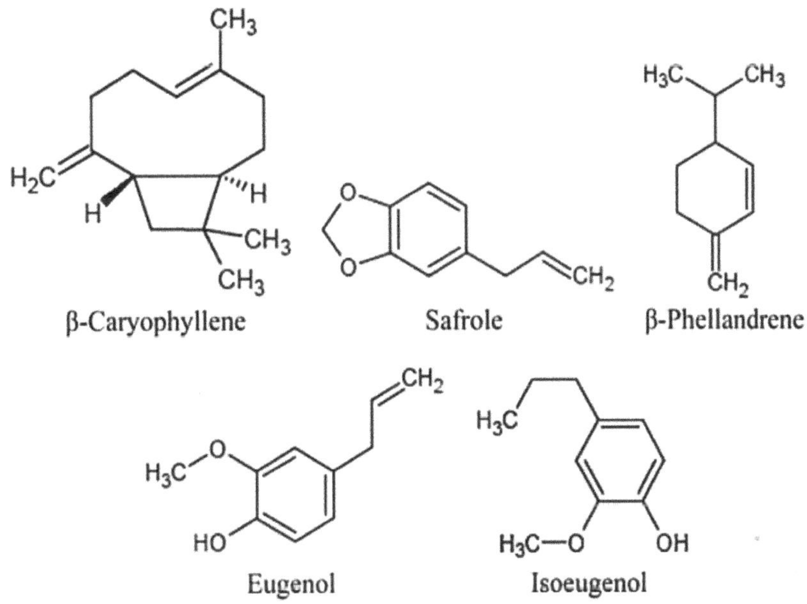

Lignan is another important class of secondary metabolites present in nutmeg kernels. Previous studies have reported the isolation of numerous lignans from nutmeg (Duan et al., 2009, Nguyen et al., 2010). There are many important commercial products which can be obtained from *Myristica fragrans* or nutmeg, as shown the figure 3.

Figure 3. The principal commercial products obtained from Myristica fragrans or nutmeg (Singh et al., 2003)

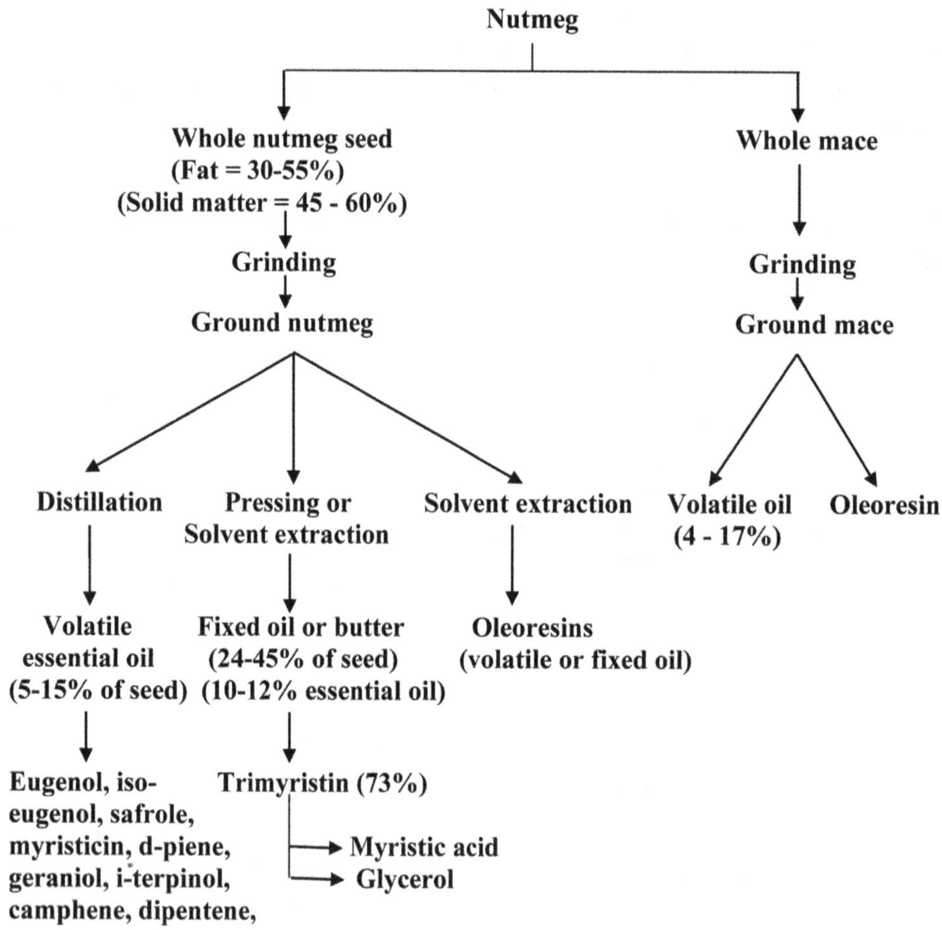

Acceptable Daily Intake (ADI)

No noticeable neurological or physiological response was observed when nutmeg is consumed in low doses, whereas large doses of nutmeg intoxication may cause delirium, amnesia, anxiety, dry mouth, nausea, confusion, sweating, inattentiveness, hallucination and in severe cases body pain. Central nervous system (CNS) effects were induced after consuming 1 to 2 mg/kg b.wt. of nutmeg, and toxic overdose occurs after consuming 5g. In pregnancy and lactation very small doses may be used safely. It is generally recognized safe when used as a flavoring agent in food products (De Milto and Frey, 2005).

Pharmacological Actions

Many bioactive constituents are present in the nutmeg, which plays a significant role in the medicinal world as traditional medicine and has been suggested in the treatment of many chronic and non-chronic diseases.

Antioxidant

The body requires an abundant amount of antioxidants to prevent oxidative damage caused by reactive oxygen species (ROS) and chronic inflammation. Research studies have shown that oils of mace and nutmeg contain potent antioxidants. The main antioxidant compounds present in nutmeg include methoxy-eugenol, eugenol and isoeugenol, lignans, carvacrol, α, and β-pinene, p-cymene, and β-caryophyllene. These antioxidants inhibit the production of nitric acid, metal chelation, decrease oxidation of LDL or inhibition of lipid peroxidation, scavenging nitric oxide (NO) and quenching singlet oxygen. The free radical scavenging activity of nutmeg is around 462uM BHT and 656uM α-tocopherol. Nutmeg is considered as a natural source of antioxidants, which may reduce the risk of developing pathogenic microorganisms (**Gupta and Rajpurohit, 2011**).

Antimicrobial Activity

Nutmeg possesses potential anti-microbial properties due to the presence of high phenolic content. In the case of oral health, nutmeg is considered as the king of spice in traditional medical applications. The bioactive antibacterial constituents present in nutmeg is very effective against bad breath (halitosis), toothache, cavities, and bleeding gums. Incorporating nutmeg in food is beneficial for oral health. Extracts of nutmeg can kill bacteria (*Streptococcus mutans*), causing cavities, but harmless bacteria remain unaffected. The non-pathogenic strains of *E. coli* were not sensitive to nutmeg extract, whereas 157 *E. coli* pathogenic strains were sensitive (Kadhim et al., 2013). Nutmeg is effective against aching gums and toothaches due to its antiseptic nature.

Antidiabetic Activity

The petroleum extract of nutmeg at dose of 200 mg Kg-1 was administered in alloxan-induced diabetic rats. It shows a significant ($P<0.05$) decline in the plasma blood glucose levels from 145.75±9.65 to 81.5±4.03 mg% in oral glucose tolerance test (OGTT) after 30 min when compared to control group of glucose-fed rats. In alloxan-induced diabetic rats, when petroleum ether extract of *Myristica fragrans* was given daily for two weeks, the blood sugar level reduced significantly from 326.25±7.05 to 268.0±9.6 mg% (**Somani, 2008**). The hypoglycaemic effect of nutmeg attributed to its ability to enhance insulin sensitivity and improved lipid metabolic disorders by activating peroxisome.

Anti-inflammatory Activity

It was observed that the anti-inflammatory effect of nutmeg is similar to those of non-steroidal anti-inflammatory drugs (Olajide et al., 2000). It was suggested that myristicin is an active compound present in essential oil, was responsible for the anti-inflammatory effect. According to studies, the anti-inflammatory effect of myristicin was due to inhibition of chemokines, cytokines, nitrous oxide, and growth factors in double-stranded RNA (dsRNA) stimulated macrophages via the calcium pathway (Lee and Park, 2011). In this support another study also reported that ethanolic extract of nutmeg seed exhibit high anti-inflammatory activity by inhibiting the inflammatory cytokines and nitric oxide production.

Hepatoprotective Activity

Research studies have shown that nutmeg can fight hepatotoxicity due to the presence of a specific bio-active compound named myrislignan, which protects the liver against damage. Myristicin is an active constituent of nutmeg that was reported to show potent hepatoprotective effects (Morita et al., 2003) and inhibits tumor necrosis factor (TNF)-alpha release from macrophages. The mechanism behind the protective effects of nutmeg was studied in the mouse animal model of liver toxicity; it was seen through metabolomics analyses that liver damage is possibly protected by nutmeg as it helps in restoring mice to additional healthy levels of different acylcarnitines and lipids. Nutmeg also modulated peroxisome proliferator-activated receptor alpha (*PPARα*) as shown by gene expression studies.

Antidepressant Activity

In general, approximately 5% population is affected with depression, basically characterized by melancholia, mood swings, lack of interest in the surroundings, and psychomotor retardation. Worldwide, depression is the fourth leading cause of disability, as reported by World Health Organization (WHO, 2001). Nutmeg has been used for centuries in curing psychoactive properties like hallucination and anxiogenic as it can modulate the physiology central nervous system (Forrester, 2005). The anti-depressant effect of the n-hexane extracts of *M. fragrans* seeds was studied in mice using the tail suspension test (TST) and forced swim test (FST). The mice were subjected to three different oral doses of 5, 10, and 20 mg/kg body weight. When compared with control, the highly potent dose was found to be 10 mg/kg body weight, and at this dose significant decline in the immobility of mice was observed. Moreover, the selected dose showed equivalent strength to fluoxetine (20 mg/kg) and imipramine (15 mg/kg), thus extract of nutmeg seeds showed antidepressant effect in mice (Dhingra and Sharma, 2006).

Cardioprotective Activity

In ancient times it was reported that nutmeg possesses cardio tonic property and prevents oxidative stress. Hypercholesterolemic rabbits were administered with *Myristica fragrans* seed extract and results showed that there was a significant reduction in the Low-density lipoproteins (LDL) and serum cholesterol. Nutmeg extract also increases the excretion of phospholipids and cholesterol through fecal matter and also prevents the accumulation of cholesterol, phospholipids, and triglycerides in the liver, heart, and aorta with the termination of atheromatous plaque in the aorta (**Sharma et al., 1995**). In albino rats' platelets, anti-aggregatory and hypolipidaemic activities of *Myristica fragrans* were studied, an oral dose of 500 mg/kg of ethanolic extract of Nutmeg was given to albino rats for 60days. It was observed that there was a significant reduction in the total cholesterol, Low-density lipoproteins (LDL), and very-low-density lipoproteins (VLDL) levels along with an increase in high-density lipoprotein (HDL) cholesterol. According to toxicity studies, no adverse effect was seen on different biochemical and hematological parameters (Ram et al., 1996).

Interactions

A theoretical interaction was reported to occur in nutmeg/mace due to anxiogenic properties. In rat model studies, it was shown that nutmeg interactions can occur with buspirone, diazepam, and ondansetron. Simultaneous ingestion of huge quantities of nutmeg and flunitrazepam results in death (Stein et al., 2001)

CONCLUSION

In earlier days, *Myristica fragrans* or nutmeg was used for different medicinal purposes due to its curative, aromatic, and aphrodisiac properties. In general, it will improve the overall health, which is contributed by some important bioactive compounds (macelignan, carvacrol, myristicin, β-caryophyllene, β-pinene, α-pinene, p-cymene and eugenol) present in it. A potential therapeutic mode of applications was shown by the seed/mace extract of nutmegs such as antioxidant, antimicrobial, hepatoprotective, anticancer, antidepressant, anti-inflammatory, and cardioprotective activity. To better understand the broad spectrum of scientific applications of nutmeg, more efforts are required to validate its activity and the mechanism of action.

REFERENCES

Chelladurai, P. K., & Ramalingam, R. (2017). *Myristica malabarica*: A comprehensive review. *Journal of Pharmacognosy and Phytochemistry*, *6*, 255–258.

De Milto, L., & Frey, R. J. (2005). Nutmeg. In Gale Encyclopedia of Alternative Medicine (2nd ed. vol. 3). Detroit, MI: Thomson Gale.

Dhingra, D., & Sharma, A. (2006). Antidepressant-like activity of n-hexane extract of nutmeg (Myristica fragrans) seeds in mice. *Journal of Medicinal Food*, *9*(1), 84–89. doi:10.1089/jmf.2006.9.84 PMID:16579733

Duan, L., Tao, H. W., Hao, X. J., Gu, Q. Q., & Zhu, W. M. (2009). Cytotoxic and antioxidative phenolic compounds from the traditional Chinese medicinal plant, *Myristica fragrans. Planta Medica*, *75*(11), 1241–1245. doi:10.1055-0029-1185506 PMID:19326328

El-Alfy, A., Wilson, L., ElSohly, M. A., & Abourashed, E. A. (2009). Towards a better understanding of the psychopharmacology of nutmeg: Activities in the mouse tetrad assay. *Journal of Ethnopharmacology*, *126*(2), 280–286. doi:10.1016/j.jep.2009.08.026 PMID:19703539

Everett, T. H. (1981). *Myristica. In Illustrated Encyclopaedia of Horticulture*. New York: Garland Publishing Inc.

Forrester, M. B. (2005). Nutmeg intoxication in Texas, 1998-2004. *Human and Experimental Toxicology*, *24*(11), 563–566. doi:10.1191/0960327105ht567oa PMID:16323572

Gupta, A. D., Bansal, V. K., Babu, V., & Maithil, N. (2013). Chemistry, antioxidant and antimicrobial potential of nutmeg (*Myristica fragrans* Houtt). *Journal of Genetic Engineering and Biotechnology*, *11*(1), 25–31. doi:10.1016/j.jgeb.2012.12.001

Gupta, A. D., & Rajpurohit, D. (2011). Antioxidant and Antimicrobial Activity of Nutmeg (Myristica fragrans). In V. R. Preedy, R. R. Watson, & V. B. Patel (Eds.), Nuts & Seeds in Health and Disease Prevention (pp. 831-839). London, UK: Academic Press is an imprint of Elsevier.

Kadhim, M., & Ibrahim, R. K. (2013). Abd-Sahib Antibacterial Activity of Nutmeg (*Myristica fragrans*) Seed Extracts Against Some Pathogenic Bacteria. *Journal of Al-Nahrain University*, *16*(2), 188–192. doi:10.22401/JNUS.16.2.29

Kokate, C. K., Purohit, A. P., & Gokhale, S B. (2010). Text Book of Pharmacognosy. *Nirali prakashan, 46*(1-2), 80.

Krishnamoorthy, B., & Rema, J. (2001). Nutmeg and mace. In K. V. Peter (Ed.), *Hand Book of Herbs and Spices* (pp. 239–248). Cambridge, UK: Woodhead Publishing Limited.

Latha, P. G., Sindhu, P. G., Suja, S. R., Geetha, B. S., Pushpangadan, P., & Rajasekharan, S. (2005). Pharmacology and chemistry of *Myristica fragrans* Houtt. a review. *Journal of Spices and Aromatic Crops*, *14*, 94–101.

Lee, J. Y., & Park, W. (2011). Anti-inflammatory effect of myristicin on RAW 264.7 macrophages stimulated with polyinosinic-polycytidylic acid. *Molecules (Basel, Switzerland)*, *16*(8), 7132–7142. doi:10.3390/molecules16087132 PMID:21991618

Min, B. S., Cuong, T. D., Hung, T. M., Min, B. K., Shin, B. S., & Woo, M. H. (2011). Inhibitory Effect of Lignans from *Myristica fragrans* on LPS-induced NO Production in RAW264.7 Cells. *Bulletin of the Korean Chemical Society*, *32*(11), 4059–4062. doi:10.5012/bkcs.2011.32.11.4059

Morita, T., Jinno, K., Kawagishi, H., Arimoto, Y., Suganuma, H., Inakuma, T., & Sugiyama, K. (2003, March). Hepatoprotective effect of myristicin from nutmeg (Myristica fragrans) on lipopolysaccharide/d-galactosamine-induced liver injury. *Journal of Agricultural and Food Chemistry*, *51*(6), 1560–1565. doi:10.1021/jf020946n PMID:12617584

Naikodi, M. A. R., Waheed, M. A., Shareef, M. A., Ahmad, M., & Nagaiah, K. (2011). Standardization of the Unani drug, *Myristica fragrans* Houtt. (Javetri) with modern analytical techniques. *Pharmaceutical Methods*, *2*(2), 76–82. doi:10.4103/2229-4708.84438 PMID:23781434

Nguyen, P. H., Le, T. V., Kang, H. W., Chae, J., Kim, S. K., Kwon, K. I., ... Oh, W. K. (2010). AMP-activated protein kinase (AMPK) activators from *Myristica fragrans* (nutmeg) and their anti-obesity effect. *Bioorganic & Medicinal Chemistry Letters*, *20*(14), 4128–4131. doi:10.1016/j.bmcl.2010.05.067 PMID:20541406

Olajide, O. A., Makinde, J. M., & Awe, S. O. (2000). Evaluation of the pharmacological properties of nutmeg oil in rats and mice. *Pharmaceutical Biology*, *38*(5), 385–390. doi:10.1076/phbi.38.5.385.5976

Pal, M., Srivastava, M., Soni, D. K., Kumar, A., & Tewari, S. K. (2011). Composition and anti-microbial activity of essential oil of *Myristica fragrans* from Andaman Nicobar Island. *International Journal of Pharmacy and Life Sciences*, *2*, 1115–1117.

Piaru, S. P., Mahmud, R., Abdul Majid, A. M., Ismail, S., & Man, C. N. (2012). Chemical composition, antioxidant and cytotoxicity activities of the essential oils of *Myristica fragrans* and *Morinda citrifolia. Journal of the Science of Food and Agriculture*, *92*(3), 593–597. doi:10.1002/jsfa.4613 PMID:25520982

Qiu, Q., Zhang, G., Sun, X., & Liu, X. (2004). Study on chemical constituents of the essential oil from *Myristica fragrans* Houtt. by supercritical fluid extraction and steam distillation. *Zhong Yao Cai*, *27*, 823–826. PMID:15810588

Ram, A., Lauria, P., Gupta, R., & Sharma, V. N. (1996). Hypolipidaemic effect of *Myristica fragrans* fruit extract in rabbits. *Journal of Ethnopharmacology*, *55*(1), 49–53. doi:10.1016/S0378-8741(96)01473-0 PMID:9121167

Saxena, R., & Patil, P. (2012). Phytochemical Studies on Myristica fragrance Essential Oil, Biological Forum –. *International Journal (Toronto, Ont.)*, *4*, 62–64.

Sharma, A., Mathur, R., & Dixit, V. P. (1995). Prevention of hypercholesterolemia and atherosclerosis in rabbits after supplementation of *Myristica fragrans* seed extract. *Indian Journal of Physiology and Pharmacology*, *39*, 407–410. PMID:8582756

Singh, R. H., Sankat, C. K., & Mujaffar. (2003). *The nutmeg and spice industry in grenada: innovations and competitiveness- A Case Study*. Workshop on the Role of Science, Technology and Innovation in Increasing Competitiveness in the Productive Sector, Organized by The Office of Science and Technology (OS&T) of the Organization of American States (OAS) and the Secretariat of Science, Technology and Productive Innovation (SeCYT).

Somani, R. S., & Singhai, A. K. (2008). Hypoglycemic and antidiabetic activities of seeds of Myristica fragrans in normoglycemic and alloxan-induced diabetic rats. *Asian Journal of Experimental Sciences*, *22*, 95–102.

Stein, U., Greyer, H., & Hentschel, H. (2001). Nutmeg (myristicin) poisoning— Report on a fatal case and a series of cases recorded by a poison information centre. *Forensic Science International*, *118*(1), 87–90. doi:10.1016/S0379-0738(00)00369-8 PMID:11343860

Wahab, A., Ul Haq, R., Ahmed, A., Khan, R. A., & Raza, M. (2009). Anticonvulsant activities of nutmeg oil of *Myristica fragrans*. *Phytotherapy Research*, *23*(2), 153–158. doi:10.1002/ptr.2548 PMID:19067329

WHO. (2001). *The World health report: Mental health: new understanding*. Geneva: New Hope.

Yang, X. W., Huang, X., & Ahmat, M. (2008). New neolignan from the seed of *Myristica fragrans. Zhongguo Zhongyao Zazhi*, *33*, 397–402. PMID:18533495

Chapter 5
Traditional Uses, Phytochemistry, and Pharmacological Properties of *Zingiber officinale* Essential Oil and Extracts

Kaliyaperumal Ashokkumar
Cardamom Research Station, Kerala Agricultural University, India

Thiravidamani Sathyan
Cardamom Research Station, Kerala Agricultural University, India

Muthusamy Murugan
Cardamom Research Station, Kerala Agricultural University, India

Surya Raj
Cardamom Research Station, Kerala Agricultural University, India

M. K. Dhanya
Cardamom Research Station, Kerala Agricultural University, India

Nimisha Mathews
Cardamom Research Station, Kerala Agricultural University, India

ABSTRACT

Ginger (Zingiber officinale) has been traditionally employed in south East Asia as well as India and China for treatment of nausea, asthma, fever, vomiting, cough, constipation, pain, arthritis, inflammation, etc. This chapter discusses the phytochemical composition and pharmacological studies of ginger extracts, ginger essential oil (GEO), and active bioactive constituents. The essential oil of fresh and dry ginger was ranged between 0.2% - 2.62% and 0.72% - 4.17% respectively. The bioactive constituent zingiberene, β-sesquiphellandrene, curcumene, β-bisabolene, β-farnesene, camphene, and gingerol and shogal are the major constituents in ginger extracts. These compounds are chief bioactive substances responsible for pharmacological activities such antioxidant, antidiabetic, anticancer, anticoagulant, antiradiation, anti-inflammatory, gastrointestinal, antimicrobial, cardiovascular, anti-obesity, and weight loss effects. Future research needs to investigate the suitable duration, maximum dosage of ginger, concerns of over-dosage, and its side effects in animal models and humans.

DOI: 10.4018/978-1-7998-2524-1.ch005

INTRODUCTION

Ginger (*Zingiber officinale* Roscoe) belongs to the family Zingiberaceae and it was used in traditional medicine to treat illness almost 5000 years ago (Bode and Dong, 2004). The word ginger originated from the English word *gingivere*, while in Tamil it is known as *Ingii*, in Hindi, *adarakah*, in Chinese, *jiang* and in Arabic, *zanjabli*. Ginger is widely grown in the tropics with foremost exporting countries such as India, Nigeria, Australia, China and Jamaica. In India, ginger is cultivated in the states of Kerala, Karnataka, Orissa, Arunachal Pradesh, West Bengal, Sikkim and Madhya Pradesh. Kerala is the largest ginger producing state, which accounts for 30-40% of total production in India. Indian ginger has two popular varieties in the global market, namely Cochin Ginger and Calicut Ginger (Kubra and Rao, 2012). Dry ginger is mostly used for export purposes and fresh ginger as a vegetable.

The ginger rhizomes have a potent aroma and are extensively used as a spice and as medicine. Ginger and its extract are extensively used in beverage, food, and confectionery industries for manufacturing products such as ginger beer, ginger wine, pickles, Jam and biscuits (Wohlmuth et al., 2005). Ginger essential oil(GEO) and oleoresins are also used in several food products, especially in soft beverages and likewise various sorts of pharmaceutical formulations. It has various potential pharmacological effects in modern medicine such as anti-inflammatory, antifungal, and anticancer activities (Khan et al., 2010). In traditional medicine, ginger has been used for curing several diseases which includes cough, cold, asthma, nausea, travel sickness, morning sickness arthritis and gastrointestinal complaints (Grontved et al., 1988; Bone et al., 1990; But and Sultan, 2011; Khaki and Fathiazad, 2012).

The world health organization (WHO) has projected that nearly 80% of the global population depended on plant-based preparations as medicines to cure their health problems (WHO, 1991).

Plant-based food products are storehouses of various bioactive components like phenolics, flavonoids, carotenoids (Ashokkumar et al., 2013; Muthukrishnan et al., 2014; Ashokkumar et al., 2014; Ashokkumar et al., 2015; Ashokkumar & Shunmugam, 2016; Ashokkumar et al., 2018a; Ashokkumar et al., 2008b), folates (Jha et al., 2015; Ashokkumar et al., 2018c), terpenes (Ashokkumar et al., 2019b). These constituents have been evaluated for their potential biological effects. However, the dried ginger rhizomes contain 5 - 8% of oleoresin, and 1.5 - 3% essential oil depends upon the variety, country of origin, and quality (Zarate and Yeoman, 1996; Kayaardi et al., 2005). Also, the ginger rhizome possess significant concentration of essential nutrients, minerals and bioactive compounds such as flavonoids, terpenoids, carotenoids, essential oils, gingerols, zingiberene,zingerone, shogaolsand paradols(But and Sultan, 2011; Baliga et al., 2011; Ashokkumat et al., 2019). The pungency of ginger rhizome is mainly due to the presences of gingerols and shogaol, are key bioactive constituents of fresh ginger and it has various pharmacological effects including anticancer activity (Wohlmuth et al., 2005).However, zingiberene (10.5-16.6%), e-citrol (7.4 - 12.0%), ar-curcumene (2.9-9.8%),β-farnesene (5.1 - 8.4%), camphene (4.9 - 7.6%), β-sesquiphellandrene(5.8 - 7.2%) and citrol (5.3 - 7%) arethe major essential oil compoundsin dry ginger (Raina et al.,2005). The concentration of these compounds differs significantly depending upon the storage, country of origin, maturity stage of rhizome and preparation of ginger extract/product. The aim of this chapter is to highlight the key phytochemicals and pharmacological applications of ginger extracts and ginger essential oil (GEO) on human health.

BOTANICAL DESCRIPTION OF GINGER

Ginger (*Zingiber officinale* Roscoe), belongs to the Zingiberaceae family. The basic chromosome number x=11 and somatic chromosome number is 2n=22, it is sterile diploid in nature. The botanical classification of ginger has been shown in Table 1. Ginger is a perennial, herbaceous, rhizomatous plant and has an erect stem, grown up to 1 meter in height. It has a fibrous root and aerial shoots. Leaves are simple, alternate, linear-lanceolate, and sheathing at the base. Shoots are originated from multiple bases and wrap around one another. Moreover, the leaf type of ginger is narrowed lanceolate to linear-lanceolate, and leaves die each year (Toader, 2014). The inflorescence is spiked; irregular and bisexual flowers are densely arranged and subtended by a persistent bract. Flowers have three yellowish-orange petals with a lip-like structure (Ravindran et al., 2005). Calyx is tubular 3 lobed, bilabiate corolla; 3 stamens in one whorl; tricarpel ovary,syncarpous; inferior; axile placentation; filiform style, subglobose type stigma. The rhizome is brown, thick lobed, branched with scaly structures. The morphological differences between the fresh and dried rhizome of ginger were shown in Figure 1.

Table 1. Botanical classification of ginger

Kingdom		**Plantae**
Sub-kingdom	:	Tracheobionta – Vascular plants
Division	:	Angiosperms (Seeded plants)
Class	:	Monocotyledons
Sub class	:	Zingiberidae
Order	:	Zingiberales
Family	:	Zingiberaceae (Ginger family)
Genus	:	*Zingiber*
Species	:	*officinale*

Figure 1. The fresh and dried rhizomes of ginger (Zingiber officinale Roscoe)

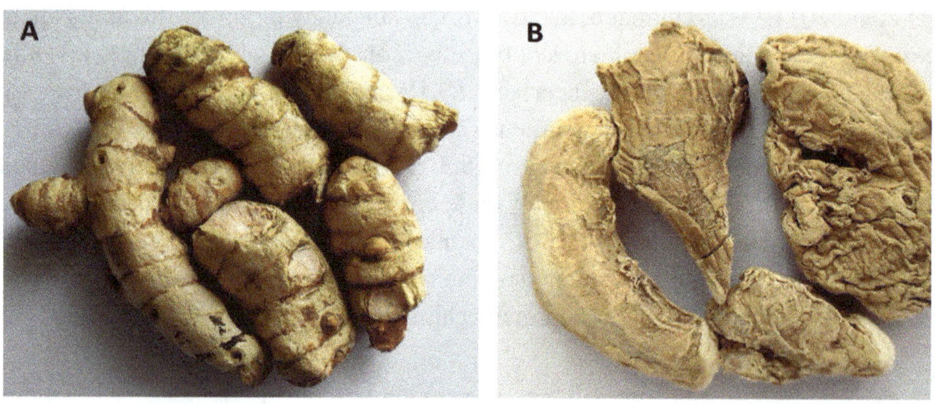

Traditional Uses of Ginger

In India, the ginger rhizome has been used for folk medicine from the Vedic period (Vasala, 2004). Ginger is an essential part of the preparation of various medicinal formulations in Ayurveda medicine. The rhizome of ginger and its extracts plays a key role in Ayurvedic, Chinese, African and Arabic folk medicines to cure headaches, cough, colds, flu, nausea, rheumatism, arthritis, muscular discomfort and inflammation (Baliga et al., 2011; Dehghani et al., 2011; Khaki and Fathiazad, 2012; Semwal et al., 2015). Several traditional medicines reported that ginger is a potential agent for antiinflammatory, carminative, antispasmodic, diaphoretic, appetite and peripheral circulatory stimulant (Vasala, 2004; Ali et al., 2008).

In Burma, peoples used to cure the flu by consumption of a mixture of ginger and palm tree juice. Ginger beer has been used to settle stomach upsets. However, in Colombia, ginger mixed with hot panela was used for the treatment of colds and flu (Semwal et al., 2015). In China, powdered ginger with scrambled eggs is taken as a home remedy to relieve a cough. Mango juice added with ginger is considered a panacea (medicine to cure all) in Congo. External application of ginger paste to cure headaches and oral administration to reduce colds in India and Nepal (Khaki and Fathiazad, 2012). Ginger is believed to reduce fatigue and increase digestion in Indonesia. Philippians had taken ginger to sooth asore throat, while the Japanese used ginger to improve blood circulation. In India, the southern states of Tamil Nadu and Kerala crushed ginger rhizomes and boiled it with tea and water to impart a pleasant aroma to tea, which is locally called "*Ingi tea*(ginger tea)" and which has been used to relieve tiredness and depression. The powdered ginger rhizome mixed with pulverized cloves, cardamom and caraway has been used for digestive ailments (Ashokkumar et al., 2020).

CHEMICAL COMPOSITION

Proximate and Mineral Composition

The proximate composition of fresh and dry ginger rhizome was summarized in Table 2. It includes moisture, ash, crude protein, crude fat, crude fiber, vitamin C, ascorbic acid and carbohydrates. The crude protein content of fresh and dried ginger rhizome was ranged between 3.1 - 12.3% and 7.9 - 34.1%, respectively (Agu et al., 2016;Sultan et al., 2005;Shahid and Hussain, 2012; Latona et al., 2012). Fresh ginger has significant level of crude fat and fibre with 2.1-11.7% and 1.4 -15% correspondingly (Ajayi et al., 2013;Sultan et al., 2005;Onimawo et al., 2019). Dry ginger has 1.04 -3.75%, in vitamin-C and 68.2 - 72.8% (Latona et al., 2012; Shahid and Hussain, 2012).

The serving of 100g dried ginger rhizome contains substantial levels of calcium (34.5- 280 mg), phosphorus (26.7 mg), Sodium (39 mg), manganese (18.9 mg) and other micronutrients with traces amount (Latona et al., 2012; Ogbuewu et al., 2014; Adel and Prakash, 2010; Onimawo et al., 2019), (Table 2). These are essential mineral elements for normal day-to-day physiological activities of humans. Ashokkumar et al. (2019) reported nutritionally important metabolites including flavonoids (catechin and myricetin,) and carotenoids (lutein and β-carotene) in rhizomes of fresh ginger (Table 2).

Table 2. Proximate, mineral and metabolite content of fresh and dry rhizome of ginger

	Fresh	Dry	Reference
Proximate composition (%)			
Moisture	70.1 - 89	6.4 - 13.7	Aguet al. (2016); Sultan et al. (2005); Otunola et al. (2010); Latona et al. (2012)
Ash	0.81 - 2.54	1.74 - 7.64	Onimawo et al. (2019); Odebunmi et al. (2010); Shahid and Hussain (2012); Latona et al. (2012)
Crude protein	3.1 – 12.3	8.6 – 34.1	Aguet al. (2016); Sultan et al. (2005); Shammari (2018);Latona et al. (2012)
Crude fat	2.1 – 11.7	4 – 6.4	Ajayi et al. (2013); Onimawo et al. (2019); Latona et al. (2012); Shammari (2018)
Crude fibre	1.4 - 15	0.9 - 3.2	Onimawo et al. (2019); Sultan et al. (2005);Otunola et al. (2010)
Vitamin- C	-	1 – 3.8	Latona et al. (2012); Shahid and Hussain (2012)
Carbohydrates	2 – 16.7	68.2 – 72.8	Onimawo et al. (2019); Ajayi et al. (2013); Otunola et al. (2010); Shammari (2018)
Minerals (mg/100g)			
Calcium	88.4 -182.7	34.5 - 280	Latona et al. (2012); Ogbuewu et al. (2014); Adel and Prakash (2010); Onimawo et al. (2019)
Phosphorus	174	26.7	Adel and Prakash (2010);Ogbuewu et al. (2014)
Sodium	7.3	39	Onimawo et al. (2019); Ogbuewu et al. (2014)
Iron	8 – 9.7	1.59	Adel and Prakash (2010); Onimawo et al. (2019); Ogbuewu et al. (2014)
Copper	0.55	0.86	Ogbuewu et al. (2014); Adel and Prakash (2010)
Manganese	9.1	18.9	Ogbuewu et al. (2014); Adel and Prakash (2010)
Zinc	5	4.2	Ogbuewu et al. (2014); Adel and Prakash (2010)
Metabolites (µg/g)			
Flavonoids			
Catechin	757.9	-	Ashokkumar et al. (2019)
Myricetin	35.5	-	Ashokkumar et al. (2019)
Total flavonoids	793.4	-	Ashokkumar et al. (2019)
Carotenoids			
Lutein	0.2	-	Ashokkumar et al. (2019)
β-carotene	0.5	-	Ashokkumar et al. (2019)
Total carotenoids	0.7	-	Ashokkumar et al. (2019)

Ginger Essential Oil (GEO) and its Composition

The yield of GEO varied from 0.2% - 2.62% and 0.72% - 4.17% on a wet and dry basis, respectively, depending on the variety and extraction methods summarized in Table 3. Recent studies claim that the yield of dry ginger essential oil (GEO) was greater when using a hydro-distillation method (1.10% - 4.17%) compared to steam distillation (2.1%) and Ionic liquid based microwave assisted extraction (0.72%) methods (Pinoet al. 2004; Kiran et al., 2013; Stoyanova et al., 2006; Stoyanova, et al., 2006;

Guo et al., 2017). Among the hydro-distillation extraction, dry ginger yielded higher oil content than fresh ginger (Table 3).

Table 3. Yield of essential oil from ginger rhizomes by various extraction methods

Technique or method	Rhizome	Oil yield (%)	References
Ionic liquid-based microwave assisted extraction	Dry	0.72	Guo et al. (2017)
Steam distillation	Dry	2.1	Stoyanova et al. (2006)
Super critical fluid extraction	Fresh	0.24 - 2.62	Mesomoet al (2013)
Hydro-distillation	Dry	1.10- 4.17	Raina et al. (2005); Pino et al (2004); Kiran et al. (2013); Stoyanova et al. (2006)
Hydro-distillation	Fresh	0.20- 1.79	Gurib-Fakim et al. (2002); Mesomo et al. (2013); Héritier et al. (2018)

Figure 2. Molecular structures of major bioactive molecules isolated from ginger essential oil and extracts

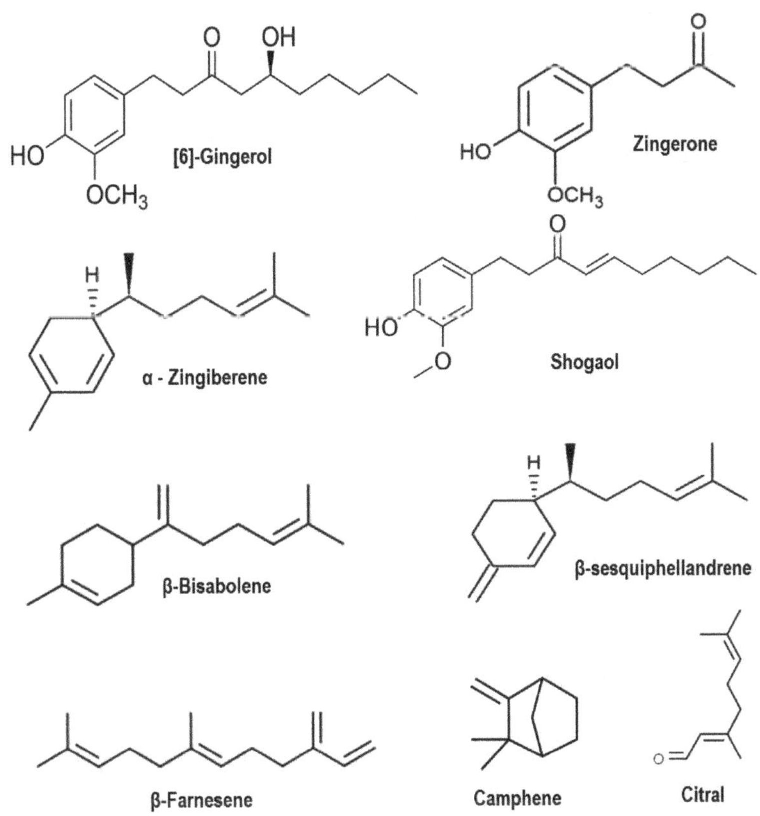

Table 4. Major essential oil constituents of ginger from various origins

Origin	Rhizome	Constituents	Yield (%)	Authors
Nigeria	Dry	Zingiberene	29.54	Onyenekwe & Hashimoto (1999)
		β-Sesquiphellandrene	18.42	
		Farnesene	6.46	
China	Fresh	Zingiberene	22.76	An et al. (2016)
		β-phellandrene	12.40	
		Geranial	14.50	
		b-Sesquiphellandrene	7.01	
		β-Bisabolene	3.25	
Mauritius	Fresh	Geranial	16.3	Gurib-Fakim et al. (2002)
		Neral	10.3	
		Zingiberene	9.5	
		p-sesquiphellandrene	6.3	
		ar-Curcumene	5.1	
India, North East	Dry	Zingiberene	20.98	Kiran et al. (2013)
		Geranial	12.36	
		Camphene	8.49	
		β-sesquiphellandrene	7.96	
		Neral	4.95	
India	Fresh	Zingiberene	46.71	Sharma et al. (2016)
		Citronellyl n-butyrate	19.34	
		Valencene	7.61	
		β-phellandrene	3.70	
Cuba	Dry	ar-Curcumene	22.1	Pino et al. (2004)
		Cadina-1,4-diene	12.5	
		Zingiberene	11.7	
		β-bisabolene	11.2	
India, North	Semi dry	Zingiberene	10.5-16.6	Raina et al. (2005)
		e-Citral	7.4- 12.0	
		ar-Curcumene	2.9-9.8	
		β-Farnesene	5.1 - 8.4	
		Camphene	4.9- 7.6	
		β-Sesquiphellandrene	5.8 - 7.2	
		z-Citral	5.3- 7.0	
Vietnam	Dry	ar-Curcumene	12.6	Stoyanova et al. (2006)
		α-Zingiberene	10.3	
		β-Bisabolene	8.1	
		β-Sesquiphellandrene	7.4	

The chemical composition of major ginger essential oils across the countries and regions is presented in Table 4. The EO of fresh ginger from India predominantly exhibited zingiberene (46.71%), citronellyl n-butyrate (19.34%), valencene (7.61%) and β-phellandrene (3.70%), (Sharma et al., 2016). Kiran et al. (2013) indicated that rhizomes of dry ginger collected from across the ginger growing region of north east India chiefly contain zingiberene, geranial, camphene, β-sesquiphellandrene and neral with percentages of 20.98, 12.36, 8.49, 7.96, and 4.95, respectively (Table 4). Profiling of EO of fresh ginger rhizomes from China showed zingiberene (22.76%), β-phellandrene (12.40%), geranial (14.50%) and sesquiphellandrene (7%) as principal compounds (An et al., 2016). The molecular structure of major bioactive constituents isolated from gingeressential oil and extracts is shown in Figure 2. The yield of minor constituents of GEO from fresh ginger includes, 1,8-cineole (5.08%), camphor (0.16%), δ-3-carene (0.03%), citronelly lacetate (0.58%), copanene (0.21%), α-elemene (0.12%), β-elemene (0.30%), 2-farnesene (0.13%), myrcene (1.75%), sabinene (0.17%), terpinolene (0.29%)and 2-undecanone (0.40%),(Qin and Xu, 2008).

Biological Activities

The GEO and ginger extracts have various biological effects including antioxidant, antibacterial, anti-cancer insecticidal and other miscellaneous activities that are summarized in Table 5. The schematic representation of biological activities of ginger rhizome extract, GEO and active constitutes were presented in Figure 3.

Figure 3. Schema depiction of biological activities of ginger rhizome extract, essential oil, gingerol and Shogaol

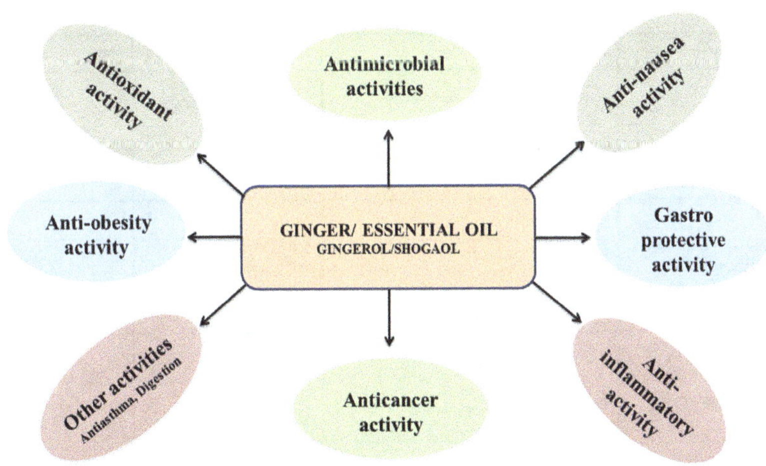

Antioxidant Activity

Oxidative stress is one of the major health problems in humans, for which several therapies are utilized and where medicinal plants offer a favorable alternative. The rhizome of ginger possesses a rich source of antioxidants that are used to scavenge free radicals and associated health problems. Gingerols is the major bioactive metabolite, which has potent antioxidant activity determined by various antioxidant

Table 5. Biological activities of ginger rhizome extract, essential oil and bioactive compounds

Pharmacological activities	Studyextract/ GEO	In vitro/ In vivo	Target/ Model	IC 50/ Dosage	Control	Reference
Antimicrobial activity	GEO	*In vitro*	*Bacillus subtilis*	MIC:10.0µl/ml	Positive: Tetracycline Negative: DMSO	Sharma et al. (2016); Sasidharan, & Menon (2010)
Antimicrobial activity	GEO	*In vitro*	*Staphylococcus aureus*	MIC: 8.7 mg/ml	-	Bellik, (2014)
Antimicrobial activity	Aqueous extract	*In vitro*	*Helicobacter pylori*	MIC: 300µg/ml	Positive: Lansoprazole	Nanjundaiah et al. (2011)
Antimicrobial activity	Ethanol extract	*In vitro*	*E. col*	MIC: 75.6 µg/ml	Positive: Ciprofloxacin	Karuppiah, and Rajaram (2012)
	Ethanol extract	*In vitro*	*Klebsiella* sp.*Enterobacter* sp.	MIC: 185.6µg/ml	Positive: Ciprofloxacin	
	Ethanol extract	*In vitro*	*S. aureus* *Bacillus sp.* *Proteus sp.*	MIC: 68.4 µg/ml MIC: 74.5 µg/ml MIC: 70.2µg/ml	Positive: Ciprofloxacin	
Antimicrobial activity	Oleoresin	*In vitro*	*S. aureus*	MIC: 50 mg/ml	-	Bellik, (2014)
Antimicrobial activity	GEO	*In vitro*	*Vibrio vulnificus* *V. parahaemolyticus* *Pseudomonas aeruginosa &* *Yersinia enterocolitica*	MIC: 31.2 µl/ml MBC:31.3µl/ml MIC: 31.3µl/ml MBC:125 µl/ml MIC: 31.3 µl/ml MBC: 62.5 µl/ml	Positive: Ampicillin Negative: DMSO	Debbarma et al. (2013)
	GEO	*In vitro*	*Salmonella typhimurium* *S. paratyphi* *E. coli*	MIC: 62.5µl/ml	Positive: Ampicillin Negative: DMSO	
Antimicrobial activity	GEO	*In vitro*	*Candida albicans*	MIC:10.0µl/ml	Positive: Fluconazole Negative: DMSO	Sharma et al. (2016)
Antimicrobial activity	Ethanol	*In vitro*	*C. albicans*	MIC: 6.3 mg/ml MBC: 25 mg/ml	Negative: Sterile water	Lucky et al. (2017)
	Aqueous extract	*In vitro*	*C. albicans*	MIC: 6.3 mg/ml MBC: 25 mg/ml	Negative: Sterile water	Lucky et al. (2017)
Antimicrobial activity	Oleoresin	*In vitro*	*Penicilliumspp.*	MIC: 2mg/ml	-	Bellik (2014)
Antimicrobial activity	GEO	*In vitro*	*Fusarium verticillioides*	MIC: 2500µl/ml	-	Yamamoto-Ribeiro et al. (2013)
Antimicrobial activity	GEO	*In vitro*	*Botrytis cinerea* *Alternaria panax* *F. oxysporum*	MIC: 0.3%	-	Hussein, & Joo (2018)
Antimicrobial activity	Methanol extract	*In vitro*	*E. coli* *S. aureus* *E. faecalis* *C. albicans* *M. smegmatis* *S. mutans*	MIC:125 mg/ml MIC:62.5mg/ml MIC: 250 mg/ml	-	Agrawal et al. (2018)
	Chloroform extract	*In vitro*	*E. faecalis* *S. mutans* *C. albicans* *M. smegmatis* *E. coli* *S. aureus*	MIC:125 mg/ml MIC: 62.5mg/ml MIC: 250 mg/ml	-	
	Ethyl acetate extract	*In vitro*	*S. aureus* *S. mutans* *E. faecalis* *C. albicans* *E. coli* *M. smegmatis*	MIC:125 mg/ml MIC: 250 mg/ml MIC: 62.5 mg/ml	-	
	Petroleum ether extract	*In vitro*	*S. aureus* *C. albicans* *S. mutans* *E. coli* *E. faecalis*	MIC:250 mg/ml MIC:125 mg/ml	-	

continued on following page

Table 5. Continued

Pharmacological activities	Studyextract/ GEO	In vitro/ In vivo	Target/ Model	IC 50/ Dosage	Control	Reference
Antimicrobial activity	Aqueous extract	*In vitro*	*K. pneumoniae* *Proteus vulgaris* *P. mirabilis* *B. subtilis* *C. albicans* *E. coli*	MIC:156.3 µg/ml MIC:39.1 µg/ml	Positive: Amracin (for bacteria) Nystatin (for yeast)	Švarc-Gajić et al. (2017)
	Subcritical extract	*In vitro*	*K. pneumoniae* *Proteus vulgaris* *P. mirabilis* *B. subtilis* *C. albicans* *E. coli*	MIC:78.1 µg/ml MIC:19.5 µg/ml	Positive: Amracin (for bacteria) Nystatin (for yeast)	Švarc-Gajić et al. (2017)
Antimicrobial activity	Methanol extract	*In vitro*	*B. subtilis* *K. pneumoniae* *P. mirabilis* *S. aureus* *P. aeruginosa* *E. coli*	MIC: 8.17µg/ml MBC:30.0 µg/ml MIC: 16.4µg/ml MBC:61.8µg/ml MIC: 20.5 µg/ml MBC:74.3µg/ml MIC: 18.2µg/ml MBC:64.5µg/ml MIC: 16.3µg/ml MBC:44.9µg/ml MIC: 26.3µg/ml MBC:86.5µg/ml	-	Chakraborty et al. (2014)
Antimicrobial activity	Ethanol extract	*In vitro*	*B. subtilis* *K. pneumoniae* *P. mirabilis* *S. aureus* *P. aeruginosa* *E. coli*	MIC: 10.6µg/ml MBC:36.8µg/ml MIC: 17.6µg/ml MBC:66.4µg/ml MIC: 23.5µg/ml MBC:83.2µg/ml MIC: 20.3µg/ml MBC:67.5µg/ml MIC: 18.9µg/ml MBC:52.8µg/ml MIC: 34.0µg/ml MBC:84.3µg/ml	-	Chakraborty et al. (2014)
	Acetone extract	*In vitro*	*B. subtilis* *K. pneumoniae* *P. mirabilis* *S. aureus* *P. aeruginosa* *E. coli*	MIC: 10.5µg/ml MBC:40.8µg/ml MIC: 21.5µg/ml MBC:77.8µg/ml MIC: 27.9µg/ml MBC:94.2µg/ml MIC: 28.2µg/ml MBC:75.9µg/ml MIC: 11.5µg/ml MBC:40.2µg/ml MIC: 13.3µg/ml MBC:50.5µg/ml	-	Chakraborty et al. (2014)
	Aqueous extract	*In vitro*	*B. subtilis* *K. pneumoniae* *P. mirabilis* *S. aureus* *P. aeruginosa* *E. coli*	MIC: 11.5µg/ml MBC:45.6µg/ml MIC: 15.8µg/ml MBC:42.7µg/ml MIC: 19.3µg/ml MBC:65.7µg/ml MIC: 13.1µg/ml MBC:45.7µg/ml MIC: 21.3µg/ml MBC:55.9µg/ml MIC: 20.2µg/ml MBC:78.2µg/ml	-	Chakraborty et al. (2014)
Antimicrobial activity	Ethanol extract	*In vitro*	*P. aeruginosa* *B. subtilis*	MIC:12.5 mg/ml MBC: 50mg/ml MIC: 6.3 mg/ml MBC: 25 mg/ml	Negative: Sterile water	Lucky et al. (2017)
Antifungal activity	GEO	*In vitro*	*Fusarium verticillioides*	MIC: 5000mg/ml	-	Yamamoto-Ribeiro et al. (2013)
Antifungal activity	GEO	*In vitro*	*Aspergillus niger* *M. hemalis* *F. oxysporum*	MIC: 70µg/ml MIC: 75µg/ml	-	El-Baroty et al. (2010)

continued on following page

Table 5. Continued

Pharmacological activities	Studyextract/ GEO	In vitro/ In vivo	Target/ Model	IC 50/ Dosage	Control	Reference
Antifungal activity	GEO	*In vitro*	*Aspergillus flavus Penicillium expansum*	MIC: 500μg/ml	-	Sharma et al. (2013)
Antioxidant activity	Aqueous extract	*In vitro*	*Rats*	IC_{50}: 6.8 μg/ml	-	Nanjundaiah et al. (2011)
Gastro protective activity	Aqueous extract	*In vivo*	*Ulcer induced rats by ethanol/ swim stress*	200 mg/kg body weight	Positive: Lansoprazole	Nanjundaiah et al. (2011)
Gastro protective activity	Zingerone	*In vivo*	*Ethanol-induced gastric ulcers in rats*	200 mg/kg body weight	Positive: Ranitidine	Karampour et al. (2019)
Antidiabetic activity	Aqueous Extract	*In vivo*	Streptozotocin (STZ)-induced type I diabetic rats	4 ml/ kg, p.o. daily for 6 weeks	Negative: Sterile water	Akhani et al. (2004)
Antidiabetic activity	Ethanolic Extract	*In vivo*	STZ-induced diabetic rats	200 mg/kg p.o daily for 20 days	Positive: Gliclazide	Bhandari et al. (2005)
Cytotoxic activity	Subcritical water extracts	*In vitro*	Hep2c cells RD cells L2OBcells	IC_{50}: 9.82 μg/ml IC_{50}: 13.81 μg/ml IC_{50}: 6.88 μg/ml	-	Švarc-Gajić et al. (2017)
Cardioprotective activity	Ethanol extract	*In vivo*	Wistar rats	400 mg/kg body weight	-	Amran et al. (2015)
Antiproliferative activity	Aqueous extract	*In vitro*	A549 cells HeLa cells	IC_{50}: 239.4μg/ml IC_{50}: 253.4μg/ml	Control: Untreated	Choudhury et al. (2010)
Insecticidal activity	GEO	*In vivo*	*Culex theileri*	1 ml	-	Madreseh-Ghahfarokhi et al. (2018)

Note: GEO, Ginger essential oil, MIC, Minimum inhibition concentration; MBC, Minimum bactericide concentration; $LC_{50,}$ Lethalconcentration; IC_{50}, Inhibitory concentration

studies (Kikusaki and Nakatani, 1993; Dugasani et al., 2010). Increasing antioxidant activity of the human body will undoubtedly protect against the oxidative stress (Shukla and Singh, 2007). Bellik, (2014) reported that ginger oleoresin has greater antioxidant activity (IC_{50} =1.82mg/ml) compared to essential oil (IC50 =110.14 mg/ml). The bioactive molecule [6]-Gingerol is the major pungent constituent that has considerable antioxidant activity. [6]-Gingerol have greater scavenging activity compared to ethanol extract of ginger against 1,1-diphenyl-2-picrylhydrazyl and 2,2-diphenyl-1-picrylhydrazyl (DPPH) radical at lower concentrations (<100 μg/ml). However, both the ginger extract and [6]-gingerol displayed same antioxidant potential at higher doses (100–1000 μg/ml) (Harliyansyah et al. 2007). Ginger extracts also protect the DNA from lipopolysaccharide-induced oxidation damage in rats (Tchombé et al., 2012). Ginger oil can act as a scavenger of oxygen radical and could be used as antioxidant (Yadav et al., 2016). The alcoholic extracts of ginger have shown effective antioxidant effects and can prevent lipid peroxidation (Shobana and Naidu, 2000).

Antimicrobial and Antifungal Activity

Ginger extracts have significant antimicrobial activity against *Bacillus subtilis, Escherichia coli,Staphylococcus aureus, Salmonella typhimurium, Bacillus cereus, Candida albicans*and*B. subtilis* (Thongson et al., 2005; Natta et al., 2008; Singh et al. 2008; Bellik, 2014) and antifungal activity against *Fusarium*sp., *Pseudomonas aeruginosa* and *Aspergillus Niger* (Sa-Nguanpuag et al., 2011;Auta et al. 2011; Bellik, 2014; Riaz et al., 2015).The active biomolecule [6]-gingerol and [12]-gingerol revealed potential antibacterial effects against gram negative bacteria, *Porphyromonas gingivalis,P. endodontalis* and *Prevotella intermedia.* However, another bioactive molecule, [10]-gingerol showed antibacterial activity against *Mycobacterium avium* and *M. tuberculosis* (Hiserodt et al., 1998). Furthermore, several antimicrobial studies were summarized in Table 5.

Anticancer Activity

Worldwide, researchers are interested in identifying plant derived bioactive constituents that have the capacity to interfere with carcinogenic processes. Several spices and medicinal plants are known to possess an array of pharmacological properties including anticarcinogenic and antimutagenic activities. Tumor induction is strictly linked to oxidative stress, a constituent that exhibits antioxidant properties might be act as antitumorogenic agent. Masuda et al. (2004) isolated more than 50 antioxidants from the rhizomes of ginger. Among them topical application of [6]-gingerol to DMBA initiated skin cancer in SENCAR mice contributed a substantial protection against skin canceras reported by Katiyar et al. (1996). Glioblastoma multiforme (GBM) is the most lethal, destructive and malignant astrocytoma of primary brain tumors in adults. Lee et al., 2008 reported the [6]-Gingerol induced tumor necrosis factor-related apoptosis-inducing ligand (TRAIL) mediated apoptosis of glioblastoma. The previous study reports noticed that the bioactive molecule [6]-gingerol had been induced apoptosis of gastric cancer cells by increasing caspase-3/7 activation (Prasad and Tyagi, 2015). The other bioactive constituent gingerdione has been demonstrated as a potential antitumor agent in human leukemia cells(Hsu et al., 2005).

In another study, the methanolic extract of ginger inhibited the growth of 19 *Helicobacter pylori* (HP) strains with a minimum inhibitory concentration (MIC) range of 6.25-50µg/ml (Mahady et al., 2003). Yusof et al. (2009) demonstrated that oleoresin of ginger has chemopreventive activity against liver cancer in rats. The ginger extract also remarked that suppression of cell cycle progression and prompted the death of human pancreatic cancer cell lines (Akimoto et al. 2015). Tahir et al. (2015) observed that fresh ginger extract contains a high level of gingerols, and it is used to induce cell death of colon cancer cells.

Anti-inflammatory Activity

The anti-inflammatory activity of ginger has been well known for centuries. However, the scientific evidence confirmed it mostly in animal models more than humans, Wei et al. (2005). Anti-inflammatory potential of gingerols was evidenced by the inhibitory effects of prostaglandins and leukotrienes synthesis in Rat Basophilic Leukemia -1 (RBL-1) cells (Kiuchi et al., 1982). The ginger rhizome contains bioactive constituents such as [6]-gingerol and [6]-paradol which has been reported to have durable anti-inflammatory effects and suppress the production of TNF α in TPA- treated female ICR mice (Surh et al., 1999).Ramadan et al. (2011) reported that oral administration of ginger (200 mg/kg) suppressed the incidence and severity of adjuvant-induced arthritis by increasing the production of anti-inflammatories and decreasing pro-inflammatory cytokines in rat.

OTHER ACTIVITIES

Anti-nausea Activity

The consumption of ginger may be a safe and effective option for the treatment of nausea and vomiting in the pregnancy period (Borrelli et al., 2005). Maitre et al. (2011) evaluated four randomized controlled trials (RCTs) on the use of ginger for pregnancy-induced nausea, and vomiting (PINV) which were sourced from MEDLINE, TRIP CINAHL, and the Cochrane library. All the trials noticed that orally administered ginger was significantly more effective for reducing vomiting and nausea. Additionally, in the U.K, the National Institute of Health and Clinical Excellence, has included a list of ginger acceptable therapies to cure nausea and vomiting during early pregnancy.

Anti-respiratory Diseases Activity

Ginger rhizome has been used for centuries in treating respiratory diseases. Gingerols remarkably reduced the eosinophils in the lungs of ovalbumin-sensitized mice and suppressed the allergen-induced Th2 cell-drivenn airway inflammation (Ahui et al., 2008). Ingestion of 6-, 8- gingerols, and 6-shogaol reduced asthma disease at doses ranged between 100 to 300 μM, by prompt relaxation of precontracted airway smooth muscle (Townsend et al., 2013).

Anti-diabetic and Anti-obesity Activity

The oral administration of ethanolic ginger extract significantly decreased fasting blood glucose levels in streptozotocin (STZ) - treated type 1 diabetic rat model (Ojewole, 2006). Okamoto et al. (2011) reported that [6]-gingerol reduce body weight and fat accumulation in mice. In another study, [6]-gingerol inhibits rosiglitazone-induced adipogenesis through suppressing oil droplet accumulation and reduces the oil droplet size in 3T3-L1 cells (Tzeng and Liu, 2013).

Cardio Protective and Lipid-Lowering Activity

Cardiovascular activity of ginger reported that ginger extract has an antioxidative potent, and it can scavenge the superoxide anion and hydroxyl radicals (Fuhrman et al., 2000). *In vitro* and *in vivo*, studies with animal models showed that ginger extract possessed antioxidant activity, and it might be triggering the anti-inflammatory response and protect against cardiovascular disease (Masuda et al., 2004). The ethanol extract of ginger at 400 mg/kg body weight of Wistar rats showed a significant decrease in all the cardiac enzyme activities. (Amran et al., 2015).The aqueous ginger extract also exhibited durable inhibitions against low-density lipoprotein (LDL) and platelet aggregation (Saputri and Jantan, 2011). Ethanolic *Zingiber officinale* extract (200 mg/kg)p.o. for 20 days is substantially lowering the lipids in streptozotocin (STZ) - induced diabetic rats (Bhandari et al., 2005).

Antithrombotic Activity

Earlier studies reported that ginger extract was found to possess antithrombotic activity as a result of inhibiting platelet aggregation and thromboxane-B2(TXB2)*in vitro*. Whereas, effect of *in vivo* experiments, oral administration of high doses of ginger extract in rats substantially reduced the level of TXB2andprostaglandin-E2 (PGE2) production (Srivastava and Mustafa, 1989;Thomson et al., 2002).

CONCLUSION

Nowadays, plant based nutraceutical compounds have increased wider acceptance as chosen alternatives to several synthetic medicines, mainly for cancer and diabetes. Also, people are aware that long term uses of synthetic drugs are connected with various side effects. The rhizome of ginger is well known for its medicinal value and flavor-enhancing agent. Gingerol is the key pungent constituent, it is a major bioactive compound accumulated in the rhizome of fresh ginger. Presently, ginger is mainly used for the prevention of travel sickness and chemoprevention of cancer. Several studies are extensively investigated for discovering the therapeutic potential of ginger extracts, GEO and its bioactive compounds such as α-zingiberene, gingerol and shogaol in humans and animal models.

Various results accounted that ginger has antibacterial, antifungal, anticancer, anti-inflammatory, antidiabetic, insecticidal, and other miscellaneous activities. Future research should focus on the genetic variability of GEO and bioactive constituents from various cultivated varieties as well as the country of origin. GEO contains major active constituents such as zingiberene, geranial, camphene, β-sesquiphellandrene, neral, citrol, farnesene, bisabolene, and ar-curcumene. The presence of these biologically active molecules as major constituents in ginger essential oil can be used in food, aroma, cosmetics and pharmaceutical domains. Additionally, future research needs attention on the influence of environmental factors attributed to ginger and its active compounds.

Further studies on determining the various pharmacological potential of the ginger extracts, GEO, gingerol, shogaol and other active compounds should include human intervention clinical trials to investigate the activity against humans from various diseases. Future research should also focus on the suitable duration, maximum dosage of ginger, concerns of overdosage and its side effects. Furthermore, future investigations also are required to study the genetic diversity of phytochemicals among various ginger germplasm lines grown across the world or country for improving GEO or particular bioactive constituents, which are essential for developing varieties with higher beneficial bioactive constituents.

REFERENCES

Adel, S. P. R., & Prakash, J. (2010). Chemical composition and antioxidant properties of ginger root (Zingiber officinale). *Journal of Medicinal Plants Research*, *4*(24), 2674–2679. doi:10.5897/JMPR09.464

Agrawal, P., Kotagiri, D., & Kolluru, V. C. (2018). Comparative analysis of antimicrobial activity of herbal extracts against pathogenic microbes. *Current Trends in Biomedical Engineering & Biosciences*, *16*, 1–7.

Agu, C. S., Igwe, J. E., Amanze, N. N., & Oduma, O. (2016). Effect of oven drying on proximate composition of ginger. *American Journal of Engineering Research*, *5*(8), 58–61.

Ahui, M. L., Champy, P., Ramadan, A., Pham Van, L., Araujo, L., Brou André, K., ... Herbelin, A. (2008). Ginger prevents Th2-mediated immune responses in a mouse model of airway inflammation. *International Immunopharmacology*, *8*(12), 1626–1632. doi:10.1016/j.intimp.2008.07.009 PubMed

Ajayi, O. B., Akomolafe, S. F., & Akinyemi, F. T. (2013). Food value of two varieties of ginger (Zingiber officinale) commonly consumed in Nigeria. *ISRN Nutrition*. doi:10.5402/2013/359727

Akhani, S. P., Vishwakarma, S. L., & Goyal, R. K. (2004). Anti-diabetic activity of Zingiber officinale in streptozotocin-induced type I diabetic rats. *The Journal of Pharmacy and Pharmacology*, *56*(1), 101–105. doi:10.1211/0022357022403 PubMed

Akimoto, M., Iizuka, M., Kanematsu, R., Yoshida, M., & Takenaga, K. (2015). Anticancer effect of ginger extract against pancreatic cancer cells mainly through reactive oxygen species-mediated autotic cell death. *PLoS One*, *10*(5). doi:10.1371/journal.pone.0126605

Ali, B. H., Blunden, G., Tanira, M. O., & Nemmar, A. (2008). Some phytochemical, pharmacological and toxicological properties of ginger (Zingiber officinale Roscoe): A review of recent research. *Food and Chemical Toxicology*, *46*(2), 409–420. doi:10.1016/j.fct.2007.09.085 PubMed

Amran, A. Z., Jantan, I., Dianita, R., & Buang, F. (2015). Protective effects of the standardized extract of Zingiber officinale on myocardium against isoproterenol-induced biochemical and histopathological alterations in rats. *Pharmaceutical Biology*, *53*(12), 1795–1802. doi:10.3109/13880209.2015.1008147 PubMed

An, K., Zhao, D., Wang, Z., Wua, J., Xu, Y., & Xiao, G. (2016). Comparison of different drying methods on Chinese ginger (Zingiber officinale Roscoe): Changes in volatiles, chemical profile, antioxidant properties, and microstructure. *Food Chemistry*, *197*, 1292–1300. doi:10.1016/j.foodchem.2015.11.033 PubMed

Ashokkumar, K., Arjun, P., Murugan, M., Dhanya, M. K., Sathyan, T., Sivakumar, P., & Surya, R. (2018a). Simple and rapid extraction method for determination of carotenoids in the edible parts of Vitis vinifera, Vaccinum sect. cyanococcus, Ipomoea batatas and Capsicum annum. Advances in Research, 17(4), 1–8. doi:10.9734/AIR/2018/45132

Ashokkumar, K., Diapari, M., Jha, A. B., Tar'an, B., Arganosa, G., & Warkentin, T. D. (2015). Genetic diversity of nutritionally important carotenoids in 94 pea and 121 chickpea accessions. *Journal of Food Composition and Analysis*, *43*, 49–60. doi:10.1016/j.jfca.2015.04.014

Ashokkumar, K., Elayabalan, S., Shobana, V. G., Sivakumar, P., & Pandiyan, M. (2018b). Nutritional value of cultivars of Banana (Musa spp.) and its future prospects. *Journal of Pharmacognosy and Phytochemistry*, *7*(3), 2972–2977.

Ashokkumar, K., Kumarakurubaran, S., & Saradha Devi, S. M. (2013). Reverse phase-high performance liquid chromatography-diode array detector (RP-HPLC-DAD) analysis of flavonoids profile from curry leaf (Murraya koenigii L). *Journal of Medicinal Plants Research*, *7*, 3393–3399. doi:10.5897/JMPR2013.5150

Ashokkumar, K., Murugan, M., Dhanya, M. K., Surya, R., & Kamaraj, D. (2019b). Phytochemical variations among four distinct varieties of Indian cardamom Elettaria cardamomum (L.) Maton. Natural Product Research, 1–4. doi:10.1080/14786419.2018.1561687

Ashokkumar, K., Murugan, M., Dhanya, M. K., & Warkentin, T. D. (2020). Botany, traditional uses, phytochemistry and biological activities of cardamom [Elettaria cardamomum (L.) Maton] - A critical review. *Journal of Ethnopharmacology*, *246*, 112244. doi:10.1016/j.jep.2019.112244 PubMed

Ashokkumar, K., Pandian, A., Murugan, M., Dhanya, M. K., Sathyan, T., Sivakumar, P., . . . Warkentin, T. D. (2019). Profiling bioactive flavonoids and carotenoids in select south Indian spices and nuts. Natural Product Research, 1–5. doi:10.1080/14786419.2018.1557179

Ashokkumar, K., & Shunmugam, A. S. K. (2016). Curry leaf (Muraya koenji L. Spreng): its phytochemistry and pharmacological properties - A review. Medicinal Plants: Phytochemistry. *Pharmacology & Therapeutics*, *4*, 375–390.

Ashokkumar, K., Sivakumar, P., & Saradha Devi, M. (2018). Identification and determination of naturally occurring folates in grains of rice (Oryza sativa L.) by UPLC-MS/MS analysis. *Natural Product Research*, *32*(14), 1733–1737. doi:10.1080/14786419.2017.1392957 PubMed

Ashokkumar, K., Tar'an, B., Diapari, M., Arganosa, G., & Warkentin, T. D. (2014). Effect of cultivar and environment on carotenoid profile of pea and chickpea. *Crop Science*, *54*(5), 2225–2235. doi:10.2135/cropsci2013.12.0827

Auta, K. I., Galadima, J. U., Olowoniyi, O. D., Moses, O. O., & Yako, A. B. (2011). Antimicrobial properties of the ethanolic extracts of Zingiber officinale (Ginger) on Escherichia coli and Pseudomonas aeruginosa. *Research Journal of Biological Sciences*, *6*(1), 37–39. doi:10.3923/rjbsci.2011.37.39

Baliga, M. S., Haniadka, R., Pereira, M. M., D'Souza, J. J., Pallaty, P. L., Bhat, H. P., & Popuri, S. (2011). Update on the chemopreventive effects of ginger and its phytochemicals. *Critical Reviews in Food Science and Nutrition*, *51*(6), 499–523. doi:10.1080/10408391003698669 PubMed

Bellik, Y. (2014). Total antioxidant activity and antimicrobial potency of the essential oil and oleoresin of Zingiber officinale Roscoe. *Asian Pacific Journal of Tropical Disease*, *4*(1), 40–44. doi:10.1016/S2222-1808(14)60311-X

Bhandari, U., Kanojia, R., & Pillai, K. K. (2005). Effect of ethanolic extract of Zingiber officinale on dyslipidaemia in diabetic rats. *Journal of Ethnopharmacology*, *97*(2), 227–230. doi:10.1016/j.jep.2004.11.011 PubMed

Bode, A. M., & Dong, Z. (2004). Ginger. In L. Packer, C. N. Ong, & B. Halliwell (Eds.), Herbal and traditional medicine: molecular aspects of health (pp. 131–156). New York: Marcel Dekker; doi:10.1201/9780203025901.ch8.

Bone, M. E., Wilkinson, D. J., Young, J. R., McNeil, J., & Charlton, S. (1990). Ginger root, a new antiemetic. The effect of ginger root on postoperative nausea and vomiting after major gynaecological surgery. *Anaesthesia*, *45*(8), 669–671. doi:10.1111/j.1365-2044.1990.tb14395.x PubMed

Borrelli, F., Capasso, R., Aviello, G., Pittler, M. H., & Izzo, A. A. (2005). Effectiveness and safety of ginger in the treatment of pregnancy induced Nausea and vomiting. *Obstetrics and Gynecology*, *105*(4), 849–856. doi:10.1097/01.AOG.0000154890.47642.23 PubMed

Butt, M. S., & Sultan, M. T. (2011). Ginger and its health claims: Molecular aspects. *Critical Reviews in Food Science and Nutrition*, *51*(5), 383–393. doi:10.1080/10408391003624848 PubMed

Chakraborty, B., Nath, A., Saikia, H., & Sengupta, M. (2014). Bactericidal activity of selected medicinal plants against multidrug resistant bacterial strains from clinical isolates. *Asian Pacific Journal of Tropical Medicine*, *7*, S435–S441. doi:10.1016/S1995-7645(14)60271-6 PubMed

Choudhury, D., Das, A., Bhattacharya, A., & Chakrabarti, G. (2010). Aqueous extract of ginger shows antiproliferative activity through disruption of microtubule network of cancer cells. *Food and Chemical Toxicology*, *48*(10), 2872–2880. doi:10.1016/j.fct.2010.07.020 PubMed

Debbarma, J., Kishore, P., Nayak, B. B., Kannuchamy, N., & Gudipati, V. (2013). Antibacterial activity of ginger, eucalyptus and sweet orange peel essential oils on fish-borne bacteria. *Journal of Food Processing and Preservation*, *37*(5), 1022–1030. doi:10.1111/j.1745-4549.2012.00753.x

Dehghani, I., Mostajeran, A., & Asghari, G. (2011). In vitro and in vivo production of gingerols and zingiberene in ginger plant (Zingiber officinale Roscoe). *Indian Journal of Pharmaceutical Sciences*, *7*, 129–133.

Dugasani, S., Pichika, M. R., Nadarajah, V. D., Balijepalli, M. K., Tandra, S., & Korlakunta, J. N. (2010). Comparative antioxidant and anti-inflammatory effects of [6]-gingerol, [8]-gingerol, [10]-gingerol and [6]-shogaol. *Journal of Ethnopharmacology*, *127*(2), 515–520. doi:10.1016/j.jep.2009.10.004 PubMed

El-Baroty, G. S., El-Baky, H. H. A., Farag, R. S., & Saleh, M. A. (2010). Characterization of antioxidant and antimicrobial compounds of cinnamon and ginger essential oils. *African Journal of Biochemistry Research*, *6*, 167–174.

Fuhrman, B., Rosenblat, M., Hayek, T., Coleman, R., & Aviram, M. (2000). Ginger extract consumption reduces plasma cholesterol, inhibits LDL oxidation and attenuates development of atherosclerosis in atherosclerotic, apolipoprotein E-deficient mice. *The Journal of Nutrition*, *130*(5), 1124–1131. doi:10.1093/jn/130.5.1124 PubMed

Grontved, A., Brask, T., Kambskard, J., & Hentzer, E. (1988). Ginger root against seasickness: A controlled trial on the open sea. *Acta Oto-Laryngologica*, *105*(1-2), 45–49. doi:10.3109/00016488809119444 PubMed

Guo, J. B., Fan, Y., Zhang, W. J., Wu, H., Du, L. M., & Chang, Y. X. (2017). Extraction of gingerols and shogaols from ginger (Zingiber officinale Roscoe) through microwave technique using ionic liquids. *Journal of Food Composition and Analysis*, *62*, 35–42. doi:10.1016/j.jfca.2017.04.014

Gurib-Fakim, A., Maudarbaccus, N., Leach, D., Doimo, L., & Wohlmuth, H. (2002). Essential oil composition of zingiberaceae species from Mauritius. *The Journal of Essential Oil Research*, *14*(4), 271–273. doi:10.1080/10412905.2002.9699850

Harliyansyahm, H., Murad, N. A., & Wan Ngah, W. Z. (2007). Antiproliferative, antioxidant and apoptosis effects of Zingiber officinale and 6-gingerol on HepG2 cells. *Asian Journal of Biochemistry*, *2*(6), 421–426. doi:10.3923/ajb.2007.421.426

Héritier, V. N. V., Arthur, D. N., Augustin, M. M., Nadège, N. K., & Roger, K. V., Eric et, S. Z. L. P., & Jude-Thaddée, M. N. (2018). Article. *J. Pharmacogn.Phytochem.*, *7*(1), 643–648.

Hiserodt, R. D., Franzblau, S. G., & Rosen, R. T. (1998). Isolation of 6-, 8-, and 10-gingerol from ginger rhizome by HPLC and preliminary evaluation of inhibition of Mycobacterium avium and Mycobacterium tuberculosis. *Journal of Agricultural and Food Chemistry*, *46*(7), 2504–2508. doi:10.1021/jf9709481

Hsu, M. H., Kuo, S. C., Chen, C. J., Chung, J. G., Lai, Y. Y., & Huang, L. J. (2005). 1-(3,4-Dimethoxy-phenyl 3,5-dodecenedione (I6) induces G1 arrest and apoptosis in human promyelocytic leukemia HL-60 cells. *Leukemia Research*, *29*(12), 1399–1406. doi:10.1016/j.leukres.2005.04.014 PubMed

Hussein, K. A., & Joo, J. H. (2018). Antifungal activity and chemical composition of ginger essential oil against ginseng pathogenic fungi. Current Research in Environmental & Applied Mycology, 8(2), 194–203. doi:10.5943/cream/8/2/4

Jha, A. B., Ashokkumar, K., Diapari, M., Ambrose, S. J., Zhang, H., Tar'an, B., ... Purves, R. W. (2015). Genetic diversity of folates profiles in seeds of common bean, lentil, chickpea, and pea. *Journal of Food Composition and Analysis*, *42*, 134–140. doi:10.1016/j.jfca.2015.03.006

Karampour, N. S., Arzi, A., Rezaie, A., Pashmforoosh, M., & Kordi, F. (2019). Gastro protective effect of zingerone on ethanol-induced gastric ulcers in rats. Medicina, 55(3), 64. doi:10.3390/medicina55030064

Karuppiah, P., & Rajaram, S. (2012). Antibacterial effect of Allium sativum, cloves and Zingiber officinale rhizomes against multiple-drug resistant clinical pathogens. *Asian Pacific Journal of Tropical Biomedicine*, *8*(8), 597–601. doi:10.1016/S2221-1691(12)60104-X PubMed

Katiyar, S. K., Agarwal, R., & Mukhtar, H. (1996). Inhibition of tumor promotion in SENCARmouse skin by ethanol extract of Zingiber officinale rhizome. *Cancer Research*, *56*(5), 1023–1030. PubMed

Kayaardi, S., Durak, F., Kayacier, A., & Kayaardi, M. (2005). Chemical characteristics of kavurma with selected condiments. *International Journal of Food Properties*, *8*(3), 513–520. doi:10.1080/10942910500269568

Khaki, A., & Fathiazad, F. (2012). Diabetic nephropathy-using herbals in diabetic nephropathy prevention and treatment - the role of ginger (Zingiber officinale) and onion (Allium cepa) in diabetics' nephropathy. In A. Bhattacharya (Ed.), A Compendium of Essays on Alternative Therapy (pp. 207–232). Rijeka, Croatia: InTech Publisher; doi:10.5772/34953.

Khan, I., Pandotra, P., Gupta, A. P., Sharma, R., Gupta, B. D., Dhar, J. K., ... Gupta, S. (2010). RP-thin layer chromatographic method for the quantification of three gingerol homologs of ultrasonic-assisted fresh rhizome extracts of Zingiber officinale collected from North Western Himalayas. *Journal of Separation Science*, *33*(4-5), 558–563. doi:10.1002/jssc.200900629 PubMed

Kikusaki, H., & Nakatani, N. (1993). Antioxidant effect of some ginger constituents. *Journal of Food Science*, *58*(6), 1407–1410. doi:10.1111/j.1365-2621.1993.tb06194.x

Kiran, C. R., Chakka, A. K., Padmakumari Amma, K. P., Menon, A. N., Sree Kumar, M. M., & Venugopalan, V. V. (2013). Essential oil composition of fresh ginger cultivars from North-East India. *The Journal of Essential Oil Research*, *25*(5), 380–387. doi:10.1080/10412905.2013.796496

Kiuchi, F., Shibuya, M., & Sankawa, U. (1982). Inhibitors of prostaglandin biosynthesis from ginger. *Chemical & Pharmaceutical Bulletin*, *30*(2), 754–757. doi:10.1248/cpb.30.754 PubMed

Kubra, I. R., & Rao, L. J. M. (2012). An impression on current developments in the technology, chemistry, and biological activities of Ginger (Zingiber officinale Roscoe). *Critical Reviews in Food Science and Nutrition*, *52*, 651–688.

Latona, D. F., Oyeleke, G. O., & Olayiwola, O. A. (2012). Chemical analysis of ginger root. IOSR Journal of Applied Chemistry, 1(1), 47–49. doi:10.9790/5736-0114749

Lee, H. S., Seo, E. Y., Kang, N. E., & Kim, W. K. (2008). [6]-Gingerol inhibits metastasis of MDS-MB-231 human breast cancer cells. *The Journal of Nutritional Biochemistry*, *19*(5), 313–319. doi:10.1016/j.jnutbio.2007.05.008 PubMed

Lucky, E., Igbinosa, O. E., & Jonahan, I. (2017). Antimicrobial activity of Zingiber officinale against multidrug resistant microbial isolates. *Health Science Research*, *4*, 76–81.

Madreseh-Ghahfarokhi, S., Pirali, Y., Dehghani-Samani, A., & Dehghani-Samani, A. (2018). The insecticidal and repellent activity of ginger (Zingiber officinale) and eucalyptus (Eucalyptus globulus) essential oils against Culex theileri Theobald, 1903 (Diptera: Culicidae. *Annals of Parasitology*, *64*(4), 351–360. PubMed

Mahady, G. B., Pendland, S. L., Yun, G. S., Lu, Z. Z., & Stoia, A. (2003). Ginger (Zingiber officinale Roscoe) and the gingerols inhibit the growth of Cag A+ strains of helicobacter pylori. *Anticancer Research*, *23*, 3699–3702. PubMed

Maitre, S., Neher, J., & Safranek, S. (2011). FPIN's clinical inquiries: Ginger for the treatment of nausea and vomiting in pregnancy. *American Family Physician*, *84*, 1–2. PubMed

Masuda, Y., Kikuzaki, H., Hisamoto, M., & Nakatani, N. (2004). Antioxidant properties of gingerol related compounds from ginger. *BioFactors (Oxford, England)*, *21*(1-4), 293–296. doi:10.1002/biof.552210157 PubMed

Mesomo, M. C., Corazza, M. L., Ndiaye, P. M., Santa, O. R. D., Cardozo, L., & Scheer, A. P. (2013). Supercritical CO2 extracts and essential oil of ginger (Zingiber officinale R.): Chemical composition and antibacterial activity. *The Journal of Supercritical Fluids*, *80*, 44–49. doi:10.1016/j.supflu.2013.03.031

Muthukrishnan, S. D., Ashokkumar, K., & Annapoorani, S. (2014). Identification and determination of flavonoids, carotenoids and chlorophyll concentration in Cynodon dactylon (L.) by HPLC analysis. *Natural Product Research*, *29*(8), 785–790. doi:10.1080/14786419.2014.986125 PubMed

Nanjundaiah, S. M., Annaiah, H. N. M., & Dharmesh, S. M. (2011). Gastroprotective Effect of Ginger Rhizome (Zingiber officinale) Extract: Role of Gallic Acid and Cinnamic Acid in H+, K+-ATPase/H. pylori Inhibition and Anti-Oxidative Mechanism. *Evidence-Based Complementary and Alternative Medicine*. doi:10.1093/ecam/nep060

Natta, L. K., & Orapin, N., Krittika, & Pantip, B. (2008). Essential oil from five Zingiberaceae for anti-food-borne bacteria. *International Food Research Journal*, *15*, 337–346.

Odebunmi, E. O., Oluwaniyi, O. O., & Bashiru, M. O. (2010). Comparative proximate analysis of some food condiments. *Journal of Applied Sciences Research*, *6*(3), 272–274.

Ogbuewu, I. P., Jiwuba, P. D., Ezeokeke, C. T., Uchegbu, M. C., Okoli, I. C., & Iloeje, M. U. (2014). Evaluation of phytochemical and nutritional composition of ginger rhizome powder. *International Journal of Agriculture & Rural Development*, *17*(1), 1663–1670.

Ojewole, J. A. O. (2006). Analgesic, antiinflammatory and hypoglycaemic effects of ethanol extract of Zingiber officinale (Roscoe) rhizomes (Zingiberaceae) in mice and rats. *Phytotherapy Research*, *20*(9), 764–772. doi:10.1002/ptr.1952 PubMed

Okamoto, M., Irii, H., Tahara, Y., Ishii, H., Hirao, A., Udagawa, H., ... Shimizu, I. (2011). Synthesis of a new [6]- gingerol analogue and its protective effect with respect to the development of metabolic syndrome in mice fed a high-fat diet. *Journal of Medicinal Chemistry*, *54*(18), 6295–6304. doi:10.1021/jm200662c PubMed

Onimawo, I. A., Esekheigbe, A., & Okoh, J. E. (2019). Determination of Proximate and Mineral Composition of Three Traditional Spices. *Acta Scientific Nutritional Health*, *3*, 111–114.

Onyenekwe, P. C., & Hashimoto, S. (1999). The composition of the essential oil of dried Nigerian ginger (Zingiber officinale Roscoe). *European Food Research and Technology*, *209*(6), 407–410. doi:10.1007/s002170050517

Otunola, G. A., Oloyede, O. B., Oladiji, A. T., & Afolayan, A. J. (2010). Comparative analysis of the chemical composition of three spices - Allium sativum L. Zingiber officinale Rosc.andCapsicum frutescens L. commonly consumed in Nigeria. *African Journal of Biotechnology*, *9*(41), 6927–6931.

Park, M., Bae, J., & Lee, D. S. (2008). Antibacterial activity of [10]-gingerol and [12]-gingerol isolated from ginger rhizome against periodontal bacteria. *Phytotherapy Research*, *22*(11), 1446–1449. doi:10.1002/ptr.2473 PubMed

Pino, J. A., Marbot, R., Rosado, A., & Batista, A. (2004). Chemical composition of the essential oil of Zingiber officinale Roscoe L. from Cuba. *The Journal of Essential Oil Research*, *16*(3), 186–188. doi:10.1080/10412905.2004.9698692

Prasad, S., & Tyagi, A. K. (2015). Ginger and Its Constituents: Role in Prevention and Treatment of Gastrointestinal Cancer. Gastroenterology Research and Practice. doi:10.1155/2015/142979

Qin, F., & Xu, H. (2008). Active compounds in gingers and their therapeutic uses in complimentary medication. *Medicinal and Aromatic Plant Science and Biotechnology*, *2*(2), 72–78.

Raina, V. K., Kumar, A., & Aggarwal, K. K. (2005). Essential oil composition of ginger (Zingiber officinale Roscoe) rhizomes from different place in india. *Journal of Essential Oil-Bearing Plants*, *8*(2), 187–191. doi:10.1080/0972060X.2005.10643442

Ramadan, G., Al-Kahtani, M. A., & El-Sayed, W. M. (2011). Anti-inflammatory and anti-oxidant properties of Curcuma longa (turmeric) versus Zingiber officinale (ginger) rhizomes in rat adjuvant-induced arthritis. *Inflammation*, *34*(4), 291–301. doi:10.1007/s10753-010-9278-0 PubMed

Ravindran, P. N., Nirmal Babu, K., & Shiva, K. N. (2005). Botany and crop improvement of ginger. In P. N. Ravindran & K. Nirmal Babu (Eds.), *Ginger: The Genus Zingiber* (Vol. 41, pp. 15–85). Boca Raton, FL: Medicinal and Aromatic Plants-Industrial Profiles.

Riaz, H., Begum, A., Raza, S. A., Khan, Z. M.-U.-D., Yousaf, H., & Tariq, A. (2015). Antimicrobial property and phytochemical study of ginger found in local area of Punjab, Pakistan. International Current Pharmaceutical Journal, 4(7), 405–409. doi:10.3329/icpj.v4i7.23591

Sa-Nguanpuag, K., Kanlayanarat, S., Srilaong, V., Tanprasert, K., & Techavuthiporn, C. (2011). Ginger (Zingiber officinale) oil as an antimicrobial agent for minimally processed produce: A case study in shredded green papaya. *International Journal of Agriculture and Biology*, *13*, 895–901.

Saputri, F. C., & Jantan, I. (2011). Effects of selected medicinal plants on human low-density lipoprotein oxidation, 2,2-diphenyl-1-picrylhydra-zyl (DPPH) radicals and human platelet aggregation. *Journal of Medicinal Plants Research*, *5*, 6182–6199.

Sasidharan, I., & Menon, A. N. (2010). Comparative chemical composition and antimicrobial activity fresh & dry ginger oils (Zingiber officinale Roscoe). *International Journal of Current Pharmaceutical Research*, *2*, 40–43.

Semwal, R. B., Semwal, D. K., Combrinck, S., & Viljoen, A. M. (2015). Gingerols and shogaols: Important nutraceutical principles from ginger. *Phytochemistry*, *117*, 554–568. doi:10.1016/j.phytochem.2015.07.012 PubMed

Shahid, M., & Hussain, F. (2012). Chemical composition and mineral contents of Zingiber officinale and Alpinia allughas (Zingiberaceae) rhizomes. *International Journal of Chemical and Biochemical Science*, *2*, 101–104.

Shammari, A. M. N. A. (2018). Protective effect of ginger (Zingiber officinale) consumption against kidney damage in rats. *Life Science Journal*, *15*(1), 80–85.

Sharma, N., Tiwari, R., & Srivastava, M. P. (2013). Zingiberofficinale Roscoe. Oil: A preservative of stored commodities against storage Mycoflora. *International Journal of Current Microbiology and Applied Sciences*, *2*, 123–134.

Sharma, P. K., Singh, V., & Ali, M. (2016). Chemical composition and antimicrobial activity of fresh rhizome essential oil of Zingiber officinale Roscoe. *Pharmacognosy Journal*, *8*(3), 185–190. doi:10.5530/pj.2016.3.3

Shobana, S., & Naidu, K. A. (2000). Antioxidant activity of selected Indian spices. *Prostaglandins, Leukotrienes, and Essential Fatty Acids*, *62*(2), 107–110. doi:10.1054/plef.1999.0128 PubMed

Shukla, Y., & Singh, M. (2007). Cancer preventive properties of ginger: A brief review. *Food and Chemical Toxicology*, *45*(5), 683–690. doi:10.1016/j.fct.2006.11.002 PubMed

Singh, G., Kapoor, I. P. S., Singh, P., De Heluani, C. S., De Lampasona, M. P., & Catalan, C. A. N. (2008). Chemistry, antioxidant and antimicrobial investigations on essential oil and oleoresins of Zingiber officinale. *Food and Chemical Toxicology*, *46*(10), 3295–3302. doi:10.1016/j.fct.2008.07.017 PubMed

Srivastava, K. C., & Mustafa, T. (1989). Spices: Antiplatelet activity and prostanoid metabolism. *Prostaglandins, Leukotrienes, and Essential Fatty Acids*, *38*(4), 255–266. doi:10.1016/0952-3278(89)90129-4 PubMed

Stoyanova, A., Konakchiev, A., Damyanova, S., Stoilova, I., & Suu, P. T. (2006). Composition and antimicrobial activity of ginger essential oil from Vietnam. *Journal of Essential Oil-Bearing Plants*, *9*(1), 93–98. doi:10.1080/0972060X.2006.10643478

Sultan, M., Bhatti, H. N., & Iqbal, Z. (2005). Chemical analysis of essential oil of ginger (Zingiber officinale). *Pakistan Journal of Biological Sciences*, *8*(11), 1576–1578. doi:10.3923/pjbs.2005.1576.1578

Surh, Y. J., Park, K. K., Chun, K. S., Lee, L. J., Lee, E., & Lee, S. S. (1999). Anti-tumor-promoting activities of selected pungent phenolic substances present in ginger. *Journal of Environmental Pathology, Toxicology and Oncology*, *18*, 131–139. PubMed

Švarc-Gajić, J., Cvetanović, A., Segura-Carretero, A., Linares, I. B., & Maškovic, P. (2017). Characterization of ginger extracts obtained by subcritical water. *The Journal of Supercritical Fluids*, *123*, 92–100. doi:10.1016/j.supflu.2016.12.019

Tahir, A. A., Abdul Sani, N. F., Morad, N. A., Makpol, S., Ngah, W. Z., & Yusof, Y. A. (2015). Combined ginger extract and gelam honey modulate Ras/ERK and P13/AKT pathway genes in colon cancer HT29 cells. *Nutrition Journal*, *14*(1), 31. doi:10.1186/s12937-015-0015-2 PubMed

Tchombé, N. L., Louajri, A., & Benajiba, M. H. (2012). Therapeutic effects of ginger (Zingiber officinale). *ISESCO Journal of Science and Technology*, *8*, 64–69.

Thomson, M., Al-Qattan, K. K., Al-Sawan, S. M., Alnaqeeb, M. A., Khan, I., & Ali, M. (2002). The use of ginger (Zingiber officinale Rosc.) as a potential anti-inflammatory and antithrombotic agent. *Prostaglandins, Leukotrienes, and Essential Fatty Acids*, *67*(6), 475–478. doi:10.1054/plef.2002.0441 PubMed

Thongson, C., Davidson, P. M., Mahakarnchanakul, W., & Vibulsresth, P. (2005). Antimicrobial effect of Thai spices against Listeria monocytogenes and Salmonella Typhimurium DT104. *Journal of Food Protection*, *68*(10), 2054–2058. doi:10.4315/0362-028X-68.10.2054 PubMed

Toader, O. R. (2014). Study of the effects of Zingiber officinale (ginger) on spermatogenesis in mice. *Annals of West University of Timisoara. Series of Biology*, *17*, 145–152.

Townsend, E. A., Siviski, M. E., Zhang, Y., Xu, C., Hoonjan, B., & Emala, C. W. (2013). Effects of ginger and its constituents on airway smooth muscle relaxation and calcium regulation. *American Journal of Respiratory Cell and Molecular Biology*, *48*(2), 157–163. doi:10.1165/rcmb.2012-0231OC PubMed

Tzeng, T. F., & Liu, I. M. (2013). 6-Gingerol prevents adipogenesis and the accumulation of cytoplasmic lipid droplets in 3T3-L1 cells. *Phytomedicine*, *20*(6), 481–487. doi:10.1016/j.phymed.2012.12.006 PubMed

Vasala, P. A. (2004). Ginger. In K. V. Peter (Ed.), *Handbook of Herbs and Spices* (Vol. 1, pp. 195–206). Cambridge, UK: Woodhead.

Wei, Q. Y., Ma, J. P., Cai, Y. J., Yang, L., & Liu, Z. L. (2005). Cytotoxic and apoptotic activities of diarylheptanoids and gingerol-related compounds from the rhizome of Chinese ginger. *Journal of Ethnopharmacology*, *102*(2), 177–184. doi:10.1016/j.jep.2005.05.043 PubMed

WHO. (1991). *Traditional medicine and modern health care: progress report by the director general document A 44(10)*. World Health Organization.

Wohlmuth, H., Leach, D. N., Smith, M. K., & Myers, S. P. (2005). Gingerol content of diploid and tetraploid clones of ginger (Zingiber officinale Roscoe). *Journal of Agricultural and Food Chemistry*, *53*(14), 5772–5778. doi:10.1021/jf050435b PubMed

Yadav, S., Sharma, P. K., & Alam, M. A. (2016). Ginger medicinal uses and benefits. *European Journal Pharmaceutical and Medical Research*, *3*, 127–135.

Yamamoto-Ribeiro, M. M. G., Grespan, R., Kohiyama, C. Y., Dias, F., Galerani, S. A., Leite, E., ... Machinski, M. (2013). Effect of Zingiber officinale essential oil on Fusarium verticillioides and Fumonisin production. *Food Chemistry*, *141*(3), 3147–3152. doi:10.1016/j.foodchem.2013.05.144 PubMed

Yusof, Y. A. M., Ahmad, N., & Das, S. (2009). Chemopreventive efficacy of ginger (Zingiber officinale) in ethionine induced rat hepatocarcinogenesis. *African Journal of Traditional, Complementary, and Alternative Medicines*, *6*, 87–93. PubMed

Zarate, R., & Yeoman, M. M. (1996). Changes in the amounts of [6]-gingerol and derivatives during a culture cycle of ginger, Zingiber officinale. *Plant Science*, *121*(1), 115–122. doi:10.1016/S0168-9452(96)04512-8

Chapter 6
Pharmacological Applications of Saffron (*Crocus sativus*): A Review

Priyanka Singh
Centre of Food Technology, University of Allahabad, India

ABSTRACT

Saffron spice also known as Crocus sativus (Saffron crocus) belongs to the family of iridaceae. Many studies have proved its potential role in disease eradication. It has been reported to possess the attributes of a sedative, an anti-asthma, an emmenagogue, an expectorant, and an adaptogenic agent. Crocin, crocetin, and safranal are the most important biochemically active ingredients that were found in different parts of the plants in varying proportions like the peels, fruits, seeds, and rind of Crocus sativus. The in vitro and in vivo studies showed that saffron has got its therapeutic implication in health management via anti-oxidant, anti-microbial, hepatoprotective, and anti-tumour activity. This review attempts to reveal the potential pharmacological properties of Crocus sativus. It also draws attention towards the use of herbs and spices in various ailments without facing the harmful side effects of chemically derived medicine.

INTRODUCTION

Crocus sativus L. is a stemless perennial herb belonging to the family Iridaceae. The word saffron was derived from the Latin word safranum that means "yellow. It is the native Mediterranean to western China, although cultivated in many countries such as Turkey, Morocco, Iran, Italy, Spain, Greece, Israel, Azerbaijan, Egypt, China, India and Mexico. It is commonly known as Red Gold in producer countries as it is the most expensive spice for its characteristic aroma, color and aphrodisiac properties. The botanical name of saffron is Crocus sativus L and in Hindi, it is called Keshar.

Saffron are dried red stigma (25-30 mm long) of the colored flower of *C. sativus* L. The flower of C. sativa is light purple containing three stigmas. For Centuries, it has been used in food for its bright orange-yellow color and intense flavor and aroma. Crocetin and crocin are the degraded carotenoids

DOI: 10.4018/978-1-7998-2524-1.ch006

Table 1. Classification

Kingdom	Plantae
Clade	Angiosperms
Clade	Monocots
Order	Asparagales
Family	Iridaceae
Genus	*Crocus*
Species	*C. sativus*
Botanical name	*Crocus sativus* L.

responsible for the yellow color and the sweet fragrance of saffron is due to the presence of a specific essential oil in the flower. In folklore medicine, it has been useful in treating many digestive disorders, as a nerve sedative with anticatarrhal, antispasmodic, emmenagogue, eupeptic, and expectorant properties (Rıos et al., 1996).

The stigmas of the saffron flower contain a number of chemical substances, including carbohydrates, minerals, musilage, vitamins B1 & B2, pigments, and carotenoids. In addition, it contains small amounts of the pigment anthocyanin; oil-soluble pigments including alpha-carotene, betacarotene and zegxantin. A phytochemical investigation of Saffron has been an isolated variety of biologically active constituents, including crocin, picrocrocin, and safranal, which is responsible for its distinct color, aroma, and medicinal properties. Safranal is the major principle of active compounds constituting around 70% of total essential oil. . Saffron contained more than 150 volatile and several nonvolatile compounds and approximately 40–50 constituents have been detected thus far (Bolhasani et al., 2005; Caballero-Ortega et al., 2007). This review article aims to summarize the pharmacological/biological activities of saffron and its bioactive constituents with possible therapeutic applications.

Botanical Description

C. sativus L. is a stemless plant with subsoil corn approximately 3-5 cm in diameter. At the base of the corn short sprinkle roots grow, and above the soil it holds 6-8 leaves, a flowering stalk, bract, and bracteole. The yellow colored flower has three petals and three sepals. In the center of the flower, there is a single-ovule ovary, which grows to 10-30 cm long and is light yellow in color, has a long thin style, and ends in the 2-3cm long bright orange-red triple stigma. It multiplies by means of corms, since flowers do not produce any seeds (**Srivastava et al., 2010**).

Ethnomedicinal Importance

Saffron has long been used as both a spice and medicine over 3,600 years ago. It is an important medicinal plant that has been used in ethnomedicine against several health ailments in many cultures. Saffron is employed to prevent fever, inflammation, expectorant, asthma, melancholia, hysteria, leucorrhoea, enlarged liver, diabetes, high blood pressure, heart ailments, and cancer. Research studies have shown that this herb is a dense source of carotenoid, riboflavin, and folate and is beneficial in regulating and promoting menstrual periods and also reducing lumbar pains.

Figure 1. The Principle Bioactive compounds of saffron

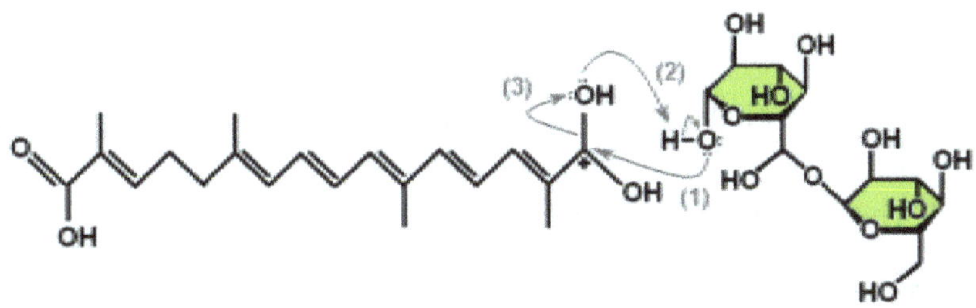

Crocin (8,8-diapo-8,8-carotenoic acid)

Phytochemistry

Chemical analysis of the stigmas of the saffron flower revealed that they are rich in proteins, fats, carbohydrates, minerals, vitamins and some pigments along with some bioactive compounds. The saffron stigma is a mixture of various components, and such constituents have therapeutics important in health management through the modulation of various biological pathways. It has documented that the therapeutic benefits of this plant are attributed to several phytochemical compounds like carotene, zigzantin, lycopene, crocetin, crocin, safranal 2,6,6-trimethyl 1,3-cyclohexadiene-1-carboxaldehyde, 2-hydroxy-4,4,6-trimethyl 2,5-cyclohexadiene-1-one, terpenes, cineol, and pinene.

Carotenoid compounds comprise more than 10% of the dry saffron's mass. The hydrolysis and degradation of saffron yields several active constituents including crocetin, crocetin glucosidic derivatives, crocins, picrocrocin, and safranal (**Pitsikas et al., 2007, Rubio-Moraga, et al, 2010**). Picrocrocin is a breakdown of products of carotenoids and imparts a characteristic bitter flavor to saffron. It comprises up to 4% of dry saffron and yields glucose and safranal on hydrolysis. Safranal is the principle that constitutes for the saffron aroma and may comprise up to 70% of the dry saffron's volatile fractions although other volatile constituents responsible for aroma were also present in a low concentration range of 0.3–2% of the total aroma fraction.

PHARMACOLOGICAL ATTRIBUTES

Anti-inflammatory

Aqueous and ethanolic extracts of petals and stigmas of saffron were shown to exhibit anti-inflammatory properties. In mice, the aqueous extract of saffron at doses 50, 100 and 200 mg/kg were injected intraperitoneally three times per week alone or with DZN (20 mg/kg/day, orally) for 4 weeks to assess the antiinflammatory activities. It has been reported that active compounds, mainly crocin and crocetin, are attributed for these activities and are active against many pro-inflammatory cytokines and radical oxygen species(**Poma et al., 2012**). In this support, Rathore et al (2015) reported extract of *C. sativus* reduces pro-inflammatory cytokines (IL-1β and TNF-α) in adjuvant-induced arthritic mice.

Immunomodulatory Effect

Earlier investigations support the role of saffron in improving immunity. It is also suggested that active constituents of saffron also modulate humoral immunity and cell-mediated immunity responses by enhancing the antioxidant capacity (Boskabady and Farkhondeh 2016). Saffron increased the IgG level and decreased the IgM level as compared to the baseline and placebo groups.

Antidepressant Activity

Many clinical and preclinical studies report that petal and stigma of *C. sativus* have antidepressant effects. The two major constituents of saffron crocin and safranal have been suggested for antidepressant activity. Previous studies have evaluated the efficacy of saffron in mild to moderate depression and found that saffron was more effective and equivalent to therapeutic doses of fluoxetine and imipramine (Sarris 2007; Siddiqui et al. 2011). Similar results were seen. In a double-blind and randomized trial study conducted for more than 6 weeks, it showed the extract of saffron is equally efficient to the drug imipramine.

Anticonvulsant Activity

In Iranian folklore medicine, saffron had been used as an anticonvulsant remedy (Zhang et al 1994). C. sativus has also proven its role in the treatment of related memory impairment and neurodegenerative disorders. Crocetin and crocin are the two main bioactive compounds that were identified for improving learning and memory skills in mice (Sigiura et al 1995). Alcoholic extract of *C. sativus* shows a sedative effect that is responsible for the anticonvulsant effect by increasing the sleeping time. Hosseinzadeh and Talebzadeh 2005 evaluated crocin and safranal for anticonvulsant activity in mice and reported anticonvulsant activity of safranal at 0.15 and 0.35 ml/kg dose whereas crocin (200 mg/kg, i.p.) does not show anticonvulsant activity

Anti tumor Activity

The anti-proliferative effect of Crocus sativus extract is well documented by previous studies, and its chief constituent crocin was shown to possess important antiproliferative properties. Another major bioactive component safranal attributed to the co-mutagenic effect. In this regard, numerous findings based on animal models confirmed that saffron and its active constituents perform an important role in the inhibition of tumor development and progression. The ethanolic extract of saffron reported antiproliferative and cytotoxic effects against human prostate cancer (D'Alessandro et al., 2013). Similarly, the ethanolic extract of saffron decreased cell viability in malignant cells and IC50 values against the lung cancer cell line were determined as 1500 and 565 μg/ml after 24 and 48 h, respectively. Research studies suggest that extract of saffron and its active constituents (safranal, crocin, and crocetin) selectively kill cancer cells and may have cancer-preventive functions. On the other hand, saffron and its constituents are non-toxic or non-genotoxic to normal cells. Crocetin or crocin was shown to have cancer-preventive or anticancer effects in animal models.

Glucoregulation

Global estimates indicate about 300 million or more are likely to have diabetes mellitus by the year 2025 (Alberti et al., 2004). Previous studies had shown that the ethanolic extract of saffron reduced blood glucose level and glycosylated serum protein levels in alloxan diabetic rats at 20, 40, 80 mg Kg-1 doses. Further, it is supported by another study reported that the administration of *C. sativus* stigma extract protects the vital tissues of the pancreas and reduced the cause of diabetes. Earlier investigations concluded extract of saffron effective in reducing fasting blood glucose in mild diabetic and in severely diabetic rats (Mohajeri et al. 2008)

Cardiovascular Effect

Previous studies elicited that the cardio-protective activity includes lowering the triglyceride and cholesterol levels and the inhibition of platelet aggregation. Ethanol and aqueous extract of saffron reduces systolic blood pressure at 400mg/d dose but not diastolic blood pressure. (Modaghegh et al, 2008). Similarly, administration of 200mg/kg of saffron shows an antiarrhythmic effect, but it was not as effective as amiodarone (Joukar and Dehesh, 2015).

Hepatoprotective Effect

The hepatoprotective effect of saffron has been reported by several studies. The saffron extract was shown to possess hepatoprotective effects on acetaminophen-induced hepatic damage in mice. Previous studies elicited the hepato-protective activity of plants by the significant increase in AST and ALT activities against the carbon tetrachloride (CCL4). Extract of Crocus sativus petals normalize the level of serum proteins and interfere with the increase in aminotransferases (Omidi, 2014).

Aphrodisiac Activities

Saffron also plays an important role in improving fertility and increases libido when consumed. Results have revealed that crocin and its aqueous extract, particularly at doses of 160-320 mg/kg b.w. increased mounting and erection frequency behaviors and in addition to this reduced ejaculation, intromission, and mount latency parameters.58

CONCLUSION

Medicinal plants are the most recent alternatives of medicines nowadays because they posses no side effects to our body while the treatment of diseases and are cheaper to afford by the maximum population. Different constituents of Saffron contains a mixture of various phytochemicals and has therapeutics importance in health management through the reformulation of various biological pathways. Antioxidant, antibacterial, anti-inflammatory, anti-diabetic, and various other therapeutic benefits have proved the potential of saffron in disease control and prevention. Studies on animal models also have shown a prospective matter of research in this area and explore more potential benefits of using saffron in eradication of different types of fatal ailments.

Table 2. Extracts with their biological activities and findings

Extract	Biological activity	finding/outcome	References
Whole saffron extract	Anti-tumorr	cytotoxic effect on HepG-2 (IC50 of 400 μ g/ml) and Hep-2 and L929 cells did not respond to any extract concentrations	Parade et al 2011
Stigma extract	Antioxidant	Saffron stigma showed antioxidant activity.	[14]
Extract of *C. sativus*	Lower serum inflammatory markers	Lower serum inflammatory markers includes serum levels of endotheline-1 (ET-1) and total protein (TP)	Gholamnezhad et al 2013
Aqueous extract	lower blood pressure	Lowered blood pressure from 133.5 ± 3.9 to 117 ± 2.1 (mmHg).	Fatehi et al. 2003
Capsule		No significant difference in plasma level of fibrinogen, factor VII (as coagulant agent), C and S protein (as anti-coagulant agent),	Ayatollahi et al. 2014
Isolated Safranal	Anticonvulsant	reduced the seizure duration, delayed the onset of tonic convulsions	Hosseinzadeh 2005
crocin and safranal	Anti-inflammatory	Study finding reported that crocin and safranal showed role in the suppression of inflammatory pain responses and decreased the the number of neutrophils.	Tamanddofard et al., 2013
C.sativus extract	Antibacterial	Strong activity against bacteria and fungi was noted.	Vahid et al., 2011
Safranal	Guinea pigs.	Reduce the number of coughs	Hosseinzadeh 2006
Whole petal	Antioxidant	decrease in lipoprotein oxidation susceptibility	Verma and Bordia, 1998
petals	Hepatoprotective	Finding demonstrated that petals ameliorate acute liver injury	36
Safranal	Protective effect against nephrotoxicity	Safranal has a protective effect against nephrotoxicity.	Boroushak et al., 2007
Saffron and crocin	Anti-obesity and anorectic	Result concluded that saffron has anti-obesity and anorectic effects and lowered leptin level	Kianbakht et al., 2015
Saffron and safranal	Cardio-protective	Result revealed that myocardial injury preserved nearly normal tissue architecture with saffron or safranal pretreatment.	Mehdizadeh et al, 2013
saffron extract, crocin and safranal	Anti-hyperglycemic	significantly reduced the fasting blood glucose levels but significantly increased the blood insulin levels in the diabetic rats compared with the diabetic control rats.	Kianbakht et al.,2011

REFERENCES

Bolhasani, A., Bathaie, S. Z., Yavari, I., Moosavi-Movahedi, A. A., & Ghaffari, M. (2005). Separation and purification of some components of Iranian saffron. *Chemistry, an Asian Journal*, *17*, 725–729.

Boroushaki, M. T., Mofidpour, H., & Sadeghnia, H. (2007). Protective effect of safranal against hexachlorobutadiene-induced nephrotoxicity in rat. *Iranian Journal of Medical Sciences*, *32*, 173–176.

Caballero-Ortega, H., Pereda-Miranda, R., & Abdullaev, F. I. (2007). HPLC quantification of major active components from 11 different saffron (*Crocus sativus* L.) sources. *Food Chemistry*, *100*(3), 1126–1131. doi:10.1016/j.foodchem.2005.11.020

D'Alessandro, A. M., Mancini, A., Lizzi, A. R., Simone, A. D., Marroccella, C. E., Gravina, G. L., ... Festuccia, C. (2013). Crocus sativus stigma extract and its major constituent crocin possess significant antiproliferative properties against human prostate cancer. *Nutrition and Cancer*, *65*(6), 930–942. doi: 10.1080/01635581.2013.767368 PMID:23909737

Hosseinzadeh, H., & Talebzadeh, F. (2005). Anticonvulsant evaluation of safranal and crocin from *Crocus sativus* in mice. *Fitoterapia*, *76*(7–8), 722–724. doi:10.1016/j.fitote.2005.07.008 PMID:16253437

Hosseinzadeh, H., Ziaee, T., & Sadeghi, A. (2008). The effect of saffron, Crocus sativus stigma, extract and its constituents, safranal, and crocin on sexual behaviors in normal male rats. *Phytomedicine*, *15*(6-7), 491–495. doi:10.1016/j.phymed.2007.09.020 PMID:17962007

Joukar, S., & Dehesh, M. M. (2015). The safety assessment of saffron (*Crocus sativus* L.) on sympathovagal balance and heart rate variability; a comparison with amiodarone. *Autonomic & Autacoid Pharmacology*, *35*(4), 46–50. doi:10.1111/aap.12040 PMID:27329172

Karimi, E., Oskoueian, E., Hendra, R., & Jaafar, H. Z.Stigma Phenolic and Flavonoid Compounds and Its Antioxidant Activity. (2010). Evaluation of Crocus sativus L.stigma phenolic and flavonoid compounds and its antioxidant activity. *Molecules (Basel, Switzerland)*, *15*(9), 6244–6256. doi:10.3390/molecules15096244 PMID:20877220

Kianbakht, S., & Hajiaghaee, R. (2011). Anti-hyperglycemic effects of saffron and its active constituents, crocin and safranal, in alloxan-induced diabetic rats. *Faslnamah-i Giyahan-i Daruyi*, *3*(39), 82–89.

Kianbakht, S., & Hashem, D. F. (2015). Anti-obesity and anorectic effects of saffron and itsconstituent crocin in obese Wistar rat. *Faslnamah-i Giyahan-i Daruyi*, *1*(53), 25–33.

Mehdizadeh, R., Parizadeh, M. R., Khooei, A. R., Mehri, S., & Hosseinzadeh, H. (2013). Cardioprotective Effect of Saffron Extract and Safranal in Isoproterenol-Induced Myocardial Infarction in Wistar Rats. *Iranian Journal of Basic Medical Sciences.*, *16*(1), 56–63. PMID:23638293

Modaghegh, M. H., Shahabian, M., Esmaeili, H. A., Rajbai, O., & Hosseinzadeh, H. (2008). Safety evaluation of saffron (Crocus sativus) tablets in healthy volunteers. *Phytomedicine*, *15*(12), 1032–1037. doi:10.1016/j.phymed.2008.06.003 PMID:18693099

Mohajeri, D., & Amouoghli, T. B. (2008). Mousavi Gh, Mesgari M. Antidiabetic activity of Crocus sativus L. (saffron) stigma ethanolic extract in alloxan-induced diabetic rats. *Research Journal of Biological Sciences*, *3*(9), 1102–1108.

Omidi, A., Riahinia, N., Montazer, T. M., & Behdani, M. (2014). Hepatoprotective effect of Crocus sativus (saffron) petals extract against acetaminophen toxicity in male Wistar rats. *Avicenna Journal of Phytomedicine*, *4*(5), 330–336. PMID:25386395

Omidi, A., Riahinia, N., Montazer, T. M., & Behdani, M. (2014). Hepatoprotective effect of Crocus sativus (saffron) petals extract against acetaminophen toxicity in male Wistar rats. *Avicenna Journal of Phytomedicine*, *4*(5), 330–336. PMID:25386395

Pitsikas, N., Boultadakis, A., Gergiadou, G., Tarantilis, P. A., & Sakellaridis, N. (2008). Effects of the active constituents of Crocus sativus L. in an animal model of anxiety. *Phytomedicine*, *15*, 1135.

Poma, A., Fontecchio, G., Carlucci, G., & Chichiricco, G. (2012). Anti-Inflammatory Properties of Drugs from saffron crocus. *Anti-Inflammatory & Anti-Allergy Agents in Medicinal Chemistry*, *11*(1), 37–51. doi:10.2174/187152312803476282 PMID:22934747

R’ıos, J. L., Recio, M. C., Ginger, R. M., & M’a˜nez, S. (1996). An updated review of saffron and its active constituents. *Phytotherapy Research*, *10*(3), 189–193. doi:10.1002/(SICI)1099-1573(199605)10:3<189::AID-PTR754>3.0.CO;2-C

Rathore, B., Jaggi, K., Thakur, S. K., Mathur, A., & Mahdi, F. (2015). Anti-inflammatory activity of Crocus sativus extracts in experimental arthritis. *International Journal of Pharmaceutical Sciences and Research*, *6*(4), 1473–1478.

Rubio-Moraga, A., Trapero, A., Ahrazem, O., & Gomez-Gomez, L. (2010). Crocins transport in Crocus sativus: The long road from a senescent stigma to a new born corm. *Phytochemistry*, *71*, 1506–1513.

Sarris, J. (2007). Herbal medicines in the treatment of psychiatric disorders: A systematic review. *Phytotherapy Research*, *21*(8), 703–706. doi:10.1002/ptr.2187 PMID:17562566

Siddiqui, M. J., Saleh, M. S., Basharuddin, S. N. B., Zamri, S. H. B., Mohd Najib, M. H., Che Ibrahim, M. Z., ... Khatib, A. (2018). Saffron (Crocus sativus L.): As an antidepressant. *Journal of Pharmacy & Bioallied Sciences*, *10*(4), 173. doi:10.4103/JPBS.JPBS_83_18 PMID:30568374

Sigiura, M., Saito, H., & Abe, K. (1995). Ethanol extract of Crocus sativus L.antagonizes the inhibitory action of ethanol on hippocampal long-term potentiation in vivo. *Phytotherapy Research*, *9*(2), 100–104. doi:10.1002/ptr.2650090204

Srivastava, R., Ahmed, H., Dixit, R. K., Dharamveer, & Saraf, S. A. (2010). Crocus sativus L: A comprehensive review. *Pharmacognosy Reviews*, *4*(8), 200. doi:10.4103/0973-7847.70919 PMID:22228962

Tamaddonfard, E., Farshid, A. A., Eghdami, K., Samadi, F., & Erfanparast, A. (2013). Comparison of the effects of crocin, safranal and diclofenac on local inflammation andinflammatory pain responses induced by carrageenan in rats. *Pharmacological Reports*, *65*(5), 1272–1280. doi:10.1016/S1734-1140(13)71485-3 PMID:24399723

Vahidi, H., Kamalinejad, M., & Sedaghati, N. (2002). Antimicrobial Properties of Crocus sativus L. *Iranian Journal of Pharmaceutical Research*, *1*, 33–35.

Zhang, Y., Shoyama, Y., Sugiura, M., & Saito, H. (1994). Effect of Crocus sativus L. On the ethanol-induced impairment of passive avoidance performances in mice. *Biological & Pharmaceutical Bulletin*, *17*, 217–221.

Chapter 7 Phytochemistry and Ethanopharmacology of *Illicium verum* (Staranise)

Priyanka Singh
Centre of Food Technology, University of Allahabad, India

Neha Mishra
Sam Higginbottom University of Agriculture, Technology, and Sciences, India

Ena Gupta
Department of Home Science, University of Allahabad, India

ABSTRACT

Illicium verum, as a spice and pharmaceutical treatment of many harmful diseases, has been widely used in most Asian countries. The Ministry of Health of the People's Republic of China considered it as both food and medicine due to its non-toxicity towards human health. In the present study, the review focuses mainly on food and medical applications of I. verum. The fruits are commonly used as an ingredient of the traditional "five-spice" powder of Chinese cooking, and the essential oil of I. verum can be used as flavoring. The extraction from I. verum has carminative, stomachic, stimulant, and diuretic properties, and is used as a pharmaceutical supplement. Shikimic acid extracted from I. verum is one of the main ingredients in the antiviral drug Tamiflu, which is used to fight avian influenza. It has also been reported to possess antimicrobial and antioxidative properties as well as significant anticancer potential. This review presents a detailed compilation of the literature on phytochemicals and pharmacological properties of Illicium verum.

DOI: 10.4018/978-1-7998-2524-1.ch007

INTRODUCTION

The Schisandraceae family contains the sole genus *Illicium*. It consists of forty-two species of evergreen small trees and shrubs. The species is native of the tropical and subtropical regions of South Eastern North America, Eastern and South Eastern Asia and the West Indies. The most frequently occurring species are *Illicium dunnianum,, Illicium verum, Illicium anisatum,* and *Illicium griffithii.* Commonly *Illicium verum* is known as star anise or star aniseed or Chinese star anise.(Kumar et al.,2012) It is a spice that very similar to anise in flavor, obtained from the star-shaped pericarp of the plant. It is a medium-sized native evergreen small or medium-sized plant of subtropical and temperate regions. They consist of star-shaped fruits, which are reddish-brown in color and contain 6–8 carpels attached in a whorl arrangement. The shape and size of the carpel is boat-shaped and 10 mm long, also contain a seed. The seeds are brown colored, ovoid shaped, and posses smooth, shiny, and brittle texture. This plant is propagated by its seeds for its application in different types of medicines, perfume, and as a culinary spice in southern China and Vietnam. The fruits are harvested before they ripen, and sun drying is done for further use. Anethole, is the main ingredient found in Star anise, that gives the unrelated anise its flavor, hence it has become a less expensive substitute for anise in baking as well as in liquor production, most distinctively in the production of the liquor Galliano. The fruits are commonly used as a spice, and the seeds are sometimes chewed after the meals to aid the digestion. Star anise has many culinary uses like, enhances the flavor of meat, the major component of *garam masala* and used as a spice in the preparation of *biryani* and *masala chai*. Traditionally, dried seedless fruit is used as incense. It is used for sweet fragrance while preparing butter-salted tea or sugar tea. Besides these properties, it is also gaining importance in the natural health world due to the medicinal values of phytochemicals present in the fruits. These plants have been extensively used for the treatment of infectious diseases in Iranian traditional medicine. The fruit consists of essential, as well as volatile oil. Traditionally, the fruit has been used as carminative, digestive, dyspepsia, antispasmodic, stimulant, antirheumatic, and diuretic. The paste/powder of Star anise is used to treat rheumatism and nostalgia, and is also used as an antiseptic. They are also used as medicine to treat cough, toothache, and sinusitis and to improve the strength of local alcohol. The fruit is considered as carminative, stomachic, and galactagogic. It is also used in curing vomiting, abdominal pain, dyspepsia, and food poisoning.

The star anise is a major source of chemical compound, such as shikimic acid, a primary precursor in the pharmacological synthesis of anti influenza drugs namely Oseltamivir (Tamiflu).There is a growing demand for star anise as a source of shikimic acid for the manufacture of anti-viral drugs widely used in the treatment and prophylaxis of avian flu (commonly bird flu). Shikimic acid is the starting compound utilized for the manufacture of the anti-viral drug oseltamivir. It is also a warming spice that contains powerful terpene antioxidants ie. Linalool and limonene. Linalool is capable of protecting the lipid bilayer present in the cell membranes, which protects the arteries and improves blood flow. Limonene shows strong anticancer activity within the body. These components also have the property of improving the energy levels and as an expectorant to remediate the mucous associated with bronchitis, asthma, common cold, and whooping cough. Chinese use fruits to treat some skin problems (Lai *et al.*, 1997). Star anise has been reported to have antifungal, antibacterial, carminative, analgesic, anticarcinogenic, sedative, and antioxidant properties.

The similar variety known as Japanese star anise (I. anisatum L.), is a closely resembling species but is not edible as it contains shikimitoxin and posses high toxicity. It can cause illness like serious neurological problems, "such as seizures". Many cases of illness have been reported after using star anise tea, e.g. serious neurologic and gastrointestinal toxicities such as convulsions, diarrhea and vomiting, (Biessels et al., 2002). Japanese star anise also contains anisantin, which are the main cause of severe inflammation of the kidneys, urinary tract and digestive organs, it's toxicity is caused due to its content in a potent neurotoxins (anisantin, neoanisantin and pseudoanisantin), because of their response as non-competitive antagonists of GABA receptor.

Apart from its toxicity for internal use, Japanese star anise was found useful in treating various types of skin complications in traditional medicine (Lai et al., 1997). It was also reported that Chinese star anise which is a widely known spice as well as safe food but sometimes could be found contaminated with highly toxic Japanese star anise (Lee et al., 2003a; Biessels et al., 2002; Ize-Ludlowet al., 2004; Vandenberghe et al., 2003;Johanns et al., 2002). It is therefore very important that *I. verum* fruits should be identified and differentiated from the fruits of the toxic species of *Illicium*, especially in powdered samples of *I. verum*. The difference between *I. lanceolatum* and *I. verum* could be noticed by the number of follicles. Star anise fruit usually contains eight follicles, while *I. lanceolatum* has ten to thirteen follicles in it.(Figure 1).

Figure 1. Morphological difference between star anise (I. verum) and poisonous star anise (I. lanceolatum).

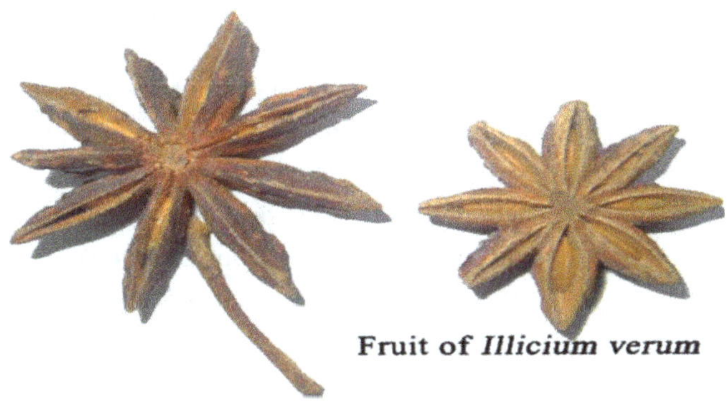

GENERAL FEATURES

Star anise is comprised of volatile oil, resin, and a high amount of fixed oil (Meisner, 1818). The fruit contains volatile oil, fat, resin, tannin, mucilage, and pectin. The volatile oil (*oil of star-anise*) is almost identical with *oil of anise* (from *P. Anisum*, Linné) and is amounts to about 4–5%. Star-anise oil from Chinese fruit has a specific gravity at 15°C (59°F) of 0.980–0.990, and its known constituents are anethol, phellandrene, safrol and hydro-quinone-ethyl-ether (Flückiger, 1879).Anethole contributes a large component of the distinctive flavors of star anise (Illiciaceae) an organic compound that is commonly used as a flavoring component. It is a type of aromatic compound and a derivative of phenylpropene, which occurs in essential oils naturally,. It is a colorless, fragrant, mildly volatile liquid. I. verum also provides lignans and seco-prezizaane-type sesquiterpenes in high quantity (Lee et al., 2003a,b;Okuyamaet al., 1993;Nakamuraet al., 1996; Song et al., 2007; Sy and Brown, 1998a,b). Illicium species contains unique structural types of these compounds which occur purely in Illicium species and they could be identified as characteristic chemical markers of *Illicium* species (Chang et al., 2010). These constituents were found to possess various biological activities as well as neurotoxic and neurotrophic effects (Huang et al., 2001b, 2002).

Table 1. Proximate Analysis of Star Anise

Nutritional composition	Harsha et al. 2003	Das et al (Acetone extract	Das et al (ethyl acetate extract)	R Dinesha et al. 2014
Carbohydrates	+	NA	NA	NA
Proteins & amino acids	++	--	--	1.23+.07mg/gm
Reducing sugar	+	--	--	1.63+.09mg/gm
Total Sugar	NA	NA	NA	54.2+4.92mg/gm

+ shows the presence, ++ shows the abundance and – shows the absence

CHEMICAL COMPOSITION

Medicinal plants have great importance in human health. Many studies have been done to analyze the particular phytochemicals present in star anise, which could be the marker of the purity of the beneficial species. The studies revealed that Chinese star anise contains about 5% volatile oil (ca. 10% in follicles and 2.5% in seeds), lignans, catechins, phenylpropanoid glucosides, and proanthocyanidins,. It also contains *trans*-anethole, which accounts as 80–90% as its major component. Estragole, β-farnesene, α-copaene, 1,4-cineole, β-bisabolene, (−)- and *trans*-α-bergamotene, nerolidol, methylanisoate, caryophyllene, *trans*-methylisoeugenol, cadinene, foeniculin, phellandrene, α-terpineol, 3-carene, *d*-α-pinene, hydroquinine, traces of *cis*-anethole, and safrole, are the other constituents found in it although the presence of safrole is disputed.

The fruit of *illicium verum* contains higher bitter principle, tannins, and essential oil (9-10%), consisting of anethole (85-90%), limone, β-phellandrene, α-terpineol, α-pinene, farnesol and safrol (Tuan et al. 1997,Dramic et al. 2009). There are 14 hydrocarbons components and 22 oxygenated hydrocarbon derivatives and small amount of nitrogenous compounds ρ-ally anisole, ρ- cumicaldehyde, anisaldehyde linoleic acid (1-4 methoxyphenyl)-prop-2-one, ρ-allylpen, anisylacetone, foeniculin and palmitic acid. (Yamada et al. 1965,Yan et al. 2002,Wang et al. 2007).The new phenylpropanoid glucosides, known phenylpropanoid, alkylglucosides and Seco-Cycloartane;3,4seco(242)cycloartane4(28),24(diene)3,26-dioic acid.26, methyl ester of nigranoic acid from the dichloromethane extract from leaves of *illicium verum* was identified.(Lee et al 2003,Lai et al 1998).

Forty-four compounds were identified from methyl alcohol (MA), Ethyl acetate(EA), and Petroleum ether (PE) extracts by GCMS, yielding 70.5%, 82.9%, and 92.7%, respectively, of the whole composition of the extracts. Results of GC-MS analysis found to have almost same composition in the three extracts. The most abundant component found was trans-anethole. Although, some minor components were different. For example, the methyl alcohol extract contained more of 4-ethyl benzaldehyde (3.4%) and 1-(4-methoxyphenyl)-2-propanone (3.7%); the Ethyl acetate extract contained more of cis-3,5-dimethoxy-β-methyl-β-nitrostyrene (4.2%),1-(3-methyl-2-butenoxy)-4-(1-propenyl)benzene (6.2%), hexadecanoic acid(4.1%), and Benzyl alcohol(4.0%); whereas the Petroleum ether extract contained more of 1-(3-methyl-2-butenoxy)-4-(1-propenyl) benzene (4.7%) and benzyl alcohol(2.8%) (Wei *et al* 2014).

The GC-MS pattern of fruit volatile oil of star anise shows the presence of 25 components, which account for 99.9% of the total amount. The major components identified were *trans*-anethole (93.9%), estragole (1.05%) and limonene (1.05%). Fifteen components are identified from its acetone extract, accounting for 80.27% of the total amount. *Trans*-Anethole (51.81%) is found as a major component, along with linoleic acid (11.6%), 1-(4-methoxyphenyl)-prop-2-one (6.71%), foeniculin (5.29%) and palmitic acid (1.47%) (Padmashree*et al.*, 2007).

Various extracts analyzed, like the ethanol extracts fractionated by hexane, ethyl ether, chloroform and ethyl acetate, and supercritical CO2 extracts. Amongst all of them, eight major components were identified by GC-MS analysis. Trans-anethole, anisyl alcohol, anisyl aldehyde, and anisyl acetone were present in a higher concentration than other phytoconstituents. As reported in the literature, (*E*)-anethole was the most abundant component in *I. verum* and proved to possess antimicrobial properties (Yang *et al.* 2010).

On the basis of different researches on extraction techniques and identification of volatile compounds the phytochemistry of *Illicuim Verum* describes that it contains essential oils, prenylated C6–C3 compounds,sesquiterpenes, lignans and flavonoids.

Table 2. Phytochemical compounds in star anise

Phytochemical Compounds	Harsha et al 2013	Das et al (Acetone extract)	Das et al (ethyl acetate extract)
Glycosides	--	--	--
Steroids	--	+	+
Alkaloids	--	+	+
Flavanoids	+	+	--
Saponins	--	--	--
Anthraquinones	+	--	--
Tannins	--	+	+
Terpenoids	+	+	--
Anthocynins	--	NA	NA
Leucoanthocynins	--	NA	NA
Coumarins	--	NA	NA
Emodins	+	NA	NA

+ Shows the presence of phytochemicals, --Shows the absence of phytochemicals

Seco-prezizaane-type Sesquiterpenes

Seco-prezizaane-type sesquiterpeneson can be isolated from the *Illicium* species. Sesquiterpenes can be classified into the three structurally unique skeletal classes like Seco-prezizaane, anislactone and allo-cedrane (Yamada et al.,1968; Kubo et al., 2009; Kouno et al., 1990; Huang et al., 2001a;Fukuyama et al., 1995; Schmidt et al., 2001). Seco-prezizaane-type sesquiterpenes on the basis of their carbon skeletons can be characterized into four subgroups like anisatin-type, pseudoanisatin-type, majucin-type, and minwanensin-type (Fukuyama et al., 1997; Yamada et al., 1968;Kouno et al., 1983; Yang et al., 1988,

1990). Anislactone-type sesquiterpenes have a different carbon skeleton from seco-prezizaane-type sesquiterpenes with two_-lactone.

Phenylpropanoids and Lignans

A characteristic component of *Illicium* species, Phenylpropanoids, are biosynthesized from shikimic acid. Anisoxide was also isolated from star anise oil extracted from the seeds of *I. verum* (Jackson and Short, 1937). A potential insecticide and as a sweetening substance (E)-anethole, which is a simple volatile phenylpropanoid, was isolated from the fruits of I. verum (Miyazawa et al., 1993; Hussainet al., 1990; Ho et al., 1997). It is found that star anise oils usually contain over 80% anethole.

Flavonoids and Other Constituents

Most of the commonly occurring flavonols in the plant kingdom were also extracted from the fruits of *I. verum* (Knackstedt and Herrmann, 1981). Kaempferol, and its glycosides and quercetin and its glycosides were the main flavanoids found from it. A ring of A-cleaved seco-cycloartane, which is the 26-methyl ester of nigranoic acid was yielded by the dichloromethane extract of the leaves of l. verum (Sy andBrown, 1998a).

THERAPEUTIC POTENTIALS OF STAR ANISE

Antioxidant Activity

Oxidation is one of the most important process for the production of free radical and these free radicals induces many of the defects in human body like arthritis, atherosclerosis, ischemia and reperfusion injury of many tissues, gastritis, cancer, central nervous system injury and AIDS (Kumpulainen and Salonen, 1999; Cook and Samman,1996). Free radicals developed due to environmental pollutants, chemicals, toxins, radiation, deep-fried and spicy food, as well as physical stress, cause weakening of immune system antioxidants, change in gene expression and induce abnormal proteins. Due to the depletion of immune system natural antioxidants in different maladies, consuming antioxidants as free radical scavengers may be necessary. But the synthetic antioxidants like BHT and BHA etc does possess harmful effects also hence now a day's many researches are going on for the identification of antioxidant properties of medicinal plants, spices, and herbs. The extract of star anise exhibited excellent activity for the inhibition of primary and secondary oxidation in rapeseed oil and could be acclaimed as a natural antioxidant, which may be used for the chemoprevention of diseases occurring due to oxidative deterioration (Anon., 1992). Anethole is the main component responsible for antioxidant activity, which is more than 80% (Padmashree*et al.*,2007). The antioxidant activity of star anise oil is due to the high percentage of anethole(more than 80%).

Yang et al 2011 has reported the antioxidant properties of the ethanol extracts fractionated by hexane, chloroform, ethyl ether and ethyl acetate, and supercritical CO2 extracts of the plant which were examined using 1,1-diphenyl-2-picryhydrazyl (DPPH) radical scavenging effect, the total equivalent antioxidant capacity and a reducing power assay. The amount of total phenolic content and the flavonoid content were also determined. The ethyl acetate fractions contained substantially higher levels of total phenolics and total flavonoids than the other extracts and possessed significant antioxidant activities. Due to their hydrogen donating ability or radical scavenging activity, the antioxidants show DPPH radical scavenging. Higher antioxidant activity can be indicated by lower IC50 value. The extracts obtained from the ethyl ether fractions and the ethyl acetate fractions showed a remarkable antioxidant activity with IC50 values of only 57.43 and 38.60 ppm, respectively. The decolorization of ABTS+ radicals exhibits the ability of an antioxidant to donate electrons or hydrogen atoms to inactivate the radicals. The neutralizing ability of ABTS+ radicals for the extracts of ethanol, the hexane, ethyl ether, chloroform, ethyl acetate and the aqueous fractions were found 15.82, 0.12, 26.75, 25.73, 26.95 and 18.24 mmol Trolox/100 g DW, respectively(**Table3,4**).

Table 3. Antioxidants content in star anise

References	TPC(mg/g)	Flavanoids(mg/g)	Ascorbic acid(mg/g)	α tocopherol (mg/g)
R Dinesha et al. (2014)(Ambient temperature water extract)	7.31+0.61	0.65+.02	5.16+0.41	0.51+.12
Boiling water extract	9.28+0.52	0.57+0.04	Nil	0.84+0.53
K Srinivasa et al (2012)MSA	271.2+0.93	14.64	NA	NA
SSA	289+0.78	13.98	NA	NA
Yang et al(2011) Ethanol crude extract	3.19+0.21	6.63+0.10	NA	NA
Hexane fraction	0.45+0.07	--	NA	NA
Ethyl ether fraction	4.19+0.53	4.84+0.11	NA	NA
Chloroform fraction	3.29+0.02	0.91+.01	NA	NA
Ethyl acetate fraction	4.49+0.12	28.63+0.87	NA	NA
Aqueous fraction	--	--	NA	NA

Table 4. Antioxidants activities of star anise

References	DPPH (μg/ml)	ABTS (μg/ml)	Hydroxyl radical (μg/ml)	Nitric oxide assay(μg/ml)	Lipid peroxide inhibition assay	Superoxide scavenging activity
R Dinesha et al. $$(2014) (Ambient temperature water extract)	37%	NA	37%	NA	55%	41%
Boiling water extract	39		39		52	48
K Srinivasa et al (2012)MSA(μg/ml)	0.508	0.714	18.65	266.09		
SSA	0.534	0.726	18.71	267.80		

Antifungal Activity

Star anise oil is a potent antifungal agent (Dzamic et al., 2009.) Because of anethole, the main component of star anise oil, it has been reported to possess antifungal activity (Hitokoto et al., 1980; Huang et al., 2010). It is also effective against dermatitis, and the oil does not give cross-reactions and pseudo-cross-sensitivity (Rudzki and Grzywa, 1976). Anethole itself is effective against the fungus gnat*Lycoriellaingenua* (Sciaridae) and the mold mite*Tyrophagusputrescentiae.* The recent findings of Singh *et al.* (2006) showed that the volatile oil inhibited the growth of *Fusarium moniliforme* completely at 6 µl dose. In the case of extract, 50% mycelial zone inhibition was obtained for *Penicillium citrinum* and *P. viridicatum.* Moreover, the volatile oil was found to be effective for controlling the growth of *F. moniliforme*and *Aspergillus niger*, whereas the extract has been found to be highly effective for *A. flavus.* The extracts from the star anise plant, Illiciumverum, showed significant promise as a natural anti-fungal agent ("Korean Journal of Medical Mycology,"). Candida albicans is a yeast,a form of fungi that is present naturally in the human mouth, intestines, throat, and genitourinary tract. When the body's balance of microflora is disturbed or immune system is somehow weakened, the uncontrolled growth of this yeast can lead to serious infection, known as candidiasis. Studies of South Korean researchers found that extracts and essential oils of star anise had shown strong antifungal properties when tested against *Candida albicans.*

A study showed that *I. verum* fruit extracts have high antifungal properties. The *I. verum* extract at a concentration of 4mg/ml inhibited the growth of *E. flucosum*and *T. mentagrophytes.* The extracts of *I. verum* at 16 mg/ml controlled all dermatophyte fungi tested. The *I. verum* fruits extract inhibited growth of *A. niger*, one of the most important saprophytic fungus known to be associated with mycotoxin production in agricultural products and foods at 16 mg/ml (Yazdani et ai 2009). The dominant component in *I. verum* oil is *trans*-Anethole, which has been shown to possess insecticidal, larvicidal, and antimicrobial activities.In order to compare the antifungal activity of *trans*-anethole with that of *I. verum* essential oil, *trans* anethole was detected to display similar inhibitory activity on the test fungi with IC50 values closed to those of the oil (Table 2), which suggested that *trans*-anethole was a major contributor to the antifungal properties of *I. verum* essential oil(Yongfu Huang et al 2010).

Antifungal activity was examined by in vitro mycelial radial growth inhibition assay, spore germination inhibition assay, and vapor contact assay. In this study, the IC50 values of the oil was found from 0.07 to 0.25 mg/mL against mycelia growth of eleven plant pathogenic fungi. On testing the growth of all test fungi, the IC50 values of the oil were ranged from 0.06mg/mL to 0.25 mg/mL. it was found that the positive control procymidone or carbendazim inhibited the growth of all test fungi completely at a dose of 5_g/mL.

Antibacterial Property

The spice has got potent antimicrobial properties. Chemical studies indicate that a major portion of this antimicrobial property is due to anethole, present in the dried fruit. Anethole (anise camphor) is an organic compound that is widely used as a flavoring substance. It is a derivative of phenylpropene, a type of aromatic compound that occurs widely in nature, in essential oils. It contributes a large component of the distinctive flavors of anise Anethole is an aromatic, unsaturatedether related to lignols . Anethole has potent antimicrobial properties and studies with isolated anethole (comparedwith standard anethole) indicated that itwas effective against bacteria, yeast and fungalstrains (De *et al.*, 2002). The extracth as shown better activity for *Staphylococcus aureus* and *Bacillus cereus* in comparison with commercial bactericide,i.e. Ampicillin. Phenylpropanoid glucosides from the fruits are preventive agents against sepsis(Lee *et al.*, 2003b). De et al. have identified anethole as an important antiseptic component, isolated from I. verum. It showed a minimum inhibitory concentration (MIC) of 5–50_g/mL against 12 bacteria and 15 fungi (De et al., 2002). Standard agar cup plate method was applied to examine the antiseptic activity of the isolated anethole using different microorganisms.

Table 5. Antibacterial activities of star anise

References	*E Coli*	*Salmonella*	*Pseudomonas aeruginos*	*Bacillus subtilis*	*S aureus*	*Proteus mirabilis*	*Bacillus cereus*
Shahnaz hamid et al 2003 (0.1ml extract)	10	NA	None	NA	None	None	
Gurdipsingh et al 2006(0.01ml extract)	18.7	--	25.0	--	--	NA	19.0
SaraswathyAriamuthu et al 2013(.04ml)	--	NA	--	--	--	--	12.0

(--) ineffective

Table 6. Minimum Inhibitory Concentration (MIC) of Star Anise (mg/ml)

Spicies	**Anushreechowdhury et al 2013**	**Parasa et al. 2012**	**SaraswathyArimuthu et al. 2013**
Vibrio cholera	12.5	NA	
Shigelladysenteriae	12.5	NA	
Vibrio fluvalis	12.5	NA	
Vibrio parahaemolyticus	12.5	NA	
E coli	12.5	NA	0.7
Salmonella typhi	12.5	NA	
Aeromonashydrophila	12.5	NA	
Proteus mirabilis	12.5	NA	0.7
A. Hydrophila	NA	1.56	
A .salmonicida	NA	0.78	
E. tarda	NA	0.78	
B.cereus	NA	NA	1.75
S.areus			1.05

Chemopreventive Property

Two phenylpropanoids having prenyl group, 4-allyl-2-methoxy-6-(3-methyl-2-butenyl) phenol and 4-allyl-2,6-dimethoxy-3-(3-methyl-2-butenyl) phenol,showed more potent activities as anti-tumour promoters. The presence of a prenyl moiety in the phenylpropanoids plays an important role in antitumor-promoting activity. Hence, the prenylated phenyl propanoids might be valuable as potential cancer chemopreventive agents. The sulphorhodamine B (SRB) assay, was used to check the cytotoxicity of the methanol extracts of I. verum and the IC50 concentration, which has reduced B16 cells growth percentage by 50% was found to be 43.68 and 37.59_g/mL, respectively. The study can postulate that the antitumor action of I. verum is due to its antiangiogenic activity, rather than its cytotoxicity.

Insecticidal Property

Star anise was found to possess insecticidal activity due to thirteen seco-prezizaaneterpenoids isolated from it (Kuriyama*et al.*, 2002). The insecticidal activities of Anisatin and pseudoanisatin was checked against German cockroaches (*Blattellagermanica* L.). phenylpropene, (*E*)-anethole, derived from the fruit of star anise, was found to have insecticidal activity against adults of *B. germanica* (Chang and Ahn, 2002). *I. verum* fruit-derived components being naturally occurring insect-control agents, are useful in controlling the population of *B. germanica.* Insecticidal properties of star anise were also observed in non-polar crude extracts, against eggs, larvae, and adults of *Triboliumcastaneum* (Herbst) and *Sitophilus zeamais*Motsch (Ho *et al.*, 1995).Anethole also is found to be a promising insecticide. Several oils formulae consisting a high amount of anethole are found to have insecticidal action against larvae of the mosquitos *Ochlerotatuscaspius* and Aedesaegypti.

Insecticidal activity of star anise was observed against fruit flies (Drosophila melanogaster) and D. (Miyazawa et al., 1993). The insecticidal activity of (E)-anethole was found against adults of Blattellagermanica (Chang and Ahn, 2002). The methanol extract of I. verum fruit found to have appreciable insecticidal activity against Lasiodermaserricorne adults on applying at 3.5mg/cm2 in a filter paper diffusion method (Kimet al., 2003). Insecticidal properties against Botrytis cinerea, Callosobruchuschinensis, T. castaneum, and Colletotrichumgloeosporioides were also observed in essential oil from the fruit of I. verum (Chaubey 2008; Shukla et al., 2008; Lee et al., 2007). The toxicity of star anise oil was also reported against , C. chinensis, T. castaneum and golden snail by Maini and Morallo-Rejesus (1992).

Analgesic, Sedative and Convulsive Activity

According to modern pharmacological studies, crude extracts and active compounds of star anise acquire a wide variety of pharmacological benefits, particularly in antimicrobial, antioxidant, insecticidal, analgesic, sedative and convulsive activities.

The methanol extract and ethyl acetate extract of star anise indicated hypothermia at an oral dose of 3 g/kg and 100 mg/kg respectively. The methanolic extract also exhibited 23% writhing inhibition at an oral dose of 500 mg/kg, while the ethyl acetate extract, administration at a dose of 500 mg/kg caused convulsions and lethal toxicity in mice. Three active components from the extracts, were isolated namely, veranisatins A, B, and C. On administration of these compounds orally at 3mg/kg was able to produce convulsions and lethal toxicity in mice and also shown a hypothermic effect without convulsions at lower doses such as 0.5 or 1mg/kg. Out of these compounds, veranisatin A was further examined for its analgesic and sedative effects. It exhibited analgesic effects at an oral dose of 0.1 mg/kg (Okuyama et al., 1993; Nakamura et al., 1996).

Digestive Aid

Star anise also gets its distinctive sweet licorice flavor from its major chemical compound anethole. Anethole has been proved helpful for digestion and improvement of symptoms of colic in babies and irritable bowel syndrome in adults. It is thought that it activates enzymes within the body, which improve the digestive process of proteins and fats. Due to this, it reduces gas and bloating and improves nutritional absorption. Consuming star anise tea after meals helps treat digestive ailments such as bloating, gas, indigestion, and constipation. Star anise tea is consumed widely after meals in china and other south east asian countries and also in US as it helps to treat digestive ailments, such as bloating, abdominal cramps, gas, indigestion and constipation and also found to activate the metabolic enzymes. **Alt**hough in India, the consumption of star anise tea is not very high, but it is an important ingredient of *masala chai*. Intake of such tea may help to overcome the digestive problems.

Improve Hormone Function in Women

To boost the mother's immunity and increases milk secretion star anise was given to women during pregnancy and lactating period in traditional Chinese medicine. This was also scientifically studied in recent times and it has been reported that star anise has an estrogenic effect due to the presence of a substance, anethole, which stimulates the hormonal function in women. The compounds including diantheole and photoantheole present in star anise, are responsible for promoting lactation in nursing mothers. They also increase libido and help reduce symptoms associated with premenstrual syndrome. However, this herb should not be used during pregnancy due to its effect on female hormone levels and the potential for complications.

CONCLUSION

Star anise is widely used as a culinary as well as a medicinal fruit and commonly used in most of the indigenous medicines. It was found to consist of potential phytochemicals with which it can be developed into natural therapeutic aid against various diseases. The fruit is a very important source of essential and volatile oil. Traditionally the fruit has been utilized as digestive, carminative, antispasmodic, dyspepsia, stimulant, antirheumatic, and diuretic. Many preclinical studies indicate the therapeutic potential of oil of I. verum fruit in the treatment of microbial diseases, as well as antifungal and antioxidant. Different studies have shown the presence of shikimic acid as a precursor of Tami flu, anethole, anisylacetone, limonene, linoleic acid, anisaldehyde, and palmitic acid and presence of seco-cycloartane in leaves. The therapeutic potential of this plant still remains as the area of investigation for researchers. Thus for applying it in ayurvedic medicine, more clinical trial and novel drug delivery systems must be developed to improve its medicinal benefits.

REFERENCES

Anon. (1992). Les agentsantioxygenes. *Pour la Science*, *179*, 10–12.

Chang, K. S., & Ahn, Y. J. (2002). Fumigant activity of (E)-anethole identified in Illiciumverum fruit against Blattellagermanica. *Journal of Pest Management Science*, *58*(2), 161–166. doi:10.1002/ps.435 PMID:11852640

Cook, N. C., & Samman, S. (1996). Flavonoids- chemistry, metabolism, cardioprotective effects, and dietary sources. *Nutritional Biochemistry*, *7*(2), 66–76. doi:10.1016/0955-2863(95)00168-9

De, M., De, A. K., Sen, P., & Banerjee, A. B. (2002). Antimicrobial properties of star anise (Illicium-verum Hook f). *Journal of Phytotherapy Research*, *16*(1), 94–95. doi:10.1002/ptr.989 PMID:11807977

Flückinger, F. A. (1879). *Pharmacographia: A History of the Principal Drugs of Vegetable Origin, Met with in Great Britain and British India*. London: Macmillan.

Goodman, P. S. (2005). *Star Rises in Fight Against Bird Flu. Demand for a Chinese Fruit 2Skyrockets*. Washington Post Foreign Service.

Hitokoto, H., Morozumi, S., Wauke, T., Sakai, S., & Kurata, H. (1980). Inhibitory effects of spices on growth and toxin production of toxigenic fungi. *Applied and Environmental Microbiology*, *39*(4), 818–822. doi:10.1128/AEM.39.4.818-822.1980 PMID:6769391

Ho, S. H., Ma, Y., Goh, P. M., & Sim, K. Y. (1995). Star anise, Illiciumverum Hook f. as a potential grain protectant against Ttiboliumcastaneum (Herbst) and Sitophilus zeamaisMotsch. *Postharvest Biology and Technology*, *6*(3-4), 341–347. doi:10.1016/0925-5214(95)00015-X

Itoigawa, M., Ito, C., Tokuda, H., Enjo, F., Nishino, H., & Furukawa, H. (2004). Cancer chemopreventive activity of phenylpropanoids and phytoquinoids from *Illicium plants. Cancer Letters*, *214*(2), 165–169. doi:10.1016/j.canlet.2004.05.005 PMID:15363542

Kumpulainen, J. T., & Salonen, J. T. (1999). *Natural Antioxidants and Anticarcinogens in Nutrition. In Health and Disease* (pp. 178–187). The Royal Society of Chemistry. doi:10.1533/9781845698409

Kuriyama, T., Schmidt, T. J., Okuyama, E., & Ozoe, Y. (2002). Structure–activity relationships of secoprezizaaneterpenoids in gamma-aminobutyric acid receptors of houseflies and rats. *Bioorganic & Medicinal Chemistry*, *10*(6), 1873–1881. doi:10.1016/S0968-0896(02)00011-1 PMID:11937345

Lai, M., Yao, W., Yang, M., Huang, P., Liu, B., & Zheng, X. (1997). Studies on the pharmacognosy of Cortex Illicii and its adulterants. *Zhong Yao Cai*, *20*(12), 601–604. PMID:12572500

Lee, S. W., Li, G., Lee, K. S., Jung, J. S., Xu, M. L., Seo, C. S., ... Son, J. K. (2003). Preventive agents against sepsis and new phenylpropanoid glucosides from the fruits of *Illiciumverum. Planta Medica*, *69*(9), 861–864. doi:10.1055-2003-43210 PMID:14598217

Lee, S. W., Li, G., Lee, K. S., Song, D.-K., & Son, J.-K. (2003). A new phenylpropanoid glucoside from the fruits ofIllicium verum. *Archives of Pharmacal Research*, *26*(8), 591–593. doi:10.1007/BF02976705 PMID:12967191

Meisner, W. (1818). Beitragzur Geschichte des Chrom. *Annalen der Physik*, *60*(12), 366–394. doi:10.1002/andp.18180601204

Padmashree, A., Roopa, N., Semwal, A. D., Sharma, G. K., Agathian, G., & Bawa, A. S. (2007). Star-anise (*Illiciumverum*) and black caraway (*Carumnigrum*) as natural antioxidants. *Food Chemistry*, *104*(1), 59–66. doi:10.1016/j.foodchem.2006.10.074

Rizvi, S. S. H., Benado, A. L., Zollweg, J. A., & Daniels, J. A. (1986). Supercritical fluid extraction operating principles and food applications. *Food Technology (Chicago)*, *40*(7), 57–64.

Rudzki, E., & Grzywa, Z. (1976). Sensitizing and irritating properties of star anise oil. *Contact Dermatitis*, *2*(6), 305–308. doi:10.1111/j.1600-0536.1976.tb03065.x PMID:1032123

Singh, G., Maurya, S., Marimuthu, P., Murali, H. S., & Bawa, A. S. (2007). Antioxidant and Antibacterial investigations on essential oils and acetonc extracts of some spices. *Journal of Natural Product Radiance*, *6*(2), 114–121.

Vijayakumar, A., Duraipandiyan, V., Jeyaraj, B., Agastian, P., Raj, M. K., & Ignacimuthu, S. (2012). Phytochemical analysis and in vitro antimicrobial activity of Illicium griffithii Hook. f. & Thoms extracts. *Asian Pacific Journal of Tropical Disease*, *2*(3), 190–199. doi:10.1016/S2222-1808(12)60045-0

Wei1a, L., Hua, R., Lilc, M., Huan, Y., Lile, S., He1f, Y., & Shen, Z. (2014). Chemical composition and biological activity of star anise *Illiciumverum*extracts against maize weevil, *Sitophilus zeamais*adults. *Journal of Insect Science*, *14*.

Yamada, K., Takada, S., Nakamura, S., & Hirata, S. (1965). The structure of noranisatin, an oxidation product of anisatin. *Tetrahedron Letters*, *52*(52), 4785–4794. doi:10.1016/S0040-4039(01)89035-3

Yan, J. H., Xiao, X. X., & Huang, K. L. (2002). Component analysis of volatile oil from Illicium Verum Hook. f. *Journal of Central South University of Technology*, *9*(3), 173–176. doi:10.100711771-002-0021-3

Yang, C. H., Chang, F. R., Chang, H. W., Wang, S. M., Hsieh, M. C., & Chuang, L. Y. (2011). Investigation of the antioxidant activity of *Illiciumverum* extracts. *Journal of Medicinal Plants Research*, *6*(2), 314–324.

Yazdani, D., Rezazadeh, S., Amin, G., Zainal Abidin, M.A., Shahnazi, S., & Jamalifar, H. (2009). Antifungal Activity of Dried Extracts of Anise *(PimpinellaanisumL.)* and Star anise (*IlliciumverumHook.* f.) Against Dermatophyte and Saprophyte Fungi. *Journal of Medicinal Plans*, *8*(S5).

Chapter 8
Pharmacological Activity and Nutritional Potential of *Buchanania lanzan Spreng*

Akanksha Awasthi
Babu Banarasi Das Northern India Institute of Technology, India

Nisha
Central University of Rajasthan, India

ABSTRACT

The plant science that studies the historical and current uses of plants is called ethnobotany. Spices and herbs have since medieval times been categorized as having medicinal properties. India is a land of spices, and several spices have been grown in the country. Buchanania lanzan Spreng, commonly known as char, achar, and chironji, is one among these spices. It has been referred to as one having immense value and medicinal use. The chapter discusses the cultivation, uses, chemical constituents, and therapeutic activities of Buchanania lanzan Spreng and emphasizes the need for and importance of pharmacognostic study.

INTRODUCTION

The plant science that studies the historical and current uses of plants is termed as ethnobotany. Since medieval times, spices and herbs have been categorized as having medicinal properties. India is a land of spices, and several spices, such as Buchanania lanzan Spreng,are grown in the country. Buchanania lanzan Spreng is commonly known as char, achar, and chironji. Francis Buchanan-Hamilton, M.D. (1762-1829), was a physician and made significant contributions as a geographer and botanist, is said to have been the first person to describe this plant in 1798. It belongs to the family of anacardiaceae. It is a wild plant, which grows in India's tropical deciduous forests. It mainly grows in the northern, central, and western parts of India. It is mainly cultivated in Chhattisgarh, Jharkhand, Madhya Pradesh, and in the Varanasi and Mirzapur districts of Uttar Pradesh. Apart from India, it is also found in several tropical

DOI: 10.4018/978-1-7998-2524-1.ch008

countries, including Asia, the Pacific Islands,and Australia. As an Indian spice it has been referred to as one possessing immense value and medicinal use (Singh, Gupta, Kumar, Singh, & Tiwari,2018). Traditional indigenous knowledge reveals that almost all the parts of the plant possess some pharmacological properties, be it the roots, leaves, fruits, seeds, or the gum. However,today, the spice, having numerous medicinal properties,has made its way into the *Red Data Book* published by the International Union for Conservation of Nature and Natural Resources,(IUCN) as one among the valuablespices (Kirtikar,1935). Nutritionally the spice is found to be a good source of protein with43.24% protein, 38% fat, 18.50% crude fibre,% and 2.20% minerals,which include several minerals ranging from phosphorus, zinc, calcium, iron, copper, magnesium, manganese, to aluminium, boron, barium, tin, and more (Khatoon, Gupta & Tyag, 2015). The oil extracted from this spice has been considered as good as almond oil and is often used as its replacement (Kumar, Vengaiah, Srivastava & Bhowmick.,2012).The chemical constituents of the oil extracted from the spice are 8-cineole, A-pinene, B-pinene, camphene,myrcene, triglycerides (dipalmito-1-olein and triolein), Y-terpinene, and sabinene. The spice has also been found to contain tannins, saponins, glycosides, steroids, flavonoids, and phenol (Kodati, Pareta, & Patra, 2010).

Buchanania lanzan Spreng have been reported to have several pharmacological activity such as antioxidant, antimicrobial and anti-inflammatory activity. The plant is used in Ayurveda and the Unani systems of medicine as a nervine tonic, anti-cough, anti-leprotic, and oleation. It has also been found to possess antioxidant and anti-inflammatory activity. Tribes of Chhattisgarh and Jharkhand mainly use it for wound healing, anti-diarrhoeal, analgesic, and anti-ulcer activity (Kodati et al, 2010). In India, the plant has well-known traditional uses and its seeds are used as an expectorant and tonic. The oil extracted from the kernels is applied to soothe skin diseases and also to remove spots and blemishes from the face. The root is used as an expectorant, in biliousness, and also for curing blood diseases. The juice of the leaves is digestive, expectorant, aphrodisiac, and purgative. The rhizome of B. lanzan finds an important place in indigenous medicine as an expectorant, diuretic, and carminative. Sushma et al. (2013) also found it to have anti-cancer, anti-hypertensive, larvicidal, anti-diabetic properties and antibacterial activity. It have been reported that B. lanzan also have broad-spectrum antimicrobial activity and could be a potential source of new classes of antibiotics that could serve as selective agents for infectious diseases and chemotherapy.

The present study discusses the cultivation, uses, chemical constituents, and therapeutic activities of Buchanania lanzan Spreng as well as emphasizes the need and importance of a pharmacognostic study of Buchanania lanzan Spreng. One of the well-established and universally accepted facts is that spices possess medicinal properties, and so are an integral and indispensable part of the traditional system of medicine practiced worldwide, because of their economic viability, easy accessibility, and century's old experience. As nature's gifts, spices are considered to be biocompatible, environment-friendly, non-toxic, much cheaper, and quite freely available in comparison to synthetic substances. They are also amongst the richest renewable source of biopolymers, having enormous potential for uses and applications in numerous industries, such as food, cosmetics, pharmaceuticals, and a host of others. Buchanania lanzan has a high socio-economic value for providing a livelihood to the tribal population of the area besides possessing enormous potentials as a commercial horticulture species. Unfortunately, due to over-exploitation and indiscriminate harvesting (lopping and cutting), a considerable reduction in the population of Buchanania lanzan has been recorded in the recent past, leading to a very severe threat to its becoming extinction, which calls for urgent conservation efforts at all levels.

Table 1. Botanical origin and vernacular names of Buchanania lanzan

Botanical Origin	Vernacular Names
Kingdom: Plantae Order: Spindales Family: Anacardiaceae Sub-family: Anacardioideae Genus: Buchanania Species: BuchananialanzanSpreng	Bengali: Chironji Hindi: Achar, Char, Baruda, Priyala Gujarati & Marathi: Charoli, Pyalchar Kannada: Charpoppu Malyalam: Mungapper Oriya: Charu Sanskrit: Priyalam, Char, Rajadana, Dhanu. Tamil: Morala Telugu: Saarachettu, Morichettu

Cultivation and Distribution

Buchanania lanzan Spreng, also known as Chironjee,is thought to have originated in India. The tree has been observed as a wildly growing one in the tropical deciduous forests of India. It is primarily found in the states of Bihar, Orissa, Jharkhand, Chhattisgarh, Madhya Pradesh, Andhra Pradesh, Maharashtra, Gujarat, and Rajasthan. It has also been found in the sub-Himalayan regions upto an elevation of about 1200 m. It has also been found in neighbouring countries, such as Burma, Nepal, other tropical Asian countries, Australia, and the Pacific Islands. Two varieties have been reported to yield edible fruits among the seven different species that have been found in the country. These edible fruits occupy the lower to middle canopy in the dry deciduous forests, and they are commonly associated with plants like sal, teak, salai, etc.

The tree generally grows to a height of 18 m, the bark of the tree is roughly 10-12 mm thick and is black or dark brown in colour, rough, and tessellate, the cracks being deep and narrow, so that the bark almost resembles the hide of a crocodile. The leaves are alternate, simple and estipulate; petiole-is 12-22 mm, stout, glabrous; laminais 10-23.5x 5-12 cm, broadly oblong, with a round or acute base; obtuse or emarginate apex, margin entire, glabrous above, and densely tomentose beneath, coriaceous; lateral nerves 10-20 pairs, pinnate, prominent, pubescent, secondary laterals prominent, intercostal reticulate, prominent.

The flowers are bisexual in nature, greenish-white in colour, sessile, in pubescent terminal and axillary panicles; calyx has five lobes, persistent; petals are oblong, reflexed, pilose, and also are five in number; 10 stamens are inserted at the base of the fleshy disc; filaments are glabrous, free, disc cupular, pilose, and five-lobed; carpels are generally tomentose, superior, free and are generally 5-6 in number, and one free ovule, which is pendulous, style is lateral, and stigma is truncate. The fruit is a drupe, about 10–13mm x 8 mm in size, laterally compressed, oblong, brownish-black to black in colour, with a hard stone that is two valved with one seed(Gupta, Sharma, & Tandon,2004).

Chemistry

The Chironjee tree has been reported to be a source of varied, unknown, phyto-chemicals. Several researchers have reported the fact that the leaf, bark, and seed are an important source of phytochemicals that possess pharmacological activity. Studies revealed that leaves contain tannins, triterpenoids, saponins, flavonoids, kaempferol-7-o'glucosides, quercetin-3-rahmnoglucoside, quercetin, gallic acid, kaemferol, and reducing sugars, including a new glycoside, and myricetin-3'-rhmnoside-3-galactoside.Epinitol, vomicine, and celidoniol are the major compounds that were obtained from the methanolic extracts of the leaves after undergoing several chemical tests and spectral analysis. Tannins, alkaloids, and saponins, have been mainly found in the bark, whereas the seed has been reported to be a good a source of dietary fibre, carbohydrates, fats, vitamins, such asthiamine, riboflavin, niacin,as well as minerals like calcium, chlorine, copper, magnesium, iron, potassium, phosphorus, sulphur, sodium, β-amyrin, and fatty oil. Chironjioil contains53.7% oleic acid, 33.4% palmitic acid,6.3% stearic acid,6.0% linoleic acid, and 0.6% myristic acid. The special characteristic of B. lanzan seed oil is its content of 22.7% of dipalmito-1-olein, 31% of dioleopalmitin,and 11.3% of triolein (Gupta, Sharma, & Tandon,2004).

Nutrients

B. lanzan is not only a source of food and nutrients for the tribal's residing around the Dnyanganga Wildlife Sanctuary, but is also a source of their livelihood, as they earn their bread by selling the spice. B. lanzan contains about 3% moisture, 12.1% carbohydrates; it is a rich source of lipids and proteinsi.e. 59% and 19.0%to 21.6%, respectively, and it contains 37-47% fatty oil. It is also a good source of minerals such as calcium (279 mg), phosphorus (528 mg), and iron (8.5 mg). A high Calcium content does not only play a mandatory role in providing rigidity to the skeleton, but is also vital for blood clotting and many other metabolic processes (Reid, Ames, Evans, Gamble, & Sharpe, 1993) Phosphorous plays a vital role in the maintenance of healthy bones and teeth and is an important part in energy metabolism. These minerals play a crucial role in several body metabolisms and, thus, have vital therapeutic significance. Vitamins like thiamine (0.69 mg), riboflavin (0.53 mg), niacin (1.50 mg), and ascorbic acid (5.0 mg) are also present in this plant. It is also a fair source of fibre, about 3.8% (Khatoon, Gupta & Tyagi 2015). While the seed is generally used as an expectorant and tonic, the oil extracted from the kernels is used for removing blemishes and spots from the face and in curing skin diseases. The gum of the plant is used as an analgesic after being mixed with goat's milk, while the juice extracted from the leaves is a digestive, expectorant, aphrodisiac, and purgative.

PHARMACOLOGY

B.lanzanoccupies an important place in the history of plants with medicinal value and has been traditionally used in the treatment of several diseases. This plant has a long history of folk use in tribal societies across the tropical regions of the world. It is used in the treatment of intrinsic hemorrhage and bloody diarrhoea, both in the form of a decoction and as a tonic. During weaning of a child, it should be given sweet bolus prepared of B. lanzan kernels, madhuka (glycyrrhiza glabra) honey, parched paddy, and sugar candy. In the case of fever and burning sensations, the powder of the kernel is given along with milk as a treatment. According to Warokar, Ghante, Duragkar, &Bhusari (2010) in case of bloody dysentery, the powder of the bark is given along with honey.

Wound Healing

For use in wound healing, B.lanzan plants were collected and then shade dried. The fruits were then crushed into small pieces and powdered. The powder was extracted viasoxhlet extractor with 95% ethanol. Then extract was concentrated under reduced pressure at a temperature of 50^0C to a thick viscid consistency, then dried and used as medication. B. lanzan extract administered orally and intramuscularly, once daily, from 0-9 days, showed healing. The process of mobilizing healthy skin around the wound to cover the denuded area while healing of the wound took place iis called wound contraction.Since B. lanzan enhances wound contraction by increasing contractile properties of myofibroblasts or increases the number of myofibroblasts collected at the wound area, it assistsin wound healing(Chitra, Dharani, Pavan, and Narayana 2009).

Analgesic & Anti-inflammatory

Studies conducted by Patsnaik Kodati, Pareta, Patra,& Harwansh (2016) demonstrated that at a dosage of 400 mg per kg of BuchananialanzanSprenga, positive analgesic response was observed among acetic acid-induced analgesia, when compared to control group animals. Even for carrageenan-induced acute inflammation produced by injecting 0.1.ml of (1%) carrageenan into the plantar surface of rat's hind paw. B. lanzan extract reduced the paw edema.

Antioxidant

Patra et al.(2011) reported that B.lanzancontains a fairly good amount of phenolic compounds that possess potential oxidation value and are an efficient oxidative radical scavenger. They can scavenge free radicles and, thus, act as potent antioxidants. The root's methanolic and acetone extract, as estimated by folin-ciocalteu reagent method, portrayed that it contained 510.79±8.308 and 475.03±7.290 mg gallic acid equivalent per 100 gm, respectively. The plants play a more crucial role in the human diet, as they assist in the prevention of many human diseases. These preventive properties of the plants have been credited to the presence of flavonoids and other polyphenolic compounds, which may exert their effects as a result of antioxidant activity; the greater the phenol and flavonoid content, the stronger the antioxidant activity.

Anti-Diabetic

The lack of the secretion of insulin from the beta cells of the pancreas langerhens and hyper-glycaemic conditions due to an abnormality in carbohydrate, lipid, and protein metabolism, induce diabetes. The leaves, air-dried, powdered, and extracted with 99% methanol, at the dose of 100mg/kg and 200mg/kg, are shown to reduced blood glucose levels (Sushma et al.,2013).

Anti-Hyperlipidaemic

Metabolic abnormality creates a hyperlipidaemic condition that results in diabetes and obesity. The leaves, air-dried, powdered, and extracted, with 99% methanol, at the dose of 100mg/kg and 200mg/kg are shown to reduced blood glucose levels (Sushma et al.,2012).

Adaptogenic Activity

The methanolic extract was prepared from the dried powder of the leaves using a soxhlet apparatus. Rats, when forced to swim in a restricted space, become immobile after a certain period of vigorous activity, which indicates a state of mental depression. An increase in total swimming time indicates better stress tolerance. Adaptogens of plant origin reduce the reactivity of the host defense system and decreases the damaging effects of the different stressors due to increased basal levels of mediators that are involved in the stress response. In conclusion, the present study provides scientific support for the antistress (adaptogenic) activity of the methanolic extract from the leaf of Buchanan lanzan(Mehta-Nayeem, & Bains, 2011).

Antiulcer Activity

Excessive production of gastric juice and/or reduction in the production of gastric mucosa might result in a peptic ulcer. Patil and Rothe (2017), and Kodati, Pareta, & Patra (2010) observed that ethanol-induced ulcers in mice, and pylorus ligation-induced ulcer in rats, at a concentration of 200-400 mg per kg of B. lanzan extract helped in treatment, and showed both preventive and therapeutic action on the gastric ulcer.

Memory Booster

The human brain is made of billions of neurons, which connect together to form a network and are engaged in performing numerous activities, such as hearing, thinking, reading, etc. Neurons work as small industrial plants that receive supplies, generate energy, construct equipment, get rid of unwanted signals, process stored information, and communicate to other cells. For the proper and smooth running of impulse transmission, proper coordination, an ample amount of fuel and oxygen are required. Researchers have revealed that beta-amyloid peptide, especially with 39-42 amino acid residues play a major role in the development of Alzheimer. Even though, to date, no cure has been found for the disease, it can still be managed to some extent with the help of drugs. Studies have demonstrated that foods with natural antioxidants like vitamin E, beta-carotene, and vitamin C may help in scavenging the free radicals generated during initiation and disease progression. Lack or shortage of acetylcholine, a neurotransmitter, is considered to be an important cause of memory loss. The amount of acetylcholine in the brain can be increased by inhibiting the activity of an enzyme i.e. acetylcholinesterase, which catalyses the breakdown of acetylcholine, thereby delaying the development of the disease.

Chironji seeds extract at an oral dosage of 500 mg per kg was studied for its neuro-psychopharmacological effect on experimental rats.The activity of seeds extract on memory acquisition, and retention showed positive results(Patil and Rothe 2017).

Anti-Venom Activity

Chironji has been listed among the plants that possess anti-snake venom properties. Minu, Harsh, Ravikant, Paridhi, Noopur (2012) documented that the fruit and the bark of the tree are used in and around the Chhattisgarh region in the treatment of snakebite by the tribals. Several in vitro and in vivo studies of the ethanolic extracts of the bark have revealed a positive result against snake venom. Patil and Rothe (2017) evaluated the effect of the extract against toxicity induced by Naja Kaouthia snake venom. The author studied the effect on neutralization of lethality, myotoxicity, phospholipase A2 activity, and human red blood cell lysis, produced via snake venom. Results revealed that at a dosage of 200-400 mg per kg, the extract had the ability to neutralize the lethality produced by the snake venom at different concentrations. A decrease in the creatine phosphokinase level characteristically demonstrated a decrease in the myotoxicity level. Haemolytic activity was also found to decline significantly with the extract in vitro model.

Diuretic Activity

Diuretic activity means the ability of any substance to form urine or to help in its formation. According to Patil and Rothe (2017), alcoholic extracts and n-hexane extracts of B. lanzanat a dosage level of 500 mg per kg produced a significant diuretic effect, which was comparable to furosemide, a standard diuretic drug. However, studies still need to be conducted to isolate the active phytochemical constituent that plays a major role in inducing the mechanism of diuresis; also the exact site of its action needs to be explored.

CONCLUSION

In the present era where herbs are once again looked upon as possible solutions to existing diseased conditions, in-depth research is needed to establish the pharmacological properties of foods and novel sources scientifically. In the present review, an attempt has been made to document the global efforts made by several studies to explore and establish the pharmacological and nutritional potential of Buchanania lanzanSpreng.

REFERENCES

Chitra, V., Dharani, P. P., Pavan, K. K., & Alla, N. R. (2009). Wound healing activity of alcoholic extract of Buchanania lanzan in Albino rats. *International Journal of Chemtech Research*, *1*(4), 1026–1031.

Khatoon, N., Gupta, R. K., & Tyagi, Y. K. (2015). Nutraceutical potential and phytochemical screening of Buchanania lanzan, an underutilized exotic Indian nut and its use as a source of functional food. *Journal of Pharmacognosy and Phytochemistry*, *4*(1).

Kirtikar, K.R. (1935). *Indian medicinal plants: Lalit mohan basu*. Allahabad, India: Academic Press.

Kodati, D., Pareta, S., & Patra, K. C. (2010). Antiulcer activity of ethanolic extract of B. lanzan Spreng roots. *Annals of Biological Research*, *1*(4), 234–239.

Kumar, J., Vengaiah, P. C., Srivastava, P. P., & Bhowmick, P. K. (2012). Chironji nut (Buchanania lanzan) processing, present practise and scope. *Indian Journal of Traditional Knowledge*, *11*(1), 202–204.

Mehta, K. S., Nayeem, N., & Bains, N. (2011). Adaptogenic activity of methanol extract of B. Lanzanleaves an experimental study in rat model. *Der Pharmacia Sinica*, *2*(3), 107–112.

Minu, V., Harsh, V., Ravikant, T., Paridhi, J., & Noopur, S. (2012). Medicinal plants of chhattisgarh with anti-snake venom property. *International Journal of Current Pharmaceutical Research*, *3*(2), 1–10.

Patil, R. N., & Rothe, S. P. (2017). Buchanania lanzan: An enormous medicinal value. *International Journal of Advance Research and Innovative Ideas in Education*, *3*(1), 2395–4396.

Patra, K. C., Pareta, S. K., Harwansh, R. K., & Kumar, J. (2011). Antioxidant activity of B. lanzan spreng. *Pharmacologyonline*, *1*, 733–739.

Patsnaik, A. K., Kodati, D., Pareta, S. K., Patra, K. C., & Harwansh, R. K. (2011). Analgesic and anti-inflammatory activities of BuchananialanzanSpreg. roots. *Research Journal of Pharmaceutical, Biological and Chemical Sciences*, *2*(1), 419–425.

Pattnaik, A., Sarkar, R., Sharma, A., Yadav, K. K., Kumar, A., Roy, P., ... Sen, T. (2013). Pharmacological studies on Buchanania lanzan Spreng.-A focus on wound healing with particular reference to anti-biofilm properties. *Asian Pacific Journal of Tropical Biomedicine*, *3*(12), 967–974. doi:10.1016/S2221-1691(13)60187-2 PMID:24093788

Reid, I. R., Ames, R. W., Evans, M. C., Gamble, G. D., & Sharpe, S. J. (1993). Effect of calcium supplementation on bone loss in postmenopausal women. *The New England Journal of Medicine*, *328*(7), 460–464. doi:10.1056/NEJM199302183280702 PMID:8421475

Singh, R. B., Gupta, D., Kumar, S., Singh, K., & Tiwari, C. (2018). Buchanania lanzan spreng (Chironji): A vulnerable multipurpose tree species in Vindhyam region. *Journal of Pharmacognosy and Phytochemistry*, *7*(5), 833–836.

Sushma, N., Smitha, P. V., Gopal, Y. V., Vinay, R., Reddy, N. S., Mohan, M., & Raju, B. (2013). Antidiabetic, antihyperlipidaemic, antioxidant activities of Buchanania lanzan Spreng methanol leaf extract in streptozotocin induced Types I & II diabetic rats. *Tropical Journal of Pharmaceutical Research*, *12*(2), 221–226.

The wealth of India: A dictionary of Indian raw materials and industrial products. (2000). New Delhi: National Institute of Science Communication.

Warokar, A. S., Ghante, M. H., Duragkar, N. J., & Bhusari, K. P. (2010). Anti-inflammatory and antioxidant activities of methanolic extract of Buchananialanzan Kernel. *Indian Journal of Pharmaceutical Education*, *44*(4), 363–368.

Chapter 9
Nutritional and Pharmacological Properties of Bay Leaves (*Laurus nobilis L.*)

Rashmi Srivastava
Centre of Food Technology, University of Allahabad, India

ABSTRACT

Laurus nobilis L., commonly known as bay leaves, is native to the southern Mediterranean region. It is a small tree belonging to the genus Laurus of the family Lauraceae. The essential oils created from the different parts of this plant, such as the leaves and flowers, have been used in the food, drug, and cosmetic industries. The essential oil chiefly consists of 1,8-cineole, sabinene, α-pinene, and p-Cymene. Researchers have reported that bay leaves possess various biological and pharmacological properties, such as antibacterial, antifungal, antioxidant, insecticidal, and nematicidal activities. Pharmacological studies found that bay leaf oil could be a promising candidate with the potential for designing new drugs. The goal of this review is to summarize the ethnomedicinal importance, phytochemistry, and wide spectrum of pharmacological and therapeutic applications of bay leaves, which will be useful to researchers for further study.

INTRODUCTION

The olfactory quality of food has been improved by spices for many centuries. Spices are natural flavours, aroma enhancers, along with food preservatives. Spices are also considered safe and effective against certain clinical manifestations, and some researchers also state that they possess therapeutic properties, such as being antidiabetic, antihypertensive, antiulcerative, antialergic, antibiotic, etc. (Abu-zaid, Al-opidi, &El-Sehrawy, 2013). Bay leaves possesses many bioactive compounds, including anthocyanins, isoflavones, and flavonoids (Al-Hadi, 2011). Many spices show therapeutic potential, such as turmeric, which has traditionally been referred to as anti-infectious, anti-inflammatory, and as having a cholesterol lowering effect.

DOI: 10.4018/978-1-7998-2524-1.ch009

Laurus nobilis, or bay leaf, belongs to the Lauraceae plant family. It is a tropical and subtropical tree that grows in the Himalayas at an altitude of 900 to 2500 meters(Garg, Siddiqui, &Agarwal, 1992). It is also grown in Asia, Australia, the Pacific region, and South Asia. It is a native spice of India and grown in Uttarakhand and Himanchal Pradesh, along with Sikkim, Assam, Mizoram, and Meghalaya, and also in the Western Himalayan region(Dighe, Gursale, Sane, Menon, & Patel, 2005). Preferably, it is grown in a warm region of the world, such as Southern Europe, and around the shores of the Mediterranean Sea (Lewis, 1984). It is a small tree with small flowers that are four-lobed. The ripe fruit is 10-15 mm in size, ovoid, and black when ripe. The leaves are plucked and dried under shade for use as a flavouring material in a variety of meal preparations. The leaves are as a seasoning for soups and condiments. In some studies, bay leaf oil showed anti-bacterial activity against Salmonella enteric and E. coli.

The bay leaves are a traditional ingredient of French cuisines. They are also characteristic of the cuisines of India, Germany, and Eastern Europe. The leaves are used to add a pleasing aromatic flavour to many different dishes, such as chicken, sauces, soups, and bland vegetables. Due to its unique aroma, bay leaves are commonly also used in soaps and in the perfume industry. Despite increasing the flavour, aroma, and palatability of foods, they also have many therapeutic properties, such as being anti-inflammatory, antioxidant, antifungal, and anti-bacterial. Bay oils are used for bruises and sprains. In traditional medicine, bay leaves and their oil have been used primarily for curing digestive problems, which include flatulence, bloating, and other gastrointestinal complaints. The pharmacological and therapeutic properties of bay leaves and its fruits are due to the presence of bioactive constituents, such as alkaloids, alkaloids (kaempferol, myricetin), flavanol (apigenin and luteolin), glycosylated flavonoids, and sesquiterpene lactones. The present chapter focuses on the pharmacological as well as traditional properties of bay leaves.

Taxonomy, Botany and Chemical Composition of Bay Leaves

Taxonomic Classification

Kingdom: Plantae
Division: Magnoliophyta
Class: Magnoliopsida
Order: Laurales
Family: Lauraceae
Genus: Laurus S
Species: Nobilis

Botanical Description

Laurus nobilis L. is a small, hardly multi-branched tree, attaining a height of 20-30 feet (Said &Hussein 2014). The trees have small, four-lobed flowers that are pale yellow-green in colour and approximately one centimetre in diameter. The ripe fruit is 10-15 mm, ovoid, black, and single-seeded. The leaves are alternate, smooth, narrowly oblong-lanceolate, and about 2.5-8 cm (1 to 3 inches) long. When fresh, the leaves are shiny and dark green on top with lighter undersides. When dried, the bay leaf is a matte olive green in colour. The leaves are plucked and dried under shade for use as flavouring in a variety of cuisines and culinary preparations, and especially in French cuisine. The fragrant leaves are sold commercially as bay leaf, a seasoning ingredient (The Columbia Encyclopedia, 2005). The dried leaves are used extensively in cooking as the naturally occurring essential oil enhances the flavour of foods. Its aromatic bark is used occasionally for medicinal tea and its pulverized leaves for soups and condiments.

Chemical Composition of Bay Leaves

The chemical composition of bay leaf essential oil varied with the plant part from which it was extracted such, as seed, leaf, and flower. The chemical analysis of bay leaf shows it is rich in protein(7.62%), oil (8.5%), ash (3.63%) and carbohydrates(50.83%) along with minerals, such as calcium (Ca is 7958,92mg/kg), phosphorus, potassium (6665,92± 495,36 mg/Kg), iron (s 162,12± 17,19 mg/Kg), copper (20,37± 1,84 mg/Kg), magnesium (1605,97 ± 33,70 mg/Kg), manganese (10,95 ± 0,30 mg/Kg), and zinc (32,88 ± 1,80 mg/Kg), as well as vitamins such as riboflavin (45.33 mg/g) and ascorbic acid (2 mg/g).

Bay leaves are pungent and have a sharp, bitter taste. Compared to other spices, the fragrance of the bay leaf is more noticeable than its taste. A chemical analysis of Laurus nobil is showed that the characteristic aroma and the flavour of bay leaves were due to the presence of volatile and non-volatile compounds. The fragrance of the leaves was due to the presence of a specific compound called myrcene, which is a component of essential oils used in perfumes and in the soap industry. Bay oil showed a high value in unsaturated fatty acids (55%), includingoleic, linoleic, and linolenic, withsaturated fatty acids at 45%,includinglauric, meristic, palmitic, and stearic.The main components of the essential oil were cineol (44.12%), eugenol (15.16%), sabinene (6.20%), 4-terpineol (3.60%),a-pinene (2.74%), methyl eugenol (2.48%),terpineol(2.19%), and b-pinene (2.05%) (AL-Hashimi & Mahmood, 2016).

THERAPEUTIC POTENTIAL OF BAY LEAVES

Around the world concern has risen about the use of medicinal plants as antibiotics. In this context, bay leaves have received attention due to their antimicrobial, antifungal, and antioxidant properties. Recently, numerous studies have shown the therapeutic properties possessed by bay leaves, which have been proven to be effective against many ailments.

Antioxidant

The potential antioxidant activity of the essential oil and the extract from the Laurus nobilis has been extensively investigated by employing DPPH free radical scavenging, hydroxyl radical scavenging], superoxide radical inhibition, hydrogen peroxide scavenging, lipid peroxidation inhibition, and β-carotene/linoleic acid tests (Ozcan, Esen, Sangun, Coleri, & Caliskan,2010). Different solvents at different concentrations have been used to extract the antioxidants. The rates of antioxidant activity and reducing power increase as the concentrate of solvent increased (Al-Hashimi &Mahmood,2016). It was found among all solvents, that the acetone and ethyl acetate extract of bay leaves exhibited the largest free radical scavenging capacity in the neutralization of DPPH, NO, O2and OH radicals (Kaurinovic, Popovic, &Vlaisavljevic, 2010). Deepa, Ayesha, Nishtha, and Thankamani(2013) reported that bay leaves showed a greater amount of phenols and higher antioxidant activity compared to cardamom and coriander extracts.

Table 1. Variation in the chemical composition of bay leaf essential oil

Components(%)	Maghtader & Salari (2012))	Choudhary et al. (2013))	Vardapetyan etal. (2013))	Said &Hussein,(2014)	Shokoohinia et al.(2014)
1,8 Cineole	25.7	0.29	66.01	60.50	-
Tricyclene	2.27	-	-	-	0.29
Limonene	3.47	-	-	2.00	-
γ-Terpinene	3.48	-	0.12	0.68	3.23
Sabinene	8.7	-	-	6.63	5.74
α-Pinene	5.25	1.39	6.92	3.72	5.17
Eugenol	1.69	-	-	-	2.47
Linalool	1.56	42.61	-	0.62	1.78
***p*-Cymene**	0.31	1.09	-	1.57	-
α-Terpineol	3.79	0.50	-	3.36	2.06

Insecticidal

The essential oil of bay leaves was found to be more active as insecticide in polar solvents as compared to non-polar solvents and also showed repellent activity against Lasioderma serricorne, commonly referred to as the cigarette beetle, cigar beetle, or tobacco beetle(Chahal,Bansal, &Kaur,2016; Jemaa, Tersim, &Khouja, 2011). . It has shown better insecticidal activity compared to Tunisian and Algerian oilsT. castaneum (Jeama, Tersim, Toudert, &Khouja,2012). Repellenceand toxicity of the essential oil from bay leaves against the rust-red flour beetle were reported by researchers Andronikashvili and Reichmuth (2003). Aromatic plants from the families Lauraceae, Myrtaceae Poaceae,and Lamiaceae can protect againstP. vulgaris, a bacterium that inhabits the intestinal tracts of animals and humans. The leaves can have eithera direct or delayed insecticidal effect, and they have been shown to increase adult mortality as well as inhibition of the bacteria's reproduction. The results revealed that this action was due to the lipid,phenolic, non-protein amino acids, or flavonoids (Regnault-Roger &Hamraoui, 1995; Mackeen et al., 1997). The protective effect of bay leave and sage essential oils was also analyzed against the larvae of the Trogoderma granarium insect, also known as the Khapra beetle, one of the world's most destructive pests of grain products and seeds(Tayoub, Odeh, & Ghanem,2012). The study revealed that vapours of bay leaf essential oil at a concentration of 60 μl/160 cm3 for 48 hours resulted in about 98% mortality of the larvae and bay leaf oil also showed a higher lethal activity of than that of sage oil.

Antibacterial Activity

Both seed oil and extract of seed oil showed remarkable antibacterial activity against gram-positive bacteria and gram-negative bacteria(Ozcan et al.,Esen, Sangun, Coleri, &Caliskan, 2010).The antibacterial activity of essential oils of theL. nobilis L., Rosmarinus officinalis L., and Ocimum basilicum L. against 20bacterial strains was evaluated by Ouibrahim et al. (2013) researchers. Laurel oil showed the highest sensitivity among the three oils against Shigella sp., and the lowest against E. faecalis ATCC 29212, Enterobacter sp., S. aureus, and S. Epermidis (0.25%), etc. (El-Sawi, Ibrahim, &Ali, 2009).

The antibacterial activities of the essential oil were determined by disc diffusion and minimum inhibitory concentration methods. The antimicrobial activity of the essential oils from bay leaves was tested against food spoiling bacteria: S.aureus, E.coli and S. typhimurium (El, Karagozlu, Karakaya, &Sahın,2014). The findings of the study showed that minimum concentration values of essential oil were 125-2000 µg/ml for all tested bacterial strain. Previous studies revealed the antimicrobial activity of bay leaves essential oils against E. coli O157:H7, Candida albicans ATCC 16231, Salmonella enteritidis ATCC 13076, and L. monocytogenesATCC 7644,with MIC values of 125, 250, and 500 g/ml, respectively (Dias, Luzia, &Jorge,2013). Antibacterial activity of bay leaves might be presence of high contents of eugenol, methyl eugenol and fatty acids (Ivanovic, Misic, Ristic, Pesic, &Zizovic, 2010;Marzouki et al.,2008).

Antifungal Activity

The antifungal effects of bay leaf essential oil was found against the growth of some fungi, particularly Bacillus megaterium, Mycobacterium smegmatus, Yersinia enterocolitica, S. aureus and L. monocytogenes (Bag &Chattopadhyay, 2015). The essential oil of the bay leaf was analyzed in vitro against two food-borne fungi belonging to the dominant mycobiota of stored rice, Fusarium culmorum and F. verticillioides, and it was found that bay essential oil revealed great potential to control both fungal pathogens (Rosello, Sampere, Sans-Berzosa, Amparo, & Santamarina,2015). The extracts of L. nobilis showed the highest antifungal activity against A. niger and C. albicans with inhibition zone diameters of 20-32 mm/15ml (Erturk, 2006). In another study by Hassiotis (2010) found that30 and 60 mg/l of essential oil showed significant inhibition in mycorrhiza development and restriction of host growth. Bay leaf essential oil was more effective at pH 5, losing their activity as the pH increased (Guynot, Marin, Setu, Sanchis, &Ramos,2005). Previous researches reported the potential of bay leaf essential oils against species belonging to Eurotium, Aspergillus and Penicillium genus (Geeta &Reddy 1990; Guynotet al., 2003).It were reported that ethanolic extract of bay leaf exhibited highest antifungal towardsA. niger with 25 mm and 0.5 mg MIC.

Antiviral Activity

The essential oils of L. nobilis have shown inhibitory activity against SARS-CoV, with an IC (50) value of 120 µg /ml. β-ocimene, 1,8-cineole, alpha-pinene, and beta-pinene were found as the main biologically active compounds responsible for the antiviral activity (Loizzo et al., 2008).

Anti-Diabetic Effect

The hypoglycemic effects of different extracts of L. nobil is were observed in several studies. Indrianingsiha et al. (2015) observed that methanolic extract reduced the postpone glucose absorption by inhibiting the enzyme α-glucosidase, which is a digestive enzyme that hydrolyzes carbohydrates. Several possible mechanisms have been suggested for the hypoglycemic actions of L. nobilis, such as an increasing the release of insulin, enhancing the synthesis of glycogen, activatingthe PPAR-γ, and reducing the absorption of intestinal glucose. Previous studies demonstrated that consumption of bay leaves, 1 to 3 g/d for 30 days, decreased risk factors for diabetes and cardiovascular diseases, and suggested that bay leaves may be beneficial for people with Type 2 diabetes. Finding in a study by Alfanso et al.(2017) suggested that1,8-cineole, 1-(S)-α-pinene, and R-(+)-limonene were the major bioactive metabolites, which had potential hypoglycemic activity.

Cytotoxic Effect

Free radicals can cause healthy cells to mutate into cancerous cells, and bay leaves are particularly adept at preventing this activity. The leaves and fruits of the L. nobilis plant are the most extensively studied parts of the plant for anticancer activity. Both polar and non-polar extracts of L. nobilis exhibit significant anti-tumour activity. Although, fresh essential oil exhibited maximum growth and greater inhibitory effects on all cell lines than did stored essential oil. The in vitro cytotoxic activity of three different extracts of bay leaves was evaluated against human peripheral blood mononuclear cells, and three human cancer cell lines (lung: A549, breast: MCF-7, and colon: COLO 205) by sulforhodamine B assay. The results revealed that methanol extract was found to be significantly more active and potent against all the cancer cell lines compared to petroleum ether and the aqueous extract of bay leaves, but all three crude extracts lacked cytotoxic effects on normal human cells (Thanekar, Dhodi, &Juvekar, 2013). It was also reported that methanolic extracts were rich in phenols, flavonols, and flavonoids, and would be the biologically active compounds responsible for the anti-tumour effect. Researchers, Samejima, Kanazawa, Ashida, and Danno (1998),analyzed ethyl acetate extract from bay leaves and identified 3-kaempferyl-p-coumarate as the major mutagenic compound. In another study, catechins, linalool, and parthenolide were found to be present in bay leaves, which demonstrated the ability to stop the proliferation of cervical cancer cells, and also the ability help to protect the body from the effects of free radicals(Samejima et al., 1998).

Other Activities

There are several organic compounds found in bay leaves, including caffeic acid and rutin. Rutin strengthens capillary walls of the heart, while caffeic acid can help eliminate LDL or bad cholesterol from the cardiovascular system. Bay leaves are extremely beneficial during the preconception period by providing sufficient folic acid content. Linalool is often associated with thyme and basil, but it is also present in bay leaves and can help lower the level of stress hormones in the body, primarily when used in aromatherapy (Loizzo et al., 2008).

Regular consumption of bay leaves in the form of a spice mix or tea can provide good amounts of vitamin C, folic acid, vitamin A, natural antioxidants, dietary fibber, and B-vitamins, such as niacin, pyridoxine, pantothenic acid, and riboflavin. Regular consumption of 4 to 5 bay leaves will help in nervous system function, enzyme synthesis, and regulating body metabolism. However, they remain unpleasantly stiff even after thorough cooking, and if swallowed whole or in large pieces, they may pose a risk of harming the digestive tract or causing choking. Hence the leaves should be ground well before consumption or they should be removed from the food before serving. The anticonvulsant effect can be due to components such as methyleugenol, eugenol, and pinene, present in the bay essential oil (Sayyah, Valizadeh, & Kamalinejad,2002).

CONCLUSION

The essential oil of bay leaves is seen in a wide range of biologically active compounds. The major compounds present in bay seed essential oil were 1,8-cineole, sabinene, limonene, eugenol, and α-pinene. Bay leaf essential oil exhibits many pharmacological properties, such as antimicrobial, insecticidal, antioxidant, anticonvulsant, etc. The presence of a variety of diverse constituents in bay leaf essential oil may be responsible for the wide spectrum of biological activities of the plant. Bay leaves are slightly bitter, so they are added to various dishes while they are cooking, to add aromatic flavour, but they are removed before the dish is served..From the many studies reviewed, it is apparent that bay leaves, the fruit of the plants, and the oil derived from the plant provide many beneficial uses besides being used as a cooking spice. Study results from numerous researchers' works revealed a wide range of medicinal properties and application, and suggested that the bay leaf plant may have the potential to prevent and/ or treat serious diseases in the future, however, more research is needed on the subject.

REFERENCES

Abu-zaid, A. A., Alopidi, M. A., & El-Sehrawy, M. H. (2013). *In vitro* antibacterial, anticancer and antioxidant properties of some oil plant extract. *The Journal of American Science*, *9*(11), 83–94.

Al-Hadi, L. M. (2011). The antibacterial activity of aqueous extract of peppermint and bay leaf against Staphylococcus aureus. *Journal of Baghdad College of Dentistry*, *23*(2), 146–150.

al-Hashimi, A. G., & Mahmood, S. A. (2016). The nutritional value and antioxidant activity of bay leaves *(laurusn obilis L.). Magallat al-Basrat Li-l-Abhat al-Baytariyyat*, *15*(4), 10–23.

Al-Hashimi, A. G., & Mahmood, S. A. (2016). The nutritional value and antioxidant activity of bay leaves (Laurus nobilis L.). *Magallat al-Basrat Li-l-Abhat al-Baytariyyat*, *15*(2), 246–259. doi:10.33762/ bvetr.2016.124310

Alfonso, A. A., Altarejos, J., & Salido, S. (2017). Phytochemicals and Biological Activities of Laurel Tree (Laurus nobilis). *Natural Product Communications*, *12*(5), 743–757. PMID:30496684

Andronikashvili, M., & Reichmuth, C. H. (2003), Repellency and toxicity of essential oils from Ocimum gratissimum (Lamiaceae) and Laurus nobilis (Lauraceae) from Georgia against the rust-red flour beetle Tribolium castaneum (Herbst.) (Coleoptera: Tenebrionidae). *Proceedings of the 8th International Working Conference of Stored Product Protection*, 749-762.

Bag, A., & Chattopadhyay, R. R. (2015). Evaluation of synergistic antibacterial and antioxidant efficacy of essential oils of spices and herbs in combination. *PLoS One*, *10*(7), 1–17. doi:10.1371/journal. pone.0131321 PMID:26132146

Chahal, K. K., Bansal, R., & Kaur, R. (2016). Chemistry and insecticidal potential of bay leaf essential oil against stored grain pest of wheat. *Journal of Applied and Natural Science*, *8*(4), 2049–2054. doi:10.31018/jans.v8i4.1085

Choudhary, D., Kala, S. P., Todaria, N. P., Dasgupta, S., Kinhal, G., & Kollmair, M. (2013). Essential oil from bay leaves in India and Nepal: An analysis for quality oriented value chain development. *International Journal of Medicinal and Aromatic Plants*, *3*(1), 11–17.

Deepa, G., Ayesha, S., Nishtha, K., & Thankamani, M. (2013). Comparative evaluation of various total antioxidant capacity assays applied to phytochemical compounds of Indian culinary spices. *International Food Research Journal*, *20*(4), 1711–1716.

Dias, L. S., Luzia, D. M. M., & Jorge, N. (2013). Physicochemical and bioactive properties of *Hymenaea courbaril* L. pulp and seed lipid fraction. *Industrial Crops and Products*, *49*, 610–618. doi:10.1016/j.indcrop.2013.06.005

Dighe, V. V., Gursale, A. A., Sane, R. T., Menon, S., & Patel, P. H. (2005). Quantitative determination of eugenol from Cinnamomum tamala nees and eberm: Leaf powder and polyherbal formulation using reverse phase liquid chromatography. *Chromatographia*, *61*(9-10), 443–446. doi:10.136510337-005-0527-6

El, S. N., Karagozlu, N., Karakaya, S., & Sahın, S. (2014). Antioxidant and antimicrobial activities of essential oils extracted from Laurus nobilis L. leaves by using solvent-free microwave and hydrodistillation. *Food and Nutrition Sciences*, *5*(02), 97–106. doi:10.4236/fns.2014.52013

El-Sawi, S. A., Ibrahim, M. E., & Ali, A. M. (2009). In vitro cytotoxic, antioxidant and antimicrobial activities of essential oil of leaves of Lauras nobilis L. grown in Egypt and its chemical composition. *Medicinal and Aromatic Plant Science and Biotechnology*, *3*(1), 16–23.

Erturk, O. (2006). Antibacterial and antifungal activity of ethanolic extracts from eleven spice plants. *Section Cellular and Molecular Biology*, *61*(3), 275–278. doi:10.247811756-006-0050-8

Garg, S. N., Siddiqui, M. S., & Agarwal, S. K. (1992). New fatty acid esters and hydroxyl ketones from fruits of Laurus nobilis. *Journal of Natural Products*, *55*(9), 1315–1319. doi:10.1021/np50087a023

Geeta, G. S., & Reddy, T. K. R. (1990). Aspergillus flavus link and its occurrence in relation to other mycoflora on stored spices. *Journal of Stored Products Research*, *26*(4), 211–213. doi:10.1016/0022-474X(90)90024-M

Guynot, M. E., Marin, S., Setu, L., Sanchis, V., & Ramos, A. J. (2005). Screening for antifungal activity of some essential oils against common spoilage fungi of bakery products. *Food Science & Technology International*, *11*(1), 25–32. doi:10.1177/1082013205050901

Guynot, M. E., Ramos, A. J., Seto, L., Purroy, P., Sanchis, V., & Marin, S. (2003). Antifungal activity of volatile compounds generated by essential oils against fungi commonly causing deterioration of bakery products. *Journal of Applied Microbiology*, *94*(5), 893–899. doi:10.1046/j.1365-2672.2003.01927.x PMID:12694455

Hassiotis, C. N. (2010). Evaluation of essential oil antifungal activity against mycorrhizal fungi: The case of Laurus nobilis essential oil. *Israel Journal of Ecology & Evolution*, *56*(1), 35–54. doi:10.1560/IJEE.56.1.35

Indrianingsih, A., Tachibana, S., & Itoh, K. (2015). In vitro evaluation of antioxidant and α-glucosidase inhibitory assay of several tropical and subtropical plants. *Procedia Environmental Sciences*, *28*, 639–648. doi:10.1016/j.proenv.2015.07.075

Ivanovic, J., Misic, D., Ristic, M., Pesic, O., & Zizovic, I. (2010). Supercritical carbon dioxide extract and essential oil of bay (Laurus nobilis L.): Chemical composition and antibacterial activity. *Journal of the Serbian Chemical Society*, *75*(3), 395–404. doi:10.2298/JSC090303003I

Jemaa, J. M. B., Tersim, N., & Khouja, M. L. (2011). Composition and repellent efficacy of essential oil from Laurus nobilis against adults of the cigarette beetle Lasioderma serricorne (Coleoptera: Anobiidae). *Tunisian Journal of Plant Protection*, *6*(1), 29–42.

Jemaa, J. M. B., Tersim, N., Toudert, K. T., & Khouja, M. L. (2012). Insecticidal activities of essential oils from leaves of Laurus nobilis L. from Tunisia, Algeria and Morocco and comparative chemical composition. *Journal of Stored Products Research*, *48*, 97–104. doi:10.1016/j.jspr.2011.10.003

Kaurinovic, B., Popovic, M., & Vlaisavljevic, S. (2010). In vitro and in vivo effects of Laurus nobilis L. leaf extracts. *Molecules (Basel, Switzerland)*, *15*(5), 3378–3390. doi:10.3390/molecules15053378 PMID:20657487

Lewis, Y. (1984). *Spices and herbs for the food industry*. Food Trade Press Ltd.

Loizzo, M. R., Saab, A. M., Tundis, R., Statti, G. A., Menichini, F., Lampronti, I., ... Doerr, H. W. (2008). Phytochemical analysis and in vitro antiviral activities of the essential oils of seven Lebanon species. *Chemistry & Biodiversity*, *5*(3), 461–470. doi:10.1002/cbdv.200890045 PMID:18357554

Mackeen, M. M., Ali, A. M., El-Sharkawy, S. H., Manap, M. Y., Salleh, K. M., Lajis, N. H., & Kawazu, K. (1997). Antimicrobial and cytotoxic properties of some Malaysian vegetables (Ulam). *International Journal of Pharmacognosy*, *35*(3), 174–178. doi:10.1076/phbi.35.3.174.13294

Maghtader & Salari. (2012). Comparative survey on the essential oil composition from the leaves and flowers of Laurus nobilis L. from Kerman province. *Journal of Ecology and the Natural Environment*, *4*(6), 150–153.

Marzouki, H., Piras, A., Marongiu, B., Rosa, A., & Dessì, M. A. (2008). Extraction and separation of volatile and fixed oils from berries of *laurus nobilis* l. by supercritical co_2. *Molecules (Basel, Switzerland)*, *13*(8), 1702–1711. doi:10.3390/molecules13081702 PMID:18794780

Ouibrahim, A., Tlili-Ait-kaki, Y., Bennadja, S., Amrouni, S., Djahoudi, A. G., & Djebarl, M. R. (2013). Evaluation of antibacterial activity of Laurus nobilis L, Rosmarinus officinalis L. and Ocimum basilicum L. from Northeast of Algeria. *African Journal of Microbiological Research*, *7*(42), 4968–4973. doi:10.5897/AJMR2012.2390

Ozcan, B., Esen, M., Sangun, M. K., Coleri, A., & Caliskan, M. (2010). Effective antibacterial and antioxidant properties of methanolic extract of Laurus nobilis seed oil. *Journal of Environmental Biology*, *31*(5), 637–641. PMID:21387914

Regnault-Roger, C., & Hamraoui, A. (1995). Fumigant toxic activity and reproductive inhibition induced by monoterpenes on acanthoscelides obtectus (Say) (coleoptera), a bruchid of kidney bean (phaseolus vulgaris L.). *Journal of Stored Products Research*, *31*(4), 291–299. doi:10.1016/0022-474X(95)00025-3

Rosello, J., Sampere, F., Sans-Berzosa, I., Amparo, C. A., & Santamarina, J. M. P. (2015). Antifungal activity and potential use of essential oils against Fusarium culmorum and Fusarium verticillioides. *Journal of Essential Oil-Bearing Plants*, *18*(2), 359–367. doi:10.1080/0972060X.2015.1010601

Said, C. M., & Hussein, K. (2014). Determination of the chemical and genetic differences of Laurus collected from three different geographic and climatic areas in Lebanon. *European Scientific Journal*, *2*, 412–419.

Samejima, K., Kanazawa, K., Ashida, H., & Danno, G. (1998). Bay laurel contains antimutagenic kaempferyl coumarate acting against the dietary carcinogen 3-amino-1-methyl-5h-pyrido [4, 3- b]indole. *Journal of Agricultural and Food Chemistry*, *46*(12), 4864–4868. doi:10.1021/jf980714h

Sayyah, M., Valizadeh, J., & Kamalinejad, M. (2002). Anticonvulsant activity of the leaf essential oil of Laurus nobilis against pentylenetetrazole and maximal electroshock–induced seizures. *Phytomedicine*, *9*(3), 212–216. doi:10.1078/0944-7113-00113 PMID:12046861

Shokoohinia, Y., Yegdaneh, A., Amin, G., & Ghannadi, A. (2014). Seasonal variations of Laurus nobilis L. leaves volatile oil components in Isfahan, Iran. *Research Journal of Pharmacognosy*, *1*(3), 1–6.

Tayoub, G., Odeh, A., & Ghanem, I. (2014). Chemical composition and fumigation toxicity of Laurus nobilis L. and Salvia officinalis L. Essential oils on larvae of khapra beetle (Trogoderma granarium Everts). *Herba Polonica*, *58*(2), 26–37.

Thanekar, D., Dhodi, J., & Juvekar, A. (2013). Evaluation of in vitro cytotoxic activity of petroleum ether, methanol and aqueous extracts of Indian bay leaf, Cinnamomum tamala (Buch. -ham) T. Nees and eberm on cancer cells. *World Journal of Pharmacy and Pharmaceutical Sciences*, *3*(1), 519–533.

The Columbia Encyclopedia. (2001-2005). (6th ed.). New York: Columbia University Press.

Vardapetyan, H., Tiratsuyan, S., & Hovhannisyan, A. (2014). Antioxidant and antibacterial activities of selected armenian medicinal plants. *Journal of Experimental Biology and Agricultural Sciences*, *2*(3), 300–330.

Chapter 10
Therapeutic and Pharmaceutical Potential of Cinnamon

Neha Mishra
Sam Higginbottom University of Agriculture, Technology, and Sciences, India

Rashmi Srivastava
University of Allahabad, India

ABSTRACT

Cinnamon has been used as a spice, condiment, and aromatic plant since centuries ago. Cinnamon is a small evergreen tree belonging to the genus Cinnamomum in the family Lauraceae. There are more than 250 species of cinnamon worldwide. In India, Cinnamomum verum and Cinnamomum cassia are the most common species grown in the Himalaya region. They have been used as folk medicine for the treatment of nausea, flatulent dyspepsia, coughs, diarrhea, malaria, gastric disorder, and to alleviate pain and inflammation in rheumatic arthritis. Therapeutic properties of cinnamon are due to the presence of bioactive constituents such as p-coumaric, cinnamaldehyde, cinnamic acid, and eugenol. Cinnamaldehyde and eugenol are the major active constituents responsible for its characteristic flavor, aroma, and therapeutic properties. Pharmacological studies found that it could be a promising candidate with potential for designing new drugs. This review is aimed to summarize the ethanomedicinal importance, phytochemistry, and wide spectrum of pharmacological and therapeutic applications of cinnamon.

INTRODUCTION

Cinnamon is a medicinal plant belonging to the Lauraceae family. The bark of the plant is commonly used as a spice and an aromatic and flavoring agent since ancient times. The botanical name Cinnamomum is derived from the Hebraic and Arabic term amomon, meaning fragrant spice plant. All over the world, there are about over 250 species belonging to the genus *Cinnamomum* in the family Lauraceae; however, only a few *Cinnamomum* species are grown commercially (Sangal 2011; Vangalapati et al. 2012). Among them, four species are most commonly used as spices including *Cinnamon cassia*, *Cinnamon verum*, *Cinnamon loureiroi* and *Cinnamon burmanni* Blume (Ravindran 2004).

DOI: 10.4018/978-1-7998-2524-1.ch010

Cinnamon is native to South Asia, although now it is distributed all over the world. These are evergreen trees and shrubs, and most of the species are aromatic. *Cinnamomum verum* and *Cinnamomum cassia* is the most common species of India and Sri Lanka (USDA-ARS, 2009). In India, it generally cultivated in the upper Himalayas at altitudes of 900 meters to 2500 meters. Different parts of cinnamon, especially bark and leaves, have been used as spices since Ayurvedic times. In India, dry bark is known as dalchin and leaves known as bay leaves. It is used as a folk medicine for the treatment of nausea, flatulent dyspepsia, coughs, diarrhea, malaria, gastric disorder, and to alleviate pain and inflammation in rheumatic arthritis. Around the world it is commonly used as a flavoring agent in a wide variety of cuisines, confectionery, sweets, snack foods, beverages, and chewing gums. In addition, they are commonly used in the soap and perfume industry due to its unique fragrance and aroma. Bark and leaves of the plant are a good source of aromatic essential oil that contains more than 80 phytochemical compounds and commonly used as spices. The primary constituents of the essential oil are cinnamaldehyde (65–80%) and less amount of eugenol (5-10%). It also contains mucilage, starch, and tannins (Trease and Evans 1989). The characteristic aroma and flavor of cinnamon derive from the principal component, cinnamaldehyde, and *trans*-cinnamaldehyde (Cin) present in essential oil (*Yeh et al 2013).* The pungent taste is attributed to cinnamic aldehyde, whereas sweetness in cinnamon arises from mannitol. This is well established that it also contributes to various biological activities such as anti-inflammatory, antioxidant, anti-ulcer, anti-microbial, hypoglycemic and hepatoprotective activities (Lin et al. 2003). The pharmacological and therapeutic properties of cinnamon are due to the presence of bioactive constituents such as vanillic, caffeic, gallic, protocatechuic, *p*-coumaric, ferulic acids, cinnamaldehyde, cinnamate, cinnamic acid and eugenol. It is also documented that it is active against many pathogenic gram-positive and gram-negative bacteria. It could serve as an ideal preservative agent as it would increase the safety and shelf life of food products by acting against foodborne pathogens and spoilage bacteria. Cinnamon is being practiced in Ayurvedic medicine, unani medicine, traditional Chinese medicine for cold, diarrhea, digestive disorder and as an appetizer. In European, it is approved by German health authorities for the same. Several types of research have been done on exploring its biological activities since last two decades. The aim of this review article is to summarize the ethnomedicinal importance, phytochemistry and wide spectrum of pharmacological and therapeutic applications of Cinnamon.

Taxonomic Tree

Domain: Eukaryota
Kingdom: Plantae
Phylum: Spermatophyta
Subphylum: Angiospermae
Class: Dicotyledonae
Order: Laurales
Family: Lauraceae
Genus: Cinnamomum
Species: Cinnamomum verum

Figure 1. Parts of Cinnamon used for spices

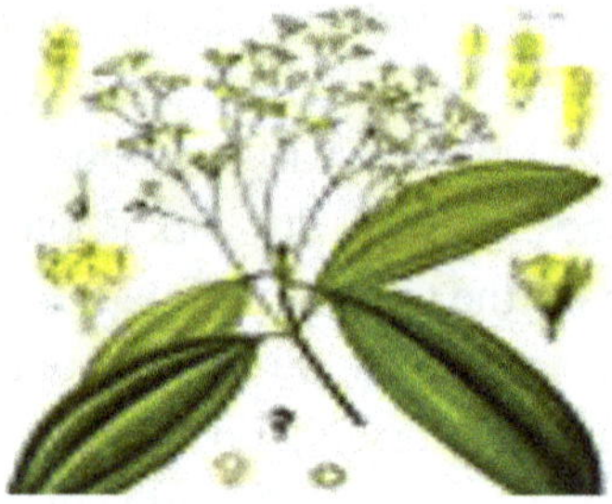

Whole plant

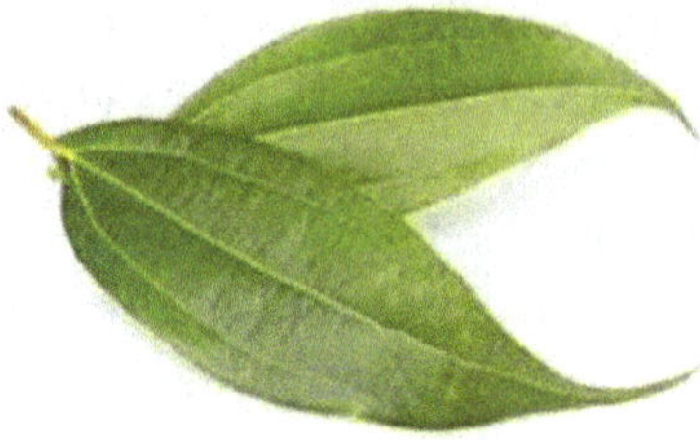

Leaves

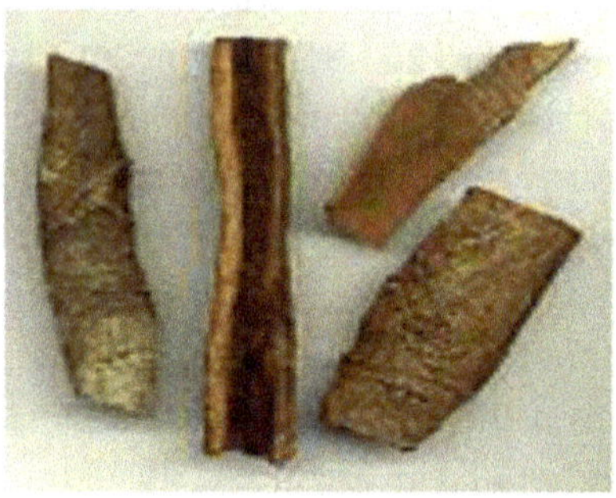

Cinnamonquills

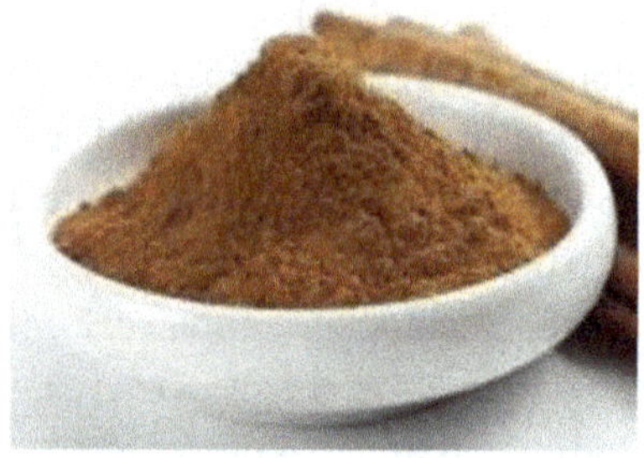

Cinnamon powder

Botanical Description

Cinnamon is the small evergreen tree that can grow up to 18 m long. The plants possess oval lanceolate 4–14 cm long, glossy green, rough-textured oppositely arranged leaves. The fruit is 1 cm long and one-seeded ovoid-shaped. They have small yellowish-white flowers with a disagreeable odor (Hakima, 2009). The bark is about 10 mm thick and strongly aromatic Cinnamon is the dried bark which is yellowish-brown externally while the inner surface is darker. The aromatic odor is warm, sweet, and fragrant due to the presence of active constituents in oil cells located in the phloem.

Ethnomedicinal Importance

The bark and leaf of the plant have been used as spice, condiments and flavoring agent in foods and beverages since prehistoric times due to its intense flavor and aroma. It is also used as a folk medicine for the treatment of nausea, flatulent dyspepsia, coughs, diarrhea, malaria and to alleviate pain and inflammation in rheumatic arthritis patients. The powdered bark is also employed to in alleviating gastric disorders, particularly reducing the risk of colon cancer and dysmenorrheal. Earlier researches have shown that this plant is a dense source of bioactive compounds that contributes to significant antioxidant (Mathew, 2006), anti-inflammatory (Tung et al 2010) and anticancer (Kwon et al 2010). It exhibits remarkable antimicrobial properties and is an ideal food preservative that will aid in prolonging the shelf life of foods (Gende et al 2008). Cinnamon has also been traditionally used in tooth powder to treat toothaches, dental problems, oral microbiota, and bad breath (Jakhetia et al 2010; Gupta, 2010).

Phytochemistry

Cinnamon is a valuable medicinal and aromatic plant that has characteristic aroma and flavor. Polyphenol and the volatile essential oil is the main active constituent of cinnamon. Among polyphenols, cinnamon contains bioactive compounds, including vanillic, caffeic, gallic, protocatechuic, *p*-coumaric, and ferulic acids as shown in figure 2. The chemical compounds in essential oils, including cinnamaldehyde, cinnamate, cinnamic acid, are responsible for its characteristic aroma, flavor and therapeutic properties (Singh et al 2006). Its taste, fragrance, and flavor were due to the presence of active constituents in essential oil. The major bioactive constituents vary in a different part of the plant i.e. bark, leaves, and root is shown in table 1.

Table 1. Major bioactive constituents is vary in different part of plant (*Vangalapati et al., 2012*)

Party of Plant	Major bioactive constituents
Leaves	Cinnamaldehyde: 1-5% Eugenol: 70-95%
Bark	Cinnamaldehyde: 65-80% Eugenol: 5-10%
Root	Camphore: 60%

In bark essential oil, cinnamaldehyde is the major substance (90% to 62%–73%,) depending on the type of extraction (Muchuweti et al 2007). The steam distillation and solvent extraction is a common method used to obtain phytochemical compounds. Steam distillation is more efficient than soxhlet extraction (Wong et al 2014).

Bio-Synthetic and Biotransformation Pathway

Cinnamaldehyde is an important phytochemical compound that occurs in the bark of cinnamon trees responsible for its flavor and odor. It is an organic compound with chemical formula is $C_6H_5CH{=}CHCHO$ and naturally present as *trans* (*E*) isomer predominantly. It is a phenylpropanoid that is naturally synthesized by the shikimate pathway.

Figure 2. Major bioactive compounds present in Cinnamon (Nabavi, 2015)

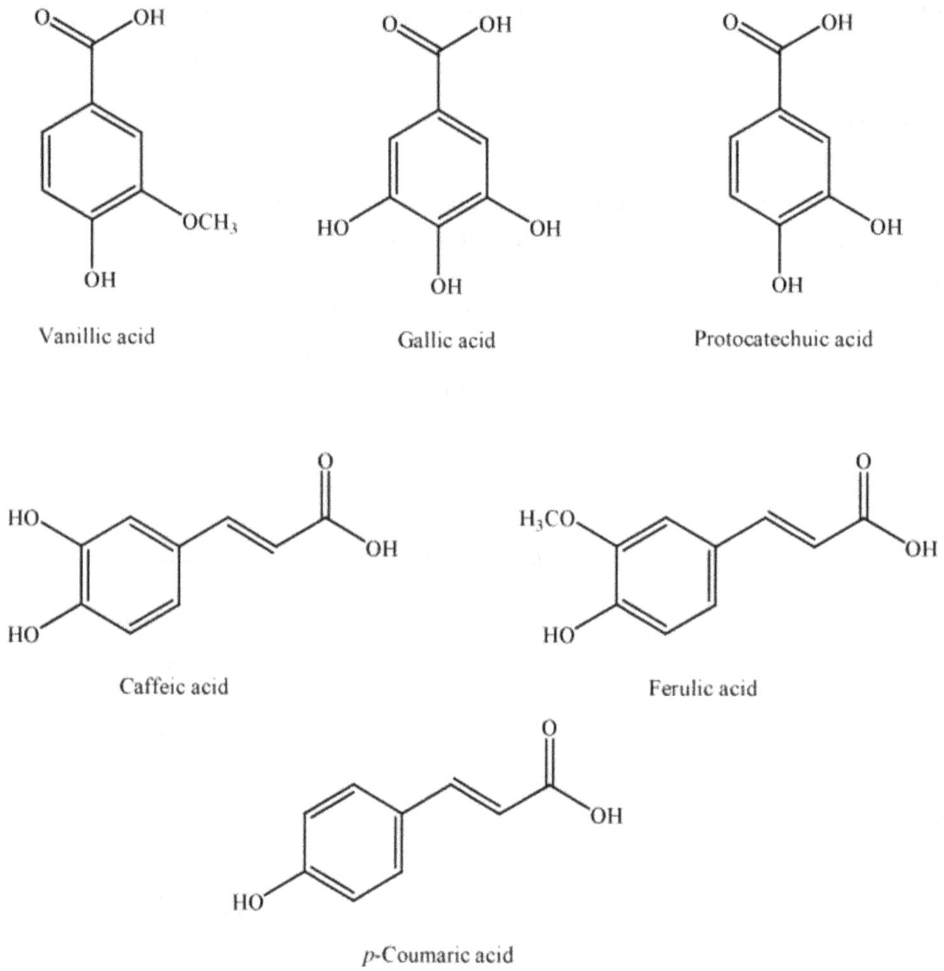

The most accepted theory for the biosynthesis of cinnamaldehyde is started with the deamination of L-phenylalanine. As shown in Figure 3, L-phenylalanine gives cinnamic acid by the action of phenylalanine ammonia lyase (PAL). This reaction is called as non-oxidative deamination(Bang et al 2016). The deamination relies on the MIO prosthetic group of PAL(Kong, 2015). The cinnamic acid is then converted into cinnamoyl-CoA by 4-coumarate–CoA ligase (4CL) as shown in figure. In acid–thiol ligation reaction, 4CL uses ATP to catalyze the formation of cinnamoyl-CoA. Cinnamoyl-CoA is reduced by NADPH catalyzed by CCR (cinnamoyl-CoA reductase) to form cinnamaldehyde.

In the body, this compound is quickly oxidized to cinnamic acid, which in turn is converted to benzoic or hippuric acid and excreted in the urine. It is estimated that over 90% is eliminated this way, with only a small amount being stored long-term in fat reserves.

Figure 3. Pathway for the biosynthesis of trans-cinnamaldehyde

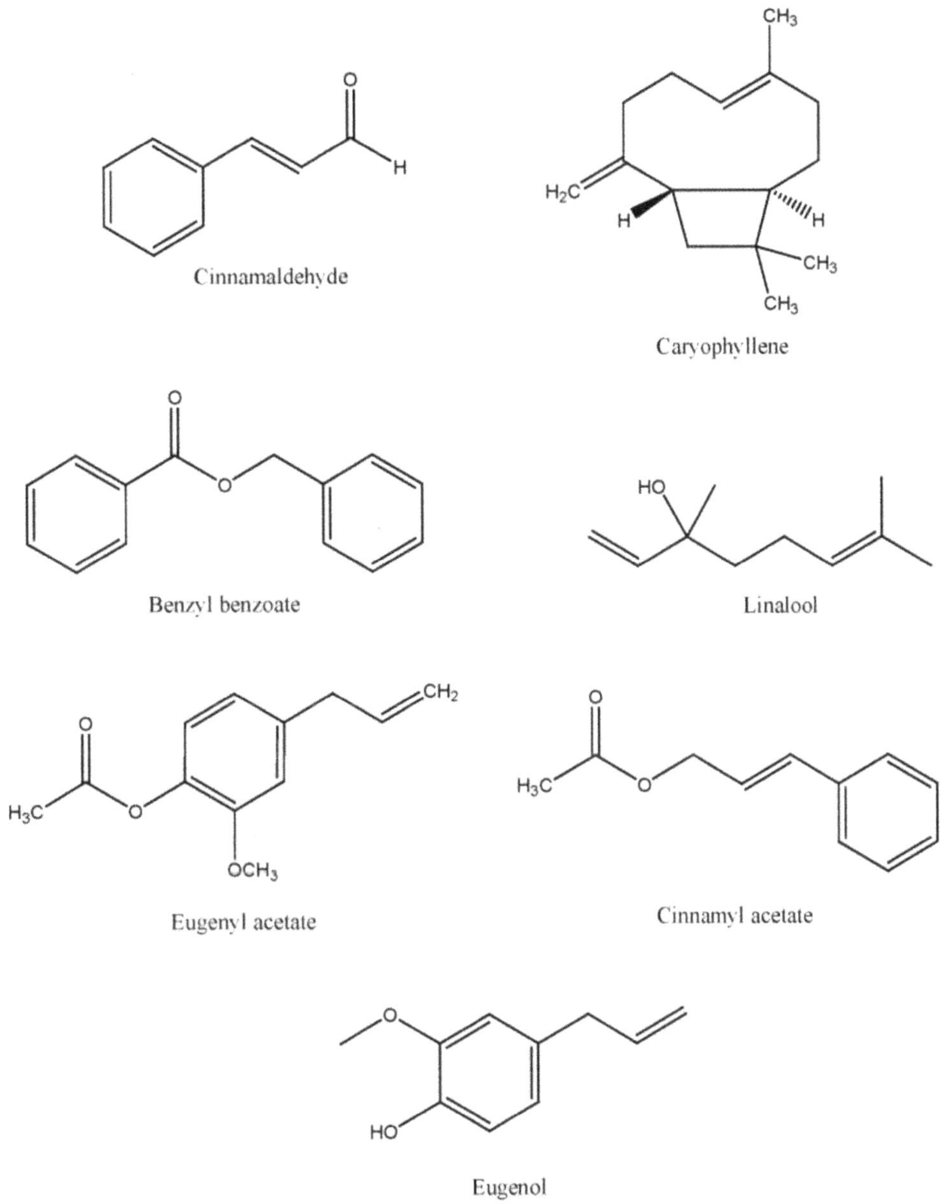

Biological Activities

Cinnamon is a medicinal plant and has been used as a traditional remedy around the world (Gupta 2010). There have been numerous investigations on identifying the bioactive compounds for exploring its possibilities as alternatives for modern medications (Alu'datt et al 2016). The potential pharmacological effects of cinnamon in modern medicine such as anti-inflammatory, antifungal, and anticancer activities are summarized in table 2 and has discussed here:

Table 2. Pharmacological action of Cinnamon

Extract	Experimental model	Doses	Experimental Finding	References
Antioxidant activities				
Aqueous and alcoholic extract (1 : 1)	In vitro		Significantly inhibits fatty acid oxidation and lipid peroxidation	Shobana S, Naidu 2000
Bark powderof C. verum	rat	10% for 90 days	Enhance the cardiac and hepatic antioxidant enzymes, lipid conjugate dienes, and glutathione (GSH)	Dhuley 1999
Cardio-protective				
Cinnamon extract	rats	200 mg/kg body weight) for 6 weeks.	Lowered blood concentration of TG and total cholesterol	Kim et al 2006
Cinnamic acid	rats	37.5, 75, 150 mg/kg)	decreased serum levels of creatine kinase (CK), lactate dehydrogenase (LDH), tumor necrosis factor-α (TNF-α), interleukin-6 (IL-6),and increase the serum nitric oxide (NO) activity.	Song et al2013
cinnamic aldehyde	rats	22.5, 45, 90 mg/kg	increased SOD activity and decreased MDA content in myocardial tissue	Song et al2013
Antimicrobial				
Essential oils of *C. cassia*	invitro	0.05%	effectively inhibit the growth of *E. coli*	Sheng, L.; Zhu2014
cinnamon essential oils	invitro	---	antibacterial effects against *H. pylori.*	Dugoua et al 2007
ethyl acetate, acetone and methanol,	invitro	30 μL	inhibition zone, ranges from 7 to 18 mm aganist *Klebsiella pneumonia* 13883, *Bacillus megaterium* NRS, *Pseudomonas aeruginosa* ATCC 27859, *Staphylococcus aureus* 6538 P, *Escherichia coli* ATCC 8739, *Enterobacter cloacae* ATCC 13047, *Corynebacterium xerosis* UC 9165, *Streptococcus faecalis* DC 74,	*Keskin and, Toroglu 2011*
Anti-diabetes				
Aqueous extract	Mice	500 mg/d for 12 weeks	decreased oxidative stress and improved impaired fasting glucose	Roussel et al 2009
Capsule of saffron	Women aged 20–45 years	5, 10, and 20 mg/kg	relieving symptoms of PMS.	Agha-Hosseini et al 2008
Anti-inflammatory				
ethanolic extract of C. cassia	invivo	---	activation of Src/spleen-tyrosine-kinase-(Src/Syk-) mediated NF-κB	Youn et al 2008; Yu et al 2012
aqueous extract	invivo	---	lipopolysaccharide-induced tumor necrosis factor-α levels in the serum	Hong et al 2012

Antioxidant

During oxidative stress, large amounts of ROS reactive oxygen species (ROS), such as superoxide anion radical, hydroxyl radical and hydrogen peroxide is produced and which can attack numerous molecules, including proteins and lipids and reported to contribute cellular aging, coronary heart disease cancer.

Recently, extensive studies have conducted to explore the antioxidant activity of the spices. Several previous studies have reported significant antioxidant activity in various extracts of cinnamon, such as ether, aqueous, and methanolic extracts (Mancini-Filho et al. 1998). The aqueous and alcoholic extract (1 : 1) of cinnamon exhibit a higher percentage of inhibition of fatty acid oxidation and lipid peroxidation in vitro. Lin et al 2003 reported that ethanolic extract of *C. cassia* exhibited significant inhibition (96.3%) compared to the natural antioxidant α-tocopherol (93.74%). The essential oils and some of the major compounds present in cinnamon, including (E)-cinnamaldehyde, eugenol, and linalool, is the major bioactive metabolite, which has potent antioxidant activity determined against peroxynitrite-induced nitration and lipid peroxidation. Shan et al. (2005) conducted a study to compare antioxidant activity among 26 spices and found the highest antioxidant activity in cinnamon.

Anti-Inflammatory

Anti-inflammatory activity of cinnamon is observed in several studies. C. cassia bark showed an inhibitory effect on the production of nitric oxide by inhibiting the activation of the nuclear factor kappa-beta cell (NF-κB), (Lee et al 2005). 2¢-hydroxycinnamaldehyde isolated active compound from *C Cassi.* A study was conducted to analyze the anti-inflammatory activity among 20 traditional herbs of Indonesia. The result found the highest inflammatory activity in *C. burmannii* . Coumarin and 2-hydroxy-cinnamaldehyde are isolated to have anti-inflammatory effects and exhibited good soybean lipoxygenase (SLO) inhibitory activity (IC_{50} = 60 μM).

Antidiabetic

It has been reported that cinnamon extract has anti-diabetic potency since they have the stimulatory effect of increasing the release of insulin, enhancing the synthesis of glycogen, activating the PPAR-γ and reduce the absorption of intestinal glucose, (Mueller and Jungbauer et al 2009). The finding suggested that cinnamaldehyde is the major bioactive metabolite, which has potential hypoglycemic activity. The possible mechanism for hypoglycemic action is its ability to regulate glucose metabolism and repair pancreatic beta cells (Li, et al 2013). When cinnamon extract administrated in mice shows decline blood glucose and increase of insulin level. Inconsistent of the study, Ping et al (2010) reported a similar result after applying 100 mg/kg of cinnamon essential oil (containing cinnamaldehyde 78.51%) to KK-Ay mice. In another study, 50 μM *C. cassia* bark extract showed the antidiabetic nephropathy activity, and sesquiterpenoids are suggested for this nephropathy activity (Yan et al 2015) .

Antimicrobial Activity

Earlier studies reported cinnamon has significant antimicrobial activity aganist different bacterial (*Pediococcus halophilus and Staphylococcus aureus*), fungal (*Aspergillus flavus, Mucor plumbeus, Penicillium roqueforti, and Eurotium sp.*), and yeast species (*Candida lipolytica, Pichia membranaefaciens, De-*

baryomyces hansenii, and Zygosaccharomyces rouxii)(Matan et al 2006). Cinnamaldehyde is a biologically active component extracted from *C.Cassia*, which shown a potent inhibition against *Clostridium perfringens* and *Bacteroides fragilis*, but no inhibitory activity was obtained against *Bifidobacterium longum* or *Lactobacillus acidophilus*(Lee and Ahn, 1998).In consistent, the extract of *C. cassia* shown antibacterial activity against *Escherichia coli* and *Salmonella infantis* at the highest Minimum Inhibitory Concentration (2640 mg) (Alzoreky and Nakahara,2003).

Anti-Tumor

Studies reported the anti-neoplastic activity of the aqueous cinnamon extract. Research studies suggest that the extract of cinnamon and its active constituents (cinnamic aldehyde) selectively kills cancer cells. The bioactive molecule cinnamic aldehyde inhibits the activity of NF-κB and the production of tumor necrosis factor alpha (TNFα-) in A375 cells [Cabello et al 2009]. Similarly, the potential of trans-cinnamaldehyde in restraining tumor cell growth and in enhancing tumor cell apoptosis was observed (Fang et al 2004). *Cinnamomum cassia* showed cytotoxicity to the colon (HCT-116), liver (HepG2), and breast (MCF-7) cancer cells. The leaves of *Cinnamon tamala* exhibit strong anticancer activity against human ovarian cancer cells (Dumbre 2014).

Cardio-Protective Effects

Cinnamon plays important in maintaining the blood lipid profile. Several studies have reported the cardio-protective activities of Cinnamon. One of the active components Cinnamophilin, an important lignans isolated from *C. philippinensis* reported to have thromboxane A2 (TXA_2) receptor blocking activity in animal model (Yu et al 1994). A recent study showed that cinnamaldehyde shows hypotensive effects mainly due to vasodilatory function. The cinnamon extract at 200 mg/kg body weight of rats showed a significant decrease in all the cardiac enzyme activities (Kim et al 2006). It also significantly lower the serum triglyceride and lipoprotein level and increases the high-density lipoprotein (HDL)levels. Polyphenol and cinnamaldehyde are active compounds responsible for the hypolipidemic effects of cinnamon.

Hepatoprotective Activity

The extract of Cinnamon has reported to have significant hepatoprotective activity, which is attributed to its free radical scavenging activity. The extract of cinnamon shown to reduce the hepatic lipid accumulation and significant hepatoprotective activity against alcohol and carbon tetrachloride. Cinnamon AX, a polysaccharide isolated from the dried bark of C. cassia found as an active constituent for hepato-protective action (kanari et al. 1989). The aqueous and ethanolic extract of cinnamon (200 mg/kg) was administrated orally in mice for 7 days. The result found more effective hepatoprotective action of ethanolic extract than water extract and it might be extract by lowering the malondialdehyde (MDA) level and elevating the activities of the antioxidant enzymes, superoxide dismutase (SOD) and catalase (CAT) (Moselhy and Ali, 2009)

CONCLUSION

Cinnamon is an important spice in the culinary kitchen all over the world. In Ayurveda and the folklore system of medicine, the whole plant is used as a remedy for the treatment of a range of diseases such as loss of appetite, indigestion, flatulence, gastritis, arthritis, toothache. Over the last two decades, several pharmacological studies reported the diverse bioactive compounds in a different part of the plant, which could be utilized for the development of drugs and functional foods. It also has incredible antimicrobial activities and the ability to prevent oxidation. Therefore, it could be used as a drug, functional ingredient, and preservative in food.

REFERENCES

Sangal, A. (2011). Role of cinnamon as beneficial antidiabetic food adjunct: A review. *Advances in Applied Science Research*, *2*(4), 440–450.

Vangalapati, M., Satya, N. S., Prakash, S. D. V., & Avanigadda, S. (2012). A review on pharmacological activities and clinical effects of cinnamon species. *Research Journal of Pharmaceutical, Biological and Chemical Sciences*, *3*(1), 653–663.

Ravindran, P., Shylaja, M., Nirmal Babu, K., & Krishnamoorthy, B. (2004). Botany and crop improvement of cinnamon and cassia. In P. N. Ravindran & K. N. Babu (Eds.), *Cinnamon and Cassia—The Genus Cinnamomum*. CRC Press.

USDA-ARS. (2009). Germplasm Resources Information Network (GRIN). Online Database. Beltsville, MD: National Germplasm Resources Laboratory. https://npgsweb.ars-grin.gov/gringlobal/taxon/taxonomysearch.aspx

Alu'datt, M. H., Rababah, T., Alhamad, M. N., Gammoh, S., Ereifej, K., Johargy, A., ... Rawashdeh, M. (2016). Optimization of Phenolic Content, Antioxidant, and Inhibitory Activities of α-Glucosidase and Angiotensin Converting (AC) Enzymes from *Zingiber Officinale* Z. *International Journal of Food Properties*, *19*(6), 1303–1316. doi:10.1080/10942912.2015.1063066

Alzoreky, N. S., & Nakahara, K. (2003). Antibacterial activity of extracts from some edible plants commonly consumed in Asia. *International Journal of Food Microbiology*, *80*(3), 223–230. doi:10.1016/S0168-1605(02)00169-1 PMID:12423924

Bang, Lee, Kim, Sung, & Jeong. (2016). Metabolic engineering of *Escherichia coli* for the production of cinnamaldehyde. *Microbial Cell Factories*, *15*(1), 16.

Cabello, C. M., Bair, W. B. III, Lamore, S. D., Ley, S., Bause, A. S., Azimian, S., & Wondrak, G. T. (2009). The cinnamon-derived Michael acceptor cinnamic aldehyde impairs melanoma cell proliferation, invasiveness, and tumor growth. *Free Radical Biology & Medicine*, *46*(2), 220–231. doi:10.1016/j.freeradbiomed.2008.10.025 PMID:19000754

Dhuley, J. N. (1999). Anti-oxidant effects of cinnamon (Cinnamomum verum) bark and greater cardamon (Amomum subulatum) seeds in rats fed high fat diet. *Indian Journal of Experimental Biology*, *37*(3), 238–242. PMID:10641152

Dugoua, J. J., Seely, D., Perri, D., Cooley, K., Forelli, T., Mills, E., & Koren, G. (2007). From type 2 diabetes to antioxidant activity: A systematic review of the safety and efficacy of common and cassia cinnamon bark. *Canadian Journal of Physiology and Pharmacology, 85*(9), 837–847. doi:10.1139/Y07-080 PMID:18066129

Dumbre, R. K., Kamble, M. B., & Patil, V. R. (2014). Inhibitory effects by ayurvedic plants on prostate enlargement induced in rats. *Pharmacognosy Research, 6*(2), 127. doi:10.4103/0974-8490.129031 PMID:24761116

Fang, S. H., Rao, Y. K., & Tzeng, Y. M. (2004). Cytotoxic effect of trans-cinnamaldehyde from cinnamomum osmophloeum leaves on Human cancer cell lines. *International Journal of Applied Science and Engineering, 2*(2), 136–147.

Gende, L. B., Floris, I., Fritz, R., & Eguaras, M. J. (2008). Antimicrobial activity of cinnamon (*Cinnamomum zeylanicum*) essential oil and its main components against paenibacillus larvae from argentine. *Bulletin of Insectology, 61*(1), 1–4.

Gupta, M. (2010). Pharmacological Properties and Traditional Therapeutic Uses of Important Indian Spices: A Review. *International Journal of Food Properties, 13*(5), 1092–1116. doi:10.1080/10942910902963271

Hong, J. W., Yang, G. E., Kim, Y. B., Eom, S. H., Lew, J. H., & Kang, H. (2012). Anti-inflammatory activity of cinnamon water extract in vivo and in vitro LPS-induced models. *BMC Complementary and Alternative Medicine, 12*(1), 237. doi:10.1186/1472-6882-12-237 PMID:23190501

Jakhetia, V., Patel, R., Khatri, P., Pahuja, N., Garg, S., Pandey, A., & Sharma, S. (2010). Cinnamon: A pharmacological review. *International Journal of Advances in Scientific Research, 1*(2), 19–23.

Kanari, M., Tomoda, M., Gonda, R., Shimizu, N., Kimura, M., Kawaguchi, M., & Kawabe, C. (1989). A reticuloendothelial system-activating arabinoxylan from the bark of Cinnamomum cassia. *Chemical & Pharmaceutical Bulletin, 37*(12), 3191–3194. doi:10.1248/cpb.37.3191 PMID:2632069

Keskin, D., & Toroglu, S. (2011). Studies on antimicrobial activities of solvent extracts of different spices. *Journal of Environmental Biology, 32*(2), 251–256. PMID:21882663

Kim, S. H., Hyun, S. H., & Choung, S. Y. (2006). Anti-Diabetic Effect of Cinnamon Extract on Blood Glucose in Db/Db Mice. *Journal of Ethnopharmacology, 104*(1), 119–123. doi:10.1016/j.jep.2005.08.059 PMID:16213119

Kong, J.-Q. (2015). Phenylalanine ammonia-lyase, a key component used for phenylpropanoids production by metabolic engineering. *RSC Advances, 5*(77), 62587–62603. doi:10.1039/C5RA08196C

Kwon, H. K., Hwang, J. S., So, J. S., Lee, C. G., Sahoo, A., Ryu, J. H., ... Park, Z. Y. (2010). Cinnamon extract induces tumor cell death through inhibition of NFκB and AP1. *BMC Cancer, 10*(1), 392. doi:10.1186/1471-2407-10-392 PMID:20653974

Lee, H. S., & Ahn, Y. J. (1998). Growth-inhibiting effects of Cinnamomum cassia bark-derived materials on human intestinal bacteria. *Journal of Agricultural and Food Chemistry, 46*(1), 8–12. doi:10.1021/jf970548y PMID:10554188

Lee, H. S., & Ahn, Y. J. (1998). Growth-inhibiting effects of Cinnamomum cassia bark-derived materials on human intestinal bacteria. *Journal of Agricultural and Food Chemistry*, *46*(1), 8–12. doi:10.1021/jf970548y PMID:10554188

Li, R., Liang, T., Xu, L., Li, Y., Zhang, S., & Duan, X. (2013). Protective Effect of Cinnamon Polyphenols against STZ-diabetic Mice Fed High-Sugar, High-Fat Diet and Its Underlying Mechanism. *Food and Chemical Toxicology*, *51*, 419–425. doi:10.1016/j.fct.2012.10.024 PMID:23127600

Lin, C.-C., Wu, S.-J., Chang, C.-H., & Ng, L.-T. (2003). Antioxidant activity of *Cinnamomum cassia*. *Phytotherapy Research*, *17*(7), 726–730. doi:10.1002/ptr.1190 PMID:12916067

Mancini-Filho, J., van-Koiij, A., Mancini, D. A. P., Cozzolino, F. F., & Torres, R. P. (1998). Antioxidant activity of cinnamon (Cinnamomum zeylanicum, breyne) extracts. *Bollettino Chimico Farmaceutico*, *137*(11), 443–447. PMID:10077878

Matan, N., Rimkeeree, H., Mawson, A. J., Chompreeda, P., Haruthaithanasan, V., & Parker, M. (2006). Antimicrobial activity of cinnamon and clove oils under modified atmosphere conditions. *International Journal of Food Microbiology*, *107*(2), 180–185. doi:10.1016/j.ijfoodmicro.2005.07.007 PMID:16266767

Mathew, S., & Abraham, T. E. (2006). Studies on the antioxidant activities of cinnamon (*Cinnamomum verum*) bark extracts, through various in vitro models. *Food Chemistry*, *94*(4), 520–528. doi:10.1016/j.foodchem.2004.11.043

Moselhy, S. S., & Ali, H. K. (2009). Hepatoprotective effect of cinnamon extracts against carbon tetrachloride induced oxidative stress and liver injury in rats. *Biological Research*, *42*(1), 93–98. doi:10.4067/S0716-97602009000100009 PMID:19621136

Muchuweti, M., Kativu, E., Mupure, C. H., Chidewe, C., Ndhlala, A. R., & Benhura, M. A. N. (2007). Phenolic composition and antioxidant properties of some spices. *American Journal of Food Technology*, *2*, 414–420. doi:10.3923/ajft.2007.414.420

Mueller, M., & Jungbauer, A. (2009). Culinary plants, herbs and spices – A rich source of PPARγ ligands. *Food Chemistry*, *117*(4), 660–667. doi:10.1016/j.foodchem.2009.04.063

Nabavi, S. F., Di Lorenzo, A., Izadi, M., Sobarzo-Sánchez, E., Daglia, M., & Nabavi, S. M. (2015). Antibacterial effects of cinnamon: From farm to food, cosmetic and pharmaceutical industries. *Nutrients*, *7*(9), 7729–7748. doi:10.3390/nu7095359 PMID:26378575

Ping, H., Zhang, G., & Ren, G. (2010). Antidiabetic Effects of Cinnamon Oil in Diabetic KK-Ay Mice. *Food and Chemical Toxicology*, *48*(8), 2344–2349. doi:10.1016/j.fct.2010.05.069 PMID:20561948

Roussel, A. M., Hininger, I., Benaraba, R., Ziegenfuss, T. N., & Anderson, R. A. (2009). Antioxidant effects of a cinnamon extract in people with impaired fasting glucose that are overweight or obese. *Journal of the American College of Nutrition*, *28*(1), 16–21. doi:10.1080/07315724.2009.10719756 PMID:19571155

Shan, B., Cai, Y. Z., Sun, M., & Corke, H. (2005). Antioxidant capacity of 26 spice extracts and characterization of their phenolic constituents. *Journal of Agricultural and Food Chemistry*, *53*(20), 7749–7759. doi:10.1021/jf051513y PMID:16190627

Sheng, L., & Zhu, M. J. (2014). Inhibitory effect of Cinnamomum cassia oil on non-O157 Shiga toxin-producing Escherichia coli. *Food Control*, *46*, 374–381. doi:10.1016/j.foodcont.2014.05.050

Shobana, S., & Naidu, K. A. (2000). Antioxidant activity of selected Indian spices. *Prostaglandins, Leukotrienes, and Essential Fatty Acids*, *62*(2), 107–110. doi:10.1054/plef.1999.0128 PMID:10780875

Singh, G., Maurya, S., deLampasona, M. P., & Catalan, C. A. N. (2007). A comparison of chemical, antioxidant and antimicrobial studies of cinnamon leaf and bark volatile oils, oleoresins and their constituents. *Food and Chemical Toxicology*, *45*(9), 1650–1661. doi:10.1016/j.fct.2007.02.031 PMID:17408833

Song, F., Li, H., Sun, J., & Wang, S. (2013). Protective effects of cinnamic acid and cinnamic aldehyde on isoproterenol-induced acute myocardial ischemia in rats. *Journal of Ethnopharmacology*, *150*(1), 125–130. doi:10.1016/j.jep.2013.08.019 PMID:24001892

Trease, G. E., & Evans, W. C. (1989). *Pharmacognosy* (13th ed.). Bailliere Tindall Ltd.

Tung, Y.-T., Chua, M.-T., Wang, S.-Y., & Chang, S.-T. (2008). Anti-inflammation activities of essential oil and its constituents from indigenous cinnamon (*Cinnamomum osmophloeum*) twigs. *Bioresource Technology*, *99*(9), 3908–3913. doi:10.1016/j.biortech.2007.07.050 PMID:17826984

Vangalapati, M., Sree Satya, N., Surya Prakash, D., & Avanigadda, S. (2012). A review on pharmacological activities and clinical effects of cinnamon species. *Research Journal of Pharmaceutical, Biological and Chemical Sciences*, *3*(1), 653–663.

Wong, Y. C., Ahmad-Mudzaqqirand, M. Y., & Wan-Nurdiyana, W. A. (2014). Extraction of Essential Oil from Cinnamon (*Cinnamomum zeylanicum*). *Oriental Journal of Chemistry*, *30*(1), 37–47. doi:10.13005/ojc/300105

Yan, Y.-M., Fang, P., Yang, M.-T., Li, N., Lu, Q., & Cheng, Y.-X. (2015). Anti-Diabetic Nephropathy Compounds from Cinnamomum Cassia. *Journal of Ethnopharmacology*, *165*, 141–147. doi:10.1016/j.jep.2015.01.049 PMID:25725434

Yeh, H. F., Luo, C. Y., Lin, C. Y., Cheng, S. S., Hsu, Y. R., & Chang, S. T. (2013). Methods for thermal stability enhancement of leaf essential oils and their main constituents from indigenous cinnamon (Cinnamomum osmophloeum). *Journal of Agricultural and Food Chemistry*, *61*(26), 6293–6298. doi:10.1021/jf401536y PMID:23738884

Youn, H. S., Lee, J. K., Choi, Y. J., Saitoh, S. I., Miyake, K., Hwang, D. H., & Lee, J. Y. (2008). Cinnamaldehyde suppresses toll-like receptor 4 activation mediated through the inhibition of receptor oligomerization. *Biochemical Pharmacology*, *75*(2), 494–502. doi:10.1016/j.bcp.2007.08.033 PMID:17920563

Yu, S. M., Wu, T. S., & Teng, C. M. (1994). Pharmacological characterization of cinnamophilin, a novel dual inhibitor of thromboxane synthase and thromboxane A2 receptor. *British Journal of Pharmacology*, *111*(3), 906–912. doi:10.1111/j.1476-5381.1994.tb14824.x PMID:8019768

Chapter 11
Potential Health Benefits of Fenugreek With Multiple Pharmacological Properties

Akanksha Srivastava
Nutritionist and freelancer, New Delhi, India

Zoomi Singh
https://orcid.org/0000-0003-4638-142X
Centre of Food Technology, University of Allahabad, India

Vandana Verma
https://orcid.org/0000-0001-8986-7177
Centre of Food Technology, University of Allahabad, India

Tashi Choedon
Nutritionist and freelancer, New Delhi, India

ABSTRACT

Fenugreek is one of the familiar spices found in human food and has been used extensively for curing numerous disorders. It provides natural food fibers and other nutrients required in the human body. It is used in functional foods, traditional foods, and nutraceuticals as well as in physiological uses such as antidiabetic agent, antibacterial, hypocholesterolemic, hypoglycemic, antioxidant, enzymatic pathway, and modifier gastric stimulant. It has a valuable influence on digestion and also has the capability to modify food texture. In modern food technology, it is used as a food stabilizer, adhesive, and emulsifying agent due its fiber, protein, and gum content. Recent pharmocological exploration of the seed extract of this plant discovered anticancer properties. Although it has many potential effects, there are some side effects as well; therefore, there is a greater need to study the pharmacological and toxicological effects of fenugreek to examine its clinical efficacy and safety.

DOI: 10.4018/978-1-7998-2524-1.ch011

INTRODUCTION

Fenugreek is a prominent herb in the practices of Ayurvedic medicine (The Ayurvedic Pharmacopoeia of India). Fenugreek, with a diversity in its forms and modes of use, has elicited its potential health benefits as a functional food in recent years, which until now has been a part of the traditional system of curing skin conditions and many other diseases (Basch et al., 2003).

Furthermore, fenugreek seeds are currently used as an antidiabetic agent, antibacterial, antilithogenic, antiulcer, anthelmintic, immunomodulatory effect, enzymatic pathway modifier, gastric stimulant, hypocholesterolemic, hypoglycemic, antioxidant, antiulcer, antifertility, and anti-anorexia agent.

Health benefits involve curing numerous disorders, from thyroid to diabetes. Fenugreek seeds, leaves, and powder are commonly used as household spices and herbs. The family of *Fabaceae* includes a number of important food plants, and Fenugreek (*Trigonellafoenum-graecum*) is one among them, it was also named as Trigonella, meaning "little triangle" in Latin language owing to its yellowish-white triangular flowers (Flammang et al., 2004). It has its origin in Central Asia in 4000 BC (Altuntas et al., 2005).

Earlier in 1500 BC in Egypt, description and health benefits of Fenugreek had been documented in the Ebers Papyrus (one of the oldest maintained medicinal document) (Betty, 2008).

It is known as Methi (Hindi, Marathi, Punjabi, and Urdu), Hulba (Arabic), Moshoseitaro (Greek), Uluva (Malayalam), Dari (Persian), Shoot (Hebrew), while it is known as hayseed in English.

It is commercially available and grown in India, Pakistan, Afghanistan, Iran, Spain, Nepal, France, Egypt, Morocco, North Africa, Turkey, Argentina and the Middle East (Flammang et al., 2004, Altuntas et al., 2005).

For thousands of years, it was one of the ancient conventional medicinal plants cultivated in the Indian subcontinent, Middle East, Canada, North Africa, Russia, United Kingdom, Mediterranean Europe, US, Australia, and parts of West Asia (Acharya et al., 2008).

It has various potential pharmacological effects in modern medicine such as antidiabetic, antilipidemic, antioxidant, hypocholesterolemic, hepatoprotective, antifungal, anti-inflammatory, antibacterial, anticarcinogenic, antiulcer, antilithigenic and neuroprotective effects in both clinical trials in humans as well as in experimental animals (Neelkanthan et al., 2014).

Fenugreek contains 20-25% protein, 45-50% dietary fiber, 20-25% mucilaginous soluble fiber, 2-5% steroidal saponins, 6-8% fixed fatty acid, and essential oils.

Breastfeeding is important for a baby's development, but some mothers suffer to produce an adequate amount. Initial research suggests that fenugreek was conventionally advised for increasing milk production in lactating women (Ghedira et al., 2010; Bukhari et al., 2008; Damanik et al., 2004). The objective of this chapter is to highlight the key phytochemicals and pharmacological applications of fenugreek on human health.

Botanical Description of Fenugreek

Fenugreek (*Trigonellafoenum-graecum*), belongs to the *Fabaceae* family. Fenugreek is an annual legume, diploid (2n =16) plant (Ahmad et al., 1999) with no aneuploidy (Petropoulos, 2002; Trease and Evans, 2002; Flammang et al., 2004). The botanical classification of fenugreek has been shown in Table 1.

Table 1. Botanical classification of Fenugreek

Kingdom		Plantae
Sub-kingdom	:	Tracheobionta (Vascular plants)
Division	:	Magnoliophyta (Flowering plants)
Class	:	Magnoliopsida (Dicotyledons)
Sub class	:	Rosidae
Order	:	Fabales
Family	:	Fabaceae
Genus	:	Trigonella
Species	:	T. foenum-graecum

Morphologically, fenugreek is an upright, aromatic annual spice closely similar to clover with cylindrical stem grown up to 30-60 cm long. It has roots that are huge finger-like structures (Basu, 2006; Mehrafarin et al., 2011; Moradikor and Moradi, 2013). Leaves of fenugreek are pinnate trifoliate, long stalked compounds having lanceolate, toothed, stipules triangular, oblanceolate to obovate leaflets (Srinivasan, 2006; Basu, 2006). Its flowers have five petals known as wing, keel and banner. Color of the ovary is deep green and glaucous, while the pollen grains are circular to oval in shape (Basu, 2006; Montgomery, 2009; Mehrafarin et al., 2011).

Fenugreek flower exhibits yellowish brown to brownish color and 15 cm long 2–8 pods. Each pod contains 10–20 seeds per pod; seeds are 5 mm long in size, smooth, hard and vary from dull yellow to brownish-yellow in color (Altuntas et al., 2005; Moradikor and Moradi, 2013).

CHEMICAL COMPOSITION

Proximate and Mineral Composition

The proximate and mineral composition of fenugreek leaves and seeds was summarized (Table 2). Its comprised of ash, moisture, crude fat, crude protein, crude fiber, vitamin C, vitamin A and carbohydrates.

The crude protein content of fenugreek leaves and seeds ranged between 4.4 – 25.4% respectively (Montgomery, 2009; Nasri and Tinay, 2007).

Dietary fiber content was 48.0 (Brummer et al., 2003) and crude fiber in fenugreek seeds was 50.0 (Montgomery, 2009).

The serving of 100g of fenugreek contains substantial level of calcium (75 mg), phosphorus (26.7 mg), iron (25.8 mg), magnesium (42 mg), potassium (603mg), manganese (0.9mg), copper (0.9mg) and other micronutrients with trace amount (Jasass and Jasser, 2012) (Table 2). These are crucial mineral elements for the daily physiological activities of humans.

Table 2. Proximate, mineral and metabolite content of fenugreek seeds and leaves

Particulars	Content		Reference
Moisture content			
Leaves	86		Sowmya and Rajyalakshmi (1991)
Seeds	7.49		Sowmya and Rajyalakshmi (1991)
Carbohydrates	42.3		El Nasri and El Tinay (2007)
Gum (seeds)	20.9		Kakani et al (2009)
Ash (seeds)	3.38		Sowmya and Rajyalakshmi (1991)
Fiber (seeds)	50.0		Montgomery (2009)
a) Soluble 1)Raw 2)Germinated	21.7 10.3		Muralidhara et al (1999) Muralidhara et al (1999)
b) Insoluble 1)Raw 26.8 Muralidhara et al (1999) 2)Germinated 23.9 Muralidhara et al (1999) Fiber (leaves) Soluble 0.7 Altuntas et al (2005) Insoluble 4.2 Altuntas et al (2005) Dietary fiber 48.0Brummer et al (2003) Fats (seeds) 7.9 El Nasri and El Tinay (2007) Montgomery (2009) Fats (leaves) 1.0 Montgomery (2009) Protein (seeds) 25.4 El Nasri and El Tinay (2007) Protein (leaves) 4.4 Montgomery (2009) **Mineral contents (mg/100g) of fenugreek seeds**			
Potassium (K)	603.0±15.0		Al Jasass and Al Jasser, 2012).
Magnesium	42.0 ± 5.0		Al Jasass and Al Jasser, 2012).
Calcium (Ca)	75.0 ± 9.0		Al Jasass and Al Jasser, 2012).
Iron	25.8 ± 1.2		Al Jasass and Al Jasser, 2012).
Copper	0.9 ± 0.1		Al Jasass and Al Jasser, 2012).
Manganese	0.9 ± 0.1		Al Jasass and Al Jasser, 2012).
Zinc	2.4 ± 0.2		Al Jasass and Al Jasser, 2012).
Vitamins (value/100g)			
Vitamin C			
Seed	12-43 mg		Leela and Shafeekh (2008) Srinivasan (2006)
Leaves	52.0 mg		Srinivasan (2006)
β carotene			
Seed Leaves	96 μg 2.3 μg		Srinivasan (2006) Srinivasan (2006)

Table 3. Nutrients per 100 grams of the edible portion of Fenugreek leaves

Total energy	49 Kcal
Carbohydrates	6.0g
Protein	4.4g
Fat	0.9g
Calcium	395mg
Phosphorus	51mg
Iron	1.93mg

Traditional Uses of Fenugreek

In India, fenugreek has been taken as a medicinal plant since ancient times and is regarded as safe to human health. In food, fenugreek seeds are added as preservatives in pickles as they are rich in vitamin E. Also, dried leaves of fenugreek are used for flavoring vegetable dishes, fish, and meat (Yadav et al., 2014).

A traditional remedy to cure fever is an herbal tea made with fenugreek, honey and lemon. Fenugreek fiber could be effective for curing constipation and stops the growth of diverticulosis. Fenugreek has been traditionally used as a remedy for burns, eczema, abscesses, and gout. It induces childbirth as it stimulates uterine contraction. Sprouted seeds of fenugreek and microgreens are used in salads. Fenugreek seeds are rich in lysine, 1-tryptophan, and trigonelline, whereas fenugreek leaves are a rich source of vitamin K (Sinha et al., 2015).

The use of fenugreek plants for curing kidney diseases and other related conditions was recommended by traditional Chinese herbalists. The seeds of fenugreek are nourishing and consumed during convalescence and aids in weight gain (in anorexia). The soothing effect of fenugreek seeds makes them significant in healing gastric ulcers and gastritis. In China, the fenugreek seeds are used as a pessary to cure cervical cancer.

In the Middle East and the Balkans, the aerial part of the fenugreek plant is a traditional therapy for abdominal cramps. They are best remedy to ease labor pains, but it should only be used for inducing labor only after in consultation with doctor (Global herbal supplies). Fenugreek effectively cleanses the blood. The healing and calming action makes a lubricant like protective covering over inflamed areas. For proper digestion, the slightly bitter taste of the seed is favorable (Kor et al., 2013).

Nutritional Profile

Following are the nutrients per 100 grams of the edible portion of Fenugreek leaves (Gopalan, 1989 and Sharma, 1990)

Toxicological Studies

Along with potential health benefits, fenugreek possesses some mild side-effects, as well. Although it appears relatively safe at the correct dosage. Therefore, there is extensive research needed to study the pharmacological and toxicological effects of fenugreek effectively to investigate their clinical efficacy and safety.

According to a study (Sureshkumar et al., 2018), when wistar rats were supplemented at 250 to 1000 mg/d for 8-12 weeks, no adverse effects or mortality was observed when compared to control group rats. Saponin-rich standardized extract of fenugreek seeds (FHE) is safe and effective to establish hormonal balance. One 14-day acute study and another 90-day sub-chronic study assessed oral acute toxicity of FHE. In 14-day study, 40 rats were divided in four groups in which group I was untreated and remaining groups II, III, IV were administered with FHE at different concentrations at 0.5, 2.0 and 2.5 g per kg body weight respectively.

In 90 days' oral toxicity study, 60 rats were split into 6 groups with each group having 5 males and 5 female rats. Group I and II were control and control recovery respectively. Group III, group IV, group V and group VI received low dose of FHE (250mg/kg), mid dose FHE (500mg/kg), high dose FHE (1000mg/kg) and high dose recovery (1000 mg/kg) respectively. The amount of dose selected was from previous studies (Arshadi et al., 2015, Kandhare et al., 2015 and Mowla et al., 2009).

Administration of FHE did not produce any significant changes in food and water consumption, body weight and hematological or biochemical changes.

Thus, as per the present study, FHE is safe with the no-observed-adverse-effect level in an animal study (in rats) with the administration of 1000mg per kg body weight per day and can be studied in humans. But, more extensive studies with a large number of animals on genotoxicity study and reproductive toxicity using more number of strains in GLP (good laboratory practices)-certified laboratories would contribute to more reliable facts on fenugreek extracts.

Moreover, no hematological or biochemical changes were observed when post-menopausal women were supplemented at 1g/d for 12 weeks (Begum et al., 2016).

Biologically Active Compounds

Fenugreek comprises (Table 5) a fairly high amount of alkaloids, saponins, flavonoids, and antioxidants. Fenugreek endosperm has 35% alkaloids, primarily trigonelline (Jani et al., 2009). Fenugreek seeds contain 100mg/g flavonoids (Naidu et al., 2011). Such compounds are referred to as biologically active constituent as these have pharmacological effects on the human body when consumed. Their consumption should be recommended in daily diet to manage diabetes mellitus, hypercholesterolemia and cancer because they exhibit hypoglycemic, anti-carcinogenic, antilipedemic and cholagogic properties (Meghwal and Goswami, 2012). However, alkaloids and volatile oils are the two key components that result in bitter taste and bad odor, and may then be removed before use.

Recent findings on the effects of *Trigonella* in different diseases are reported in this review study (Table 5) within both experimental and clinical studies. Overview of the pharmaceutical effects of Fenugreek (Figure 1).

Antioxidant Activity

Oxidative stress is one of the major health problems in humans, for which several therapies are utilized and where medicinal plants offer a favorable alternative. Fenugreek contains phenolic and flavonoid compounds that aid in improving its antioxidant capacity (Dixit et al., 2005).

Table 4. Pharmacological and therapeutic benefits of fenugreek as recurrently reported

Disease/Disorders	Description	Reference
Anemia	Prevents red blood cell oxidation	Kaviarasan et al., 2007
Aging	Antioxidants reduces cell death and aging	Kaviarasan et al., 2007
Cancer	Polyphenolic compounds from seed possess anti-carcinogenic activities	Mohamed et al., 2015
Diabetes	4-hydroxyisoleucin (amino acid) stimulates insulin production thereby control blood sugar level. Polyphenolic compounds exhibit anti-diabetic effects. Curative effects of fenugreek seed powder is a potential neuropathic medicine in diabetes	Kaviarasan et al., 2007 and Nanjundan et al., 2009
Hypercholesterolemia	Anti-oxidants from seeds control high blood cholesterol	Srinivasan, 2006
Immunodeficiency	Natural anti-oxidants help to strengthen immune system immunomodulatory and immune stimulatory effects	Kaviarasan et al., 2004
Indigestion and flatulence	Fenugreek has been used as laxative. It stimulates appetite	Sauvare et al. (2000) Petit et al. (1993)
Inflammation	Reduces swelling and pain	Kaviarasan et al., 2007
Kidney disorders	Protects functional and histopathological abnormalities of kidney in diabetic patients. Reduces catalase (CAT) and superoxide dismutase (SOD0 activity in hypercholesterolemia patients. Inhibit accumulation of oxidized DNA to prevent kidney injuries	Xue et al., 2011
Others	Respiratory disorders, bacterial infection, epilepsy, gout, chronic cough, paralysis, dropsy, piles, heavy metal toxicity, liver disorders and arthritis	Nanjundan et al., 2009, Xue et al., 2011, Kaviarasan et al., 2007

It has a beneficial effect on the liver and pancreas; antioxidant properties are associated with health benefits of natural products. Such properties are studied with germinated fenugreek seeds which are perceived to be more beneficial than un-germinated seeds because with germination the bioavailability of different components of fenugreek increases (Balch, 2003). Pulse radiolysis and the deoxyribose system demonstrated The OH scavenging activity of the seed extract. The fenugreek seeds extract contains antioxidants and protects cellular structures from oxidative damage. An aqueous methanolic extract of fenugreek was analyzed for its antiradical and in vitro antioxidant action in varied model systems. The results obtained by different methods present some important factors associated with the antioxidant activity of fenugreek seeds (Kaviarasan et al., 2007).

Table 5. Biologically active constituents of fenugreek and their classifications

Chemical group	Compound	References
Alkaloids	Trigonelline, choline, carpaine	Lee et al. (2005) Kaviarasan et al. (2007) Rababah et al. (2011)
Amino Acids	Lysine, histidine, 4-hydroxyisoleucine, tryptophan, tyrosine, cystine, arginine	Gupta et al. (2001) Ruby et al. (2005) El Nasri and El Tinay (2007)
Coumarins	Methyl coumarin, trigocumarin, trimethylcoumarin	Raju et al. (2001)
Flavonoids	Naringenin, lilyn, kaempferol, vecenin-1, tricin 7-O-D glucopyranoside, saponaretin, isovitexin, isoorientin. Orientin, vitexin, luteolin, quercetin	Blumenthal et al. (2000) Sauvare et al. (2000) Meghwal and Goswami (2012)
Saponins	Fenugrin, foenugracin, glycoside, yamogenin, trigonoesides, smilagenin, gitogenin, sarsasapogenin, yuccagenin, hederagin, diosgenin, tigonenin, neotigogenin	Gupta et al. (2001)
Others	Vitamin A, folic acid, ascorbic acid, thiamin, riboflavin, biotin, nicotinic acid, gum	Hamden et al. (2010) Chatterjee et al. (2010)

Anti Diabetic Activity

Sauvaire et al. (1998) reported that fenugreek seeds contain a free unnatural amino acid, 4-hydroxyisoleucine, which increases glucose-induced insulin release in pancreatic islet cells of humans and rats.

In another study, fenugreek stimulates tyrosine phosphorylation of the insulin receptor and enhances glucose uptake into cells (Kumar et al., 2005).

Presence of steroids in fenugreek has been studied to minimize blood glucose levels when supplemented to diabetic rats (Hamden et al., 2010).

In STZ-induced diabetic rats, fenugreek seed mucilage has beneficial effects on intestinal and renal disaccharide activity by enhancing the reduction in maltase activity in diabetes (Kumar et al., 2005).

Lipid Lowering Activity

Fenugreek seeds lower serum triglycerides, total cholesterol and low-density lipoprotein cholesterol owing to hypolipidemic effect of fenugreek.

Figure 1. Overview of pharmaceutical effects of Fenugreek

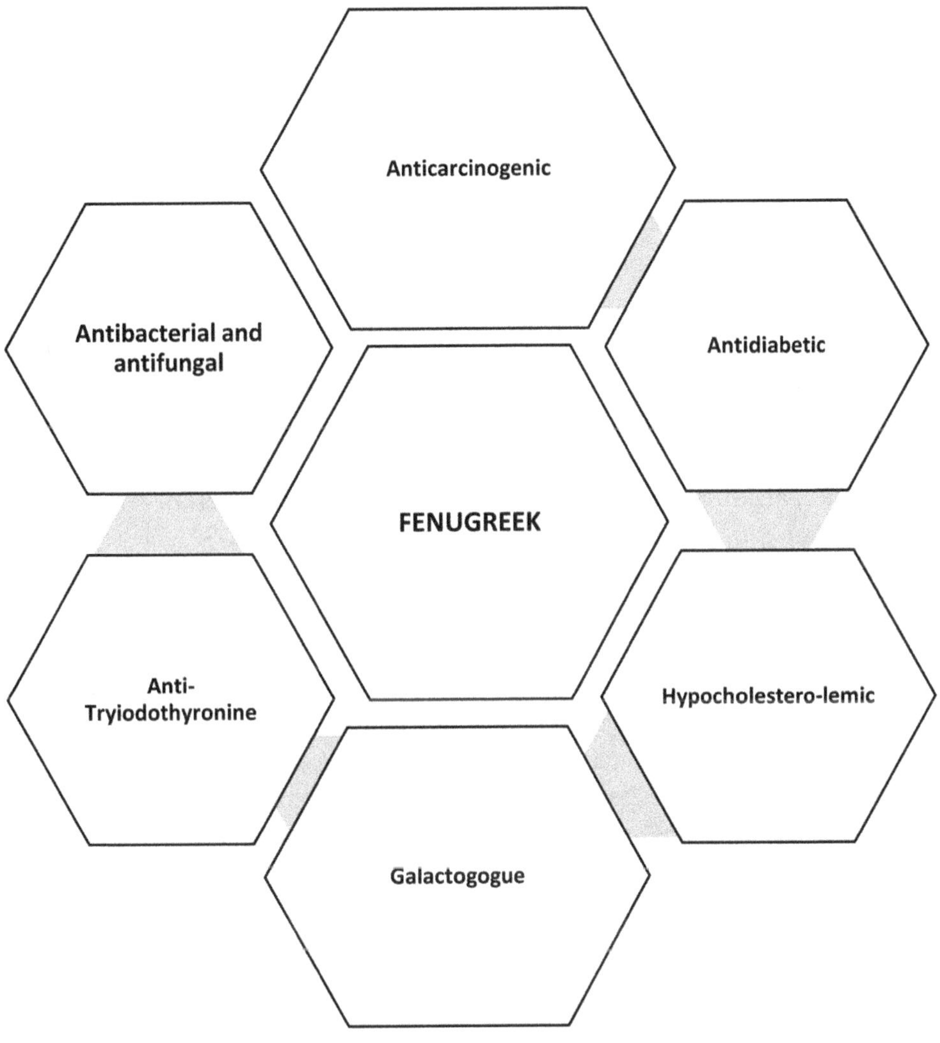

Dietary fibre (galactomannan) in fenugreek seeds is a polysaccharide that consists of a mannose backbone with galactose side chains, form a viscous gel in the intestine and inhibit lipid and glucose absorption (Hannan et al., 2007).

Anti-Tryiodothyronine Activity

The effects of fenugreek seed extract on the variations in serum thyroid hormone concentrations were reported in adult male mice and rats. Three enzymes viz., catalase (CAT), hepatic lipid per oxidation (LPO) and superoxide dismutase (SOD) were examined. As per the findings, fenugreek seed extract induced inhibition in T3 to T4 conversion is not peroxidation-mediated and hindrance in superoxide dismutase (SOD) could be the consequence of a decrease in the protein anabolic hormone, T3 (Panda et al., 1999).

Fibrinogen and Fibrinolytic Activity

In a placebo controlled trial the effect of fenugreek was analyzed on blood sugar, platelet aggregation, blood lipids, fibrinogen and fibrinolytic activity. Fenugreek does not show any effect on fibrinogen, platelet aggregation and fibrinolytic activity when administered for 3 months in dose of 2.5 gram twice daily (Bordia et al., 1997).

Anti-Carcinogenic Activity

Trigonellafoenum-graecum, possess anti-carcinogenic activity. Hibasami et al. (2003) reported that fenugreek-derived compound protodioscin exhibited a growth inhibitory action against HL-60 cells by inducing apoptotic changes. Amin et al. 2005 also showed that fenugreek seed extracts significantly inhibited7, 12-dimethylbenz (a) anthracene-induced mammary hyperplasia and decreased its incidence in rats and reported that anti-breast cancer-protective effects of fenugreek due to augmenting apoptosis.

Moreover, Verma et al., 2010 reported that alcoholic whole plant extracts of fenugreek indicated in vitro cytotoxicity in averse to various human cancer cell lines namely IMR-32, aneuroblastoma cell line, and HT29, which is a cancer cell line.

Growth inhibitory effects on breast, pancreatic, and prostate cancer cell lines are shown after the treatment with fenugreek extract, but primary prostate or immortalized prostate cells remained unaffected (Shabbeer et al., 2009). The potentiality of *Trigonella*to inhibit cancer cell growth is attributed to induce cell death, in spite of simultaneous up-regulation of growth stimulatory pathways within normal cells. Diosgenin, a steroid saponin obtained from *Trigonella,* was reported to preventazoxymethane (AOM)-induced aberrant crypt foci formation, a preneoplastic-colonic lesions in F344 rats and also induces caspase-3protein expression and inhibits bcl-2, making it potential as a colon cancer preventive element (Raju et al., 2004).

Antifungal and Antibacterial Effect

The antifungal and antibacterial effect of fenugreek is recently popular. In a study reported by (Haouala et al., 2008) aqueous extract from different parts of fenugreek plant in various solvents include petroleum ether, methanol, ethyl acetate fractions of the aerial parts and determined their action against fungal strains such as *Fusarium graminearum, Rhizoctoniasolani, Pythium aphaniderma-tum, Botrytis cinerea, and Alternaria* sp.

The presence of antifungal properties in all parts of the fenugreek is also reported, and the magnitudes of effect differ with species of fungus and plant parts. It could be propounded that fenugreek is a prime source of biologically active compounds beneficial for unfolding better and novel antifungal drugs.

Many studies described the beneficial effect of extracts derived from fenugreek against Helicobacter pylori (Mahony et al., 2005; Randhir et al., 2004; Randhir and Shetty, 2007). In a study, honey samples with the highest antibacterial activity against *Staphylococcus aureus, Pseudomonas aeruginosa* and *Escherichia coli* have more pollen from fenugreek compared to other plants (Mercan et al., 2007). The nematicidal activity was seen in the methanol soluble fraction of fenugreek extract and resulted in significant mortality of *Meloidogyne javanica* larvae, showing its prospective application against nematodes (Zia et al., 2001).

In a report by (Laroubi et al., 2007) reported the prophylaxis effect of fenugreek seeds on renal stone formation in rats. Use of fenugreek in curing patients with calcic-urolithiasis is also effective. (Chauhan et al., 2010) studied anti-inflammatory prospects of fenugreek.

Application Food Industries

It is used as spice (seeds), an herb (fresh or dried leaves), vegetable (fresh leaves) and also as a condiment in artificial flavoring of maple syrup or in the production of steroid and other hormones for the pharmaceutical, nutraceutical and functional food industries (Zandi et al., 2015). The widespread application of fenugreek in the food industry is due to the presence of dietary fiber because its galactomannan composition possesses emulsifying and stabilizing properties.

Supplementation of flour with a percentage of 8% and 10% of fenugreek dietary fiber has been used in the preparation of baked goods such as pizza, muffins bread, and cakes. Incorporation of fenugreek to flour makes it available in producing functional foods that may be widely acceptable to consumers observing western diets (Roberts, 2011).

SOLUTIONS AND RECOMMENDATIONS

Fenugreek is a well explored plant/herb by medical science for its contribution towards human health. Although it is a small part, it is of various benefits as a medicinal plant.

An extensive genomic and agronomic characterization/clustering is needed to discover the potential genes which could further assist in breeding programs along with targeted mutation and genetic advancement for abiotic stress tolerance. Moreover, fenugreek as a fodder crop and green manuring, and for soil, reclamation must be investigated and encouraged, particularly in arid agricultural systems (Ahmad et al., 2016).

Future Research Directions

Fenugreek has been shown to possess hypoglycemic potential but data is not sufficient to recommend its applicability in diabetes in the deprivation of careful supervision. Therefore, further research in this area may hold promise in this regard. A huge gap is still existing, particularly in biotechnologically facilitated breeding (Ahmad et al., 2016).

CONCLUSION

In recent years, several research studies have been done to explore the functional and medicinal properties of fenugreek seeds. The major medicinal properties of fenugreek include Antidiabetic, antioxidant, hypoglycemic and hypocholesterolemic, anticarcinogenic, activities. Fenugreek is a promising dietary supplement with versatile properties and several research studies have reported its beneficial effects. It contains vitamins such as thiamin, ribofavin, niacin, folic acid, vitamin A, C and minerals as Potassium, Calcium, Zinc, Magnesium, Iron, etc. On the basis of these health benefits, fenugreek can be recommended in our day-to-day diet and considered as functional food when incorporated in foods.

REFERENCES

Acharya, S., Thomas, J., & Basu, S. (2008). Fenugreek, an alternative crop for semiarid regions of north America. *Crop Science*, *3*(3), 841–853. doi:10.2135/cropsci2007.09.0519

Ahmad, A., Alghamdi, S. S., Mahmood, K., & Afzal, M. (2016). Fenugreek a multipurpose crop: Potentialities and improvements. *Saudi Journal of Biological Sciences*, *23*(2), 300–310. doi:10.1016/j.sjbs.2015.09.015 PMID:27307778

Ahmed, M. A., Ibrahim, O. M., & Elham, A. B. (2010). Effect of bio and mineral phosphorus fertilizer on the growth, productivity and nutritional value of fenugreek (*Trigonellafoenumgraecum* L.) in newly cultivated land. *Research Journal of Agriculture and Biological Sciences*, *6*(3), 339–348.

Al Jasass, F. M., & Al Jasser, M. S. (2012). Chemical composition and fatty acid content of some spices and herbs under Saudi Arabia conditions. *TheScientificWorldJournal*, *2012*, 1–5. doi:10.1100/2012/859892 PMID:23319888

Altuntas, E., Ozgoz, E., & Taser, O. F. (2005). Some physical properties of fenugreek (*Trigonellafoenumgraecum* L. seeds. *Journal of Food Engineering*, *71*(1), 37–43. doi:10.1016/j.jfoodeng.2004.10.015

Amin, A., Alkaabi, A., & Al-Falasi, S. (2005). Chemopreventive activities of *Trigonellafoenumgraecum* (Fenugreek) against breast cancer. *Cell Biology International*, *29*(8), 687–694. doi:10.1016/j.cellbi.2005.04.004 PMID:15936223

Arshadi, S., Azarbayjani, M.A., & Hajaghaalipor, F. (2015). Evaluation of *Trigonellafoenum-graecum* extract in combination with swimming exercise compared to glibenclamide consumption on type 2 diabetic rodents. *Food Nutr. Res.*, *59*.doi: .v59.29717 doi:10.3402/fnr

Balch, P. A. (2003). Prescription for dietary wellness (2nd ed.). Penguin Group.

Basch, E., Ulbricht, C., & Kuo, G. (2003). Therapeutic applications of fenugreek. *Alternative Medicine Review*, *8*(1), 20–27. PMID:12611558

Begum, S. S., Jayalakshmi, H. K., & Vidyavathi, H. G. (2016). A novel extract of fenugreek husk (FenuSMARTTM) alleviates postmenopausal symptoms and helps to establish the hormonal balance: A randomized, double-blind, Placebo-Controlled Study. *Phytotherapy Research*, *30*(11), 1775–1784. doi:10.1002/ptr.5680 PMID:27406028

Betty, R. (2008). *The many healing virtues of fenugreek*. Spice India.

Blumenthal, M., Goldberg, A., & Brinckmann, J. (2000). Herbal Medicine: Expanded Commission E Monographs. American Botanical Council, Integrative Medicine Communications.

Bordia, A., Verma, S. K., & Srivastava, K. C. (1997). Effect of ginger and fenugreek on blood lipids, blood sugar and platelet aggregation in patients with coronary disease Prostaglandins, Leukotrienes and Essential Fatty Acids. *Pharmacological Research*, *36*, 379–384.

Brummer, Y., Cui, W., & Wang, Q. (2003). Extraction, purification and physicochemical characterization of fenugreek gum. *Food Hydrocolloids*, *3*(3), 229–236. doi:10.1016/S0268-005X(02)00054-1

Bukhari, S. B., Bhanger, M. I., & Memon, S. (2008). Antioxidative activity of extracts from fenugreek. *Pakistan Journal of Analytical & Environmental Chemistry*, *9*(2), 78–83.

Chatterjee, S., Variyar, P. S., & Sharma, A. (2010). Bioactive lipid constituents of fenugreek. *Food Chemistry*, *1*(1), 349–353. doi:10.1016/j.foodchem.2009.05.076

Chauhan, G., Sharma, M., & Varma, A. (2010). Phytochemical analysis and anti-inflammatory potential of fenugreek, Medicinal plants. *Int. J. Phytomedicine. Rel. Ind*, *2*(1), 39–44.

Damanik, R., Wahlqvist, M. L., & Wattanapenpaiboon, N. (2004). The use of a putative lactogogue plant on breast milk production in Simalungun, North Sumatra, Indonesia. *Asia Pacific Journal of Clinical Nutrition*, *13*, S118.

Dixit, P., Ghaskadbi, S., Mohan, H., & Devasagayam, T. P. A. (2005). Antioxidant properties of germinated fenugreek seeds. *Phytotherapy Research*, *19*(11), 977–983. doi:10.1002/ptr.1769 PMID:16317656

El Nasri, N. A., & El Tinay, A. (2007). Functional properties of Fenugreek (*Trigonellafoenumgraecum*) protein concentrate. *Food Chemistry*, *2*(2), 582–589. doi:10.1016/j.foodchem.2006.09.003

Flammang, A., Cifone, M., Erexson, G., & Stankowski, L. F. Jr. (2004). Genotoxicity testing of a fenugreek extract. *Food and Chemical Toxicology*, *11*(11), 1769–1775. doi:10.1016/j.fct.2004.07.003 PMID:15350674

Ghedira, K., Goetz, P. L. J. R., & Le Juene, R. (2010). Fenugrec: *Trigonellafoenumgraecum* L. (Fabaceae ex. Leguminosae). *Phytothérapie*, *8*(3), 180–184. doi:10.100710298-010-0551-z

Gopalan, C., Ramasastri, B.V., & Balasubramaniyam, S.C. (1989). *Nutritive value of Indian food*. National Institute of Nutrition, ICMR Hydrabad.

Gupta, A., Gupta, R., & Lal, B. (2001). Effect of *Trigonellafoenum- graecum*(fenugreek) seeds on glycaemic control and insulin resistance in type 2 diabetes mellitus: A double blind placebo controlled study. *The Journal of the Association of Physicians of India*, *49*, 1057–1061. PMID:11868855

Hamden, K., Jaouadi, B., Carreau, S., Aouidet, A., El-Fazaa, S., Gharbi, N., & Elfeki, A. (2010). Potential protective effect on key steroidogenesis and metabolic enzymes and sperm abnormalities by fenugreek steroids in testis and epididymis of surviving diabetic rats. *Archives of Physiology and Biochemistry*, *116*(3), 146–155. doi:10.3109/13813455.2010.486405 PMID:20507258

Hannan, J. M. A., Ali, L., Rokeya, B., Khaleque, J., Akhter, M., Flatt, P. R., & Abdel-Wahab, Y. H. A. (2007). Soluble dietary fibre fraction of *Trigonellafoenum-graecum*(fenugreek) seed improves glucose homeostasis in animal models of type 1and type 2 diabetes by delaying carbohydrate digestion and absorption and enhancing insulin action. *British Journal of Nutrition*, *97*(3), 514–521. doi:10.1017/S0007114507657869 PMID:17313713

Haouala, R., Hawala, S., El-Ayeb, A., Khanfir, R., & Boughanmi, N. (2008). Aqueous and organic extracts of *Trigonellafoenumgraecum* L. inhibit the mycelia growth of fungi. *Journal of Environmental Sciences (China)*, *20*(12), 1453–1457. doi:10.1016/S1001-0742(08)62548-6 PMID:19209631

Hibasami, H., Moteki, H., & Ishikawa, H. (2003). Protodioscin isolated from fenugreek (*Trigonella-foenumgraecum*) induces cell death and morphological change indicative of apoptosis in leukemic cell line H-60 but not in gastric cancer line KATO III. *International Journal of Molecular Medicine*, *11*, 23–26. PMID:12469212

Jani, R., Udipi, S., & Ghugre, P. (2009). Mineral content of complementary foods. *Indian Journal of Pediatrics*, *1*(1), 37–44. doi:10.100712098-009-0027-z PMID:19391001

Kakani, R.K., Anwer, M.M., & Meena, S.S. (2009). Advance production technology of fenugreek. *NRCSS Tech. Release*, 1-24.

Kandhare, A. D., Bodhankar, S. L., Mohan, V., & Thakurdesai, P. A. (2015). Acute and repeated doses (28 days) oral toxicity study of glycosides based standardized fenugreek seed extract in laboratory mice. *Regulatory Toxicology and Pharmacology*, *72*(2), 323–334. doi:10.1016/j.yrtph.2015.05.003 PMID:25979642

Kaviarasan, S., Naik, G., Gangabhagirathi, R., Anuradha, C. V., & Priyadarsini, K. I. (2007). In vitro studies on antiradical and antioxidant activities of fenugreek (*Trigonellafoenumgraecum*) seeds. *Food Chemistry*, *103*(1), 31–37. doi:10.1016/j.foodchem.2006.05.064

Laroubi, A., Touhami, M., Farouk, L., Zrara, I., Aboufatima, R., Benharref, A., & Chait, A. (2007). Prophylaxis effect of *Trigonellafoenumgraecum* L. seeds on renal stone formation in rats. *Phytotherapy Research*, *21*(10), 921–925. doi:10.1002/ptr.2190 PMID:17582593

Lee, S. J., Umano, K., Shibamoto, T., & Lee, K.-G. (2005). Identification of volatile components in basil (*Ocimumbasilicum* L.) and thyme leaves (*Thymus vulgaris* L.) and their antioxidant properties. *Food Chemistry*, *1*(1), 131–137. doi:10.1016/j.foodchem.2004.05.056

Leela, N., & Shafeekh, K. (2008). *Fenugreek. Chemistry of Spices*. Pondicherry, India: CAB. International.

Meghwal, M., & Goswami, T. K. (2012). A review on the functional properties, nutritional content, medicinal utilization and potential application of fenugreek. *Journal of Food Processing & Technology*, *3*(09). doi:10.4172/2157-7110.1000181

Mehrafarin, A., Rezazahdeh, S. H., & Naghdi, B. H. (2011). A review on biology, cultivation and biotechnology of fenugreek (*Trigonellafoenumgraecum* L.) as a valuable medicinal plant and multipurpose. *Faslnamah-i Giyahan-i Daruyi*, *10*, 6–24.

Mercan, N., Guvensen, A., Celik, A., & Katircioglu, H. (2007). Antimicrobial activity and pollen composition of honey samples collected from different provinces in Turkey. *Natural Product Research*, *21*(3), 187–195. doi:10.1080/14786410600906277 PMID:17365707

Mohamed, W. S., Mostafa, A. M., Mohamed, K. M., & Serwah, A. H. (2015). Effects of fenugreek, Nigella, and termis seeds in nonalcoholic fatty liver in obese diabetic albino rats. *Arab Journal of Gastroenterology*, *16*(1), 1–9. doi:10.1016/j.ajg.2014.12.003 PMID:25670619

Montgomery, J. (2009). *The potential of Fenugreek (Trigonellafoenumgraecum) as a forage for dairy herds in central Alberta*. University of Alberta.

Moradi, K. N., & Moradi, K. (2013). Physiological and pharmaceutical effects of fenugreek (*Trigonella-foenumgraecum* L.) as multipurpose and valuable medicinal plant. *Global J. Med. Plant Res.*, *1*, 199-206.

Mowla, A., Alauddin, M., & Rahman, M. A. (2009). Antihyperglycemic effect of *TrigonellaFoenum-Graecum* (Fenugreek) seed extract in alloxan-induced diabetic rats and its use in diabetes mellitus: A brief qualitative phytochemical and acute toxicity test on the extract. *AJTCAM*, *6*(3), 255–261. PMID:20448850

Naidu, M. M., Shyamala, B., & Naik, J. P. (2011). Chemical composition and antioxidant activity of the husk and endosperm of fenugreek seeds. *Lebensmittel-Wissenschaft + Technologie*, *2*(2), 451–456. doi:10.1016/j.lwt.2010.08.013

Nanjundan, P., Arunachalam, A., & Thakur, R. (2009). Antinociceptive property of *Trigonellafoenum graecum*(fenugreek seeds) in high fat diet-fed/low dose streptozotocin-induced diabetic neuropathy in rats. *Pharmacology*, 24–36.

Narasimhamurthy, K., Vishwanatha, S., & Ramesh, B. S. (1999). Acute and subchronic toxicity assessment of debitterized fenugreek powder in the mouse and rat. *Food and Chemical Toxicology*, *37*(8), 831–838. doi:10.1016/S0278-6915(99)00076-9 PMID:10506006

Neelkanthan, N., Narayanan, M., & de Souza, R. J. (2014). Effect of fenugreek (*Trigonellafoenum-graecum*L.) intake on glycemia: A meta-analysis of clinical trials. *Nutrition Journal*, *13*(1), 7. doi:10.1186/1475-2891-13-7 PMID:24438170

O'Mahony, R., Al-khtheeri, H., & Weerasekera, D. (2005). Bactericidal and antiadhesive properties of culinary and medicinal plants against *Helicobactor pylori*. *World Journal of Gastroenterology*, *11*(47), 7499–7507. doi:10.3748/wjg.v11.i47.7499 PMID:16437723

Panda, S., Tahiliani, P., & Kar, A. (1999). Inhibition of Triiodothyronine production by fenugreek seeds extract in mice and rats. *Pharmacological Research*, *40*(5), 405–409. doi:10.1006/phrs.1999.0510 PMID:10527654

Petit, P., Sauvaire, Y., Ponsin, G., Manteghetti, M., Fave, A., & Ribes, G. (1993). Effects of a fenugreek seed extract on feeding behavior in the rat: Metabolic endocrine correlates. *Pharmacology, Biochemistry, and Behavior*, *2*(2), 369–374. doi:10.1016/0091-3057(93)90253-P PMID:8327543

Petropoulos, G. A. (2002). *Fenugreek, The genus Trigonella*. London: Taylor and Francis. doi:10.4324/9780203217474

Rababah, T. M., Ereifej, K. I., Esoh, R. B., Al-u'datt, M. H., Alrababah, M. A., & Yang, W. (2011). Antioxidant activities, total phenolics and HPLC analyses of the phenolic compounds of extracts from common Mediterrarean plants. *Natural Product Research*, *6*(6), 596–605. doi:10.1080/14786419.2010.488232 PMID:21409721

Raju, J., Gupta, D., Rao, A. R., Yadava, P. K., & Baquer, N. Z. (2001). *Trigonellafoenumgraecum* (Fenugreek) seed powder improves glucose homeostasis in alloxan diabetic rat tissues by reversing the altered glycolytic, gluconeogenic and lipogenic enzymes. *Molecular and Cellular Biochemistry*, *224*(1/2), 45–51. doi:10.1023/A:1011974630828 PMID:11693199

Randhir, R., Lin, Y. T., & Shetty, K. (2004). Phenolics, their antioxidant and antimicrobial activity in dark germinated fenugreek sprouts in response to peptide and phytochemical elicitors. *Asia Pacific Journal of Clinical Nutrition*, *13*, 295–307. PMID:15331344

Randhir, R., & Shetty, K. (2007). Improved alpha-amylase and *Helicobactor pylori* inhibition by fenugreek extracts derived via solid-state bioconversion using *Rhizopusoligosporous. Asia Pacific Journal of Clinical Nutrition*, *16*, 382–392. PMID:17704018

Roberts, K. T. (2011). The potential of fenugreek (*Trigonellafoenumgraecum)* as a functional food and nutraceutical and its effects on glycemia and lipidemia. *Journal of Medicinal Food*, *14*(12), 1485–1489. doi:10.1089/jmf.2011.0002 PMID:21861724

Ruby, B., Gaskill, S., Slivka, D., & Harger, S. G. (2005). The addition of fenugreek extract (*Trigonellafoenum- graecum)* to glucose feeding increases muscle glycogen resynthesis after exercise. *Amino Acids*, *1*(1), 71–76. doi:10.100700726-004-0143-z PMID:15719265

Sauvaire, Y., Petit, P., Broca, C., Manteghetti, M., Baissac, Y., Fernandez-Alvarez, J., ... Ribes, G. (1998). 4-Hydroxyisoleucine: A novel amino acid potentiator of insulin secretion. *Diabetes*, *47*(2), 206–210. doi:10.2337/diab.47.2.206 PMID:9519714

Sauvare, Y., Pett, P., & Baissao, Y. (2000). Chemistry and pharmacology of fenugreek. In G. Mazza & B. D. Oomah (Eds.), *Herbs, Botanicals and Teas* (pp. 107–129). Technomic Publishing Company Inc.

Shabbeer, S., Sobolewski, M., Anchoori, R. K., Kachhap, S., Hidalgo, M., Jimeno, A., ... Khan, S. R. (2009). Fenugreek: A naturally occurring edible spice as an anticancer agent. *Cancer Biology & Therapy*, *8*(3), 2720–278. doi:10.4161/cbt.8.3.7443 PMID:19197146

Sharma, R. D., Raghuram, T. C., & Rao, N. S. (1990). Effect of fenugreek seeds on blood glucose and serum lipids in type I diabetes. *European Journal of Clinical Nutrition*, *44*(4), 301–306. PMID:2194788

Sinha, R., Rauniar, G. P., & Panday, D. R. (2015). Fenugreek: Pharmacological actions. *World Journal of Pharmacy and Pharmaceutical Sciences*, *5*(1), 1481–1489.

Sowmya, P., & Rajyalakshmi, P. (1999). Hypocholesterolemic effect of germinated fenugreek seeds in human subjects. *Plant Foods for Human Nutrition (Dordrecht, Netherlands)*, *4*(4), 359–365. doi:10.1023/A:1008021618733 PMID:10540988

Srinivasan, K. (2006). Fenugreek (*Trigonellafoenumgraecum* L.): A review of health beneficial physiological effects. *Food Reviews International*, 2, 2013–2224.

Suresh, K. G., Shetty, A. K., & Salimath, P. V. (2005). Modulatory effect of fenugreek seed mucilage and spent turmeric on intestinal and renal disaccharidases in streptozotocin induced diabetic rats. *Plant Foods for Human Nutrition (Dordrecht, Netherlands)*, *60*(2), 87–91. doi:10.100711130-005-5104-5 PMID:16021836

Sureshkumar, D., Begum, S., Johannah, N. M., Maliakel, B., & Krishnakumar, I. M. (2018). Toxicological evaluation of a saponin-rich standardized extract of fenugreek seeds (FenuSMART): Acute, subchronic and genotoxicity studies. *Toxicology Reports*, *5*, 1060–1068. doi:10.1016/j.toxrep.2018.10.008 PMID:30416976

Trease, G. E., & Evans, M. C. (2002). Textbook of Pharmacognosy (15th ed.). London: Academic Press.

Verma, S. K., Singh, S. K., & Mathur, A. (2010). In vitro cytotoxicity of Calotropisprocera and *Trigonellafoenum-graecum* against human cancer cell lines. *Journal of Chemical and Pharmaceutical Research*, *2*, 861–865.

Vijaykumar, M. V., Singh, S., & Chhipa, R. R. (2005). The hypoglycaemic activity of fenugreek seed extract is mediated through the stimulation of an insulin signaling pathway. *British Journal of Pharmacology*, *146*(1), 41–48. doi:10.1038j.bjp.0706312 PMID:15980869

Yadav, R., Kaushik, R., & Gupta, D. (2011). The health benefits of *Trigonellafoenum- graecum*: A review. *Int. J. Engineering Research and Applications*, *1*(1), 32-35.

Zandi, P., Basu, S.K., & Khatibani, L.B. (2015). Fenugreek (*Trigonellafoenum-graecum* L.) seed: a review of physiological and biochemical properties and their genetic improvement. *Acta. Physiol. Plant.*, *37*, 1714. DOI 10.1007/s11738-014-1714-6

Zia, T., Hasnain, S. N., & Hasan, S. K. (2001). Evaluation of the oral hypoglycaemic effect of *Trigonellafoenumgraecum* L.(methi) in normal mice. *Journal of Ethnopharmacology*, *75*(2-3), 191–195. doi:10.1016/S0378-8741(01)00186-6 PMID:11297850

Chapter 12
Mustard Is a Miracle Seed to Human Health

Mamta Sahu
Department of Agricultural Biochemistry, Chandra Shekhar Azad University of Agriculture and Technology, Kanpur, India

Suman Devi
Department of Agricultural Biochemistry, Chandra Shekhar Azad University of Agriculture and Technology, Kanpur, India

Pragya Mishra
Department of Agricultural Biochemistry, Chandra Shekhar Azad University of Agriculture and Technology, Kanpur, India

Ena Gupta
Department of Home Science, University of Allahabad, India

ABSTRACT

Brassica juncea, known as Indian mustard, has been used for centuries for its nutritional and medicinal values. L. brassica is a genus of plants in the mustard family, Brassicaceae. The members of the genus are informally known as cruciferous vegetables, cabbages, or mustard plants. Among the different varieties of mustard, the three principals are Brassica hirta or Alba (yellow-white), B. nigra (black), and B. juncea (brown). In Asian countries, India ranks first in mustard production, and mustard is the primary cooking oil used. In folkloric medicine, different parts of the plants are obtained to treat a wide variety of human aliments. Mustard seed is good source of protein, fibre, minerals, vitamins, antioxidants, and phytonutrients. The plant has several health benefits acting as antimicrobial, antibacterial, anti-diabetic, antimalarial, etc. The present study aims to discuss the up to date information regarding the botany, traditional uses, phytochemistry, and pharmacological applications of mustard seed and its essential oil.

DOI: 10.4018/978-1-7998-2524-1.ch012

INTRODUCTION

India is the land of medicinal plants, which forms the basis of traditional medicinal systems, such as Ayurveda, Siddha, and Unani. In modern society, a number of drugs havebeen derived from these natural resources, which form a major backbone of the primary healthcare systems throughout the world. Brassica juncea is known as Indian mustard and has been used for centuries for its nutritional and medicinal importance.

Brassicaceae or cruciferae is a medium-sized and economically important family of flowering plants commonly known as mustard plants. Among the different varieties of mustard, the three principal ones are Brassica hirta or Alba (yellow-white), B. nigra(black), and B. juncea (brown) (Elvin-Lewis, 2001). Brassica hirta is a native of Eastern Mediterranean regions, B. nigra comes from the Middle East, and B. juncea is found in the foothills of the Himalayas (Wikipedia, 2009). Brassica juncea is known as mustard seeds, and in India, it is commonly called as Rai, Sarso, Shorshe, and Kadugu.

The plant is a winter crop that requires a temperate climate and moist soil for its growth (Wikipedia, 2009). It is an herbaceous plant having petiolate leaves and small yellow flowers. The tiny seeds are present in one flower, which is about two millimetres in diameter, and the seeds are used as spices in many countries. Among the agricultural, it is an important oilseed crop that contributes approximately 14% of the world's vegetable oil production, and it is among the third leading source of vegetable oil, after palm and soybean oil, as per data revealed by National Commodity & Derivatives Exchange Limited (NCDEX). In Asian countries, India ranks first in mustard production and mustard accounts for the main oil used in Indian cooking. The defatted mustard cake is used as fertilizer and animal fodder(John& Soba,2011).

In folkloric medicine, different parts of the plants are obtained to treat a wide range of human aliments. However, most of the traditional uses are cantered on the seed and oil. The seed has been used for the treatment of ailments such as arthritis, foot pain, cancer, vomiting, dengue, and rheumatism. Mustard seed is also a good source of protein, with a protein efficiency ratio of 2.64, which is higher when compared to soybean. The seed of this crop is also rich in fibre, minerals, vitamins, antioxidants, and phytonutrients, such as alpha-linolenic acid, erucic acid, palmitic acid, tocopherols, tocotrienols, carotene, oryzanol, squalene, and thiamine (Billman, 2013). Tocopherolsare recognized for their antioxidant activity and have been observed to be useful in treating degenerative diseases such as cancer, cataracts, cardiovascular disease, and aging. Tocopherols in oil act through several mechanisms, such as inhibiting the lipid peroxidation, chain termination, singlet oxygen quenching, and radical scavenging from deactivating free radicals that are produced during the oxidation of biomolecules (Qureshi et al., 1991).The oil from this seed has a balanced ratio of saturated fatty acids/monounsaturated fatty acids/ polyunsaturated fatty acids(SFA/MUFA/PUFA) and antioxidants. Consuming mustard oil will not compensate for a generally unhealthy diet or a lack of physical activity.

Producing mustard oil involves pressing or grinding the seeds. The presence of allyl isothiocyanate in the oil gives it its strong taste and may contribute to some health benefits. Allyl isothiocyanate is also present in foods such as horseradish and wasabi. Mustard oil may pose a serious risk because it contains high levels of erucic acid. In small doses, erucic acid is safe, but at higher levels it may be dangerous(Delisle,1984).

The market for mustard oil is huge, and it is expected to seesignificant growth in the coming years, mainly attributed to increasing applications of mustard seeds in the food and beverage industries, pharmaceutical industry, personal care industry, the cosmetic industry, and others. B. juncea seeds are a source for obtaining pharmacologically standardized phytotherapeutics, which could be potentially useful for the development of modern drugs (Dubie,Stancik, Morra, & Nindo, 2015). The present study aims to discuss the latest information regarding the botany, traditional uses, phytochemistry, and pharmacological applications of mustard seed extract and its essential oils.

BOTANICAL DESCRIPTION

The mustard plant is an herbaceous plant that grows annually up to a length of one meter. The shape of the leaves is petiolate, alternate in dark green colour. The leaves, which are present on the lower position, look rough, irregular, sinuate dentate, have a pinate shape, with a terminal lobe and also small lobes. The texture of the top leaves is smooth and moderately lobed. The flowers of these crops are small in size, have four petals, and arebright yellow in colour(Pawar,2012). The fruit of the mustard plant is known as siliqua, which is a smooth quadrangular texture with a slender beak. Commonly, black mustard is also called the true mustard and is locally known as senafich, Amcariczwariemosterd (Dutch), Moutarde noir (French),and rai (Hindi)(Uhl, 2000). Among the temperate regions in the world, the third most popular spice is mustard. Mustard originated from a mixture of sweet and old wine, combined with the powdered form of mustard seed in the paste form. The condiment belongs to the Cruciferae plant family, which has four-pedalled flower in a cross formation. The members of this family include mustards, radishes, cabbage, broccoli, turnips, cresses, and horseradish, to name a few.

ETHNOMEDICINAL IMPORTANCE

The yellow colourof the mustard seed originates from the Himalayan Mountain foothills and the mustard seed has been mentioned in ancient Sanskrit writings, dating back 5000 years,for their diverse human health benefits(Iqbal,Akhtar, Zafar, & Ali,2008). This popular spice is an excellent source of selenium, omega three fatty acids, manganese, phosphorus, copper, magnesium, and vitamin B-1. Yellow mustard seeds are also garnering interest for their anti-cancer effects, particularly against gastrointestinal tract and colorectal cancer. The seeds may also reduce the effects of asthma, rheumatoid arthritis, help lower high blood pressure, reduce the symptoms of menopause, prevent heart attack, migraine attacks, and diabetes. Yellow mustard seeds are also known to help to prevent cardiovascular disease, neurological function, and also help to control metabolic activity while maintaining the integrity of mucus and cell membranes, in addition to protecting the skin from harmful oxygen-free radicals (Bhuiyan, Begum, & Sultana, 2009).

PHYTOCHEMISTRY

Although phytochemical compounds are the secondary metabolites that are non-essential for the growth of the plant,they play an important role in protecting the plantfrom environmental stress, plant pathogens, and other predators.The edible part of the brassica family of plants consists of such pigments known as phenolics, polyphenols, phenolic acid, flavonoids, carotenoids, alkaloids, phytosterols, glucosinolates, and terpenoids(Khattab&Arntfield,2009). These pigments arealso an important source of antioxidants such as metal-reducing, metal-chelating, lipid-reducing, and free-radical-cleaning agents. The actions of this antioxidant on enzyme activity, such as glutathione peroxidase, superoxidase dismutase, catalase, and ascorbate peroxidasehelpto minimize the effects of aging in human beings.

The oilseed of the mustard is rich in phytonutrients, such as glucosinolates, which were reported in plant science in the 1990s(Yadava et al.,2011). In flowering plants, glucosinolates occurand are composed of sugar molecules. Enzymatically, glucosinolates are broken down into isothiocyanates, cyanides, and thiocyanates, which are the main bio-actives responsible for pharmacological effects. Sinigrin is a major glucosinolate found in Brassicaceae juncea (Indian mustard). Brassica junceais a rich source of nutritionally important chemical constituents such as phytate, fibre, minerals, tocopherols, vitamins, and phenolic compounds(Crozier, Jaganath, & Clifford, 2009).

Figure 1. Structure of glucosinolates
Obtained fromRadojčić Redovniković, Glivetic, Delonga, &Vorkapić-Furač(2008).

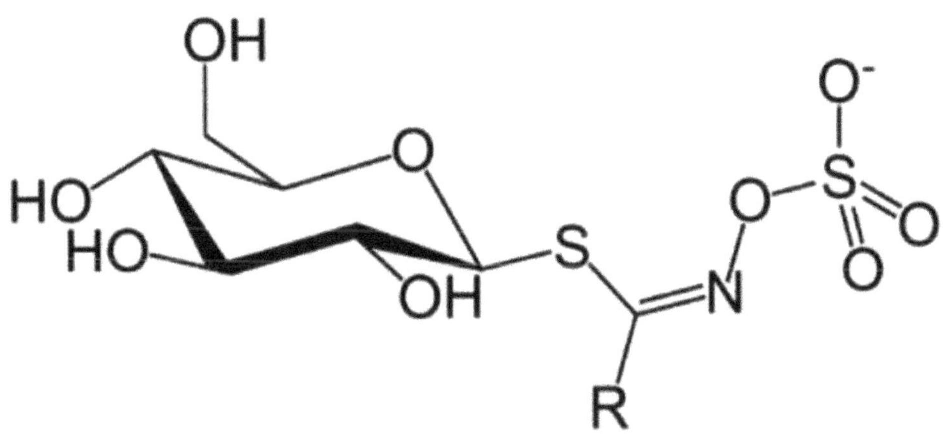

This crop has high levels of both alpha-linolenic acid and erucic acid. In abroad countries, mustard oil cannot be imported or sold for use in cooking, except for those products with exceptionally low erucic acid content. Therefore, brown mustard is being used for oil production, having low glucosinolates and low erucic acid content (Merah,2015).

There have been varying opinions in a number of studies as to the value of mustard seed oil. This oil, which is high in alpha-linolenic acid, has been thought by some researchers to protect the heart and to prevent cardiovascular disease(Desai,2005).In other studies, the mustard oil showed no protective effect on the heart, and the researchers stated that they thought the benefits of alpha-linolenic acid were outweighed by the potential harm of the erucic acid. Another study found that mustard oil had a protective effect on the heart, and the researchers' opinions were that the benefits of alpha-linolenic acid outweighed the potential harm of the erucic acid(Merah, 2015). During ancient times, the oils were used for infant massage, which one study viewed as risking damage to the skin integrity and permeability.

Figure 2. Biotransformation pathway

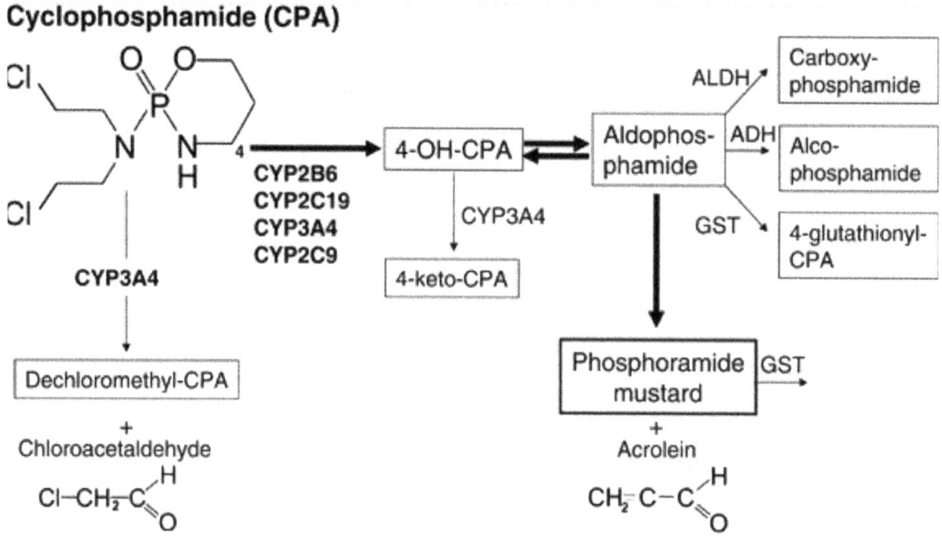

The conversion of molecules from one form to another within an organism is often associated with changed (increase, decrease, or little change) in pharmacologic activity, which refers especially to drugs and other xenobiotics. Transformation is the process by which substances that enter the body are changed from hydrophobic to hydrophilic molecules to facilitate elimination from the body. This process usually generates products with few or no toxicological effects. Biotransformation is the chemical modification made by an organism on a chemical compound. Biotransformation sometimes yields toxic metabolites, through a process known as *bio-activation*(Elvin-Lewis, 2001).The chemical reactions responsible for changing a lipophilic toxicant into a chemical form are known as *Phase I* and *Phase II biotransformations*. The two groups are defined based on the reactions that are catalysed. Phase I reactions transform hydrophobic chemicals to more polar products via oxidation, hydrolysis, or similar reactions. Phase II processes involve conjugation reactions that add polar functional groups, such as glucose or sulphate, to the Phase I products to produce what are often even more polar metabolites. Thus, these become even more water-soluble and can be readily excreted (Manohar,Pushpan, & Rohini, 2009).

Many biotransformation enzymes exhibit broad substrate specificity, providing a mechanism for enhancing the excretion of a wide range of hazardous compounds. Biotransformation is of primary importance to toxicology because the biological activity of toxicants is enhanced or decreased by this process. The biotransformation of toxicants is catalysed by enzymes that have various kinetic mechanisms of combining with substrates and releasing products. Understanding the kinetic mechanisms of the enzymes involved in xenobiotic biotransformation is important for understanding mechanisms of toxicity and designing antidotal therapy (Anuradha et al., 2012). Exposure to multiple chemicals can lead to exaggerated biological effects due to modulation of the metabolism of one toxicant by another. These modulations generally occur by inhibition of biotransformation, or by induction of enzyme activity (Yadav et al.,2013).

HEALTH BENEFITS

Since ancient times, mustard has been used as a food, and it has also illustrated medicinal benefits in Ayurvedic medicine. Mustard is a major part of the diet because of its high-energy value and because of the fat-soluble micronutrients and essential fatty acids. The balancing of fats relating to quality and quantity, affects the human diet, which helps to prevent chronic, debilitating diseases such as cardiovascular disease and rheumatoid arthritis. Among the fatty acids present in fats and oils are monounsaturated fatty acids(MUFA), or healthy fats, such as oleic acid and Essential fatty acids (EFA). Essential fatty acids are of particular interest because they are critical for human survival. EFAs are polyunsaturated and include linoleic acid (n-6 or 6 fatty acids), and α-linolenic acid (n-3 or 3 fatty acids). (Grover,Yadav, & Vats, 2003).

Inside the human body, essential fatty acids are dissolved into their long chain. They act as a precursor to prostaglandins (PGs), thromboxanes (TXs), and leukotrienes (LTs), and also give rise to lipoxins (LXs), resolvins, isoprostanes, hydroxyl, and hydroperoxy eicosatetraenoates. The enzymes affect the acetylcholine levels in the brain and increases the synthesis of endothelial nitric oxide, augments diuresis, enhances insulin action, and may function as endogenous HMG-CoA reductase inhibitors, nitric oxide enhancers, β-blockers, anti-hypertensives, and anti-atherosclerotic molecules. EFAs/metabolites have been reported to react with nitric oxide (NO) to yield respective nitroalkene derivatives that exert cell-signalling actions via ligation and activation of peroxisome proliferator-activated receptors (Thirumalai,Therasa, Elumalai, & David, 2011).

In clinical practice, conditions have been reported in which EFAs, especially the n-3 series have been shown to have synergistic effects with drugs; examples include hypertension, arthritis, psoriasis, and ulcerative colitis. In a studyby Manohar et al. (2009),sinigrin was shown to reduce the level of plasma triglycerides, hence suggesting that alkenyl glucosinolates could be an encouraging agent to prevent postprandial hypertriglyceridemia.

According to research by Nomura et al.(2005), sinigrin is known as the precursor of the myrosinase–mediated breakdown product allyl isothiocyanate, which exerts various biological effects and also has a vital role in the prevention of cancer and DNA damage caused by carcinogens. Mustard leaves consist of very low calorie and fat content, but the dark green colour of the leaves contains a huge amount of phytonutrients, vitamins, and minerals. It is rich in dietary fibre, which is also helpful in controlling cholesterol ranges with the absorption. The dietary fibre helps to treatconstipation, haemorrhoids, and colon cancer diseases.

Green mustard is rich source of calcium, magnesium, folic acid and vitamin K. Vitamin K is important for bone health and promote osteoblastic activity in the bones. The fresh leaves of green mustard crops are a good source of the B-complex group of vitamins, such as folic acid, thiamine, and riboflavin. It is also the best source of vitamin-C, which acts as powerful natural antioxidant that protects cells from free radical injury. This water-soluble vitamin also helps with DNA synthesis and cell division.

APPLICATION IN THE FOOD INDUSTRY

Mustard oils are classified on the basis of their region, distribution, and application. Pressing extraction and distillation process come under the production process. Mustard oil is used in numerous industries, including personal care, food, pharmaceutical, and aromatherapy. The food segment area is one where mustard oils show major dominance among all the sectors, thus it appears that mustard oil will become a global market in the future (Anuradha,2012). North America, Eastern Europe, Western Europe, and the Asia Pacific regions are the most identified markets of mustard, but it is in high demand in the Asia Pacific regions (India). A large amount of this oil is also used in Thailand and China.

Commonly, mustard has three varieties that are used for the extraction of oil on a commercial basis; these are: Brassica nigra or black mustard, Brassica hirta or whitemustard, and Brassica juncea or brown mustard (Qureshi,1991). The brassica species are used for the extraction of oils that have a pungent taste and bad odour. In recent times, people used this crop oil for cooking purposes and also in aromatherapy, soap production, and pharmaceuticals, etc. (Kumar, Thakur, Barothia, &Chatterjee, 2011). The oil is extracted from the seed by steam or water distillation. During aromatherapy, it helps to excrete from the sweat glands, which helps control the body's water balance and increases the glow in the skin (Malan,Walia, Saini, & Gupta,2011). Mustard oil is very useful for the skin and overall health, and it also makes an excellent cooking oil, so there is great competition to replace sunflower oil for cooking (Singh&Panda, 2005).

Derivatives of the mustard constituent allyl isothiocyanate form the basis for toxic agents, such as mustard gases and anti neoplastic drugs (e.g.bendamustine). Mustard is used as a food flavouring, for forage, as an emetic, and diuretic, as well as a topical treatment for inflammatory conditions, such as arthritis and rheumatism. Mustard also has potential pharmacological benefits to treatcardiovascular disease, cancer, and diabetes. However, there are limited clinical trials to support its use for any specific conditions other than epilepsy.

CONCLUSION

In India, Brassica juncea is among the most common oilseed crops grown for commercial purpose. For thousands of years, Indian mustard seeds and the oil derived from the seeds have been aptly used to relieve joint pain, fever, alleviate cough and colds, lessen swelling, and for cleaning cranial cavity. Mustard oil has also been used for the treatment of various skin diseases and wounds. . It has beneficial effect to the human skin. It is a miracle seed crop in the therapeutic sector, because it consists of phytochemical compounds that have therapeutic properties, such as antibacterial, antimalarial, anti-aging, antiulcer,anti-hyperglycemic,anti-hyperlipidaemia,anti-proliferative, etc. The broad spectrum of beneðcial effects of the seeds perceived with this plant warrants further exploration of B. juncea seeds as a potential source for obtaining pharmacologically standardized phytotherapeutics, which could be potentially very useful.

REFERENCES

Anuradha, M., Pragyandip, D., Murthy, P. N., Siddique, H. H., & Poonam, K. (2012). A classical review on Rajika (Brassica juncea). *Res Rev J Biol Sci*, *1*(1), 18–23.

Basha, S. K., Sudarshanam, G., & Prveen, D. (2011). Plant sources for the treatment of jaundice in the Sugali tribes of Yerramalais forest of Eastern Ghats, Andhra Pradesh, India. *Life Sciences Leaflets*, *14*, 449–457.

Bhuiyan, N. I., Begum, J., & Sultana, M. (2009). Chemical composition of leaf and seed essential oil of Coriandrum sativumL. from Bangladesh. *Bangladesh Journal of Pharmacology*, *4*(2), 150–153. doi:10.3329/bjp.v4i2.2800

Billman, G. E. (2013). The effects of omega-3 polyunsaturated fatty acids on cardiac rhythm: A critical assessment. *Pharmacology & Therapeutics*, *140*(1), 53–80. doi:10.1016/j.pharmthera.2013.05.011 PMID:23735203

Crozier, A., Jaganath, I. B., & Clifford, M. N. (2009). Dietary phenolics chemistry, bioavailability and effect on health. *Natural Product Reports*, *26*(8), 1001–1043. doi:10.1039/b802662a PMID:19636448

Delisle, J., Amiot, J., Goulet, G., Simard, C., Brisson, G. J., & Jones, J. D. (1984). Nutritive value of protein fractions extracted from soybean, rapeseed and wheat flours in the rat. *Plant Foods for Human Nutrition (Dordrecht, Netherlands)*, *34*(4), 243–251. doi:10.1007/BF01126553

Desai, U. (2005). *The Ayurvedic cookbook: A personalized guide to good nutrition and health*. New Delhi: MotilalBanarsidass.

Dubie, J., Stancik, A., Morra, M., & Nindo, C. (2013). Antioxidant extraction from mustard (Brassica juncea) seed meal using high-intensity ultrasound. *Journal of Food Science*, *78*(4), 542–548. doi:10.1111/1750-3841.12085 PMID:23488824

Elvin-Lewis, M. (2001). Should we be concerned about herbal remedies? *Journal of Ethnopharmacology*, *75*(2-3), 141–164. doi:10.1016/S0378-8741(00)00394-9 PMID:11297844

Grover, J. K., Yadav, S. P., & Vats, V. (2003). Effect of feeding murrayakoeingii and brassica juncea diet on [correction] kidney functions and glucose levels in streptozotocin-diabetic mice. *Journal of Ethnopharmacology*, *85*(1), 1–5. doi:10.1016/S0378-8741(02)00355-0 PMID:12576195

Iqbal, M., Akhtar, N., Zafar, S., & Ali, I. (2008). Genotypic responses for yield and seed oil quality of two Brassica species under semi-arid environmental conditions. *South African Journal of Botany*, *74*(4), 567–571. doi:10.1016/j.sajb.2008.02.003

John, A. A., & Soba, N. (2011). Hepatoprotective activity of Brassica juncea (L) Czernagainst carbon tertrachloride induced hepatotoxicity in albino rats. *Pharmacologyonline*, *3*, 609–621.

Khattab, R. Y., & Arntfield, S. D. (2009). Functional properties of raw and processed canola meal. *Lebensmittel-Wissenschaft + Technologie*, *42*(6), 1119–1124. doi:10.1016/j.lwt.2009.02.009

Kumar, V., Thakur, A. K., Barothia, N. D., & Chatterjee, S. S. (2011). Therapeutic potentials of Brassica juncea: An overview. *Tang*, *1*(1), 2–1. doi:10.5667/tang.2011.0005

Malan, R., Walia, A., Saini, V., & Gupta, S. (2011). Comparison of different extracts leaf of Brassica juncea Linn on wound healing activity. *European Journal of Experimental Biology*, *1*(2), 33–40.

Manohar, R. P., Pushpan, R., & Rohini, S. (2009). Mustard and its uses in Ayurveda. *Indian Journal of Traditional Knowledge*, *8*, 400–404.

Merah, O. (2015). Genetic Variability in Glucosinolates in Seed of Brassica juncea: Interest in mustard condiment. *Journal of Chemistry*.

Nomura, T., Shinoda, S., Yamori, T., Sawaki, S., Nagata, I., Ryoyama, K., & Fuke, Y. (2005). Selective sensitivity to wasabi-derived 6-(methylsulfinyl)hexyl isothiocyanate of human breast cancer and melanoma cell lines studied *in vitro*. *Cancer Detection and Prevention*, *29*(2), 155–160. doi:10.1016/j.cdp.2004.07.010 PMID:15829375

Pawar, S. (2012). Plant based folk recipes for treatment of hepatic disorders in Jalgaon district (ms) India. *International. Journal of Basic and Applied Sciences*, *1*, 109–114.

Qureshi, A. A., Qureshi, N., Wright, J. J., Shen, Z., Kramer, G., Gapor, A., ... Peterson, D. M. (1991). Lowering of serum cholesterol in hypercholesterolemic humans by tocotrienols (palmvitee). *The American Journal of Clinical Nutrition*, *53*(4), 1021S–1026S. doi:10.1093/ajcn/53.4.1021S PMID:2012010

Radojčić Redovniković, I., Glivetic, T., Delonga, K., & Vorkapić-Furač, J. (2008). Glucosinolates and their potential role in plant. *Periodicum Biologorum*, *110*(4), 297–309.

Singh, M. P., & Panda, H. (2005). *Medicinal herbs with their formulations*. New Delhi: Daya Publishing House.

Thirumalai, T., Therasa, S. V., Elumalai, E., & David, E. (2011). Hypoglycemic effect of Brassica juncea (seeds) on streptozotocin induced diabetic male albino rat. *Asian Pacific Journal of Tropical Biomedicine*, *1*(4), 323–325. doi:10.1016/S2221-1691(11)60052-X PMID:23569784

Uhl. (2000). Effects of mustard sprouts and allylisothiocyanate. *Ensuring global food safety. Exploring global harmonization*.

Wikipedia. (2009). *Mustard seed*. Available http://en.wikipedia.org/wiki/mustard_seed

Yadav, S. K., Yadava, D. K., Vasudev, S., Yadav, S., Kumar, P. R., & Nigam, R. (2013). Assessment of seed quality and oil content in different branches of Indian mustard (Brassica juncea) cultivars at different storage intervals. *Indian Journal of Agricultural Sciences*, *83*(2), 227–233.

Yadava, D. K., Giri, S. C., Vignesh, M., Vasudev, S., Yadav, A. K., Dass, B., ... Prabhu, K. V. (2011). Genetic variability and trait association studies in Indian mustard (Brassica juncea). *Indian Journal of Agricultural Sciences*, *81*(8), 712–716.

Chapter 13
Turmeric:
Biological Operations and Medicinal Applications

Mazia Ahmed
https://orcid.org/0000-0002-7006-3192
Center of Food Technology, University of Allahabad, India

Urvashi Srivastava
https://orcid.org/0000-0002-0779-155X
Center of Food Technology, University of Allahabad, India

Chitra Gupta
Center of Food Technology, University of Allahabad, India

ABSTRACT

Turmeric (Curcuma longa) is a rhizomatous crop found in tropical regions and belongs to the family Zingiberaceae. It was used in the form of a spice, flavoring substance, coloring agent, and as a therapeutic agent for the treatment of several human ailments for centuries. Turmeric, along with its extracts, has a very broad and diverse field of application. It is an exclusive and versatile naturally occurring plant product having properties of not only a spice but also food colorant, medicine or drug, and cosmetics. In ethnic delicacies, turmeric is a commonly used flavoring ingredient. It is also a popularly used natural food color. It exhibits several biological activities such as having antioxidant, anti-inflammatory, anti-carcinogenic, antimutagenic, antimicrobial, antiviral, and antiparasitic properties. It is well known as a skincare product and a healthy food ingredient. It is found to have the capability to prevent or retard a wide range of ailments.

DOI: 10.4018/978-1-7998-2524-1.ch013

INTRODUCTION

One amongst the most valuable and influential plants present on the surface of the earth is Turmeric, which was extensively used as a native conjecture by the ancient Indian population. It is a member of the Zingiberaceae family. The scientific name of turmeric is *Curcuma longa Linn.* It is cultivated expansively in Asia, mostly in the regions of India and China. It is a leafy-plant having huge, perennial, vertically rigid, and lily-like leaves ranging up to 1.2 meters in length. Its leaves are oblong and lanceolated, having tapered endings. It has yellow-colored flowers shaped like a funnel. The rhizome has been used to treat colds, coughs, diarrhea, diabetes, cancer, and inflammatory diseases in traditional and modern medicine system. The yellow colored powder is usually obtained by first boiling, cleaning, and then drying the rhizome. The dried form of *Curcuma longa* is used as the spice, which gives curry powder its distinguished yellow color. The rhizome possesses a distinct aroma like pepper and a bitter-warm taste. Turmeric is used in foods for its intense flavor and vibrant color throughout the world. Along with this, it also has an extended traditional use in the medicines of Chinese and Ayurveda systems. India has a rich history of utilizing this plant not only as a medicine but also as a dye, cosmetic, and an essential ingredient in religious ceremonies.

BACKGROUND

The medicinal use of turmeric is known for a very long period, i.e. about 4000 years ago. Its use was reported in the Indian Vedic culture as a culinary spice and also showed some sacred and religious importance. Turmeric was reported to reach China most likely by 700 AD, East Africa by about 800 years AD, West Africa by 1200 AD, and Jamaica in the 18th century. Marco Polo, in the year 1280, described and compared turmeric with saffron. He said that it exhibited the same qualities as found in saffron. The treatises of Sanskrit medical systems, Ayurveda and Unani medicine, showed the long history of turmeric's medicinal utilization in Southern Asia. The essence of Susruta's Ayurveda, which dated back to 250 BC, showed evidence of recommendations of an ointment having turmeric as an ingredient used to relieve the ill-effects of poisoned or toxic foods.

In present time, turmeric is broadly cultivated in tropical regions and holds a variety of names in different cultures and nations. Turmeric is usually called "Haldi" in the northern part of India. The word "Haldi" is a derivative of the Sanskrit word *haridra*, which means 'the one having a golden color. In South India, it is known by the name of "manjal," a word that is used very frequently in ancient Tamil literature. The name turmeric is derived from the Latin word *terra merita*, which means meritorious earth. It refers to the color of ground turmeric, resembling a pigmented mineral. In French, It is called as *Terre merite* and merely as "yellow root" in several other languages. In various cultures, the name of turmeric is based on a modern Latin word *curcuma*. In Sanskrit language, turmeric has nearly fifty-three different names.

Table 1. Nutritional factors and values of Tumeric

Nutritional factors	Values
Energy	390 kcal
Protein	8 g
Carbohydrate	69.9 g
Sugar	3 g
Dietary fiber	21 g
Total fat	10 g
Saturated fat	3 g
Cholesterol	0 mg
Calcium	0.2 g
Phosphorous	0.26 g
Sodium	10 mg
Potassium	2500 mg
Iron	47.5 mg
Thiamine	0.9 mg
Riboflavin	0.19 mg
Niacin	4.8 mg
Ascorbic acid	50 mg

COMPOSITION OF TURMERIC

Turmeric is a marvelous plant that is being used for the isolation of about a hundred different components. The major component is present in the root or rhizome in the form of volatile oil, containing a bioactive compound turmerone. Various other coloring agents are also present in turmeric called curcuminoids. Curcuminoids are made up of curcumin demethoxycurcumin, 5'-methoxycurcumin, and dihydrocurcumin, which are the naturally present antioxidants (Ruby et al. 1995; Selvam et al. 1995). On average, turmeric has moisture greater than 9%, polyphenol curcumin in the range of 5–6.6%, extraneous matter less than 0.5% by weight, mold less than 3%, and volatile oils less than 3.5%. The volatile oil of turmeric includes d-α-phellandrene, d-sabinene, cinol, borneol, zingiberene, and sesquiterpenes (Ohshiro, Kuroyanag, and Keno 1990). A wide variety of sesquiterpenes exist, like germacrene; termerone; ar-(+)-, α-, and β-termerones; β-bisabolene; α-curcumene; zingiberene; β-sesquiphellanderene; bisacurone; curcumenone; dehydrocurdione; procurcumadiol; bis-acumol; curcumenol; isoprocurcumenol; epiprocurcumenol; procurcumenol; zedoaronediol; and curlone. Some of them are specific for a specific species of turmeric. Various components accountable for the distinct aroma of spice turmeric are turmerone, ar-turmerone, and zingiberene. It is also reported that the rhizomes/roots of turmeric contain 4 novel polysaccharides such as ukonans together with stigmasterole, β-sitosterole, cholesterol, and 2-hydroxymethyl anthraquinone (Kapoor et al. 1990; Kirtikar and Basu et al. 1993).

Nutritional investigations of turmeric demonstrated that 100 gm of turmeric have the following nutritional factors (Balakrishnan 2007):

Also, turmeric is reported as a good source of omega-3 (ω-3) fatty acids and α-linolenic acid that is present in a concentration of about 2.5% (Goud, Polasa, and Krishnaswamy 1993).

Figure 1. Chemical structure of Curcumin

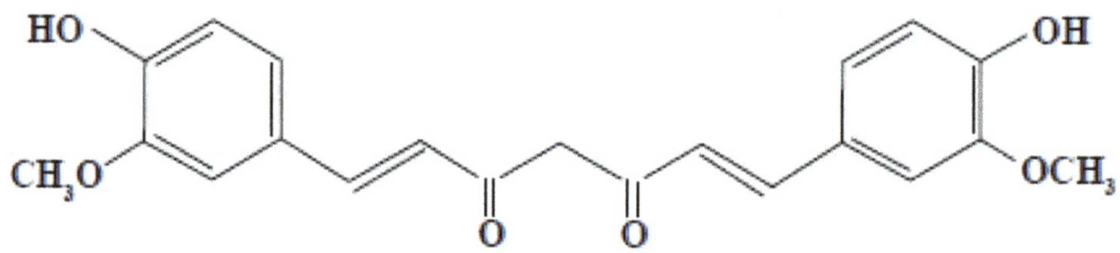

Acceptable Daily Intake (ADI) of Turmeric

Research indicates that turmeric doses of 500–2,000 mg per day may be effective.

Ethnomedicinal Importance of Turmeric

Traditionally, turmeric is widely used as a home remedy for an injury or wound healing. Turmeric also aids in treating digestive disorders, Liver ailments, cancer or sarcoma, atherosclerosis, osteoarthritis, menstrual problems in women, microbial infection, and eye diseases. Turmeric is said to be anti-inflammatory for cells of mucous membranes, which form the coating of the lungs, throat, abdomen, and intestine.

Disorders of the Digestive System

Turmeric is regarded as a digestive bitter and flatulence relieving carminative. It is added as an ingredient in food preparations, including rice and bean dishes, which facilitate in improving digestion, decrease the gas formation, and cure bloating. It is a cholagogue, which stimulates the production of bile in the liver and encourages secretion of bile from the gall bladder. Bile, in turns helps in improving one's ability to digest fatty substances. Turmeric is also recommended for treating chronic digestive flaws and congestion. It can be taken alone in the form of an extract or as digestive bitters, combining with various other bitter (sour) and carminative herbs. Turmeric is said to be beneficial for such people who experience a tiring episode soon after having meals or for people who have a problem of gas and feel bloating soon after eating. No matter in what way turmeric is used and consumed along with food, it is always advantageous to cure both the digestive ailment and liver diseases.

Hepatic Disorders

Turmeric has a beneficial and useful influence on the hepatic system (liver). Curcumin (produced by turmeric) is used widely to protect the liver. It is an indigenous molecule endowed by a variety of defensive functionalities which aids in liver protection. Turmeric has similar liver protective chemical compounds, as found in *Silybum marianum* (milk thistle) and *Cynara scolymus* (artichoke) leaves. It is reported that turmeric can shrink inflamed hepatic ducts; therefore, it can be used to treat liver diseases like hepatitis, liver cirrhosis, and icterus or jaundice.

Nervous System

A manganese complex and the antioxidants present in curcumin are reported to have a protective and positive effect on the treatment of vascular dementia (Vajragupta et al., 2003; Thiyagarajan and Sharma, 2004).

Cancer

Various recent studies proved that turmeric helps cure a lot of sarcoma diseases. They also found out that turmeric can restrain the growth and proliferation of a different kind of cancer. It is used as a medicine for treating skin cancer and pre-cancerous skin conditions. Both external application and ingesting internally are found to be beneficial.

Alzheimer's Disease

Curcumin can cross the blood-brain barrier and can lead to many improvements in Alzheimer's disease and its pathological processes.

Atherosclerosis

Turmeric may inhibit the blockage of arteries, which gradually results in causing myocardial infarction (heart attack) or strokes. Turmeric is found to make depletion in cholesterol levels and inhibits the oxidation of Low-Density Lipoprotein (LDL), also called bad cholesterol. Oxidized LDL gets deposited within the walls of arteries and veins and can contribute to forming atherosclerotic plaque. The building up of blood platelets inside the walls of a damaged vessel can also be prevented by turmeric. Platelets getting collected at the location of an injured blood vessel may cause blood to form clots which enhance the blockage of the arteries as well.

Osteoarthritis

As turmeric has got the power to decrease pain and immobility/disability, it is found helpful in relieving the symptoms and signs of osteoarthritis.

Menstruation Cycle

Turmeric acts as an antispasmodic for smooth muscles; therefore, it helps in the reduction of digestive as well as menstrual cramping. It is found to reduce the rigorousness of pain and cramps, if not relieve them completely. Surely, diet and living standards can deeply manipulate the menstrual cycle; however, turmeric is found to be an eminent addition in this regard.

Microbial (Bacterial) Infections and Wounds

Turmeric is found to be a very helpful antibiotic, when applied externally, in the prevention of infections and wounds caused by bacteria and other microorganisms. (D Bhowmik *et al.* 2008)

Biological Activities and Pharmacological Activities of Turmeric

Table 2. Biological Activity of Turmeric and its Compound

S. No.	Compound	Biological activity	Reference
1.	Turmeric Powder	Antitumor, Ant protozoan Anti-inflammatory, and Wound healing	Gujral *et al.,* (1953)
2.	Methylcurcumin	Anti-protozoan	Gomes *et al.,* (2002)
3.	Demethoxycurcumin and Bisdemethoxycurcumin	Antioxidant	Unnikrishnan *et al.,* (1995)
4.	Volatile oil	Anti-inflammatory, Antibacterial, Antifungal	Chandra et al., (1972)
5.	Curcumin	Antibacterial, Anti protozoan, Antiviral, Antitumor and Antioxidant	Lutomski et al., (1974)

Table 3. Pharmacological Activities of Turmeric

S. No.	Pharmacological activity	Mechanism of action
1.	Anti-inflammatory	Inhibit lipoxygenase and COX-2 inhibitor
2.	Anti-oxidant	It inhibits the generation of reactive oxygen species (ROS) like superoxide anion, H2O2 and nitrite radicle
3.	Anti-coagulant	It inhibits collagen and adrenaline-induced platelet aggregation.
4.	Anti-diabetic	It prevents galactose induced cataract formation at very low doses.
5.	Anti-microbial	It inhibits the growth of a variety of bacteria, parasite, and pathogenic fungi.
6.	Wound healing	Its mechanism involved an increase in the levels of beta transforming growth factor plus an increase in the activity of the enzyme nitric oxide synthase.
7.	Anti-fertility	It inhibits 5a-reductase, which converts testosterone to 5a-dihydrotestosterone, thereby inhibiting the growth of flank organs in the hamster.

Reference: Menon VP, Sudheer AR. Antioxidant and anti-inflammatory properties of Curcumin, Adv Exp Med Biol. 2007; 595:105-125.

Areas of Application

Turmeric has a huge scope in food and other industries. Along with this, the cultural importance of turmeric cannot be ruled out. It is used as a raw material for nearly all forms of cosmetic industry. Also, it is used as a medical ingredient in various medicinal appliances. Turmeric holds an essential place in the Indian medicine system as an active ingredient used in preparing many medicinal oils, ointments/creams, and poultice. Turmeric occupies an extremely high value in the Hindu culture and is widely used in several ceremonies, religious functions, and rituals. The pigment of turmeric produces a typical vibrant yellow color at a pH ranging between 2.5 to 7.0. Turmeric is an exceptional, brilliantly colored and versatile plant product having the properties of both spice or flavoring agent, and colorant as a bright yellow dye. Also, it is used in cosmetic products, as a medicine/drug, and is found helpful in various diseases. Certainly, turmeric is widely consumed as an important spice, but its utilization for different other purposes is limited.

Ayurvedic Uses

Turmeric is used everywhere in the Ayurvedic system of cooking. This multifaceted super spice is found helpful in the detoxification of the liver, balancing the levels of cholesterol, fighting allergies, stimulating digestion, boosting the immunity system, and also enhancing the skin complexion.

Culinary Uses

It is nearly impossible to even think of any Indian food with no turmeric. It imparts a rich and vibrant color and slight flavor when added in Indian foods like curry or rice. Turmeric unites well with all the other spices like chili powder, grounded coriander powder, cumin powder, and cinnamon powder. In grounded form, it is also used throughout the world as seasonings.

Food Flavor and Color

The largest quantities of turmeric are used in the majority of Asian countries as an additional food spice in the preparation of vegetables, meat, and some fish. It is utilized as a flavoring agent and as a colorant in the preparation of butter, margarine cheese, mustard, pickles, and other food items. Also, it is used to color beverages, fruit drinks, pastries/cakes, or jellies. Turmeric is also one amongst the chief ingredients of the Indian curry powder. The curry powder is a mixture of a lot of spices along with common salt.

Cosmetic Uses

The use of turmeric is very popular, especially in women's cosmetics for a very long period. The skin comprises a significant portion of our body and acts as a shielding barrier for harmful chemicals, micro-organisms, and ultraviolet (UV) radiations. The products obtained from natural plants such as turmeric is being prepared to cure and check dry skins, heal skin conditions like eczema and acne, and also help in the retardation of the process of aging.

Medicinal Uses

Turmeric is considered essential in our day-to-day life. It is found to be very helpful in healing many health-related disorders such as liver ailments, digestive disorders, as a cure for various skin diseases and as wound-healing substance. It has been greatly used in medicines to reduce inflammation. The active ingredient present in turmeric is Curcumin, which is found to have had a broad range of remedial or therapeutic effects. In the Indian system of medicine, Turmeric also has great significance and is used as an ingredient in preparing medicinal oils, creams/ointments, and poultice in the Indian system of medicine. It is called a stomachic, carminative, stimulant or tonic, vermicide, blood purifier, and an antiseptic. Along with this, it is also recommended as an alternative for anti-periodic episodes. It is helpful in relieving common cold/flu and sore throats when boiled with milk and ingested internally, or inhaled from boiling-hot water smoked by a pipe along with omum. The juice taken out from raw rhizomes is useful as an anti-parasitic drug for various skin infections. It is applied as a paste in combination with sesame oil and neem leaves in the treatment of smallpox. Burnt turmeric is used as a tooth powder, which is found helpful in relieving dental troubles. The juice of Turmeric rhizomes is believed to relieve purulent ophthalmia. Turmeric is also proved to be useful in the treatment of gall stones and other gallbladder complaints.

As Dye

In ancient times of India, turmeric was widely used as a dye for woolen materials, silk clothes, and cotton. It imparts a brilliant yellow shade when used in the acid batch. It is used in present time to also dye cotton threads or clothes. Tumeric dye is also used as a coloring agent in pharmacies, cakes and confectionery, rice milling, and various other food industries. Culturally, a considerable amount of turmeric is converted into kumkum and used as tilak for religious purposes. The use of turmeric is also reported in paint and varnish industries as a coloring material. Turmeric paper is an official reagent in British pharmacopeia for testing alkalinity. It is appropriate to use its diluted tincture as an indicator for fluorescence, even in brown and yellow solutions. Because of the phenolic nature of curcumin, turmeric acts as an anti-oxidant also.

Problems

The usage of turmeric is regarded as safe not only as a spice but also as a household remedy for centuries. Up to this date, no studies have been reported in either animals or humans to cause any toxic effect associated with turmeric (Lao et al. 2006). It is clearly demonstrated that turmeric does not act as a toxin, even in high doses. The U.S. Food and Drug Administration (FDA) has conducted its own clinical trials with turmeric and published a 300-page monograph. The FDA has given a declaration for turmeric and the active component (curcumin) present in as GRAS (Generally Regarded as Safe). Thus, in the United States of America, turmeric along with its components are widely being used in cereals, mustard, cheese, chips, butter, and various other products.

FUTURE PROSPECTS

Since prehistoric times, turmeric was used in the ayurvedic system of medicines with several biological applications. Nowadays, enthusiasm is found among researchers to treat various diseases in a natural way, employing natural products. Although some preliminary work has been done on the possible medicinal applications, not much study has been conducted for drug development yet. Curcumin is a non-toxic, highly promising natural antioxidant compound that has a wide spectrum of biological functions. Curcumin is now available in pure form, which shows a wide spectrum of biological activities. It would be easier to develop new drugs from this compound after extensive studies on its mechanism of action and pharmacological effects are conducted. It is expected that curcumin may find application as a novel drug in the near future to control various diseases, disorders, and oxidative stress.

CONCLUSION

To sum up this study, it could be concluded that turmeric is one of the medicinal as well culturally significant elements in the history of human development in India. Today, more innovation is being made in various respects, which also signifies the role of this commodity in the pharmaceutical as well as the medical world. Culturally it has occupied a pivotal role in almost all tribes and religions in India. According to all findings of turmeric, biological activities make it the right candidate for the development of pharmaceuticals, nutraceuticals, or food ingredients with functional properties.

REFERENCES

Balakrishnan, K. V. (2007). Postharvest technology and processing of turmeric. In P. N. Ravindran, K. Nirmal Babu, & K. Sivaraman (Eds.), *Turmeric: The Genus Curcuma* (pp. 193–256). Boca Raton, FL: CRC Press.

Bhowmik, D., & Jayakar, B. (2008). Turmeric. Herbal and traditional medicine. *Archives of Applied Science Research, 1*(2), 86–108.

Goud, V. K., Polasa, K., & Krishnaswamy, K. (1993). Effect of turmeric on xenobiotic metabolising enzymes. *Plant Foods for Human Nutrition (Dordrecht, Netherlands), 44*(1), 87–92. doi:10.1007/BF01088486 PMID:8332589

Kapoor, L. D. (1990). *Handbook of Ayurvedic Medicinal Plants*. Boca Raton, FL: CRC Press.

Kirtikar, K. R., Basu, B. D., Blatter, E., Caius, J. F., & Mhaskar, K. S. (1993). *Indian Medicinal Plants* (2nd ed., Vol. 2). Allahabad, India: Lalit Mohan Basu.

Lao, C. D., Ruffin, M. T. IV, Normolle, D., Heath, D. D., Murray, S. I., Bailey, J. M., ... Brenner, D. E. (2006). Ruffin4th M. T, Normolle D. Dose escalation of a curcuminoid formulation. *BMC Complementary and Alternative Medicine, 6*(1), 10–13. doi:10.1186/1472-6882-6-10 PMID:16545122

Menon, V. P., & Sudheer, A. R. (2007). Antioxidant and anti-inflammatory properties of Curcumin. *Advances in Experimental Medicine and Biology, 595*, 105–125. doi:10.1007/978-0-387-46401-5_3 PMID:17569207

Ohshiro, M., Kuroyanag, M., & Keno, A. (1990). Structures of sesquiterpenes from Curcuma longa. *Phytochemistry, 29*(7), 2201–2205. doi:10.1016/0031-9422(90)83038-3

Ruby, A. J., Kuttan, G., Babu, K. D., Rajasekharan, K. N., & Kuttan, R. (1995). Anti-tumour and antioxidant activity of natural curcuminoids. *Cancer Letters, 94*(1), 79–83. doi:10.1016/0304-3835(95)03827-J PMID:7621448

Selvam, R., Subramanian, L., Gayathri, R., & Angayarkanni, N. (1995). The anti-oxidant activity of turmeric (Curcuma longa). *Journal of Ethnopharmacology*, *47*(2), 59–67. doi:10.1016/0378-8741(95)01250-H PMID:7500637

Thiyagrajan, M., & Sharma, S. S. (2004, January 9). Neuroprotective effect of curcumin in middle cerebral artery occlusion induced focal cerebral ischemia in rats. *Life Sciences*, *74*(8), 969–985. doi:10.1016/j.lfs.2003.06.042 PMID:14672754

Vajragupta, O., Boonchoong, P., Watanabe, H., Tohda, M., Kummasud, N., & Sumanont, Y. (2003). Manganese complexes of curcumin and its derivatives: Evaluation for the radical scavenging ability and neuroprotective activity. *Free Radical Biology & Medicine*, *35*(12), 1632–1644. doi:10.1016/j.freeradbiomed.2003.09.011 PMID:14680686

Chapter 14
Pharmacology and Phytochemistry of Coriander

Sonia Singh
GLA University, Mathura, India

Nitin Agrawal
Faculty of Pharmacy, Raja Balwant Singh Engineering Technical Campus, India

Isha Mishra
GLA University, Mathura, India

ABSTRACT

Coriander, named as Coriandrum sativum Linn, belongs to the family Umbelliferae and is one of the most popular and well-known spices/condiments and herbal medicines. The essential oils and fatty oils are the two major active chemical constituents present in the plant. The other minor ingredients found to be present are monoterpenes hydrocarbons i-e limonene, γ-terpinene, α-pinene, p-cymene, borneol, citronellol, camphor, geraniol, and geraniol acetate and abd heterocyclic components such as pyrazine, pyridine, thiazole, furan and tetrahudrofuran derivatives, isocoumarins, coriandrin, dihydrocoriandrin, coriandrons A-E, flavonoids. The volatile oil from the leaf contains aromatic acids such as 2-decenoic acid, E-11-tetradecenoic acid, undecyl alcohol, tridecanoic acid, capric acid, undecanoic acid, and more. The current pharmacological research reveals the application of coriander has antibacterial and antifungal activity.

INTRODUCTION

The genus Coriandrum has included two species, the cultivated species *C. sativum* and wild species *C. tordylium*. The name 'cilantro' has been randomly as well as frequently employed in American English which is referred to as *green herb* or *dried leaves*. The origin of *Coriandrum sativum* is still unknown; even many authors and scientists have described coriander to be as a wild plant in nature. But no specific information is available about the same fact. In 1780, Linnaeus had reported coriander occurred as a

DOI: 10.4018/978-1-7998-2524-1.ch014

weed in cereals (Diederichsen, 1996).The 'Coriandrum' is coined from koros, referring to the disagreeable odor of the leaves (Shelef, 2003).

Family: *Umbelliferae Juss.* ;455 genera; 3600-3751 species
Subfamily: *Apioideae Drude*; 404 genera; 2827-2936 species
Tribe: *Coriandreae W. Koch*; 8 genera; 21 species
Genera: *Bifora F. Hoffm.*;3 species
Common Names Used Worldwide (Diederichsen, 1996).
Arab :kuzbara, kuzbura
Armenian :chamem
Chinese :yuan sui, hu sui
Czec :koriandr
Danish :koriander
Dutc :koriander
English :coriander, collender, chinese parsley
Ethiopian :dembilal
French :coriandre, persil arabe
Georgian :kinza, kindza, kindz
German :koriander, Wanzendill, Schwindelkorn
Greek :koriannon, korion
Hindi :dhania, dhanya
Hungarian :coriander
Italian :coriandolo
Japanese :koendoro
Malay :ketumbar
Persian :geshnes
Polish :kolendra
Portuguese :coentro
Rumanian :coriándru
Russian :koriandr, koljandra, ki nec, kinza, vonju ee zel'e, klopovnik
Sanskrit :dhanayaka, kusthumbari
Spanish :coriandro, cilantro, cilandrio, culantro
Swiss :chrapfechörnli, Böbberli, Rügeliкümmi
Turkish :kisnis
Vernacular Indian Names(Diederichsen, 1996).
Bengali : dhane, dhania
Gujarati : kothmiri, konphir, libdhane
Kannada : kothambri, kothmiri bija
Kashmiri : daaniwal, kothambalari
Malayalam : kothumpkalari bija, kothumpalari
Marathi :dhana, kothimber
Oriya : dhania
Punjabi : dhania
Tamil : kothamali
Telugu : dhaniyalu

HABITAT AND CULTIVATION

The plant was brought from east Egypt to Southern Europe by Romans. Now, it has been found in North Africa, Russia, USA, and India (Shelef, 2003). The crop is cultivated as *Kharif* or as *rabi* crop. It requires light to heavy black soil, followed by a drilling method. It is occasionally rotated with wheat, grain, *jowar* and onion; and even also has grown along with cotton, or sugarcane as a mixed crop (Kokate, 2007).

The germination of the plant takes place at temperatures of above 4°C. It is even optimum to grow at 17-20°C (genotypes containing small fruits) whereas it can also be at 22-27°C (genotypes with larger fruits). It requires a sufficient supply of water for sowing. It is highly resistant to drought condition, but during stem elongation, it becomes sensitive to low temperatures. Long days accelerate the generative development of coriander, but the effect is only minor. It is grown very well in tropical, subtropical and temperate regions. The soil should be sandy loam, the crop will grow well on loam as well as clay soils containing a good drainage property.

During ripening, the aldehyde content of essential oil disappears, and even the odour of fruits changes. The crop becomes ready for harvesting after a hundred days of growth (Coriandrum sativum (coriander), (Invasive species compendium, 2018).

MACROSCOPY AND MICROSCOPY DESCRIPTION

Organoleptic Characteristics

It is a cremocarp type of fruit and is found to be perennial. It attained a height of about 30–100 cm. The stems are much-branched, erect and dark green. The flowers are small, with short-stalked containing umbels of 6-10 rays. It is off white. The seeds are globular, ribed with brownish-yellow color. The size of seeds is about 5 mm(d), containing five longitudinal ridges. A cremocarp has two mericarps, where each mericarp has two surfaces:

a) A flat surface called as commissural surface, and
b) A rounded surface named as dorsal surface.

The dorsal surface shows five primary and four secondary ridges. The primary ridges are wavy, indistinct and prominent in appearance whereas secondary ridges are straight in shape.

Two varieties of coriander have distinguished, based on fruit diameter, *C. sativum* L. var. vulgare had 2–5 mm whereas *C. vulgare* L. var. microcarpum 2–4 mm (Shelef, 2003).

Figure 1. Morphology of coriander fruit

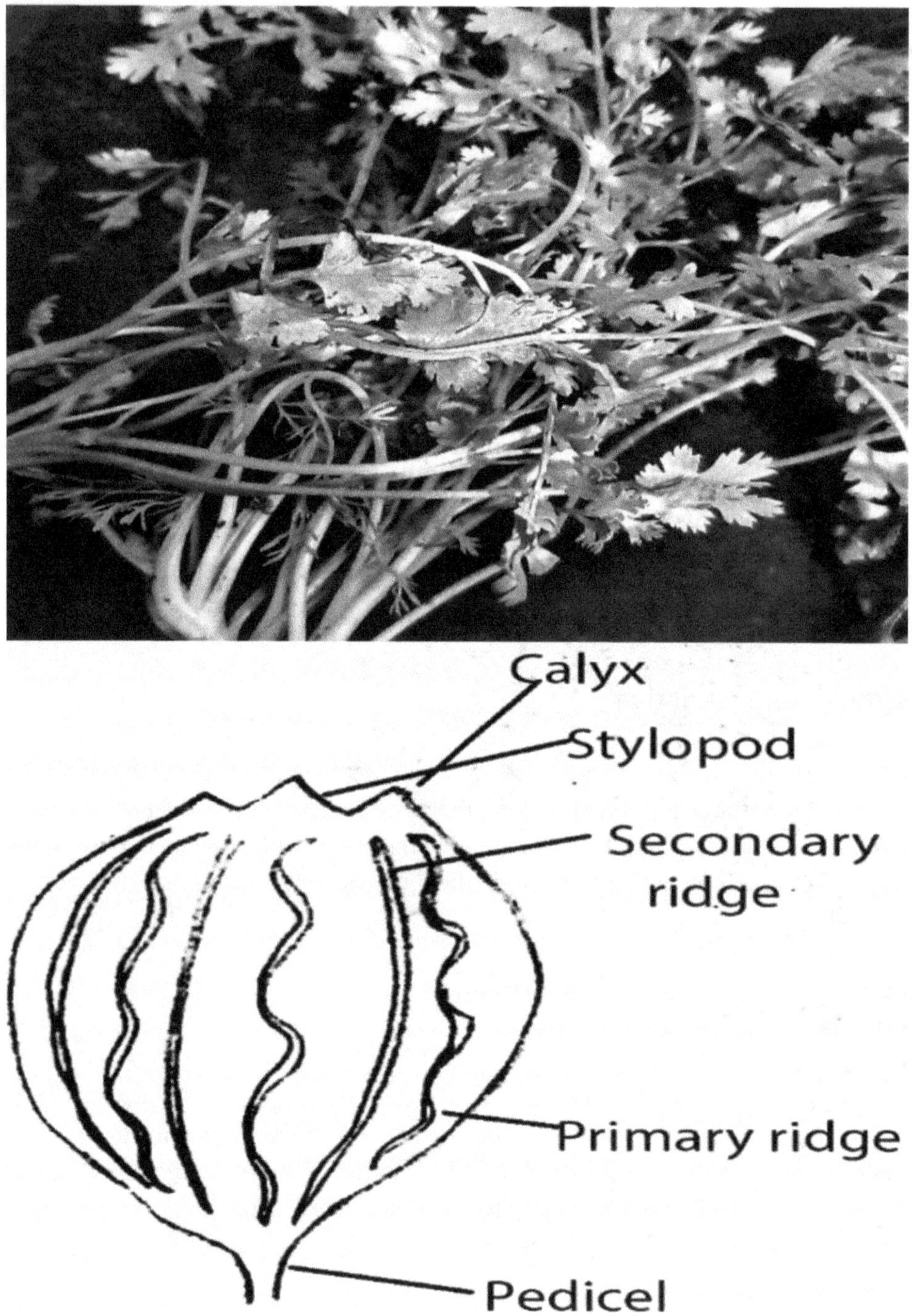

Figure 2. Transverse section of Coriander fruit (Iyengar, 1991)

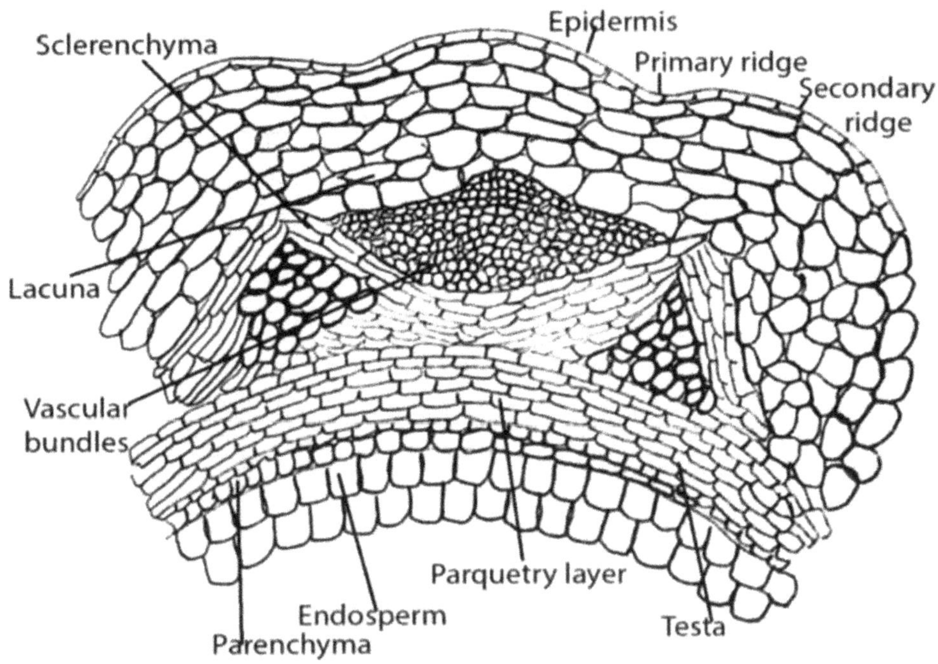

Microscopical Characteristics

A transverse section of coriander fruit shows mericarp, where two prominent distinct surfaces are present, namely, commisural and dorsal surfaces. The commisural region has a flat surface, containing two vittae with carpophore present in the middle. Whereas the dorsal surface is ridged with no vittae present. Some of the essential tissues of a mericarp are Pericarp, testa, and endosperm.

The pericarp is divided into epicarp, mesocarp, and endocarp. Epicarp consists of single-layered small thick-walled cells, in which calcium oxalate crystals is embedded in between the cells. Mesocarp may get differentiated into three regions:

a) Outer layered parenchyma cells tangentially arranged elongated in shape.
b) Middle sclerenchymatous cells, compact in nature, which is represented by longitudinally running fibers, can be seen below the primary ridges whereas the inner region comprised of tangentially running fibers corresponding to secondary ridges. Vascular bundles have seen as a crown in the sclerenchymatous region below the primary ridges, and
c) Inner layered lignified parenchymatous cells irregularly arranged polygonally in shape.

Endocarp is comprised of a parquetry layer. Testa is composed of a single-layered cell, that is yellowish. Endosperm consists of thick-walled polygonal-shaped colorless parenchymatous cells, containing aleurone grains as well as fixed oil (Iyengar, 2004).

Figure 3. Powder characteristic of Coriander fruit (Iyengar, 1997)

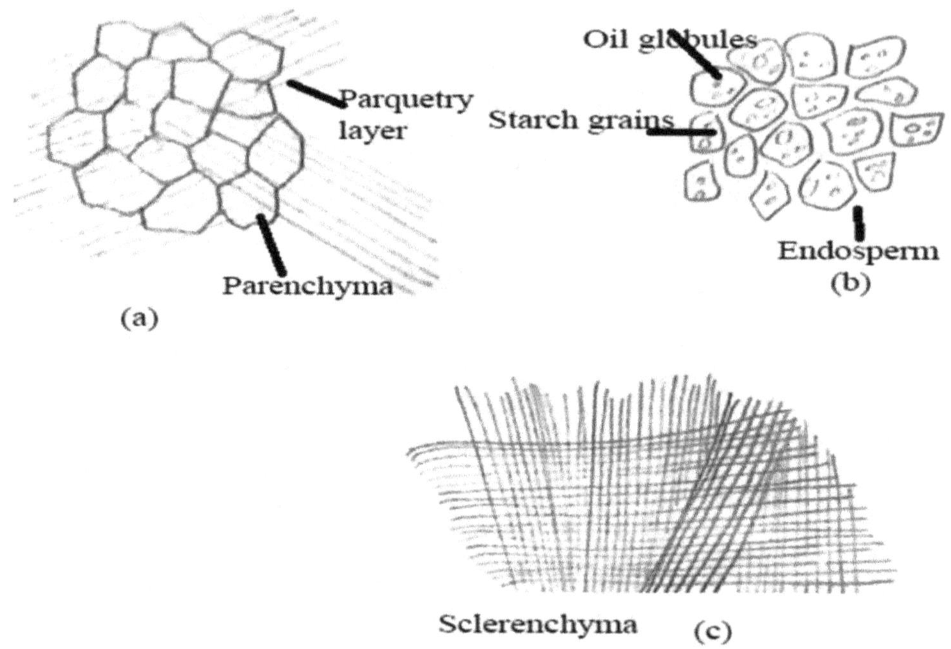

Histochemical Powder Characteristics

The powder characteristics of coriander revealed the presence of endocarp which consists of thin-walled lignified cells followed by parquetry arrangements, along with mesocarp cells.

(a) The endosperm consists of polygonal thick-walled cells, containing aleurone grains and fixed oil.
(b) The sclerenchymatous layer consists of thin-walled lignified mesocarp cells. (Iyengar, 1991).

Key Points for Determination of Different Types of Coriander Species Found in Geographical Regions of the World

1. Presence of 1-3 basal lobed leaves, pinnate. Stems are no longer than about 70 cm and not much branched; containing few leaves. Fruits are round or slightly ovate; with a minimum percentage of essential oil. It is named as **Near Eastern type as** found in North Africa, Mediterranean areas, Bhutan, Americas, and Europe.
2. Presence of ovate shaped fruits with shallow essential oil content. It has cultivated in Pakistan. It is commonly called an **Indian type.**
3. Presence of prostrate type of basal leaves with rosette shape; aromatic; medium-sized fruits with a considerable amount of essential oil; long vegetation period. It is present in Daghestan, Georgia and Armenia, called a **Central Asian type.**

4. Presence of curve-shaped leaves with ascending type without aroma flavor; small shaped fruits are containing a negligible amount of essential oil; abundant amount of fatty oil and long vegetation period. It is called a **Syrian type.**
5. Presence of most extended basal leaves with pinnate, lobed leaflets; leaflets are emarginated; an aromatic flavor; flowers contain anthocyans; fruits with essential oil content. It has found in most of the countries of the Caucasian area, Eastern Europe, Russia, Mongolia, Germany. It is called a **Caucasian type.**
6. Presence of most extended pinnate lobed shaped basal leaves, leaflets are with saw-toothed margin; the flavor of the leaves least aromatic; stems and flowers without anthocyans; fruits containing a minor amount of essential oil, called as **Ethiopian type** (Diederichsen, 1996).

PHYTOCHEMISTRY OF CORIANDER

Chemical Constituents

The green leaves have an aromatic taste and contain a high amount of volatile oil. The essential oils and fatty oils are the two major classes present in the fruit. The Georgian (Caucasus) types of leaves have a very spicy taste whereas the Syrian types have a mild flavor, considered to be suitable in salads rather than as a spice. Ethiopian accessions (based on geographical types of Coriander) have a similar tendency when compared with Syrian types, with a more aromatic flavor. Its regarded as camphor, a non-essential component (0-6.3%). The fatty oil content was found to be present in the leaves of Syrian types up to 27.7%. The leafy samples obtained from the Caucasian region (an area occupied by Armenia, Azerbaijan, Georgia and Russia) had a very high fatty oil volume. The constitution of fatty acids is found to remain in the same proportion in all of these accessions. Petroselinic acid is considered as the principal component. The percentage of essential oil present in ripe and dried fruits may vary from 0.03 -2.6%, and the amount of fatty oil from 9.9 -27.7% (Diederichsen, 1996).

Bang: Bangladesh; Alg: Algeria; Pak:Pakistan; Alt can: Atlantic canada; Tun:Tunisia; Euro:Europe; “NA”:not available.

In the Bangladesh region, the chief compounds found in oil of coriander seed were linalool (37.7%), geranyl acetate (17.6%), and γ-terpinene (14.4%) (Nazrul, 2009). De Figueiredo et al. had identified eighteen new compounds and among them only few of them were found to be present in large proportion, namely, linalool (77.48%), γ-terpinene (4.64%), α- pinene (3.97%), limonene (1.28%), geraniol (0.64%) a, α-decenal (0.16%) (De Figueiredo, 2004). Even, Pino et al. analyzed and identified about thirty-five compounds obtained from Cuba region were linalool (54.57%), α- pinene (1.14%), geraniol (6.97%), γ-terpinene (4.08%) and limonene (1.55%) (Jorge,1990). The presence of components of essential oil may vary along with different geographical regions, such as Russia, Italy, Albania, and India. These variations would be due to the presence of environmental factors including, altitude, latitude, rainfall, sunlight, soil composition, and so on. The major compounds found in Russia and Albina linalool would be different like γ- terpinene, camphor, and α-pinene (Diederichsen, 1996).

Table 1. Percentage composition of the seed oil of Coriandrum sativum obtained from the different origin of the world as reported in the literature

Chemical components	Bang	Cuba	Iran	Brazil	Alg	India	Pak	Atl can	Tun	Euro
α-Pinene	NA	1 .14	0.12	3.97	3.41	4.09	1.63	1.2-3.2	0.02	0.2–10.9
β-Pinene	1.82	NA	0.14	0.38	0.78	0.86	0.23	NA	0.05	NA
γ-Terpinene	14.42	NA	0.11	4.64	NA	NA	4.17	NA	NA	NA
α-Cedrene	NA	NA	NA	NA	NA	NA	NA	NA	NA	NA
α-Farnasene	1.22	NA	NA	NA	NA	NA	NA	NA	NA	NA
p-Cymene	NA	NA	2.52	2.16	1.76	0.45	1.12	NA	NA	NA
Limonene	0.40	NA	0.62	1.28	1.23	0.63	0.26	0.7-1.8	0.02	NA
Linalool	37.65	NA	57.57	77.48	73.11	75.30	69.60	73.11	87.54	NA
Citronellal	1.96	NA	0.39	NA	NA	0.10	0.45	NA	NA	NA
Camphor	NA	5.83	3.02	2.60	1.85	0.14	0.38	1.85	0.17	3.0–5.1
Geraniol	1.87	6.97	0.24	0.64	NA	0.81	NA	NA	NA	NA
Anethole	NA	NA	0.21	NA	NA	NA	1.15	NA	0.01	NA
Cis-dihydrocarvone	NA	NA	NA	NA	NA	NA	NA	NA	2.36	NA
p-mentha-1,4-dien-7-ol	NA	NA	NA	NA	NA	NA	NA	NA	NA	NA
Geranyl acetate	NA	4.96	NA	1.06	NA	8.12	4.99	0.9-1.6	0.83	0.2–5.4
Neryl acetate	NA	0.19	NA	NA	NA	NA	NA	NA	traces	NA
Linalyl-acetate	NA	NA	NA	NA	NA	NA	NA	NA	NA	NA
Phellandrene	NA	0.04	NA	NA	NA	NA	NA	NA	NA	NA
(E)-2-decenal	NA	NA	NA	0.16	NA	NA	NA	NA	NA	NA
Decanal	NA	0.15	NA	0.46	0.43	NA	0.14	0.5-1.2	NA	NA
Camphene	0.14	0.21	NA	0.33	NA	NA	NA	NA	NA	NA
E-Verbenol	0.27	NA	NA	NA	NA	NA	NA	NA	NA	NA
Sabinene	0.23	0.14	0.58	0.26	NA	NA	NA	NA	NA	NA
E-Ocimene	0.05	0.09	NA	NA	NA	NA	NA	NA	NA	NA
m-Cymene	1.27	NA	NA	NA	NA	NA	NA	NA	NA	NA
α-Thujene	0.04	NA	0.19	NA	NA	NA	NA	NA	NA	NA
Cyclooctanol	0.02	NA	NA	NA	NA	NA	NA	NA	NA	NA
β-Myrcene	0.55	NA	NA	0.77	NA	NA	NA	NA	NA	NA
2-Oxabicyclo[2.2.2]0ctan-6- ol,1,2,3-trimethyl	0.02	NA	NA	NA	NA	NA	NA	NA	NA	NA
Z-Ocimene	0.04	NA	0.41	NA	NA	NA	NA	NA	NA	NA
α-Campholenal	0.22	NA	NA	NA	NA	NA	NA	NA	NA	NA
Lilac alcohol	0.11	NA	NA	NA	NA	NA	NA	NA	NA	NA
α-Terpinene	0.04	0.02	NA	NA	NA	NA	NA	NA	NA	NA
Z-Verbenol	0.11	NA	NA	NA	NA	NA	NA	NA	NA	NA
Isothujol	0.04	NA	NA	NA	NA	NA	NA	NA	NA	NA
Umbellulone	0.11	NA	NA	NA	NA	NA	NA	NA	NA	NA
Borneol	0.32	1.55	1.27	0.18	NA	NA	NA	NA	NA	NA
4-Terpineol	0.06	1.38	0.14	0.14	NA	NA	NA	NA	NA	NA
Terpinyl acetate	0.31	NA	NA	NA	NA	NA	NA	NA	NA	NA
Decanal	0.14	NA	NA	NA	NA	NA	NA	NA	NA	NA
Z-verbenone	0.10	NA	NA	NA	NA	NA	NA	NA	NA	NA
Citronellol	1.31	NA	NA	NA	NA	NA	NA	NA	NA	NA
Citral	1.36	NA	NA	NA	NA	NA	NA	NA	NA	NA
Rnyrcene	NA	0.65	NA	NA	NA	NA	NA	NA	NA	NA
Eugenol	0.90	NA	NA	NA	NA	NA	NA	NA	NA	NA
Carveol	0.15	NA	NA	NA	NA	NA	NA	NA	NA	NA
Undecanal	0.58	0.10	NA	NA	NA	NA	NA	NA	NA	NA
Methyl geranate	0.17	NA	NA	NA	NA	NA	NA	NA	NA	NA
Myrtenyl acetate	0.43	NA	NA	NA	NA	NA	NA	NA	NA	NA
Citronellyl acetate	1.36	NA	NA	NA	NA	NA	NA	NA	NA	NA

continued on following page

Table 1. Continued

Chemical components	Bang	Cuba	Iran	Brazil	Alg	India	Pak	Atl can	Tun	Euro
Geranyl acetate	17.57	NA	NA	NA	NA	NA	NA	NA	NA	NA
Z-myrtenyl acetate	0.10	NA	NA	NA	NA	NA	NA	NA	NA	NA
β-Elemene	0.06	NA	NA	NA	NA	NA	NA	NA	NA	NA
Dodecenal	0.15	0.20	NA	NA	NA	NA	NA	NA	NA	NA
Caryophyllene	0.33	NA	NA	NA	NA	NA	NA	NA	NA	NA
β-Farnesene	0.07	NA	NA	NA	NA	NA	NA	NA	NA	NA
2-Dodecenal	0.18	NA	NA	NA	NA	NA	NA	NA	NA	NA
Curcumene	0.98	NA	NA	NA	NA	NA	NA	NA	NA	NA
α-Cubebene	0.13	NA	NA	NA	NA	NA	NA	NA	NA	NA
β-Bisabolene	0.80	NA	NA	NA	NA	NA	NA	NA	NA	NA
β-Sesquiphellandrene	1.56	NA	NA	NA	NA	NA	NA	NA	NA	NA
E-Nerolidol	0.13	NA	NA	NA	NA	NA	NA	NA	NA	NA
Artumerone	0.04	NA	NA	NA	NA	NA	NA	NA	NA	NA
8-Hexadecenal, 14-methyl-, (Z)	0.22	NA	NA	NA	NA	NA	NA	NA	NA	NA
α-Bisabolol	0.15	NA	NA	NA	NA	NA	NA	NA	NA	NA
n-Hexadecanoic acid	0.08	5.82	NA	NA	NA	NA	NA	NA	NA	NA
α-Cedrene	3.87	NA	NA	NA	NA	NA	NA	NA	NA	NA
α-Terpineol	2.32	NA	0.18	NA	NA	NA	NA	NA	NA	NA
Myrtenal	0.1 6	NA	NA	NA	NA	NA	NA	NA	NA	NA
citronellol + nerol	1.23	NA	NA	NA	NA	NA	NA	NA	NA	NA
Geranial	NA	0.16	1.03	NA	NA	NA	NA	NA	NA	NA
P-caryophyllene	NA	0.16	NA	NA	NA	NA	NA	NA	NA	NA
cis-linalool oxide tetradecanal (furanoid)	NA	0.18	NA	NA	NA	NA	NA	NA	NA	NA
tetradecanoic acid	NA	0.57	NA	NA	NA	NA	NA	NA	NA	NA
Bicyclogermacrene	NA	0.04	NA	NA	NA	NA	NA	NA	NA	NA
terpinolene	NA	0.53	0.17	NA	NA	NA	NA	NA	NA	NA
dillapiole	NA	0.45	NA	NA	NA	NA	NA	NA	NA	NA
octadecanoic acid	NA	0.20	NA	NA	NA	NA	NA	NA	NA	NA
Heptanol	NA	NA	0.78	NA	NA	NA	NA	NA	NA	NA
α-Terpinene	NA	NA	0.39	NA	NA	NA	NA	NA	NA	NA
l^3-Carene	NA	NA	0.11	NA	NA	NA	NA	NA	NA	NA
1,8-Cineol	NA	NA	0.97	NA	NA	NA	NA	NA	NA	NA
Cis-linalool oxide	NA	NA	0.07	NA	NA	NA	NA	NA	NA	NA
Carvone	NA	NA	1.14	NA	NA	NA	NA	NA	NA	NA
Thymol	NA	NA	0.12	NA	NA	NA	NA	NA	NA	NA
Trans-linalool oxide	NA	NA	0.83	NA	NA	NA	NA	NA	NA	NA
Nerol	NA	NA	1.98	NA	NA	NA	NA	NA	NA	NA
Neral	NA	NA	0.29	NA	NA	NA	NA	NA	NA	NA
p-Cymen-8-ol	NA	NA	0.29	NA	NA	NA	NA	NA	NA	NA
Cis-Dihydrocarvone	NA	NA	0.35	NA	NA	NA	NA	NA	NA	NA
Menthol	NA	NA	0.54	NA	NA	NA	NA	NA	NA	NA
Tetradecane	NA	NA	NA	0.05	NA	NA	NA	NA	NA	NA
Heptanal	NA	NA	NA	2.06	NA	NA	NA	NA	NA	NA

Source: (Nazrul 2009; Laribi 2015; Jorge 1990; Abbas 2012).

The composition of essential oil present in the *C. sativum* seed containing chemical compounds with different variations, including benzofuran,2,3-dihydro (15.4%); hexadecanoic acid, methyl ester (10.32%); 2,4a-epioxy-3,4,5,6,7,8-hexahydro-2,5,5,8a-tetramethyl-2h-1-benzofuran (9.35%); 2-methyoxy-4-vinyl-phenol (8.8%); 2,3,5,6-tetrafluroanisole (8.62%); 2,6-dimethyl-3- aminobenzoquinone (6.81%); dodecanoic acid (5%) in India. Generally, the major components of *C.sativum* essential oil contain different classes of chemical compounds, namely, Alcohols: Linalool (60–80%), geraniol (1.2%–4.6%), terpinen-4-ol (3%), a-terpineol (0.5%); Hydrocarbons: γ-terpinene (1–8%), r-cymene (3.5%), limonene (0.5%–4.0%),

Table 2. Percentage composition of Coriandrum sativum leaf obtained from different origin of the world as reported in the literature

Chemical components	Bangladesh	Brazil	India	Kenya	Korea	Fiji
g-Thionodecalactone	0.16	NA	NA	NA	NA	NA
1,2-Decanediol	0.45	NA	NA	NA	NA	NA
n-Cetyl alcohol	0.43	NA	NA	NA	NA	NA
2.4-Dimethylheptane	0.18	NA	NA	NA	NA	NA
2-Decenoic acid	30.82	NA	NA	NA	NA	NA
2-Dodecanal	1.32	2.9	NA	NA	9.93	1.32
2-Tridecenal, (E)	0.99	NA	NA	NA	NA	NA
2-Undecenal	3.87	NA	NA	NA	NA	NA
4-Allylphenyl acetate	0.22	NA	NA	NA	NA	NA
5-Nonanol, 5-methyl	0.28	NA	NA	NA	NA	NA
Anisle, P-allyl	0.25	NA	NA	NA	NA	NA
Benzene	0.05	NA	NA	NA	NA	NA
β-Cinene	0.10	NA	NA	NA	NA	NA
Z-Nonene	0.07	NA	NA	NA	NA	NA
Cyclododecane	2.45	NA	NA	NA	NA	NA
Cyclooctanol	0.57	NA	NA	NA	NA	NA
Decahydroazulene	0.38	NA	NA	NA	NA	NA
Decamethylene glycol	1.15	NA	NA	NA	NA	NA
Decanal	1.39	4.8	14.36	14.3	2.33	6.56
d-Limonene	0.18	NA	NA	NA	NA	NA
Dodecanal	1.25	NA	5.81	4.36	5.16	NA
Dodecanoic acid	2.63	NA	NA	NA	NA	NA
E-11-tetradecenoic acid	13.37	NA	NA	NA	NA	NA
Ethylidenecyclooctane	0.31	NA	NA	NA	NA	NA
Eucalyptol	0.30	NA	NA	NA	NA	NA
1-Pentadecene	0.08	NA	NA	NA	NA	NA
α-Caryophyllene	0.26	NA	NA	NA	NA	NA
α-Pinene	0.49	NA	NA	NA	NA	NA
m-aminoaniline	0.27	NA	NA	NA	NA	NA
Capric acid	12.71	NA	NA	NA	NA	NA
Nonanoic acid	1.17	NA	NA	NA	NA	NA
Nonanol	0.39	NA	NA	NA	NA	NA
Octanoic acid	0.60	NA	NA	NA	NA	NA
o-Cymene	0.08	NA	NA	NA	NA	NA
Oleic acid	0.64	NA	NA	NA	NA	NA
Oxirane tetradecyl	0.07	NA	NA	NA	NA	NA
Oxirane, octyl	0.27	NA	NA	NA	NA	NA
E-2-Ethyl-3-methyl thiophane	0.23	NA	NA	NA	NA	NA
E-Undecanoic acid	4.97	NA	NA	NA	NA	NA
Tridecanoic acid	5.45	NA	NA	NA	NA	NA
Undecanal	0.34	NA	NA	NA	NA	NA
Undecanoic acid	2.13	NA	NA	NA	NA	NA
Undecyl alcohol	6.42	NA	NA	NA	NA	NA
Undecylenic acid	0.28	NA	NA	NA	NA	NA
(E)-2-Decenol	NA	18	NA	NA	NA	NA
(Z)-2-Dodecenol	NA	17.6	NA	NA	NA	NA
Tetradecenol	NA	12	NA	NA	6.85	NA
Tridecanal	NA	3.0	NA	NA	NA	NA
1-Decenol	NA	24.2	NA	NA	NA	NA
(E)-2-Decenal	NA	NA	18.02	15.9	NA	NA

continued on following page

Table 2. Continued

Chemical components	Bangladesh	Brazil	India	Kenya	Korea	Fiji
Cyclododecanol	NA	NA	NA	-	23.11	NA
(E)-2-Decen-1-ol	NA	NA	NA	14.2	NA	NA
(E)-2-Undecen-1-ol	NA	NA	NA	NA	NA	NA
(E)-2--Dodecen-1-ol	NA	NA	NA	NA	NA	NA
1-Decanol	NA	NA	5.77	13.6	NA	NA
Nonane	NA	NA	NA	NA	NA	NA
Dec-9-en-1-ol	NA	NA	NA	NA	NA	NA
1-Dodecanol	NA	NA	NA	NA	NA	NA
1-Undecanol	NA	NA	NA	NA	NA	NA
Undecanol	NA	NA	NA	NA	3.37	NA
Undecanal	NA	NA	NA	NA	3.23	NA
Tridecanal	NA	3.0	NA	NA	1.16	NA
Tetradecanal	NA	NA	NA	NA	17.86	NA
n-Tetradecanol	NA	NA	6.09	NA	NA	NA

(Nazrul 2009; Laribi 2015; Freires 2019)
"NA":not available

a-pinene (0.2%–8.5%),camphene (1.4%), myrcene (0.2%–2.0%); Ketones: Camphor (0.9%–4.9%); Esters: Geranyl acetate (0.1%–4.7%),linalyl acetate (0%–2.7%) (Ramasamy, 2017)."-":not available.

(Jorge 1990; Diederichsen 1996; Nazrul 2009; Mahendra 2011; Abbas 2012; Laribi 2015; Chahal 2017; Freires 2019).

The constitution of fatty oil found to be present in the ripe fruits of the plant grown in Germany were observed to be petroselinic acid (68.8%), linoleic acid (16.6%), oleic acid (7.5%), palmitic acid (3.8%), stearic acid (>2%), vaccenic acid (>2%) and myristic acid (>2%), respectively. By extraction or by the pressing method of Coriander fruits, they may yield a reasonable amount of fatty oil which is applied as a lubricant in most of the technical processes. The fatty oil from seeds contains petroselinic acid, chemically as an isomer of oleic acid. Presence of higher amount of petroselinic acid makes the plant used in surfactants, polymers (Diederichsen, 1996).

Importance of Aldehydes in Coriander

The leaves of the plant do contain a higher percentage of aldehydes. Even the same group of aldehydes are found present in soaps or lotions. Researchers discovered the genetic factors might somewhat influence the disliked taste. Though some of the studies suggested that if coriander leaves were crushed, it would lead to a rapid breakdown of organic compounds, like aldehydes that tend to diminish the soapy taste of the plant.

The aromaticity of coriander is due to the presence of aldehyde compounds. The essential constituents in leaves are named, 2-decenoic acid, decanoic acid (also known as capric acid) and octadecenoic acid (The chemistry of coriander, 2014).

Table 3. Percentage composition of Coriandrum sativum fruit obtained from different origin of world as reported in the literature

Chemical components	Algeria	Canada	Kenya	Tunisia	India
α-Pinene	3.41	1.80	0.04	0.02	10.5
β-Pinene	0.78	NA	NA	0.05	> 2%
β-Myrcene	0.65	NA	NA	NA	> 2%
p-Cymene	1.76	1.30	NA	Traces	NA
Phellandrene	NA	2.50	NA	NA	NA
Limonene	1.23	0.70	NA	0.02	> 2%
p-mentha-1,4-dien-7-ol	6.51	NA	NA	NA	NA
p-mentha-1,8-diene	0.28	NA	NA	NA	NA
Linalool	73.11	82.00	0.32	87.54	67.7
Camphor	1.85	3.80	NA	NA	3.0
Camphene	NA	NA	NA	NA	> 2%
Borneol	NA	NA	NA	NA	> 2%
4-Terpineol	NA	NA	NA	NA	NA
Terpineol	NA	NA	NA	NA	NA
c-terpinene	NA	NA	NA	NA	NA
cis-Dihydrocarvone	NA	NA	NA	NA	NA
Decanal	NA	0.60	14.30	NA	NA
Propanal, 2-methyl-3-phenyl-	NA	NA	NA	NA	NA
Lavandulol	0.43	NA	NA	NA	NA
2E-Decenal	NA	NA	15.90	NA	NA
2E-Decen-1-ol	NA	NA	14.20	NA	NA
n-Decanol	NA	NA	13.60	NA	NA
Undecanal	NA	NA	3.23	NA	NA
Undecanol	NA	NA	-	NA	NA
Trans-2-Undecen-1-ol	NA	NA	2.12	NA	NA
n-Undecanol	NA	NA	2.38	NA	NA
Docecanal	NA	NA	4.36	NA	NA
Linalyl acetate	NA	2.90	NA	NA	NA
Geranyl acetate	NA	1.2	NA	0.83	4.0
Neryl acetate	NA	NA	NA	traces	NA
Tridecanal	NA	NA	NA	NA	NA
2E-Tridecen-1-al	NA	NA	NA	NA	NA
Tetradecanoic acid	NA	NA	NA	NA	NA
γ-terpinene p-cymol	NA	NA	NA	NA	NA
Geraniol	NA	NA	NA	NA	NA
Dipentene	NA	NA	NA	NA	NA
α-terpinene	NA	NA	NA	NA	NA
n-decylaldehyde	NA	NA	NA	NA	>2%
acetic acid esters	NA	NA	NA	NA	>2%

Source: (Diederichsen 1996; Laribi 2015; Chahal 2017; Mahendra 2011).
"NA":not available.

Figure 4. Structures of major chemical constituents present in Coriander

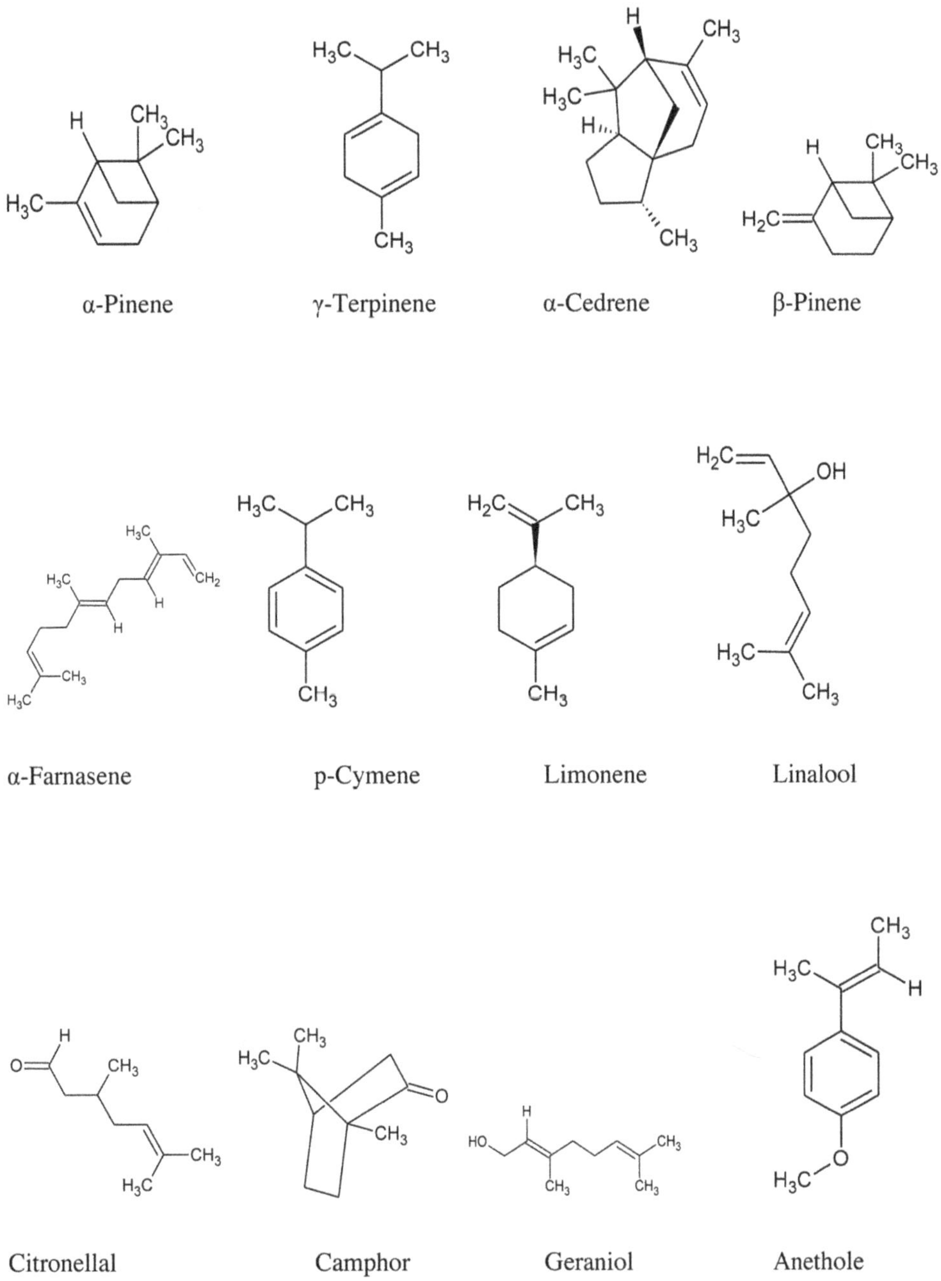

APPLICATIONS OF CORIANDER

Medicinal Uses of Coriander

The plant is found to be helpful in aiding digestion. It has been used as an aphrodisiac. It is useful in the treatment of ulcers and rheumatism, externally. The fruits are used to treat halitosis. Fruits can be used as a carminative, diuretic, tonic, stomachic, antibilious, refrigerant, and aphrodisiac. Even the fruit was given along with rhubarb and senna to rectify gripping effects of the crude drugs. The seeds are found to be more effective in the treatment of halitosis. The dried form of fruits can be used as spices in the preparation and baking of fish and meat. In India, it is a popular spice. Even in Ethiopia, it is most commonly employed in combination with "berbere" to enhance flavor; it is also used with spicy red pepper (powder form) in various meat as well as vegetarian dishes. Nowadays, it has been used in the form of curry powder. Extensively, it has been used as spices and condiments in preparation of pickles, seasonings and it is employed in the development of flavoring pastries, cookies, buns, cakes, and tobacco products. The whole plant has used in the preparation of chutneys and sauces and it is employed as a flavoring agent in several alcoholic beverages. The green leaves of the plant have been used in soups and salads in India.

Table 4. Main volatile compounds of Coriandrum sativum L. oil with their odor description

Compound	Concentration range (%)	Odor descriptors
α-Pinene	2.36–23.23	Woody, spicy, oily
Linalool	57.52–75.14	Floral, grassy, pleasant, citrusy
Terpineol	0.08–5.37	Sweet, lilac odor
Cuminal	0.13–0.54	Spicy, harsh
Citronellol	0.65–1.67	Intense floral, rose, sweet like
Geraniol	0.45–2.35	Fresh, delicious, rose-like
Geranyl acetate	8.95–24.51	Pleasant, floral rose, herbal

Source: (Ramasamy, 2007)

Table 5. Chemical composition of the coriander fruits

Chemical components	Component Content (%)
Water	11.37
Crude protein	11.49
Fat	19.15
Crude fibre	28.43
Starch	10.53
Pentosane	10.29
Sugar	1.92
Mineral constituents	4.98
Essential oil	0.84

Source: (Diederichsen, 1996)

PHARMACOLOGY ACTIVITIES

Antibacterial

It has been observed that α, β-unsaturated aldehydes present in fresh leaves of the plant, i.e aliphatic (2E)-alkenals and alkanals, possess bactericidal properties against any stage of Salmonella choat at any stage of growth (Ramasamy, 2007). Scientists investigated the synergistic effects along with the antibacterial activity between volatile oils and various antibacterial drugs, including, gentamicin, chloramphenicol, cefoperazone, ciprofloxacin, piperacillin, and tetracycline. The essential oil was evaluated for the activity with the help of a microdilution susceptibility test or by a synergistic interaction using the checkerboard method. In research studies, in vitro effectiveness was found in between the synergistic interaction along with antibacterial drugs against Acinetobacter baumannii, namely, LMG 1025 / LMG 1041(Duarte, 2012).

The antibacterial property of essential oil against gram-positive as well gram-negative has been investigated by flow cytometry. These techniques were evaluating the cellular physiology of bacteria against the antimicrobial effects of essential oils of the plant. The studies revealed the fact that coriander oil would be employed in the antibacterial formulations as they had the progressive tendency of killing pathogenic bacteria for foodborne as well as hospital infections (Filomena, 2011). Researchers found the antibacterial property of the aqueous decoction of coriander along with the incorporation of black pepper, bay leaf, and aniseed against bacteria. The hypothesis proved with the disc diffusion technique, that black pepper showed 75%, aniseed 18.8% activity at 10ml/disc concentration and an aqueous decoction of the crude drug did not possess antibacterial potential against bacteria (Chaudhry, 2006).

Antifungal

Researchers revealed the antifungal property of essential oils obtained from coriander leaves was found to be more significant against *Candida albicans*. The essential oils and its active isolated fractions tended to lower the cytotoxicity level on human cells along with the putative actions which could affect the gene expression involved in the pathways such as chemokines, MAP-kinase and some adhesion proteins (Irlan, 2014). Methanol, chloroform, hexane, petroleum ether and aqueous extracts of coriander were examined against both enterotoxigenic and enteropathogenic E.coli, Salmonella typhimurium, S. entertidis, Shigella dysentriae, S. flexineri, Candida albicans, C. tropicalis, and C. krusei, where it was analyzed that methanol, chloroform, and aqueous extracts showed significant antifungal activity. The synergistic effect of coriander oil along with amphotericin B was evaluated successfully against *C. albicans* strains, using flow cytometry evaluation, and these evaluations would be found helpful in the development of new formulations in candidiasis infections (Uma, 2009).

Antioxidant

The antioxidant activity of herbal extracts based on polarity, obtained from coriander leaves and seeds, were investigated using three different assay methods, namely, DPPH scavenging, 15-LO, and inhibition of $Fe2+$ induced porcine brain phospholipid peroxidation. It wsas concluded from the studies that leaves of coriander show potent antioxidant activity when compared with the seeds, but it is also analyzed the ethyl acetate extracts of both parts had contributed the same activity (Filomena, 2011).

Darughe, 2012 et al. analyzed and identified the different constituents of the volatile oil obtained from coriander using GC-MS. Some major chemical components were in different proportions like camphor (44.99%), cyclohexanol acetate (14.45%), limonene (7.17%) and α-pinene (6.37%). Researchers had proved the antioxidant and antifungal properties of essential oils (Darughe, 2012). Enaydede Almedia Melo recognized some of the phenolic components, namely, caffeic acid, protocatechinic acid, and glycitin containing antioxidant potential found in the aqueous extract of coriander (Enaydede, 2005).

Sedative –Hypnotic

The hydro-alcoholic extracts (100, 200, 400 and 600 mg/kg) of coriander seeds were investigated for sedative effects, using the pentobarbital-induced sleeping time method in male albino mice. The extracts of different doses were administered intraperitoneal to albino mice before 30 minutes, injecting an pentobarbital injection at a dose of 40mg/kg, where sleep duration and sleep latency were also analyzed. The observation proved the sedative and hypnotic effects of coriander seeds extracts and essential oils of the same plant (Enaydede, 2006).

Insulin-like Activity

Also, coriander has been studied for insulin-releasing and insulin-like activity, as hyperpolarized B-cells would further have enhanced the secretion of insulin in the presence of the aqueous extract of the plant (Alison, 1999).

Diuretic

The GIT stimulatory, inhibitory, and hypotensive effects of fruits, mediated in combination with cholinergic and Ca2+antagonist mechanisms, were also observed respectively (Qaiser, 2009). It has been used in hypertension because of diuretic effects (Alison, 1999).

Antiplatelet

Aqueous extracts of coriander and curry leaves were studied for antiplatelet activity against the different concentration of agonists such as ADP, epinephrine, and collagen in human platelets. Both were capable of inhibiting aggregation of human platelets (W. Jessie, 2008).

Nematicidal Activity

Researchers examined the nematicidal effects of coriander, Oriental sweetgum, and valerian against pinewood nematode, namely *Bursaphelenchus xylophilus* by GC-MS. These analyses led the identification of major chemical compounds, such as benzaldehyde, trans-cinnamyl alcohol, cis-asarone, octanal, nonanal, decanal, trans-2-decenal, undecanal, dodecanal, decanol, and trans-2-decen-1-ol which possessed higher nematicidal activity, respectively (Junheon, 2008).

Table 5. Pharmacological activities of Coriander

Pharmacological activity	Extract used	Model used	Experiment
Analgesic	Aqueous extract of seeds	Hot plate method	Possessed significant effect at 200 mg/kg with reaction time was 5.281 sec. compared to Morphine at 5 mg/kg, i.p, with reaction time 6.282 sec.
Anthelmintic	Aqueous and hydroalcoholic extracts of seeds	Sheep infected with *Haemonchus contortus;* both in vitro & in vivo	Both extracts inhibited egg hatching at a concentration > 0.5 mg/mL, in vitro completely. Whereas in vivo, both doses not able to maintain their packed cell volume and group of albendazole possessed significant increase the same.
Sedative hypnotic	Aqueous and hydroalcoholic extracts of seeds	Pentobarbital sleep-induced time test (40 mg/kg)	The hydro-alcoholic extract showed dose-dependent sedative effect. Did not showed a significant impact on sleep induction time.
Memory- enhancing	Fresh leaves	Elevated plus-maze	Dose-dependent improvement in memory scores of young as well as aged rats; even reversed memory deficits induced by the drugs.
	Fruits	Aβ(1- 42) rat model of Alzheimer's disease (in vivo)	Improved spatial memory effect in Y-maze task and radial arm-maze, significantly.
Insecticidal	Leaves, stems, flowers, and green fruits	Filter paper arena test	Effective against *T. castaneum* larvae, pupae, and adults and showed repellent activity.
	Seeds	Two stored product insects such as *Tribolium confusum, Callosobruchus maculatus* (in vitro)	Found effective against these insects.
Hypolipidemic	Aqueous extract of Seeds	Hypercaloric diet as well as forced limited physical activity in rats	Decreased total cholesterol, LDL, triglycerides, respectively.
Hypoglycemic	Powdered, aqueous and alcoholic extracts	Type-2 diabetes mellitus patients (in vivo)	Found significant activity at a higher dose, but not tolerated by some of the patients.
	The essential oil from seeds	Streptozotocin-induced diabetic rats (in vivo)	Decreased serum glucose and enhanced glutathione peroxidase level.
	Aqueous extracts of Fruits	Streptozotocin-induced diabetic rats (in vivo)	Decreased blood glucose level significantly at 500 mg/kg.
Anticancer	Aqueous, methanol extracts obtained from leaves and seeds	lymphoma cell line L5178Y-R (in vitro)	Aqueous leaf extract possessed significant activity.
	Ethyl acetate, aqueous, methanol extracts from roots, leaves, and stems	Human tumor cell lines MCF-7, MTT assay (in vitro)	Ethyl acetate extract obtained from roots observed the excellent anti-proliferative activity.
Anti-convulsant	Aqueous and ethanolic extracts of seeds	PTZ and maximal electroshock tests	Both extracts showed anticonvulsant activity at a dose of 5 mg/kg compared to phenobarbital at a dose of 20 mg/kg in the PTZ test.
	Hydroalcoholic extract of aerial parts of the plant	PTZ induced toxicity in rats	Increased the latency period of minimal clonic seizures and generalized tonic-clonic seizures
Antioxidant	Ethanol, dichloromethane, ethyl acetate, diethyl ether, butanol extracts, Aqueous residue of Seeds Leaves	DPPH assay, inhibition of 15-lipoxygenase, inhibition of $Fe^{2}+$ induced porcine brain phospholipid peroxidation.	Ethyl acetate leaf extract showed potent DPPH radical-scavenging activity and highest inhibitory activity toward 15-LO. Diethyl ether leaf extract showed potential activity. Seed oil showed minimum inhibitory activity.
Anxiolytic	Aqueous extract of seeds	Elevated plus-maze test (in vivo)	Enhanced time spent in the model used at 200 mg/kg, compared with diazepam.
Antifungal	The essential oil from leaves	Micro-dilution technique (in vitro)	Possessed weak Minimum Inhibitory Concentration and Fungicidal Inhibitory Concentration against *Candida* spp.
Anti-inflammatory	Essential oil	Ultraviolet erythema test (in vivo)	The essential oil of lipolotion decline UV-induced erythema and not effective than hydrocortisone.
	Ethanol extract of fruits	Carrageenan induced rat paw edema (in vivo)	Possessed edema inhibition at 200 mg/kg dose.
Antibacterial	The essential oil from seeds	Agar disc diffusion method; bacteria isolated from patients (in vitro)	Showed potent antimicrobial activity against three bacteria isolated from patients such as *Lactobacilli, Streptococcus salivarius*, and *Streptococcus sanguis.*
			Antibacterial activity against E. coli.
	An essential oil from fruits	Macro-dilution test(in vitro)	Showed significant antibacterial activity against bacterial strains tested, respectively.

continued on following page

Table 5. Continued

Pharmacological activity	Extract used	Model used	Experiment
Antidepressant	Diethyl ether extract of seeds	----------------------	Significant effects through adrenergic, dopamine, and GABA-ergic system.
Anti-implantation effect	Aqueous extract of leaves	The model used: oestrus cycle, implantation, foetal loss, abortion, teratogenicity, serum progesterone levels.	Decrease in serum progesterone levels, significantly.
Dermatological effect	Ethanol extract	UVB-induced skin photoaging in normal human dermal fibroblasts; in the skin of hairless mice in vivo	Reduced the levels MMP-1.
	------------------	2,4-dinitrochlorobenzene-induced CD-like skin lesions	Regulation of immune mediators.
	Leaf extract	Oxidative stress in human HaCaT keratinocytes.	Decreased cell viability by H_2O_2-induced damage.
Diuretic	Aqueous extract of seed	-------------------	Increased diuresis, electrolytes excretion, and glomerular filtration rate.
Detoxification effect	Ethanol extract	Lead deposition as lead acetate trihydrate in drinking water.	Reduced lead deposition in the femur and severe lead-induced injury in kidneys.
	Hydroalcoholic extract	Lead-induced oxidative stress in rats.	Tissue-specific amelioration of oxidative stress produced by lead.
Hepatoprotective effect	Aqueous extract of seeds	Gamma radiation-induced toxicity in rats	Reduced radiation-induced serum biochemical disorders.
	Aqueous extract of seeds	Paracetamol induced toxicity in rats	Improved significantly biochemical parameters.
	Essential oils	Carbon tetrachloride-induced toxicity in rats	Reduced stable DPPH level in a dose-dependent manner; to neutralize the hydrogen peroxide level.
	------------------	Carbon tetrachloride-induced toxicity in rats	Decreased liver weight, biochemical parameters such as SGOT, SGPT, and ALP, and direct bilirubin.
Neuroprotective effect	Methanolic extract of leaves	Ischemic-reperfusion insult in the brain.	Increased endogenous enzyme levels of superoxide dismutase, glutathione, catalase, and total protein levels, reduced cerebral infarct size, lipid peroxidation as well as calcium levels.

Source: (Laribi 2015; Safia 2010; Appian 2016; Al-Said MS 1987; Hwang 2014; Park 2014; Park 2012; Aissaoui 2008; Velaga 2014; Farag 2013; Ramadan 2013; Rodriguez 2006; Vekaria 2012).

Preservative

Studies revealed the successful usage of coriander oil as a food preservative. And it was even examined as an antimicrobial activity of coriander oil (Filomena, 2017).

Memory Enhancer

Coriander had the potential to satisfactorily reverse memory deficits induced by scopolamine and diazepam, as proved by Vasudevan Mani et al. (Vasudevan, 2009). The anti-inflammatory, cholesterol-lowering, antioxidant properties would contribute its potential in memory-enhancing properties. The investigators had the plan of exploring the plant in the treatment of Alzheimer disease (Poonam, 2011).

Anti-anxiety

Studies explored the anti-anxiety activity of hydroalcoholic extract of *C. sativum* (Linn.) using different models such as EPM, OFT, light and dark test, and the social interaction test. Different doses of fruit extract i-e 50, 100, 200 mg/kg and diazepam (0.5 mg/kg) and standard drugs were tested. The results revealed 100 and 200 mg/kg doses of the plant showed significant effects similarly to the standard drug (Poonam, 2011).

The antianxiety effect of aqueous extract was evaluated using the EPM model at different doses of 50, 100, and 200 mg/kg. All treatments had a significant increase in the time spent in the open arm parameter (Latha,2015).

The hydroalcoholic extract of the plant possessed dose-dependent effects similar to diazepam using an elevated plus maze, an open field test, the light /dark test, and the social interaction test (Mahendra, 2011). Another study showed the hydroalcoholic leaf extract was found to be more effective at 200 and 400 mg/kg in EPM and the OFT model. The doses of 200 and 400 mg/kg had increased the time spent as well as the number of entries in open arms of the EPM model whereas enhanced locomotion activity of OFT was found in mice. The lower doses of crude extract did not show any effect on the action (Harsha, 2011).

Anti-Inflammatory

Studies revealed coriander oil possessed an anti-inflammatory property in the ultraviolet erythema test in vivo. From these experiments, it has been analyzed that the lipolotion of coriander oil 0.5% reduced UV-induced erythema significantly when compared to placebo, and it did not find much useful than hydrocortisone. Also, the essential oil was found to possess an excellent skin tolerance activity (Juliane, 2008).

CONCLUSION

Still, humans have discovered numerous herbal medicines which not only cure illness but also prevent diseases; even boosting up the immune system of the body. Various chemical constituents have been isolated from coriander and a number of pharmacological activities have been conducted on the different parts of coriander. The present literature can provide information about the phytochemical and pharmacological activities of coriander. It requires more research and investigations about the undeveloped potential of the plant.

ACKNOWLEDGMENT

The authors thank Prof. Pradeep Mishra, Director, and Prof. Meenakshi Bajpai, Head of Department, Institute of Pharmaceutical Research, GLA University, for giving valuable insights. Even the authors are showing their sincere gratitude toward Mr. Himanshu Sharma, Assistant Professor, Department of Computer Science and Application, GLA University, for his amazing and excellent support through the work.

REFERENCES

Abbas, K., & Tahere, R. (2012). Composition and insecticidal activity of essential oil from *Coriandrum sativum* seeds against tribolium confusum and callosobruchus maculatus. ISRN Pharmaceutics, 5.

Aissaoui, A., El-Hilaly, J., Israili, Z. H., & Lyoussi, B. (2008). Acute diuretic effect of continuous intravenous infusion of an aqueous extract of *Coriandrum sativum* L. in anesthetized rats. *Journal of Ethnopharmacology*, *115*(1), 89–95. doi:10.1016/j.jep.2007.09.007

Al-Said, M. S., Al-Khamis, K. I., Islam, M. W., Parmar, N. S., Tariq, M., & Ageel, A. M. (1987). Post-coital antifertility activity of the seeds of *Coriandrum sativum* in rats. *Journal of Ethnopharmacology*, *21*(2), 165–173. doi:10.1016/0378-8741(87)90126-7

Alison, M. G., & Peter, R. F. (1999). Insulin-releasing and insulin-like activity of the traditional anti-diabetic plant *Coriandrum sativum* (coriander). *British Journal of Nutrition*, *81*(3), 203–209. doi:10.1017/S0007114599000392

Chahal, K. K., Singh, R., Kumar, A., & Bhardwaj, U. (2017). Chemical composition and biological activity of *Coriandrum sativum* Lin [review]. *Indian Journal of Natural Products and Resources*, *8*(3), 193–203.

Chaudhry, N. M., & Tariq, P. (2006). Bactericidal activity of black pepper, bay leaf, aniseed and coriander against oral isolates. *Pakistan Journal of Pharmaceutical Sciences*, *19*(3), 214–218.

Coriandrum sativum (coriander). (n.d.). Retrieved from https://www.cabi.org/isc/datasheet/15300

Darughe, F., Barzegar, M., & Sahari, M. A. (2012). Antioxidant and antifungal activity of coriander (*Coriandrum sativum* L.) essential oil in cake. *International Food Research*, *19*(3), 1253–1260.

De Figueiredo, R. O., Marques, M. O. M., Nakagawa, J., & Ming, L. C. (2004). Composition of coriander essential oil from Brazil. *Acta Horticulturae*, (62): 135–137. doi:10.17660/ActaHortic.2004.629.18

Diederichsen, A. (1996). *An ecogeographical study of promoting the conservation and use of underutilized and neglected crops: Coriander*. International Plant Genetic Resources Institute.

Duarte, A., Ferreira, S., Silva, F. C., & Domingues, F. C. (2012). Synergistic activity of coriander oil and conventional antibiotics against Acinetobacter baumannii. *Phytomedicine*, *19*(3–4), 236–238. doi:10.1016/j.phymed.2011.11.010

Enaydede, A. (2005). Characterization of antioxidant compounds in aqueous coriander extract (*Coriandrum sativum* L.). *Lebensmittel-Wissenschaft + Technologie*, *38*(1), 15–19. doi:10.1016/j.lwt.2004.03.011

Enaydede, A., Meloa, J. M., Filhob, N. B., Guerrac, E. G., & Heidari-Hamedani. (2006). *Sedative-hypnotic activity of extracts and essential oil of coriander seeds*. Academic Press.

Farag, M. F. S. (2013). Evaluation of radioprotective effects of coriander (Coriandrum sativum L.) in male rats. *Arab Journal of Nuclear Science and Applications*, *46*(1), 240–249.

Filomena, S., & Fernanda, C. D. (2017). Antimicrobial activity of coriander oil and its effectiveness as a food preservative. *Critical Reviews in Food Science and Nutrition*, *57*(1), 35–47. doi:10.1080/10408398.2013.847818

Filomena, S., & Susana, F. (2011). Antifungal activity of *Coriandrum sativum* essential oil, its mode of action against Candida species and potential synergism with amphotericin B. *Phytomedicine*, *19*(1), 42–47. doi:10.1016/j.phymed.2011.06.033

Filomena, S., Susana, F., & Joao, A. (2011). Essential oil: Its antibacterial activity and mode of action evaluated by flow cytometry. *Journal of Medical Microbiology*, *60*(10), 1479–1486. doi:10.1099/jmm.0.034157-0

Freires, I. D. A., Murata, R. M., Furletti, V. F., Sartoratto, A., De Alencar, S. M. D., & Figueira, G. M. (2019). *Coriandrum sativum* L. (Coriander) essential oil: Antifungal activity and mode of action on Candida spp. and molecular targets affected in human whole-genome expression. *PLoS One*, *9*(6), e99086. doi:10.1371/journal.pone.0099086

Harsha, S. N., & Anila, K. K. R. (2012). Effects of *Coriandrum sativum* extract on exploratory behavior pattern and locomotor activity in mice: An experimental study. *IJGB*, *6*(2), 157–162.

Helle, W. (2004). Antioxidant activity in extracts from coriander. *Food Chemistry*, *88*(2), 293–297. doi:10.1016/j.foodchem.2004.01.047

Hwang, E., Lee, D. G., Park, S. H., Oh, M. S., & Kim, S. Y. (2014). Coriander leaf extract exerts antioxidant activity and protects against UVB-induced photoaging of skin by regulation of procollagen type I and MMP-1 expression. *Journal of Medicinal Food*, *17*(9), 985–995. doi:10.1089/jmf.2013.2999

Irlan de Almeida, F., Ramiro, M.M., Vivian, F.F., Adilson, S., Severino, M., de Alencar, G. (2014). *Coriandrum sativum L. (coriander) essential oil: antifungal activity and mode of action on Candida spp., and molecular targets affected in human whole-genome expression*. doi:10.1371/journal.pone.0099086

Isao, Kubo, & Fujita, Kubo,& Nihei. (2004). Antibacterial activity of coriander volatile compounds against Salmonella choleraesuis. *Journal of Agricultural and Food Chemistry*.

Iyengar, M. A. (1997). *Pharmacognosy of powdered crude drugs*. Manipal, Karnataka: Manipal Power Press.

Iyengar, M. A. (2004). *Study of crude drugs*. Manipal, Karnataka: Manipal Power Press.

Iyengar, M. A., & Nayak, S. G. K. (1991). *Anatomy of crude drugs*. Manipal, Karnataka: Manipal Power Press.

Jessie Suneetha, W., & Krishnakantha, T. P. (2008). Antiplatelet activity of coriander and curry leaf spices. *Pharmaceutical Biology*, *43*(3), 230–233. doi:10.1080/13880200590928807

Jorge, A. P., Aristides, R., & Victor, F. (1990). Composition of the seed oil of *Coriandrum sativum* L. from Cuba. *The Journal of Essential Oil Research*, *8*, 97–98.

Junheon, K., Sun-Mi, S., Sang-Gil, L., & Sang-Chul, S., & II-Kwon, P. (2008). Nematicidal activity of plant essential oils and components from coriander (Coriandrum sativum), oriental sweetgum (Liquidambar orientalis), and valerian (Valeriana wallichii) essential oils against pinewood nematode (Bursaphelenchus xylophilus). *Journal of Agricultural and Food Chemistry*.

Kokate, C. K., & Gokhlae. (2007). *Text book of Pharmacognosy*. New Delhi: Nirali Prakashan.

Laribi, B., Kouki, K., M'Hamdi, M., & Bettaieb, T. (2015). Coriander (*Coriandrum sativum* L.) and its bioactive constituents. *Fitoterapia*, *103*, 9–26. doi:10.1016/j.fitote.2015.03.012

Latha, K., Rammohan, B., Sunanda, B. P., Maheswari, M. S., & Mohan, S. K. (2015). Evaluation of anxiolytic activity of aqueous extract of *Coriandrum sativum* Linn in mice: A preliminary experimental study. *Pharmacognosy Research, 7*(5Suppl 1), S47–S51. doi:10.4103/0974-8490.157996

Mahendra, P., & Bisht, S. (2011). Anti-anxiety activity of *Coriandrum sativum* assessed using different experimental anxiety models. *Indian Journal of Pharmacology, 43*(5), 574–577. doi:10.4103/0253-7613.84975

Nadeem, M., Anjum, F. M., Khan, M. I., Tehseen, S., El-Ghorab, A., & Sultan, J. I. (2013). Nutritional and medicinal aspects of coriander (*Coriandrum sativum* L.)-a review. *British Food Journal, 115*(5), 743–755. doi:10.1108/00070701311331526

Nazrul Islam, B., Jaripa, B., & Mahbuba, S. (2009). Chemical composition of leaf and seed essential oil of *Coriandrum sativum* L. from Bangladesh. *Bangladesh Journal of Pharmacology, 4*, 150–153.

Park, G., Kim, H. G., Kim, Y. O., Park, S. H., Kim, S. Y., & Oh, M. S. (2012). *Coriandrum sativum* L. protects human keratinocytes from oxidative stress by regulating oxidative defense systems. *Skin Pharmacology and Physiology, 25*(2), 93–99. doi:10.1159/000335257

Park, G., Kim, H. G., Lim, S., Lee, W., Sim, Y., & Oh, M. S. (2014). Coriander alleviates 2,4-dinitrochlorobenzene-induced contact dermatitis-like skin lesions in mice. *Journal of Medicinal Food, 17*(8), 862–868. doi:10.1089/jmf.2013.2910

Poonam, M., & Shradha, B. (2011). Anti-anxiety activity of *Coriandrum sativum* assessed using different experimental anxiety models. *Indian Journal of Pharmacology, 43*(5), 574–577. doi:10.4103/0253-7613.84975

Qaiser, J. (2009). Coriander fruit exhibits gut modulatory, blood pressure lowering, and diuretic activities. *Journal of Ethnopharmacology, 122*(1), 123–130. doi:10.1016/j.jep.2008.12.016

Ramadan, M. M., & Abd Algader, N. N. E. (2013). Chemopreventive effect of Coriandrum sativum fruits on hepatic toxicity in male rats. *World Journal of Medical Sciences, 8*(4), 322–333.

Ramasamy, R. (2007). Aroma characterization of coriander (*Coriandrum sativum* L.) oil samples. *European Food Research and Technology, 225*(3-4), 367–374. doi:10.100700217-006-0425-7

Rodriguez, L., Ramirez, M., Badillo, M., León-Buitimea, A., & Reyes-Esparza, J. (2006). Toxicological evaluation of *Coriandrum sativum* (cilantro) using in vivo and in vitro models. *The FASEB Journal, 20*, A645.

Safia, Z. (2010). Essential oil composition of *Coriandrum sativum* seed cultivated in Algeria as food grains protectant. *Food Chemistry, 122*(4), 1226–1228. doi:10.1016/j.foodchem.2010.03.119

Shelef, L. A. (2003). Herbs: Herbs of the Umbelliferae. In *Encyclopedia of Food Sciences and Nutrition*. Retrieved from https://www.sciencedirect.com/topics/agricultural-and-biological-sciences/coriandrum-sativum

Subramoniam. (2016). *Plants with Anti-Diabetes Mellitus Properties*. . doi:10.1201/978131537148

The Chemistry of Coriander. (2014). Retrieved from https://www.compoundchem.com

Uma, B., Prabhakar, K., Rajendran, S., Sarayu, Y., & Lakshmi. (2009). Antimicrobial activity and phytochemical analysis of *Coriander sativum* against infectious diarrhoea. *Ethnobotanical Leaflets*, 5.

Vasudevan, M., & Milind, P. (2009). Memory enhancing activity of Coriandrum sativum in rats. *Pharmacologyonline*, *2*, 827–839.

Vekaria, R. H., Patel, M. N., Bhalodiya, P. N., Patel, V., Desai, T. R., & Tirgar, P. R. (2012). Evaluation of the neuroprotective effect of *Coriandrum sativum* Linn. against ischemic-reperfusion on insulin in the brain. *International Journal of Phytopharmacology*, *3*(2), 86–193.

Velaga, M. K., Yallapragada, P. R., Williams, D., Rajanna, S., & Bettaiya, R. (2014). Hydroalcoholic seed extract of *Coriandrum sativum* (coriander) alleviates lead-induced oxidative stress in different regions of rat brain. *Biological Trace Element Research*, *159*(1-3), 351–363. doi:10.100712011-014-9989-4

APPENDIX

cm centimetre
mm millimetre
d diameter
kg kilogram
mg microgram
% percentage
ml millilitre
MAP-kinase mitogen-activated protein kinase
DPPH diphenylpicrylhydrazyl
LO 15-lipoxygenase
GIT gastrointestinal tract
Ca^{2+} calcium
ADP adenosine di-phosphate
EPM elevated plus maze
OFT open field test
UV ultraviolet
SGOT aspartate transaminase
SGPT alanine transaminase
PTZ pentylene tetrazole
GABA gamma-aminobutyric acid
MMP matrix metalloproteinases
LDL low-density level
ALP alkaline phosphatase
H_2O_2 hydrogen peroxide
GC-MS gas chromatography-mass spectroscopy
MCF-7 michigan cancer foundation
MTT 3-(4,5-dimethylthiazol-2-yl)-2,5-diphenyl tetrazolium bromide
ferrous form
HaCaT cells human keratinocyte cells.
CD contact dermatitis

Chapter 15
Proven Health Benefits and Uses of Coriander (*Coriandrum sativum L.*)

Suman Devi
Department of Food Science and Nutrition, University of Allahabad, India

Ena Gupta
Department of Home Science, University of Allahabad, India

Mamta Sahu
Department of Agricultural Biochemistry, University of Allahabad, India

Pragya Mishra
Department of Food Science, University of Allahabad, India

ABSTRACT

Coriander (Coriandrum sativum L) is an annual herb that belongs to the family Apiaceae (Umbelliferae) and is commonly known as dhanya. For centuries, the coriander plants and their parts, primarily their leaves and ripe seeds, have been used in folk medicines in addition to culinary uses. This plant is herbaceous and aromatic and is cultivated in several countries, including India, Italy, the Netherlands, Europe, China, and Bangladesh. The coriander plant is rich in essential oils, vitamins (vitamins C and K), minerals (calcium, phosphorous, potassium, thiamine, and niacin), and other micronutrients. The plants are extensively used in the preparation of food items. C. sativum essential oil and extracts possess various potential pharmacological properties and has been found to possess carminative, diuretic, stomachic, aphrodisiac, anti-inflammatory, antibacterial, antifungal, and anticancer activities. The present study aims to discuss the botany, traditional uses, medicinal, and industrial applications of coriander extracts and essential oils.

DOI: 10.4018/978-1-7998-2524-1.ch015

INTRODUCTION

Coriander is one of the oldest crops, and it has been used in both folk medicines and for culinary purposes for approximately 3,000 years. It is indigenous to the Mediterranean region and widely cultivated in Russia, Central Europe, North Africa, and Asia (Singh, Maurya, De Lampasona, & Catalan, 2006). It is a tropical crop and can be harvested in the Rabi season during the flowering and seedling stage. The season of sowing is from May to July during kharif, and October to January during rabi season (Farooqi, Sreeramu, & Srinivasappa, 2005). Coriandrum sativum L. is commonly known as dhaniya in India.

This plant is highly aromatic and can be used for garnishing meals and in various food preparations, such as chutney, beverages, curry, pickles, fish, and meat products. All parts of this herb are used as flavouring agents and as traditional remedies for the treatment of a wide range of human aliments.

The coriander is harvested when seeds mature and change from dark green to brown. After threshing, seeds are collected and dried in the sunlight to maintain 8 to 10%of their moisture. The dried seeds contribute to the pleasant aroma that is used in international cuisines, as well as in stews, sweetbreads, cakes, and sausages (Peter, 2004). Coriander seeds are available in the market in whole, ground, and powdered forms. The seeds are rich in essential oil (0.5-1%) and fatty oils, with a high concentration of monounsaturated fatty acids, especially petroselinic acid. The roasted powder of the seeds is used as an ingredient in curry powders, pickles, and black salts, and it is used as flavouring and thickening agent in cooking. It is also used in rasam, all curries, and chutney, as powder. It is used whole in samosa, khaman dhokla, and kachori. Coriander seeds are also a good source of biologically active metabolites, such as polyphenols, particularly phenolic acids, and flavonoids.

C. sativum L. essential oil has promising antibacterial, antifungal, and anti-oxidative activities that play a great role in maintaining the shelf-life of foods. The potential of coriander in food (as flavouring or as a preservative), in pharmaceuticals (as natural drugs), and as industry product ingredients (fragrances and lotions) has increased researchers' interest in studying this plant. This present study aims to discuss the botany, traditional uses, medicinal, and industrial applications of coriander plants, extracts, and essential oils.

Taxonomy, Botany and Chemical Composition of Coriander

Taxonomical Classifications of Coriander(Coriandrum sativum L.) per Mahendra and Bisht (2011):

Kingdom: Plantae
Subkingdom: Tracheobionta
Super Division: Spermatophyta
Division: Magnoliophyta
Class: Magnoliopsida
Order: Apiales
Family: Apiaceae
Genus: Corianderum *L.*
Species: Corianderum sativum *L.*
Botanical Name: Corianderum sativum *L.*

Botanical Description

Coriander spice, commonly called cilantro, is native to Africa and South-western Asia. This spice grows up to 25-50 cm in height, the leaves vary in shape. The fruit has a very delicate fragrance, is round in shape, with longitudinal ridges, 3-5 cm in diameter, with a pale white to light brown colour. As a schizocarp, the fruit, when divided, splits into two equal parts (mericarps) with each part having one seed. The flowers of the coriander plant are arranged in small clusters referred to as umbles; the flowers are white and asymmetrical, with petals that are 0.20-0.24-inches in length. The leaves are glabrous, lobbed, lanceolate, and green in colour. Figure 1 provides a brief overview of how the coriander looks at different stages.

Figure 1.Different parts of the coriander

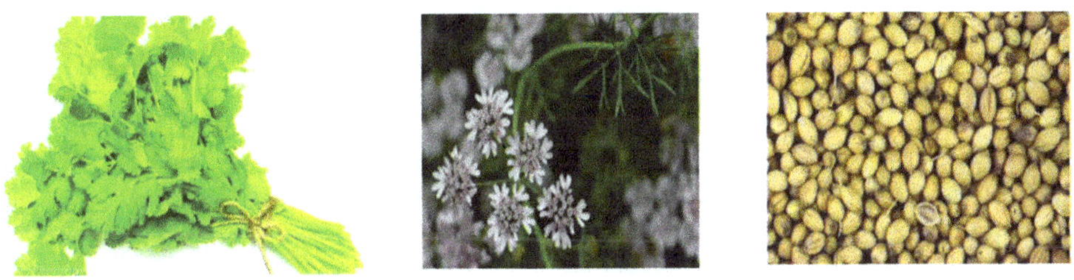

PHYTOCHEMISTRY

The leaves and seeds of the coriander are a novel source of medicine. They are rich in essential oils,which are extensively used as a flavouring agent in all types of food products, including alcoholic beverages, tobacco, candy, pickles, meat sauce, and seasonings. The spice has myriad benefits, as it possesses a wide variety of bioactive compounds,both volatile and non-volatile. The major volatile compounds in coriander seed essential oil arelinalool, γ-terpinene, α-pinene, camphor, decanal geranyl acetate, limonene, geraniol, camphene, and D-limonene.The major volatile compounds identified in the coriander leaves essential oil are(E)-2-decenal, linalool, (E)-2-dodecenal, (E)-2-tetradecenal, 2-decen-1-ol, (E)-2-undecenal, dodecanal, (E)-2-tridecenal, (E)-2-hexadecenal, pentadecenal, and α-pinene.

The major components in the oil distilled from the coriander fruit include linalool, oxygenated monoterpenes, monoterpene hydrocarbons (Bhuiyan, Begum, & Sultana, 2009). The most important constituents of the coriander fruit its essential oil and fatty oil. The major fatty acid in the essential oil of the seed is petroselinic acid, a monounsaturated fatty acid, and linalool. The biologically active compounds ofthe coriander are detailed in Figure 2, and the chemical composition of the essential oil is presented in Table 1. The essential oil has been used as both a flavouring and preservative agent. It has antibacterial, antifungal and anti-oxidative activities that extend the shelf life of food products. It is also used in pharmaceutical and beauty products, such as perfumes and lotions, as well ashaving a therapeutic action in human health (Mandal & Mandal, 2015).

Figure 2. Biologically active compounds of coriandrum sativum L.
Source: (Sharma, Jasuja, & Joshi, 2013)

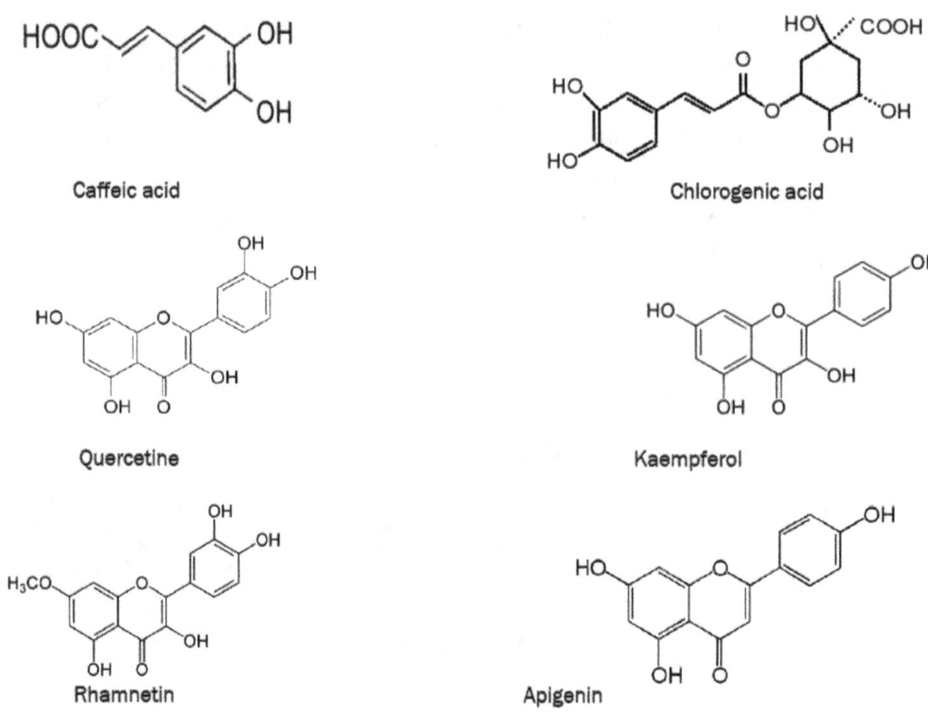

Table 1. Components of essential oil and fatty oil in the ripe fruits of the coriander plant

Components of Essential Oil in the Ripe Fruits of Coriander			Components of Fatty Oil in the Ripe Fruits of Coriander		
Components	**% of Total Essential Oil**	**Minor Component**	**Components**	**% of Total Fatty Oil**	**Minor Component**
Linalool	67.7	β-pinene	Petrosselinic acid	68.8	-
α-Pinene	10.5	Camphene	Linoleic acid	16.6	Stearic acid
γ-terpinene	9.0	Myrcene	Oleic acid	7.5	Vaccenic acid
Geramylacetate	4.0	p-cymol	Palmitic acid	3.8	Myristic acid
Camphor	3.0	Dipentene	-	-	-
Geraniol	1.9	α-terpinene	-	-	-

NUTRITIONAL ASPECTS

The most commonly used parts of the coriander plant are the green leaves and dried fruits. Like green leafy vegetables, they are also rich in Vitamin A (160 mg/100 g) and Vitamin C (12 mg/100 g). Green coriander leaves contain 84-90% water, are a good source of thiamine, zinc, and dietary fibre, and are low in saturated fat and cholesterol. Several studies reported that matured coriander leaves are rich in moisture crude protein, fat, crude fibre, and ash (Coskuner and & Karababa, 2007).The nutritional values of raw coriander leaves per 100g are shown in Table 2.

Table 2. Chemical composition of coriander per 100g

Components	Content (%)
Water	11.46
Sugar	1.93
Pentosans	10.30
Fat	11.5
Crude Fibre	19.20
Starch	28.42
Mineral Constitutes	4.97
Essential Oil	0.841

All parts of the C. sativum L. plant are edible and have been used in folk medicine and for culinary purposes for centuries. However, the fresh leaves and dried seeds of the plant are most frequently used. C. sativum L. is well known for its antioxidant properties, and some of its active components have been identified. Coriander contains active phenolic acid compounds, including caffeic and chlorogenic acid. The flavonoids include quercetin, keampferol, rhamnetin and apigenin.

Coriander is a very useful spice that has been cited as possessing healing properties, such as the ability to change the ratio of phospholipids and maintain the functions of membranes that work toreduce cholesterol levels and also improve human digestion. Dhanapakiam, Joseph, Ramaswamy, Moorthi, & Kumar (2008) reported that the administration of coriander seeds had a profound influence on the metabolism of lipids in animals fed a high cholesterol diet. Coriander has also been advocated as an anti-diabetic remedy. Most of these compounds are known to inhibit free radicals generated in the cellular system when they are obtained through the diet. Coriander is used to treat numerous digestive problems including upset stomach, loss of appetite, hernia, nausea, diarrhoea, bowel spasms, and intestinal gas. It has also been proven to have anti-inflammatory and antimicrobial properties, and is used to treat measles, haemorrhoids, toothaches, worms, joint pain, as well as infections caused by bacteria and fungus.

ACCEPTABLE DAILY INTAKE (ADI)

Coriander has some side effects, such as allergic reactions and it increases the sensitivity of the sun, which increases the risk of skin cancer, sunburn. Other side effects can include diarrhoea, stomach pain, depression, and lapse of mensuration in women. Coriander prevents intestinal spasms and also helps to improve the taste. The recommended dosage of coriander is 2.5-5 grams.

Table 3. Nutritional values of raw coriander leaves per 100g

Component	Reference		
	U. S. Department of Agriculture, Agricultural Research Service	Coskuner and Karababa, (2007)	https://www.nutritionvalue.org
	Amount (Unit)	%	Amount (Unit)
Energy (kcal)	95 KJ (23kcal)	-	-
Water	92.0%	-	-
Fibre (Total Dietary)	2.81g	28.4 to 29.1	2.8g
Fat	0.52g	17.8- 19.15	0.5g
Protein	2.13 g	11.5-21.3	2.1g
Ash	1.47g	4.9 to 6.0	
Carbohydrate	-	-	3.7
Sugar	0.87 g	-	0.9g
Potassium	0.12mg	-	
Calcium	67 mg	- -	67.00 mg
Zinc	0.5 mg	-	0.50 mg
Phosphorus	48mg	-	48.00 mg
Magnesium	26 mg	-	26.00mg
Sodium	46 mg	-	46mg
Iron	1.77 mg	-	1.77 mg
Manganese	0.426 mg	-	0.426 mg
Vitamin A	337 μg	-	337.00 mcg
Thiamine(B1)	0.067 mg	-	-
Riboflavin (B2)	0.162 mg	-	-
Niacin (B3)	1.114 mg	-	-
Pantothenic Acid (B5)	0.51 mg	-	-
Vitamin B6	0.149 mg	-	0.149 mg
Folate (B9)	62 μg	-	
Vitamin C	27 mg	-	27.0 mg
Vitamin E	2.5 mg	-	2.50 mg
Vitamin K	310 μg	-	310.0 mcg

APPLICATIONS IN THE FOOD INDUSTRY

In ancient times, the whole plant of the spice was used, but it was primarily the fresh leaves and seeds that were used. As a spice, coriander is used in cuisines throughout the world. The dry seeds have a strong citrus lemony flavour when they are crushed, which is due to the presence of terpenes, linalool, and pinene. Due to its highly aromatic nature, it is frequently used in the food industry and other industries to enhance salads, soups, sausages, chutney, and curries. This essential oil of the plant is also used in aromatherapy. After drying it, it is then added to curry powder, spice sausages, seasoning, and pickling.

It is also served as a flavouring agent for bakery preparations. The coriander seed is an important ingredient of curry powder (Ramadan & Morsel, 2002).

Occasionally, dried coriander fruit is used to mask an off-flavour, and it is one of the most important ingredients in the pickle-making industry. A high concentration of vegetable oil in the form of monounsaturated fatty acids, mainly petroselinic acid, is present in the fruits of the coriander. A variety of techniques can be used to extract the vegetable oil, such as supercritical fluid extraction, steam distillation, and organic solvent extraction (soxhlet) (Mhemdi,Rodier, Kechao, & Fages, 2011).

The extracted oil can be encapsulated in chitosan, alginates, etc., to facilitate the protection, isolation, transport, and release of its active constituents like flavours, fatty acids, antioxidants, vitamins, minerals, peptides, and enzymes (Cristian, Liliana, Petru, & Stefan,2013). The essential oil and powder of the coriander are considered as an important natural food preservative due to its antioxidant, antibacterial, and antifungal properties. Its commercial value depends on its aroma quality, physical properties, and chemical composition, which occasionally can be affected by some pests and diseases, such as stem gall, powdery mildew, and wilt (Fusarium oxysporum). According to Rohit, Kavindra, and Chintan (2011), in the Indian spice industries, the quality of essential oil can be checked by automatic quality assessment techniques, whereas image analysis is performed by morphological image operations.

This spice is abundantly found in the dried form of seeds and also in ground form. During cooking, the seeds spread the aroma of the spices and also pungency by being roasted or heated. During storage, the seeds lose their flavour and aroma. Mostly, it becomes the content of garam masala and Indian cuisine. Another common mixture of this spice is also called dhana jeera, which is coriander slightly mixed with cumin and it is also known as dhana dal and often eaten as a snack food. In the southern cities of India, two of the most popular dishes, rasam and sambhar, are prepared using this spice. The plant of the coriander is primarilyused for making chutney, salsas, baked goods, salads, sweets, sauces, beverages, chewing gums, preservatives, and curry powder. The powder made from blending the fruits is used in many products, including bakery items, curries, fish, meat, pickles, sodas, etc. Presently, in the food industries, the leaves of the coriander are processed to form different food products such as pastes and purees, which have a deep green colour and a non-spicy, intense flavour.

CONCLUSION

Coriandrum sativum L. is traditionally used as both a culinary ingredient and a therapeutic agent. Different parts of the coriander plant, such as the majorly leaves and seeds have been documented as having medicinal, nutritional, and economic value. The spice is rich in micronutrients, essential oils, and secondary metabolites, which have wide applications in different fields, including the pharmaceutical industry and the global food industry. There is a need for more research and clinical studies to assess the effect of the different parts of the plant to validate their functionality.

REFERENCES

Bhuiyan, N. I., Begum, J., & Sultana, M. (2009). Chemical composition of leaf and seed essential oil of Coriandrum sativumL. from Bangladesh. *Bangladesh Journal of Pharmacology*, *4*(2), 150–153. doi:10.3329/bjp.v4i2.2800

Coriander (cilantro) leaves, raw. (n.d.). Retrieved from https://www.nutritionvalue.org/Coriander_(cilantro)_leaves,_raw_nutritional_value.html

Coskuner, Y., & Karababa, E. (2007). Physical properties of coriander seeds (*Coriandrum sativum L.*). *Journal of Food Engineering*, *80*(2), 408–416. doi:10.1016/j.jfoodeng.2006.02.042

Cristian, D., Liliana, G., Petru, A., & Stefan, D. (2013). Encapsulation of coriander essential oil in alginate and alginate/chitosan microspheres by emulsification of external gelation method. *Inside Food Symposium*, 9-12.

Dhanapakiam, P., Joseph, J. M., Ramaswamy, V. K., Moorthi, M., & Kumar, A. S. (2008). The cholesterol lowering property of coriander seeds (*Coriandrum sativum*): Mechanism of action. *Journal of Environmental Biology*, *29*, 53–56. PMID:18831331

Farooqi, A. A., Sreeramu, B. S., & Srinivasappa, K. N. (2005). Cultivation of spice crops. Hyderabad: Universities Press (India) Private Limited.

Mahendra, P., & Bisht, S. (2011). Coriandrum sativum: A daily use spice with great medicinal effect department of pharmacology. *Pharmacognosy Journal*, *3*(21), 84–88. doi:10.5530/pj.2011.21.16

Mandal, S., & Mandal, M. (2015). Coriander (Coriandrum sativum L.) essential oil. *Chemistry and Biological Activity*, *5*(6), 421–428.

Mhemdi, H., Rodier, E., Kechaou, N., & Fages, J. (2011). A supercritical tuneable process for the selective extraction of fats and essential oil from coriander seeds. *Journal of Food Engineering*, *105*(4), 609–616. doi:10.1016/j.jfoodeng.2011.03.030

Peter, K. V. (2004). Handbook of herbs and spices. Cambridge: Woodhead Publishing Ltd.

Ramadan, M. F.&Morsel, J. T. (2002). Oil composition of coriander (Coriandrum sativum L.) fruit seeds. *European Food Research and Technology, 215*, 204-209.

Rohit, R. P., Kavindra, R. J., & Chintan, K. M. (2011, April). Image morphological operation-based quality analysis of coriander seed (Coriandrum sativum L.). In *Emerging Trends in Networks and Computer Communications (ETNCC) International Conference on* (pp. 22-24). Academic Press.

Sharma, N., Sharma, P., Jasuja, N. D., & Joshi, C. (2013). Hypocholesterolemic and Antioxidant Potentials of Some plants and herbs: A review. *Journal of Zoological Sciences, RRJZS*, *1*(2), 26–42.

Singh, G., Maurya, S., De Lampasona, M. P., & Catalan, C. A. N. (2006). Studies on the essential oils part41: Chemical composition, antifungal, antioxidant, and sprout suppressant activities of coriander (Coriandrum sativum L.) essential oil and its oleoresin. *Flavour and Fragrance Journal*, *21*(3), 472–479. doi:10.1002/ffj.1608

Chapter 16
Nano Approach:
Indian Spices as Antimicrobial Agents

Arghya Chakravorty
https://orcid.org/0000-0002-7522-8304
Vellore Institute of Technology, India

Gulzar Ahmed Rather
Sathyabama Institute of Science and Technology, India

Aarif Ali
University of Kashmir, India

Basharat Ahmad Bhat
University of Kashmir, India

Siva Sankar Sana
North University of China, China

Nalluri Abhishek
Huazhong University of Science and Technology, China

Anima Nanda
Sathyabama Institute of Science and Technology, India

ABSTRACT

The mortality rate for infectious diseases in India, in 2017, was 416.75 per 100,000 persons, which is two times more than the United States of America due to multi-drug resistant pathogens and many more social and ethical challenges. Nano formulates are an alternative, eco-friendly solution. Nano medicine development from different food material is one of the fastest growing research fields. The nano formulated phytochemicals of spices can solve the delivery issues and even shows antimicrobial properties against multi-drug-resistant microorganisms as well as through Indian daily food. In this chapter, the recent research approaches in antimicrobial activity of nano formulation of different Indian spices and active phytochemicals of spices are comprehensively discussed. The most common methods for antimicrobial determination and the minimum inhibitory concentration of modified materials are also enlisted. The size of any nano material usually is 1 to 100 nanometers. Different nano formulates of different spices show antimicrobial activity against different pathogens.

DOI: 10.4018/978-1-7998-2524-1.ch016

INTRODUCTION

Many Asian countries use different types of spices in food as a test maker, preserver, coloring agent, and for specific flavor also, and India isn't exception among them. These spices have different medicinal properties like antimicrobial, anti-inflammatory, antioxidant, and anticancer properties. A researcher has made one combination of spices with nanotechnology where it is spreading in an interdisciplinary way in association with biology, chemistry, material science, physics, medicinal science, pharmacology and engineering fields. In this chapter, we will discuss nanoparticles, i.e., Nanoformulates of some Indian spices.

We will enlist only antimicrobial properties of Indian spices nanoformulations. In this chapter, we will focus on mainly metallic nanoparticles. Actually, these are inorganic nanomaterials, and it is of three types – semiconductor nanomaterial (TiO_2, ZnO); nobel metal nanomaterial (Ag, Au, Cu); magnetic nanomaterial (Ni, Co, Fe).

Figure 1.

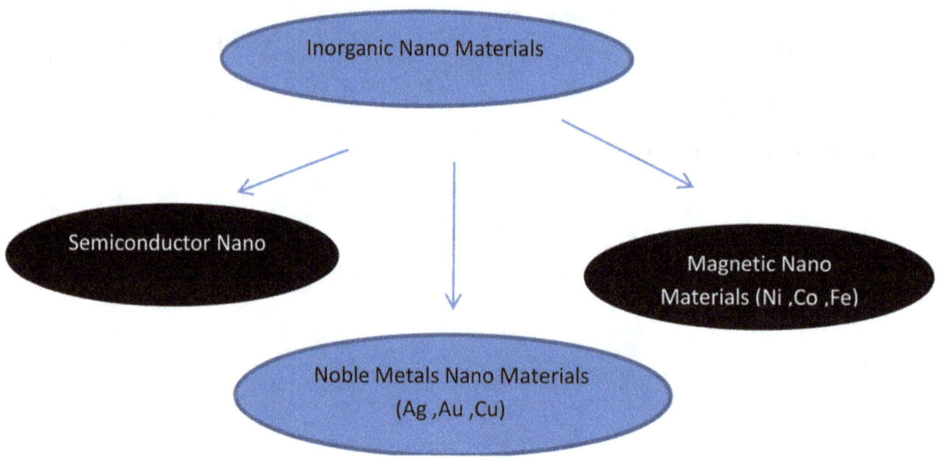

For the formation of nanoparticles, there are different types of methods used in the laboratory like physical, chemical, and biological methods. Physical and chemical methods are more expensive and deal with hazardous chemicals while the biological or green synthesis of nanoparticles is economical and eco-friendly. It is very important that is is more favorable for large scale production.

Methodology of Nanoformulates Production

Nanoparticles, due to their unique size and shape, possess various physiochemical properties like optical, thermal, magnetic, electronic, catalytic and physical that have gained much attention towards their synthesis as well as their use in different fields such as electronics, biotechnology, chemical, antimicrobial activities, DNA labelling, drug delivery, cosmetics, coatings and packaging (Rezvani et al., 2012, Kohler et al., 2001). Generally, these nanoparticles are effective and possess limited side effects. In nanotechnology, a fast growing area of research, is the biosynthesis of nanoparticles. Due to their captivating aspects over multiple fields, gold nanoparticles (AuNps) and silver nanoparticles (AgNps) are two of the most utilized metal nanoparticles. The synthesis of nanoparticles particularly gold, silver or any other material is usually done through several different methods which utilize living or non-living entities for generation of nanoparticles. There are various methods for synthesis of nanoparticles, such as co-precipitation, hydrothermal synthesis, inert gas condensation, microemulsion, ultrasound and biological synthesis. These methods have been utilized for a long time for synthesizing nanoparticles apart from the biological method which, due to its environment friendly nature, has gained much focus. The underlying basics of these methods are described below:

Figure 2.

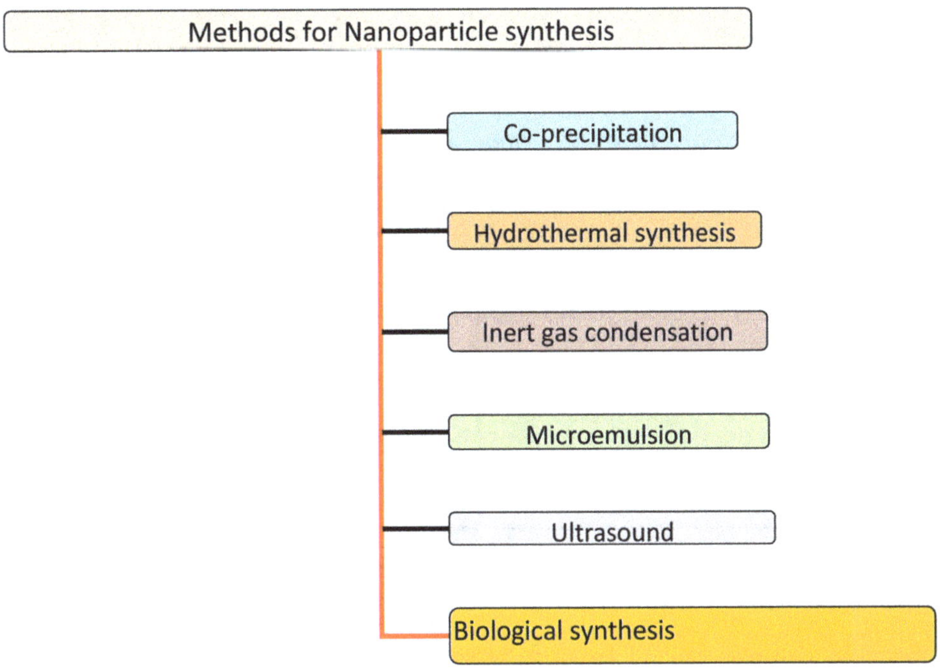

Co-precipitation

Co-precipitation reactions generally involve the processes of nucleation, growth, coarsening, and/or agglomeration, etc. Under conditions of high supersaturation, the products that are formed are usually insoluble species. The size, morphology, and properties of the products are drastically affected by secondary processes, such as Ostwald ripening and aggregation. Typical co-precipitation synthetic methods include the formation of oxides from aqueous and non-aqueous solutions, electrochemical reduction, and formation of metal chalconides by reactions of molecular precursors. The advantages and disadvantages of the co-precipitation method are shown below (Schatz et al., 2000).

Figure 3. Advantages of co-precipitation method

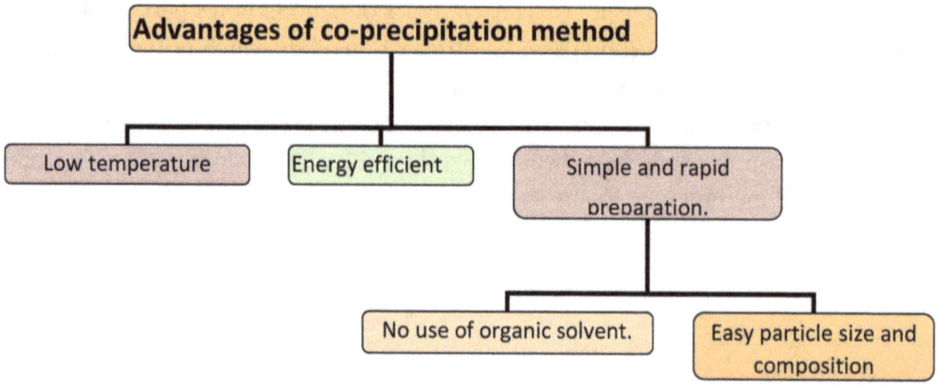

Figure 4. Disadvantages of co-precipitation method

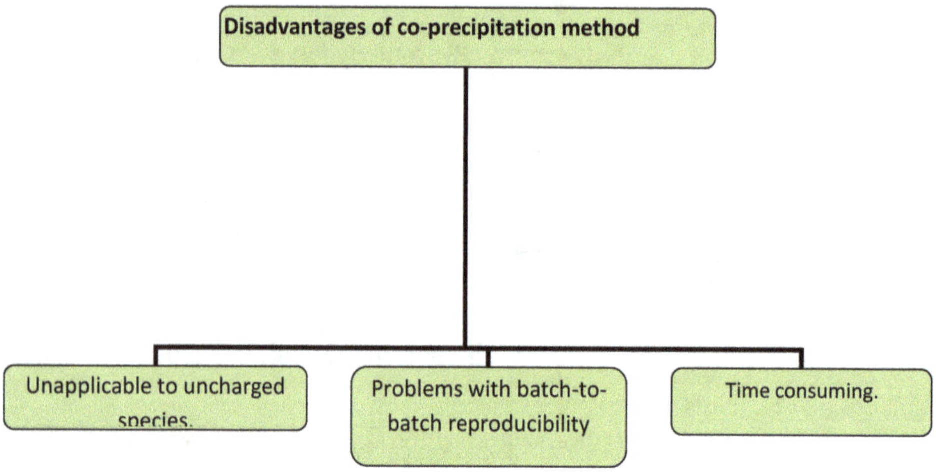

Hydrothermal Synthesis

One of the methods that has been most admired and gained attention from various disciplines is the hydrothermal technique. This technique, first of all, was described by British geologist Roderick Murchison (1792–1871) to describe the action of water at an elevated temperature and pressure that brings various changes in the crust of the earth that in turn leads to the formation of rocks and minerals. This technique has been successfully employed in the preparation of various important solids like superionic conductors, microporous crystals, chemical sensing oxides, electronically conducting solids, complex oxide ceramic magnetic materials, and luminescence phosphors. Generally, the hydrothermal technique involves chemical reactions to synthesize substances in a closed heated solution above the ambient temperature and pressure (Costa et al., 2012). Under high pressure, the solubility of minerals in hot water is important for the synthesis of single crystals, and the reaction is performed in an apparatus called an autoclave that is supplied with nutrients along with water.

Inert Gas Condensation

The most widely used technique that is used for the synthesis of metal nanoparticles is inert gas condensation (IGC). Inert gas condensation is performed in an ultrahigh vacuum chamber that is filled with inert gases like helium or argon in which metals are evaporated at very high pressure. Due to the process of evaporation, the atoms of the metals lose their kinetic energy by colliding with the gas molecules and as a result, get condensed into small particles. As a result of Brownian coagulation and Coalescence, these particles grow and develop to form nanocrystals (Hydrothermal Synthesis, n.d) the synthesis of nanocrystalline metals and alloys, gas condensation was the first method to be developed. The major advantage of IGC is the improved control of the particle size, and the disadvantage of IGC is that it is an extremely slow method and cannot be used for industrial production.

Microemulsion

An ideal method that has been used for the preparation of inorganic nanoparticles is the microemulsion method; however the mechanism for the formation of nanoparticles by this technique has not well been understood. In spite of this a mechanism for nanoparticle synthesis by microemulsion method has been suggested by some researchers. According to their view when the reactants are mixed along the microemulsion material, an exchange of reactants takes place during collision of droplets of water in the microemulsion. The exchange of reactants is too fast and in the nanodroplets there occurs a precipitation reaction. The primary particles undergo nucleation growth and coagulation to produce final nanoparticles that are surrounded by water and stabilized by which is followed by nucleation growth and coagulation surfactants. The advantages and disadvantages that are associated with microemulsion method are shown below:

Ultrasound

An important tool for the biosynthesis of nanoparticles is the ultrasound method. In this technique, ultrasonic cavitations are formed when liquids are acted upon by ultrasonic radiations. A range of physical and chemical effects is imparted by these cavitations, which provide a suitable environment for the chemical reactions to occur. In order to form nanoparticles with controllable morphologies, ultrasound method provides a unique model for generation (Synthesis of Nanoparticles… n.d.). Ultrasound is a simple, quick method and the rate of reaction is quite high to synthesize nanoparticles in a small duration of time. On the other hand, a major disadvantage associated with this method is that it is an energy-intensive process, and the yield per unit energy supplied is low.

The preparation of nanoparticles that was done through a range of physical and chemical methods was not ecofriendly and therefore, considered as environmentally benign wastages. Both of these methods were having serious drawbacks such as the presence of toxic organic solvents, generation of hazardous by-products and intermediary compounds, and high energy consumption (Jana et al., 2000). Since a wide range of conventional methods were used for synthesizing nanoparticles, however, green synthesis approaches are good competent enough over the physical and chemical techniques.

Figure 5. Advantages and disadvantages of microemulsion method

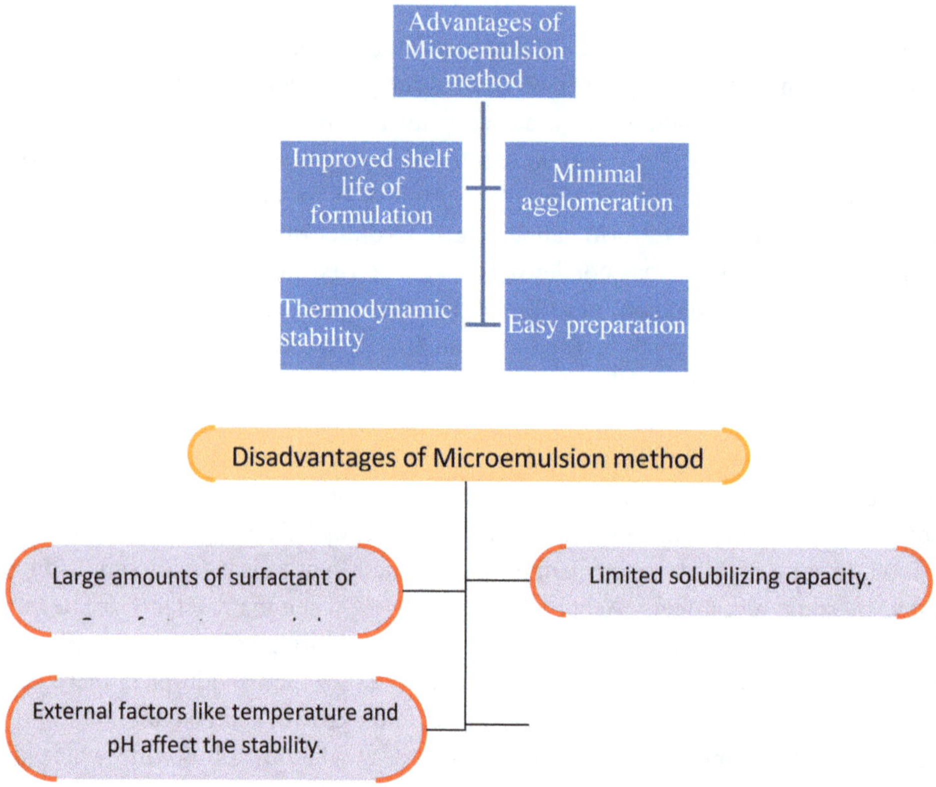

During the last few decades the use of the field of nanotechnology in research area for synthesis of nanoparticles has gained much focus because of their use in medicine and industry all round the globe and many environment friendly procedures have been developed and green chemistry has been leading field from all the way.

Biological Method

A green chemistry approach that interconnects nanotechnology and biotechnology is the biological method that synthesis nanoparticles. The rate of synthesis of nanoparticles by the biological method is slow, and the synthesized nanoparticles are not monodispersed despite being quite stable. Along with the time the synthesized macromolecules that are involved in the nucleation process their concentration varies, which in due course of time prolongs the period of nucleation. There occurs a subsequent decrease in the rate of synthesis due to polydispersity of nanoparticles. Various methods have been developed to overcome these barriers, which include microbial cultivation and the extraction techniques have been standardized, which along with combinatorial approach, such as photobiological methods, may be used. The rich diversity of plants and microbes can be utilized as potential biological materials for nanoparticle synthesis. The biological method or generally green chemistry can involve the use of living organisms or their components. The synthesis of nanoparticles through biological method has gained much attention as there is an urgent need to develop clean, non toxic, environment friendly procedures

Figure 6.

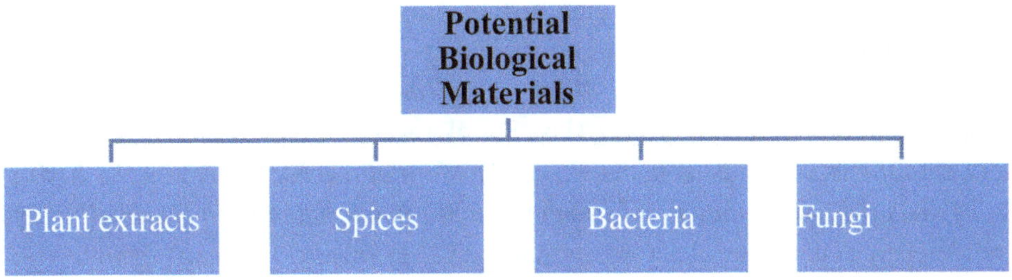

that would put an end to the use of these nontoxic hazardous substances and for that the field of green chemistry has been most successful in attaining the desired results (Bhattacharya et al., 2005; Lapkin et al., 2004). The nanopartcles that are synthesized by green chemistry approach are usually inert, biocompatible and readily bind to a large entity of biomolecules like enzymes, proteins, DNA, and amino acids etc., By immobilisation of ions of these biomolecules they expose a large surface area for binding. The limitations of the conventional methods are now covered by the green chemistry route which has now become an emerging and alternative route for synthesizing nanoparticles (Engelbrekt et al., 2009; Nadagouda et al., 2009). The main emphasis laid by green synthesis is the removal of hazardous toxic wastes, utilizing sustainable processes, implementing environmental friendly chemicals, solvents and renewable materials etc. (Salam et al., 2012; Sharma et al., 2009). The nanoparticles that are developed through biological methods are of acceptable size and morphology (Anastas et al., 1998; Matlack et al., 2001). The synthesis of nanoparticles through green chemistry has been reported by using various agents such as plant extracts, yeast, fungi, bacteria, algae, etc. Both unicellular and multicellular like yeast, fungi, and bacteria were used in synthesis methods, and they were capable of manufacturing inorganic materials either extracellular (Thomas et al., 2014) or intracellularly (Kumar et al., 2014). All of these compounds that are used for developing nanoparticles are described briefly as.

Plant Extracts

Plant extracts are the most widely used materials for synthesizing nanoparticles. A wide array of secondary metabolites with a significant proportion consisting of phenolic and flavonoid compounds are synthesized by plants (Mann et al., 1996). Various parts of the plant such as leaves, root, flower, fruits, seeds, peel and fruit pulp have been used as a basic material for nanoparticle production. By using plant or part of a plant rather than the organism is always beneficial as the organism can be pathogenic, laborious, costly, time consuming and maintaining the hygienic procedures of the cell cultures can be difficult. For efficient & quick extracellular synthesis of silver, copper, gold nanoparticles broth extracts of plants such as neem, aloe vera, tamarind, avena sativa, alfalfa, geranium, lemongrass etc., have been used successfully. Plant and spice extracts contain important phytochemical constituents such as essential oils (terpenes, eugenols etc.), polyphenols and carbohydrates. The presence of active functional groups such as hydroxyl, aldehyde, carboxyl etc. in these compounds plays a vital role in the process of reduction. The gold nanoparticles that are generated by using phytochemicals or any other extracts remain stable only for certain duration of time. The essential requirement of nanoparticles for being utilized in the biomedical application is to cross the barriers of cytotoxicity which is provided by stabilizers like plant and spices or capping with AuNps. The biomolecules that are present in plants and spices have an antimicrobial & antioxidant property which further provides excellent stability to the synthesized nanoparticles. Recently, by using several plant materials such as such as *Gliricidia sepium* (Kumar et al., 1995), *Mucuna pruriens* (Crozier et al., 2006), *Azadirachta indica* (Wei et al., 2009), *Desmodium triflorum* (Panacek et al., 2006), *Cassia fistula* (Das Shivika et al., 2013), *Cinnamomum zeylanicum* (Dias et al., 2002), *Opuntiaficus-indica* (Shankar et al., 2003), *Magnolia kobus* (Verma et al., 2010), *Coriander* (Gade et al., 2010), *Coriandrum Sativum* (Song et al., 2009), *Clerodendrum inerme* (Narayanan et al., 2008), etc. noble class of nanoparticles were synthesized. Various studies apart from the plant extracts have started using medicinal plants (Sathyavathi et al., 2010), fruits (Castellano et al., 2007; Thirum-urugan et al., 2010; Ankamwar et al., 2005), weeds (Jain et al., 2009) and spices (Ghodake et al., 2010) for the generation of new nanoparticles.

SPICES

Spices are the main ingredients that are used in all types of foods that are consumed around the world. Most of the spices possess significant antimicrobial properties due to their phytoconstituents which impart their use in traditional as well modern modes of treatment. Some of the spices that are widely used on daily basis are enlisted below:

Clove Buds

Clove buds are reported as the new face in the field of green synthesis for the production of silver nanoparticles a study reported by Singh *et al.,* (Parashar et al., 2009). As clove buds contain essential aromatic flavor compounds and 14-21% of volatile oil which accounts for 10-13% of tannin, 81- 95% of phenols (eugenol with about 3% of acetyleugenol), sesquiterpenes (α- and β-calyophyllenes) and small quantities of esters, ketones, alcohols and these compounds simultaneously reduced silver ions to silver nanoparticle (Parashar et al., 2009). Apart from this, the clover buds also contain triterpene acids, esters, and several glycosides. A potent anti-carcinogenic activity has been reported to be shown by sesqui-terpenes of cloves (Singh et al., 2010). Clove buds have been reported to have possessed anti-oxidant, anti-fungal, anti-viral, antimicrobial, anti-inflammatory, anesthetic, anti-diabetic, anti-thrombotic, pain reliving and insect repellent, anti-platelet, antistress, anti-pyretic (Singh et al., 2010).

Cardamom or Elaichi (Elettaria cardamomum)

Cardamom is a perennial herb which belongs to the family, Zingiberaceae has been considered as the 'Queen of Spices'. Cardamom is considered as the most important, easily available spices and its seeds are a great source of its aroma and flavor. A wide range of chemical compounds such as -terpineol, myrcene, subinene, limonene, cineol, α & β-pinene α-phellandrene, menthone, cis/trans-linalol oxides, trans-nerolidol, β-sitostenone, β-sitosterol, phytol, eugenyl acetate, bisabolene, borneol, citronellol, p-cymene, geraniol, geranyl acetate, stigmasterol and terpenes are present in cardamom. It has been found that cardamom by acting through cholinergic and calcium antagonist mechanisms reduced blood pressure in rats (Lyer et al., 2009; Parle et al., 2011; Shaban et al., 1987; Noleau et al., 1987). Cardamom can also serve as a good source for green chemistry for nanoparticle production.

Black Pepper or Golamaricha (Piper Nigrum)

Black pepper another spice that belongs to the family Piperaceae and has the ability to be used as source for synthesis of nanoparticle production. The major content that is present in black pepper is piperine. Besides this black pepper also contains little amounts of safrole which is known to have antioxidant properties and anticarcinogenic effects (Gopalkrishnan et al., 1990).

Cinnamon or Dal Chini (Cinnamomum Verum)

Cinnamon is another spice which can also be used in green chemistry concept for the synthesis of nanoparticles. The major phytochemical compounds present in cinnamon are doubly-linked procyanidin type-A polymers, cinnamaldehyde and esters. Cinnamon has many pharmacological properties, including antioxidant activity and antimicrobial effects (Duke et al., 1992; Lyer et al., 2009).

Crocus sativus or Saffron

Crocus sativus belongs to the Iridaceae family and is considered globally as one of the most valuable medicinal plants having red-orange tripartite stigmas (Lopez et al., 2004; Shan et al., 2004). Saffron is the native to Iran, and the major suppliers of it are the farmers from Khorasan province (Lage et al., 2009). Several attempts have been made to synthesize AuNps from *Crocus sativus* in a simple ecofriendly way. Leaf extracts of *Crocus sativus* have been used to synthesize gold nanoparticles by the green route method. Saffron has many medicinal uses and contains aroma- yielding compounds, non-volatile active compounds (carotenoids, including zeaxanthin, lycopene, a- and b-carotenes) and more than 150 volatile substances (Board et al., 2004). An important carotenoid constituent of saffron is Crocetin who has shown enormous potential as an anti-tumor agent in animal models and cell culture systems (Maggi et al., 2011). The stigma and petals of saffron are important to fight depression (Moghaddasi et al., 2010). Saffron, contains crocins and crocetin, which inhibit breast cancer cell proliferation (Gutheil et al., 2011). Due to a vast array of biological protective functions possessed by saffron, it could be an important member of the green chemistry concept. Further, the potentiality of *Crocus sativus* (saffron) in reducing and stabilizing gold nanoparticles has also emphasized its importance in the synthesis of gold nanoparticles. Thus extracts of plants and spices can serve a great and ideal source for nanoparticle synthesis because of their eco-friendly and nontoxic nature as they pose minimal threats to the environment.

Bacteria

Bacteria are also used for the production of nanoparticles in an eco-friendly manner. At present, there have been various studies in which bacteria to synthesize metal nanoparticles. For instance, *Eleutherococcuss enticosus* (Michael Bailes et al., 1997) and *Bacillus methylotrophicus* (Chryssanthi et al., 2011) have been used to synthesize AuNps and AgNps. Other microorganisms such as *Fusarium oxysporum* (Abbai et al., 2016), *Fusarium semitactum* (Wang et al., 2015; Ahmad et al., 2008), *Rhodopseudomonas* sp. (Basavaraja et al., 2008), *Megatherium* sp. (He et al., 2009), have been used for the synthesis of nanoparticles. These organisms have the ability to recover toxic metals via reduction of the metal ions.

Figure 7. Different techniques used for nanoparticle analysis

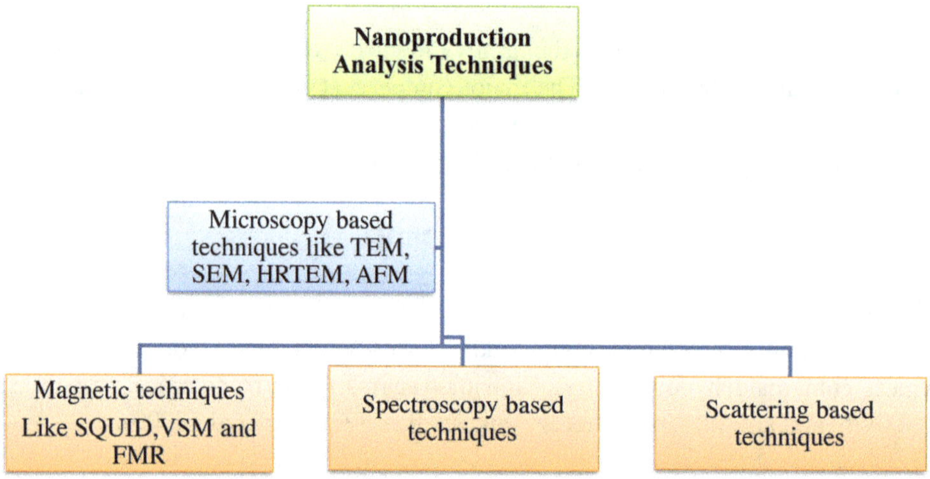

Fungi

Fungi have also been used for the synthesis of nanoparticles because most of the fungi are easy to handle, need simple nutrients, high wall binding capacity as well as capable of intracellular metal uptake etc. especially the filamentous fungi (Dias et al., 2002). Due to these unique properties that fungi possess, they show few advantages over bacteria. Till now, enough work has not been done regarding nanoparticle synthesis, particularly silver nanoparticles by the endophytic fungi, which primarily synthesize these nanoparticles. A wide range of nanoparticle options are well available, but none of them has received so much attention with regard to the silver nanoparticles because of their wide availability in medical areas (Castellano et al., 2007). The use of silver as an antimicrobial agent has been done from years; however, it has only received much attention as a therapeutic agent so as to minimize the burden of drug resistance which has resulted due to the misuse of antibiotics (Wei et al., 2009; Panacek et al., 2006; Das Shivika et al., 2013). From Geranium leaves, *Colletotrichum* sp. has been isolated, which has been utilized for the synthesis of gold nanoparticles extra-cellularly (Shankar et al., 2018). Other studies have isolated an endophytic fungus (*Aspergillus clavatus* (AzS-275) from sterilized stem tissues of *Azadirachta indica* and due to its antibacterial properties, have used it for the synthesis of silver nanoparticles (Shankar et al., 2003). In this regard, additional studies need to be carried out for using fungi as a source of nanoparticle synthesis.

CHARACTERIZATION OF NANO PRODUCTION ANALYSIS

Nanoparticle structures gained huge interest in the research field as they possess many applications the molecular level. Such properties include high surface to volume ratio, optical and other chemical properties. Now days, a range of several analytical techniques have been developed for nanoparticle analysis which include (UV, TEM, SEM, EDS, FTIR, XRD, DLS and AFM). These techniques are used to analyze the elemental composition, size, shape, morphology, crystal structure and various physical and chemical properties of nanoparticles. Until now, there was no single technique that fulfills all the requirements to analyze the nanoparticle properties completely.

Transmission Electron Microscopy (TEM)

TEM is the furthermost technique to characterize nanoparticle morphology and homogeneity. This technique provides the true nanoparticle size and captures accurate images of the sample. The procedure of TEM is that a uniform electron beam touches the specimen and diffuses through it. An image is formed upon the interaction of electrons with the specimen. This is further magnified and focused by using an imaging device. The interaction between electronic beam and sample depends upon the size, morphology, sample density and elemental composition.

TEM provides significantly higher resolution of images and is capable of visualizing very small atoms compared to any other imaging technique. TEM has been used to analyze information about the size, shape, structure, morphology and dispersion or aggregation state which is informative for nanoparticle in vitro uptake and internalization within the cell organelles. For example, Non- implanted AuNps s gathered in combinations in the vesicles while as AuNps implanted with PEG were well distributed within the intracellular vesicles in very low proportions (Verma et al., 2010). TEM not only provides information about nanoparticle size and morphology but also gives data about the interparticle distance between two metal Nps when they brought together. Due to close proximity, their plasmons couple, redshifting their plasmon band and consequently changing their color. Therefore, to analyze nanoparticle dispersion, TEM has been used for various biomedical applications such as sensing and diagnostics, therapeutic carriers, and imaging (Perrault et al., 2010). The size of the nanoparticles is calculated and expressed manually using a marking device which travels laterally along the nanoparticle. The particle length is taken as a sphere having a comparable projected area as the predictable copy of the nanoparticle. Therefore, by dividing the total length of the nanoparticles by the total number of nanoparticles counted to obtain a mean linear dimensional measure of the nanoparticles (Akbari et al., 2011). TEM, in combination with other spectroscopic techniques such as UV and DLS, it is possible to analyze the composition of the internalized nanoparticles and trace the dynamics of the individual (Laborda et al., 2016). Due to high lateral resolution, the characterization and the formation of different super-lattice nanocomposites, which can be isostructural to several atomic crystal systems, can be analyzed by TEM (Shevchenko et al., 2006). The final structure and composition of different Nps (.g. quantum dots, metals, and magnetic Nps) of these new arrangements, which are three dimensional in nature, can be measured by adapting the colloid surface charge. (Shevchenko et al., 2006) or directional bonding with DNA (Jones et al., 2010). Furthermore, the study of biodegradation of the nanoparticle polymeric coating by bacteria, which causes colloidal aggregation and affects their mobility and cytotoxicity can be studied by TEM and DLS. (Kirschling et al., 2011). Finally, TEM has also been used to assess the degree of penetration of Nps, location of Nps within a cell and also helped to understand the cell death pathways in melanoma cells (Yue et al., 2017).

Scanning Electron Microscopy (SEM)

SEM is the most widely used technique to analyze nanoscale materials. In SEM technique, the electrons are used for imaging which interacts and scans the surface of specimen to produce various signals that gives information about the nature of interaction, samples structure and composition. SEM is able to achieve resolution less than 1nm which is better than NanoSIMS which is around 50nm (Stokes et al., 2008). Furthermore, SEM has been used to copy both intact samples as well as partitioned samples (Montes et al., 2017).

X-Ray Diffraction (XRD)

X-ray diffraction is the most extensively useful and non-destructive technique to characterize Nps. This technique provides information about the crystalline structure, crystalline phase, texture, as well as the strain of nanoparticles. X-ray diffraction technique is performed usually after drying of the sample of the powdered form. The particle composition can be determined by comparing the intensity and position of the peaks obtained by using a monochromatic beam of x-rays, which diffracted at specific angles to produce different peaks. These peaks are used in detecting the periodic arrangements of minor components in the sample. This technique is not applicable to amorphous materials as it can only analyze crystalline materials.

Dynamic Light Scattering (DLS)

Dynamic light scattering (DLS) is the most widely used technique to analyze the size of Nps size and dispersion state in colloidal solutions. Nps in aqueous suspensions is in a continuous Brownian motion causes interfering both constructive as well as destructive. DLS measures light scattering intensity, which results in time-dependent oscillations to determine the hydrodynamic diameter of the solvent molecule and the Nps, which diffuse at the same rate as the colloid in the solution. The average size of the particle can be calculated from these time-dependent oscillations in scattering intensity by the use of the autocorrelation function and subsequent calculation of the exponential decay (Brar et al., 2011). In order to avoid multiple scattering effects, a low concentration of Np concentration is needed. In DLS, a relatively low Np concentration is needed so that multiple scattering effects is avoided. DLS technique is able to analyze samples having a wide scattering of species; and can also detect very small amounts of the higher mass species (Kato et al., 2012).

Energy-dispersive X-ray Spectroscopy (EDS)

The elemental composition and chemical characterization of a sample can be determined by using analytical Energy-dispersive X-ray spectroscopy (EDS) technique. In this technique, a high electronic beam is applied into the sample of interest. An electron beam focuses, and an electron excites in to the inner shell and to eject from the shell, therefore, creating an electron-hole. The energy difference between the inner shell and the outer shell release in the form of X-rays and the electron in the outer shell having higher energy fills the hole. (Goldstein et al., 2017).The electromagnetic emission spectrum of each element is unique by its distinctive number of peaks as determined by atomic structure, thus measuring the energy and the number of peaks released, we can obtain information about the elemental composition of the sample by using an EDS instrument (Goldstein et al., 2017). Therefore, EDS microanalysis facilitated in the combination of giving information about the structure and composition of such core-shell Nps (Li et al., 2004).

Fourier Transforms Infrared Spectroscopy (FTIR)

Fourier transform infrared spectroscopy (FTIR) is an analytical technique that is used to study the surface composition, molecular structure, nature of the bonds, specific functional groups, interaction and ligand binding of Nps. The technique is based on the measurement of the electromagnetic absorption spectrum with wavelengths ranging from (4000–400 cm^{-1}) (Blanco-Andujar et al., 2014).

In an experimental approach on a combination of ATR-FTIR and differential electrochemical mass spectroscopy (DEMS). These techniques used to study the volatile reaction products and also aided to review adsorbents electrochemically (Buso-Rogero et al., 2016). In another work, the combined ATR-FTIR techniques also used to determine the effect of Ag Nps content on the photocatalytic degradation of oxalic acid adsorbed on TiO_2 Nps. The process of reduction of nickel stearate synthesized Ni Nps having size 13–25 nm with hexagonal crystal structure in the presence of PEG, oleic acid and oleylamine (Tzitzios et al., 2006). The distinctive groups such as the –HC=CH– arranged in oleic acid and oleylamine present at the surface of the Nps and also the binding of the ligands on to the NP surface are also revealed by FTIR spectra (Tzitzios et al., 2006). Furthermore, there are various experimental studies on Np synthesis like NaYF4:Yb/Er upconversion nanoparticles (Duong et al., 2018) and Trioctylphosphine stabilized CdS nanorods synthesis (Chen et al., 2009). Finally, FTIR spectroscopy can be employed to assess the affinity of polymers bearing phosphate groups as surface ligands (Rithesh Raj et al., 2017).

UV-Vis Spectroscopy (UV-Vis)

UV-Vis spectroscopy (UV-Vis) is another quite simple technique and low-cost analytical technique to study the nanoparticle materials. In this technique, the intensity of light is measured which is reflected from a sample and compare with the intensity of light reflected from reference material. UV-Vis spectroscopy is a vital device to detect, analyze and investigate nanomaterial optical properties that are sensitive to size, shape, concentration, dispersion state, and refractive index near the Np surface (Rithesh Raj et al., 2017). Some nanostructures like gold and copper nanoparticles display typical UV-Vis extinction spectra due to the presence of a LPSR signal in the visible part of the spectrum. In these nanostructures, the LPSR bands are observed at the near infrared (NIR) wavelength region (Hendel et al., 2014). Due to UV-Vis, we can also measure the molar concentration and size of zerovalent Au nanoparticles (Hendel et al., 2014). The calculation of the concentration of citrate-coated silver Nps has also been successfully studied by using maximum absorbance at the UV-Vis spectroscopy (Paramelle et al., 2014). In another research study, published which is based on the use of UV-Vis spectra to determine the size and concentration of AuNps (Haiss et al., 2007). In another study, to determine the concentration of thiamine by mixing a solution of thiamine in water with AuNps solution is another use of UV-Vis spectroscopy. There is a color change in the solution from red to greenish-gray, detects the presence of thiamine. The maximum range of detection of thiamine was between 0.5 and 1 μM. Whereas the AuNps tested for this application were in the range of 20–30 nm (Zielinski et al., 2014). In another report, Au and Pt Nps prepared in an aqueous medium containing dodecyltrimethyl ammonium chloride (DTAC) and PEG by photoreduction synthesis by UV-Vis, EXAFS and other techniques (TEM, SAXS) (Harada et al., 2009). This method was also employed to determine the particle size and size distribution. Overall, this method can be considered low-cost, non-destructive and quick for the recognition of Np systems and types. Ag nanostructures have also been extensively studied by UV-Vis spectroscopy.

Atomic Force Microscopy (AFM)

Atomic force microscopy (AFM) is a microscopy technique that can generate three-dimensional images of surfaces at high intensification. It was initially developed by Gerard Binning and Heinrich Rohrer at IBM in 1986 (Binnig et al., 1986). The interacting forces between a fine probe and the sample are the basic principle of AFM technique. The probe, which is a sharp tip, is coupled to the end of a cantilever made of silicon or silicon nitride. The cantilever gets deflected when the AFM scans the sample, and as a result of the attractive or repulsive forces between the tip and the sample surface. The twisting that reflects on the cantilever backside is measured by a laser beam. The information obtained from the laser variation and the results are finally calculated by combining forces and the known cantilever stiffness. Depending on the degree of proximity between the probe and the sample, AFM can image in three different ways i.e. contact, non-contact, and tapping approach (also known as an intermediate or oscillating mode) (Vilalta-Clemente et al., 2008). The latter is the utmost common when characterizing Nps. The topological characterization of small Nps (£6 nm), such as ion-doped Y_2O_3, has been achieved by AFM without any special treatment because AFM does not involve any surface alteration or covering prior to imaging (Patel et al., 2007). Some low density materials, which show very poor results under electron microscopy, can also be characterized by AFM.

For example, to understand the formation mechanism of uniform patchy and hollow rectangular nanoplatelets made of polymer mixtures can be studied using AFM (Qiu et al., 2016). AFM provided comparable results when analyzing Np sizes in comparison between AFM and electron microscopies, i.e. SEM and TEM (Pitto-Barry et al., 2015; Hubenthal et al., 2012; Oćwieja et al., 2013). AFM allows the characterization of the nanoparticle height and copies the sample in three dimensions. Furthermore, costing much less and occupies small laboratory space and exhibits similar resolution results like SEM and TEM. Nevertheless, AFM also shows slower scanning times than any electron microscope. However, only AFM could properly analyze Nps with bimodal distribution sizes (Hoo et al., 2008). Lastly, AFM and Kelvin probe force microscopy combination can generate three-dimensional maps of nanoparticle surface potential distributions; these results were obtained by measuring the corrosion behavior of individual iron and stainless steel Nps under a sulfuric acid environment (Raj et al., 2014).

ANTIMICROBIAL PROPERTY ANALYSIS OF NANO THERAPEUTICS

It has been followed since ancient ages about finding curing properties in plants. Researchers around the globe have performed extensive research and have applied the plant properties those infused, imbibed, and in poultices of hundreds and thousands of plant species. The process of identifying the medicinal properties in plants has been believed since the prehistory and even in the present generation, many plants are used in ethnomedicine. When these antimicrobial properties are combined with nanoparticles, the healing process is proving remarkably groundbreaking. In this chapter, we discuss a few such antimicrobial properties possessed and identified in plants along with an infusion of nanoparticles by several researchers around the world (Moriz& Geszke-Mortiz, 2013). The use of nanoparticles has widespread, including food preservations. The inclusion of natural antibacterial polypeptide agent as nanoparticles is preserved in the biological activities has emphasized in antibacterial activities. The chapter mainly focuses on the antimicrobial properties of different plants and plant products as green synthesis methods

Figure 8. Versatility of antibacterial nanoparticle applications,
Source (Moriz & Geszke-Moritz, 2013)

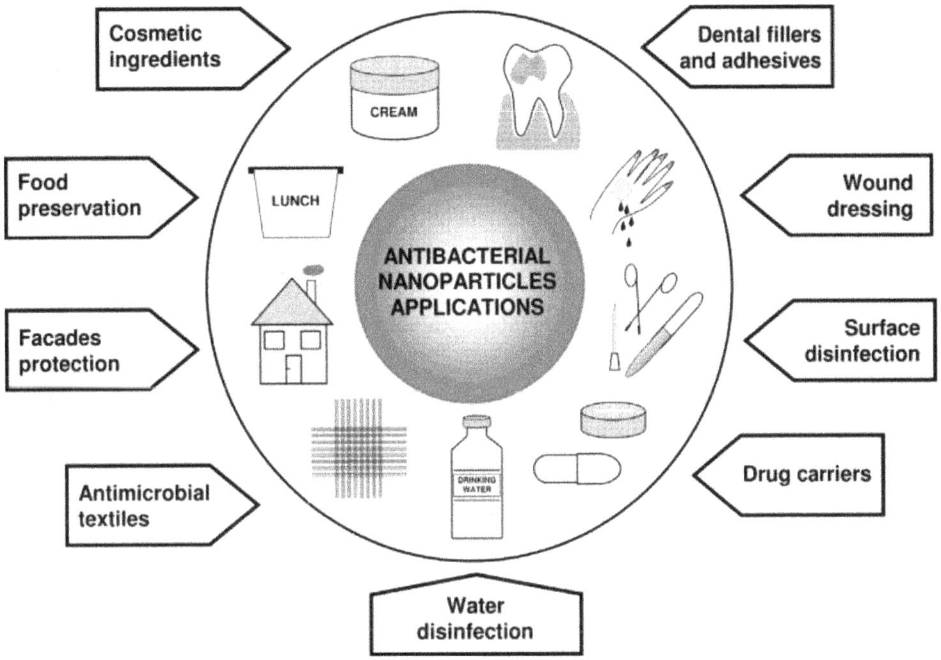

in combination with metals and chemicals. The diagrams blow explains the process and stages of the antimicrobial application with nanoparticles.

(Alsammarraie et al., 2018). As one of the many applications in food and agriculture industry that is the adaptation of AgNps green synthesis that can be utilized to inhibit the antimicrobials for pathogenic bacterial growth. The researchers used nanoparticles of Silver (AgNps) as an antioxidant and an antimicrobial in combination with Turmeric. The study proved that AgNps when combined with turmeric, the colors changed to dark brown from Yellow, showing strong antibacterial properties by shrinking the cell membranes. (Bhawana et al., 2011). The wet-milling process allows breaking the Curcumin to particle level that is the nanoparticle used to test the aqueous solubility for examining the antimicrobial properties. A gram-positive and negative test has been conducted to classify the antibacterial activities. The observations explain the pronounced antibacterial activities of gram-positive against gram-negative. The aqueous solubility of nanocurcumin showed a better in vitro efficacy for antimicrobial properties when compared to a normal curcumin solution (Robert et al., 2015). A step up from silver nanoparticles in combination with curcumin, the researchers introduce gold nanoparticles rods used as a drug delivery system in a local environment. The combination of lipophilic gold nanorods (GNRs) with polymeric nanomicelles of curcumin is proved as a novel approach to in treating at the cell level and cell membrane level (Krausz, et al., 2014). The bacterial properties are different in nature, and so are the healing properties. The curcumin nanoparticles improve the healing in an in vivo murine wound model (da Silva et al., 2018). The encapsulation of curcumin is an important and expensive process that determines the quality of the particles affecting the inhibitory values and the concentration of the particles may vary (Jayandran et al., 2015). The use of curcumin extract as a nanoparticle plays a stabilization role for Manganese nanoparticles and were tested for Gram-positive & negative along with fungus showed promising inhibition resulting in a better solution for therapeutic applications (Lertsutthiwong et al., 2011). The nanoparticles of turmeric are also preceded into oils, and the encapsulation of the oil for skin permeation has promising results, but the process of encapsulating the oil is a challenge that is overcome by adapting the chitosan addition in the encapsulation process (Govind et al., 2018). The use of *Curcuma longa* has proven its positive effects on bone recovery. The combination of eggshells, *Curcuma longa* tuber, and Na_2HPO_4 has remarkable results for treating bone infections.

By far, the discussion in the chapter was carried on turmeric particles, nanoparticles its infusion into the water, and also about the oil and roots. The entire plat of turmeric is antimicrobial in nature including the leaves. (Singh et al., 2013). The leave of *curcuma longa* is rich in secondary metabolites possessing the ability to reduce the metals. The endophytic fungus, which is produced by AgNps displays high antibacterial actives, on the whole, the Curcuma longa the turmeric as a whole also is affective anti-inflammatory when injected directly (Chainani et al., 2003) (Waidha et al., 2015). The FTIR analysis with Silver rods displays the binding of various types obtained from the green synthesis methods.

Turmeric is well known as the kitchen remedies; there is another antimicrobial that also can be found in the kitchen is *Syzygium aromaticum* i.e. clove in the generic language (Rajesh et al., 2017). The Syzygium *aromaticum* bud, when bio reduced in copper aqueous methods, shows stabilization of CuNps with Cu+ ions extraction. This application proves to be an excellent antibacterial for *Bacillus* sp. (Kaur et al., 2012). The inhibitory AgNps effects in the combination of Clove with silver nanoparticles reduced the cell growth or death of the bacterial affected cells. The next natural bioagent discussed in the cardamom also available in the kitchen (Soshnikova et al., 2018). The aqueous extraction of *Fructus Amomi* rapidly synthesizes the FA-AuNps and FA-AgNps using expensive green methods against breast cancer cells (Dhimin et al., 2014). The cardamom seeds synthesis with silver nanoparticles posse high inhibition, which results in strongly effective antibacterial in nature (Ghanajobitha et al., 2012). Silver nanoparticles with aqueously reduced seeds of Cardamom solution against *Klebsiella Planticola* and *Bacillus Subtilis* result in high efficacy antimicrobial agents.

After cardamom, the next natural agent discussed is the Cinnamon plays a natural antimicrobial pathogen (Hill et al., 2013). The nano capsulation protects the extracted spice and reduces the sensory impact by improving the efficacy (Chaudhry et al., 2006). *Cinnamomum Cassia* not only is an antimicrobial agent. This also acts as a preventive natural remedy for bacterial flora diseases (Chanda et al.). The combination of *Cinnamon Cassia* with gold nanoparticle rods displays biocompatibility in detecting the affected cells with photoacoustic signals. The combination attenuated reasonable efficiency (Huang et al., 2010). In further investigation towards identifying the antimicrobial agents, the research about essential oils has gained focus. The Fruit essential oil and the combination with trans-Anethole show strong antifungal properties for plants (Yang et al., 2010). Chemical compositions of *Illicium Verum* consist of strong antibacterial pathogens leading a pathway towards the development of antibiotic medications (Meva, et al., 2015). *Ricinodendron Heudelotti* (Bail), when combined with silver nanoparticles, result as a strongest anti-infectious microbial agent.

The green synthesis of *Pimpinella anisum* seed with nanoparticles of silver is one of the cheapest bio reductions and ecofriendly agents, proving it as the most stable antimicrobial agents (Al salhi et al., 2016). The other green synthesis discussed is ginger, as it is already proven as an anti-inflammatory nature (Zhuang et al., 2015). The GDN is not only a culinary application but is more application in medicinal applications with not much side effects on liver cells (Mathew et al., 2017). The antibacterial activities rapid the effects with sunlight effect on silver nanoparticles and *Zingiber officinale* rhizome resulting in minimal bacterial presence. (Janaki et al., 2015). Dry ginger synthesis with ZnO nanoparticles provides

Table 1. Antimicrobial property analysis of different types Nano particles of Curcuma longa (Turmeric) tuber

Sl No.	Description of Nanoparticles & Size (nm)	Zone of Inhibition (mm); MIC (µg/ml); MBC (µg/ml) against bacteria & fungus or Viable Cell count Analysis	Reference
1	AgNps synthesized by green technology; (5 – 35nm)	a) *E. coli* 0157:H7 (3log CFU/ml decreased after 4hrs incubation of AgNps at 6 & 12 µg/ml concentration) & (4log CFU/ml decreased after 4hrs incubation of AgNps at 18 µg/ml concentration) b) *Listeria monocytogenes* (3log CFU/ml decreased after 4 hrs incubation with AgNps at 6 & 12 µg/ml concentration)	**(Fouad et al., 2018)**
2	Nano curcumin formation by wet-milling technology (2 – 40nm)	a) *B. sutilis* MTCC 430(MIC 75; ZOI 20mm at 400µg/ml concentration of therapeutic.) b) *S. aureus* MTCC 99 (MIC 100; ZOI 10mm at 400µg/ml concentration of therapeutic.) c) *E. coli* MTCC 443 (MIC 250; ZOI 12mm at 400µg/ml concentration of therapeutic.) d) *P. aeruginosa* MTCC 741 (MIC 200; ZOI 14mm at 400µg/ml concentration of therapeutic) e) *A. niger* (MIC 350) f) *P. notatum* (no activity)	**(Bhawana et al., 2011**
3	Curcumin nanoparticles synthesized by sol-gel based method & in vivo application in murine model for wound healing	a) Methicilin resistance *S. aureus* (97% reduction of growth of burn wound on murine model in 24hrs) b) *P. aeruginosa* (59.2% reduction of growth of burn wound on murine model in 24hrs)	**(Aimee et al., 2014)**
4	Nano curcumin processed by wet milling technique	a) *S. aureus* MTCC 96 (MIC 100) b) *E. coli* MTCC 443 (MIC 250) c) *P. aeruginosa* MTCC 741 (MIC 250) d) *F. niger* (MIC 350)	**(Anderson et al., 2018)**
5	Nano curcumin processed by spray drying technique with Gelatin & Porous starch encapsulant	a) *B. cereus* (MIC 125) b) *B. sutilis* (MIC 125 µg/ml) c) *S. aureus* (MIC 62.5 µg/ml) d) *E. coli* (MIC 250 µg/ml) e) *Y. enterocolitica* (MIC 250 µg/ml) f) *L. monocytogenes* NR 30 (MIC 72.5 µg/ml) g) *L. monocytogenes* Scott A (MIC 173.2 ± 28.2 µg/ml)	**(Anderson et al., 2018)**
6	Nano curcumin processed by non-solvent method	a) *E. coli* ATCC 25922 (MIC 500µM with tanic acid encapsulant) b) *E. coli* ATCC 25922 (MIC 400µM with polyquaterium encapsulant) c) *E. coli* ATCC 25922 (MIC 400µM with polyvinylpyrolidon encapsulant)	**(Anderson et al., 2018)**
7	Nano curcumin processed by microeimulsification method	a) *S. epidermidis* ATCC 1228 (MIC O.86 µg/ml with myristic acid encapsulant)	**(Anderson et al., 2018)**
8	MnNps synthesized by green technology (50nm)	a) *B. subtilis* (ZOI 11mm) b) *E. coli* (ZOI 19mm) c) *S. aureus* (ZOI 18mm) d) *S. bacillus* (ZOI 17mm) e) *C. albicans* (ZOI 19mm) f) *C. lutana* (ZOI 19mm) g) *A. niger* (ZOI 18mm) h) *T. smii* (ZOI 20mm)	**(Jayandran et al., 2015)**
9	Hydroxyapatide nanorods of turmeric formed by egg shell – useful as cl source in bone infection (10 – 25nm)	a) *E. coli* (ZOI 24 ± 2mm) b) *S. aureus* (ZOI 28 ± 2mm)	**(Govindan et al., 2018)**
10	AgNps synthesized by endophytic *Penicilliumspp.* isolated from turmeric tuber (25nm)	a) *E. coli* (ZOI 13mm) b) *P. aeruginosa* (ZOI 21mm) c) *K. pneumonia* (ZOI 15mm) *d) S. typhimurium* (ZOI 14mm) *e) Enterobacter arogenes* (ZOI 14mm)	**(Dattu et al., 2013)**

Table 2. Antimicrobial property analysis of different types Nano particles of Syzygium aromaticum (Clove) budrhizome

Sl No.	Description of Nanoparticles & Size (nm)	Zone of Inhibition (mm); MIC (μg/ml); MBC (μg/ml) against bacteria & fungus	Reference
1	CuNps synthesized by Green Technology; (15nm)	a) *S. aureus* ZOI 3mm 4μl volume of therapeutic ZOI 4mm 8 μl volume of therapeutic ZOI 5mm 12μl volume of therapeutic ZOI 5mm 16μl volume of therapeutic b) *E. cloi* ZOI 4mm 4μl volume of therapeutic ZOI 5mm 8 μl volume of therapeutic ZOI 5mm 12μl volume of therapeutic ZOI 6mm 16μl volume of therapeutic c) *Pseudomonas spp.* ZOI 5mm 4μl volume of therapeutic ZOI 6mm 8 μl volume of therapeutic ZOI 6mm 12μl volume of therapeutic ZOI 7mm 16μl volume of therapeutic d) *Bacillus spp.* ZOI 6mm 4μl volume of therapeutic ZOI 7mm 8 μl volume of therapeutic ZOI 8mm 12μl volume of therapeutic ZOI 8mm 16μl volume of therapeutic e) *A. flavus* ZOI 3mm 4μl volume of therapeutic ZOI 3mm 8 μl volume of therapeutic ZOI 4mm 12μl volume of therapeutic ZOI 5mm 16μl volume of therapeutic f) *A. niger* ZOI 4mm 4μl volume of therapeutic ZOI 4mm 8 μl volume of therapeutic ZOI 5mm 12μl volume of therapeutic ZOI 5mm 16μl volume of therapeutic g) *Penicillium spp.* ZOI 4mm 4μl volume of therapeutic ZOI 5mm 8 μl volume of therapeutic ZOI 6mm 12μl volume of therapeutic ZOI 6mm 16μl volume of therapeutic	[15]
2	AgNps synthesized by Green Technology (4 – 65nm)	a) *Bacillus cereus* (Significant inhibition observed on growth)	**(Harpreet et al., 2013)**

an eco-friendly anti-bacterial property for a large-scale medicinal application (Lu et al., 2008; Aziz et al., 2018; Subhankari et al., 2013). A green and chemical synthesis combination of copper with ginger are performed to achieve the applications using non-toxic methods in order to achieve purification of water and air and also for antibacterial packaging (Velmurugan et al., 2014). Ginger, in synthesis with Gold and Silver has proven as remarkable reducing agents. The presence of AgNps demonstrates the growth of pathogens with multiplication properties and antibacterial in nature (Zhag et al., 2016). The synthetic nanoparticles with ginger improve the natural delivery mechanism with not only treatment but also with prevention benefits (Salaby et al., 2015). Silver has proven one of the strongest antibacterial properties in the green synthesis when tested against *Escherichia coli* and *Staphylococcus aureus*, leading the paths to more advanced application investigation for antibacterial agents (Azizi et al., 2016). Ginger oil and

Table 3. Antimicrobial property analysis of different types Nano particles of Zingiber officinale (Ginger) rhizome

Sl No.	Description of Nanoparticles & Size (nm)	Zone of Inhibition (mm); MIC (µg/ml); MBC (µg/ml) against bacteria & fungus	Reference
1	AgNps synthesized by physical method; (5nm)	c) *E. coli* **ZOI Quantity of therapeutic** 15.66 ± 0.33 15µg 16.33 ± 0.33 30 µg 18.00 45 µg d) *S. aureus* **ZOI Quantity of therapeutic** 16.66 ± 0.33 15µg 16.83 ± 0.33 30 µg 17.66 ± 0.33 45 µg	**(Veronika et al., 2017)**
2	AgNps synthesized by green Technology (50nm)	*B. subtilis* (ZOI 14mm)	**(Jonny et al., 2014)**
3	AgNps synthesized by phyto assisted Technology	a) *B. subtilis* MTCC 3053 **Quantity of therapeutic ZOI** 10µl 8mm 20µl 10mm 30µl 10mm 40µl 11mm 50µl 12mm b) *Klebsiella planticola* MTCC 2277 **Quantity of therapeutic ZOI** 10µl 9mm 20µl 10mm 30µl 11mm 40µl 12mm 50µl 12mm	**(Gnana Dhas et al., 2013)**

Table 4. Antimicrobial property analysis of different types of Nanoparticles of Trachysperum ammi (Carom)

Sl No.	Description of Nanoparticles & Size (nm)	Zone of Inhibition (mm); MIC (µg/ml); MBC (µg/ml) against bacteria & fungus	Reference
1	AgNps synthesized by green synthesis on carom leaves; (45 – 100nm)	a) *E. coli* **MIC ZOI** 100 µl/ml 10mm b) *Bacillus subtilis* **MIC ZOI** 6.25 µl/ml 18mm	**(Sonam et al., 2015)**

Table 5. Antimicrobial property analysis of different types of Nano particles of Cinamomum verum (Cinnamon)

Sl No.	Description of Nanoparticles	Zone of Inhibition (mm); MIC (µg/ml); MBC (µg/ml) against bacteria & fungus	Reference
1	Nanoparticle of Poly–(D, L – lactide-Co-Glycolide) (PGLA) encapsulated cinnamon bark extract produced by emulsion-solvent evaporation method	a) *Salmonella enterica* servor Typhimurium LT2 MIC 549.23µg/ml 24 & 72hrs incubation MBC >549.23 µg/ml 24 & 72hrs incubation b) *Listeria monocytogenes* ScottA MIC 549.23µg/ml 24 & 72hrs incubation MBC 549.23 µg/ml 24 & 72hrs incubation	**(Sonam et al., 2015)**

Table 6. Antimicrobial property analysis of different types of Nano particles of Myristica fragrans (Nutmeg)

S.NO.	Description of Nanoparticles & Size (nm)	Zone of Inhibition (mm); MIC (µg/ml); MBC (µg/ml) against bacteria & fungus	Reference
1.	Green synthesis of AgNps using extract of *Myristica fragrans* (NUTMEG); (7-20 nm)	a) *E. coli* {MIC;0.628; Minimum Lethal Concentration(MLC) 1.25µg/ml, in 24 hrs Incubation} b) *S. aureus* {MIC;0.0.314; Minimum Lethal Concentration(MLC) 1.25µg/ml, in 24 hrs Incubation}	**(Sharma et al., 2014)**
2	Green synthesis of AgNps (20 – 40mm)	a) ZOI of 13 different undefined strains of MDR *S. typhi* on 25 µg/ml therapeutic concentration **Sample Number ZOI (mm)** MCASMZ U1 12.13 ± 0.32 MCASMZ U2 11.13 ± o.32 MCASMZ U3 10.06 ± 0.20 MCASMZ U4 13.33 ± 0.49 MCASMZ U5 13.16 ± 0.37 MCASMZ U6 13.23 ± 0.25 MCASMZ U7 No activity MCASMZ U8 9.46 ± 0.45 MCASMZ U9 9.26 ± 0.37 MCASMZ U10 No activity MCASMZ U11 12.16 ± 0.15 MCASMZ U12 13.33 ± 0.41 MCASMZ U13 10.36 ± 0.32	**(Senthilkumar et al., 2017)**

Zinc oxide silver (ZnO-Ag) as core-shell of nanocomposite materials in a significant synthesis process, the Ag– doping has the improved antibacterial properties of ZnO-Nps.

The other spice to be discussed for its green synthesis process against the metals and deriving its antimicrobial properties is *Cuminum cyminum*. The nature of Cumin is antifungal, and when the synthesis performed for its inhibitions and efficacy towards the aflatoxin secretion and fungus, a free radical potential is identified (Kedia et al., 2013). The microbial flora can be treated with *Cuminum cyminum* and essential oils (Abbaszadegan et al., 2015). The *Cuminum cyminum* oil, when encapsulated as nanogel compared with free oils, achieves significant antifungal properties (Zhaveha et al., 2015). The introduction of nanoparticles is health, agriculture, and food industry have been proving a significant improvement in the health conditions and the quality of the produce (Zare et al., 2017). The incorporation of AgNp, AuNp and ZnO-Nps are proved to be non-toxic and safe antimicrobial agents for the process of green synthesis.

FUTURE PROSPECTS AND OTHER APPLICATIONS

This chapter has dealt with mainly an antimicrobial activity analysis of different Indian Spices. But, except this property, Nanoformulates of spices have many other activities like anti-oxidant, anti-cancer, anti-inflammatory properties. Even safranal (Saffron derivatives) a loaded solid lipid nanoparticles shows very good potential as sunscreen and a moisturizing agent. Cumin essential oil shows static and cidal activity against several microorganisms. We can enhance these activities by utilizing green synthesis technology of nanoparticles' production. For star anise seed and hing (Ferula) the future aspect is huge because till now it remains untouched on the field of Nano microbiology.

Table 7. Antimicrobial property analysis of different types Nano particles of Trigonella foeum-graecum (Fenugreek)

Sl No.	Description of Nanoparticles & Size (nm)	Zone of Inhibition (mm); MIC (µg/ml); MBC (µg/ml) against bacteria & fungus	Reference
1	CuNps of *Pleurotus ostreatus* fermented fenugreek by biogenic synthesis with gamma rays (31-36 nm)	e) *Klesiella pneumonia* **ZOI & Therapeutic Concentration** 16 mm on 62µg/ml concentration **MIC** 1.93µg/ml f) *A. calcoaceticus* **ZOI & Therapeutic Concentration** 15 mm on 62µg/ml concentration **MIC** 3.87µg/ml g) *S. aureus* **ZOI & Therapeutic Concentration** 15 mm on 62µg/ml concentration **MIC** 3.87µg/ml h) *C. albicans* **MIC** 1.93µg/ml	**(Ahmed et al., 2018)**
2	CuNps synthesized by chemical process	a) *E. coli* (MIC 3.25µg/ml) b) *S. aureus* (MIC 62.5µg/ml) c) *Salmonella typhimurium* (MIC 62.5µg/ml)	**(Ahmed et al., 2018)**
3	CuNps Synthesized at 400ºC	**Name of Organism's ZOI** *P. aeruginosa* 21mm *E. coli* 20mm *S. aureus* 22mm *B. subtilis* 24mm	**(Ahmed et al., 2018)**
4	CuONps synthesized by melanin & gamma ray	e) *E. coli* 0157: H7 (ZOI 14mm) f) *B. subtilis* (ZOI 13mm) g) *S. aureus* (ZOI 22mm) h) *A. niger* (ZOI 15mm) i) *P. citrium* (ZOI 11mm) j) *F. oxysporum* (ZOI 14mm)	**Ahmed et al., 2018**
5	Saponin conjugated AgNps useful for wound infection (4 – 15 nm)	**Name of Organism's ZOI (mm) MIC (µg/ml) MBC (µg/ml)** *E. faecalis* 9 ± 4 25 30 *S. aureus* 10 ± 0.7 10 20 *E. colacae* 8.5 ± 0.6 30 35 *E. coli* 8 ± 0.3 25 30 *K. pneumoniae* 9 ± 1 25 30 *P. aeruginosa* 7 ± 0.9 20 25 *Acinetobacter baumanii* 8 ± 0.8 25 30 *E. asburiae* 10 ± 0.99 15 20 *E. kobei* 9.5 ± 0.8 30 35 *P. mirabilis* 7.5 ± 1 30 35	**Anbarasan et al., 2017**
6	AgNps synthesized by green synthesis of fenugreek leaves (20 – 30 nm)	**Name of Organism's ZOI (mm) MIC (µg/ml) Therapeutic quantity** *S. aureus* 12.47 ± 0.31 12.5 1µl of AgNPs *E. coli* 16.27 ± 0.51 6.25 1µl of AgNPs	**Senthil et al., 2017**
7	ZnNps synthesized by gamma ray & natural polysaccharides of fermented fenugreek powder (46nm)	**Name of Organism's Zone of Inhibition (mm)** *B. subtilis* RCMB 010067 20 ± 0.2 *S. aureus* RCMB 010028 12 ± 0.513 *E. faecalis* RCMB 010075 16 ± 0.231 *E. coli* RCMB 010052 22 ± 0.3 *P. aeruginosa* RCMB 010043 17 ± 2.51 *K. pneumonia* RCMB 010093 15 ± 0.235 *C. albicans* ATCC 10231 14 ± 0.115 *C. glabrata* ATCC 15126 13 ± 0.173 *C. tropicalis* ATCC 10610 12 ± 0.154	**Ahmed et al., 2017**
8	AgNps synthesized by Green Technology t room temparature (26nm)	a) *E. coli* – Show maximum inhibition in every concentration of AgNps therapeutic b) *S. aureus* - Show lowest inhibition in every concentration of AgNps therapeutic c) *P. syringae* - Show moderate inhibition in every concentration of AgNps therapeutic	**Singh et al., 2011**

Table 8. Antimicrobial property analysis of different types Nano particles of Zingiber officinale (Ginger) rhizome

Sl No.	Description of Nanoparticles & Size (nm)	Zone of Inhibition (mm); MIC (µg/ml); MBC (µg/ml) against bacteria & fungus	Reference
1	AgNps synthesized in sunlight; (4 – 15nm)	i) *E. coli* MTCC 723 (MIC 62.5; MBC 500; ZOI 14mm in 2 hrs incubation, 16mm in 24hrs incubation) j) *S. aureus* MTCC 96 (MIC 125; MBC 250; ZOI 14mm in 2 hrs incubation, 19mm in 24 hrs incubation)	**(Xiaoying et al., 2015)**
2	ZnONps synthesized by Green Technology (23 – 26nm)	a) *Klesiella pneumonia* (MIC 62.5; ZOI 9mm) b) *S. aureus* (MIC 62.5; ZOI 9mm) c) *C. alicans* (MIC 250; ZOI 9mm) d) *P. notatum* (MIC 250; ZOI 12mm)	**(Chinnammal et al., 2015)**
3	AgNps synthesized by Green Technology at room temperature (3.86 nm average)	c) *B. subtilis* (ZOI 31mm at 200µg/ml concentration) d) *E. coli* (ZOI 30mm at 200µg/ml concentration) e) *C. albicans* (ZOI 36mm at 200µg/ml concentration)	**(Wisam et al., 2018)**
4	CuNps synthesized by Green Technology at p^H 1.91 (25 – 40nm)	k) *E. coli* (ZOI 15mm)	**(Ipsa et al., 2013)**
5	AgNps synthesized by Green Technology at 50^0 C & p^H 8 – 9 (10 – 20 nm)	h) *Staphylococcus spp.* (MIC 30 ± 14.3 µg/ml; MBC 40 ± 10.2 µg/ml; ZOI 6.5 ± 0.4mm) i) *Listeria spp.* (MIC 20 ± 12.8 µg/ml; MBC 30 ± 11.5 µg/ml; ZOI 8 ± 0.6mm)	**(Palanivel et al., 2014)**
6	AgNps synthesized by Chemical Technology at room temperature (3.1 nm average)	d) *E. coli* (ZOI 3.4mm) e) *S. aureus* (5.9mm)	**(Thanaa et al., 2015)**
7	ZnONps synthesized by Green Technology (45nm)	b) *B. subtilis* (ZOI 11.75 ± 0.49mm at 60µg/ml concentration) c) *E. coli* (ZOI 10.235 ± 0.37mm at 60µg/ml concentration)	**(Susan et al., 2016)**
8	ZnO-Ag Nano composite synthesized by Green Technology (23nm)	i) *B. subtilis* (ZOI 14.80 ± 0.35mm at 60µg/ml concentration) j) *E. coli* (ZOI 14.26 ± 0.56mm at 60µg/ml concentration)	**(Susan et al., 2016)**

Table 9. Antimicrobial property analysis of different types Nano particles of Cuminum cyminum (Cumin)

Sl No.	Description of Nanoparticles	Zone of Inhibition (mm); MIC (µg/ml or ppm); MBC (µg/ml) against bacteria & fungus	Reference
1	Chitosan – caffic acid nano gel with encapsulated cumin essential oil	**Name of Organism's MIC (ppm)** *Aspergillus flavus* 100 – 500	**(Sara et al., 2015)**
2	ZnONps synthesized by green technology	**Name of Organism's ZOI (mm) MIC (µg/ml) MBC (µg/ml)** *B. subtilis* PTCC 1023 28 ± 1 25 6.25 *L. monocytogenes* PTCC 1163 20 ± 1 12.5 6.25 *E. faecalis* PTCC 1237 22 ± 1 25 6.25 *P. aeruginosa* PTCC 1603 25 ± 1 12.5 3.12 *E. coli* PTCC 1330 22 ± 1 6.25 3.12 *P. pneumoniae* PTCC 1290 23 ± 1 12.5 6.25	**(Elham et al., 2017)**

Table 10. Antimicrobial property analysis of different types Nano particles of Crocus sativus L. (Saffron)

Sl No.	Description of Nanoparticles & Size (nm)	Zone of Inhibition (mm); MIC (µg/ml); MBC (µg/ml) against bacteria & fungus	Reference
1	AgNps synthesized by Hurdle technology	k) *E. coli* – 100% killing at 30th day on polyethylene film l) *Enterobacteriace spp.* – 100% killing at 1st day on polyethylene film m) *C. pertringens* - 100% killing at 60th day on polyethylene film	**(Hamid Sales et al., 2012)**
2	AgNps synthesized green technology with saffron wastes (12 – 20nm)	a) The Nano therapeutic show significant anti-microbial effect against *E. coli* ATCC 25922; *P. aeruginosa* ATCC 27853; *K. pneumonia* ATCC 9997; *S. flexneri* ATCC 12022; *B. subtilis* ATCC 6633 b) But don't show any activity against *S. aureus* ATCC 29213	**(Ghodsieh et al., 2017)**

Still, now much research work is done on in-vitro analysis, but for human welfare, we have to further proceed with the combination of antibiotics and for more in-vivo application analysis with exposure of pharmacodynamics & pharmacokinetics.

CONCLUSION

In case of bacterial and fungal infection, uses of inorganic nanomaterials is a promising therapeutic method. Earlier this process was applied as traditional medicine, i.e. drinking of colloidal. Nanoparticles exhibit a natural antimicrobial property and also act as transfer for therapeutic agents & directly interact with bacterial cell walls that cause disruption on that location. Some nanoparticles can cause damages on DNA and can interrupt in protein production, even in mitochondrial dysfunction.

Indian spices have very good potential as an antimicrobial agent. With the help of nano biotechnology, it can be delivered to a specific site and can treat difficult infectious conditions like urinary tract infections, infection in one, burn wound infections etc. It can be very useful in India or any other developing country for the treatment of infectious diseases and especially multidrug resistance.

ACKNOWLEDGMENT

All authors are grateful to R&D Section, SANCHARAN (A Socio-Cultural Organization) 4289/2003; Department of Clinical Biochemistry & Department of Bio Resources, University of Kashmir; Department of Biomedical Engineering, Sathyabama Institute of Science and Technology; School of Chemical Engineering and Environment, North University of China; Center for Fuel Cell Innovation, Huazhong University of Science and Technology. We express our special sincere thanks to Prof. Amar P. Garg, VC at Shobhit University, Meerut for his knowledge sharing.

REFERENCES

Abbai, R., Ramya Mathiyalagan, J. M., Kim, Y. J., Wang, C., Singh, P., Ahn, S., ... Yang, D. C. (2016). Green synthesis of multifunctional silver and gold nanoparticles from the oriental herbal adaptogen: Siberian ginseng. *International Journal of Nanomedicine*, *11*, 3131–3143. doi:10.2147/IJN.S108549 PMID:27468232

Abbaszadegan, A., Gholami, A., Ghahramani, Y., Ghareghan, R., Ghareghan, M., Kazemi, A., ... Ghasemi, Y. (2016). Antimicrobial and cytotoxic activity of Cuminum cyminum as an intracanal medicament compared to chlorhexidine gel. *Iranian Endodontic Journal*, *11*(1), 44. PMID:26843877

Abu-Zaiton, A. S. (2010). Anti-Diabetic Activity of Ferula assafoetida Extract in Normal and Alloxan-Induced Diabetic Rats. *Pakistan Journal of Biological Sciences*, *13*(2), 97–100. doi:10.3923/pjbs.2010.97.100 PMID:20415145

Ahn, T., Kim, J. H., Yang, H. M., Lee, J. W., & Kim, J. D. (2012). Formation pathways of magnetite nanoparticles by coprecipitation method. *The Journal of Physical Chemistry C*, *116*(10), 6069–6076. doi:10.1021/jp211843g

Akbari, B., Tavandashti, M. P., & Zandrahimi, M. (2011). Particle size characterization of nanoparticles–a practicalapproach. *Iranian Journal of Materials Science and Engineering*, *8*(2), 48–56.

AlSalhi, M., Devanesan, S., Alfuraydi, A., Vishnubalaji, R., Munusamy, M. A., Murugan, K., ... Benelli, G. (2016). Green synthesis of silver nanoparticles using <em>Pimpinella anisum</em> seeds: Antimicrobial activity and cytotoxicity on human neonatal skin stromal cells and colon cancer cells. *International Journal of Nanomedicine*, *11*, 4439–4449. doi:10.2147/IJN.S113193 PMID:27660438

Alsammarraie, F. K., Wang, W., Zhou, P., Mustapha, A., & Lin, M. (2018). Green synthesis of silver nanoparticles using turmeric extracts and investigation of their antibacterial activities. *Colloids and Surfaces. B, Biointerfaces*, *171*, 398–405. doi:10.1016/j.colsurfb.2018.07.059 PMID:30071481

Anastas, P. T., & Warner, J. C. (1998). Green chemistry: Theory and practice. Oxford University Press.

Ankamwar, B., Damle, C., Ahmad, A., & Sastry, M. (2005). Biosynthesis of gold and silver nanoparticles using Emblica officinalis fruit extract, their phase transfer and transmetallation in an organic solution. *Journal of Nanoscience and Nanotechnology*, *5*(10), 1665–1671. doi:10.1166/jnn.2005.184 PMID:16245525

Aranda, P., Fernandes, F. M., Wicklein, B., Ruiz-Hitzky, E., Hill, J. P., & Ariga, K. (2012). *Bioinspired materials chemistry I: organic–inorganic nanocom-posites. In Bioinspiration and biomimicry in chemistry: reverse-engineering nature* (1st ed., pp. 121–138). Hoboken, NJ: John Wiley & Sons. doi:10.1002/9781118310083.ch5

Aziz, W., & Jassim, H. A. (2018). A novel study of pH influence on Ag nanoparticles size with antibacterial and antifungal activity using green synthesis. *World Sci News*, *97*, 139–152.

Azizi, S., Mohamad, R., Rahim, R. A., Moghaddam, A. B., Moniri, M., Ariff, A., ... Namvab, F. (2016). ZnO-Ag core shell nanocomposite formed by green method using essential oil of wild ginger and their bactericidal and cytotoxic effects. *Applied Surface Science*, *384*, 517–524. doi:10.1016/j.apsusc.2016.05.052

Bagherzade, G., Tavakoli, M. M., & Namaei, M. H. (2017). Green synthesis of silver nanoparticles using aqueous extract of saffron (Crocus sativus L.) wastages and its antibacterial activity against six bacteria. *Asian Pacific Journal of Tropical Biomedicine*, *7*(3), 227–233. doi:10.1016/j.apjtb.2016.12.014

Balakrishnan, S., Sivaji, I., Kandasamy, S., Duraisamy, S., Kumar, N. S., & Gurusubramanian, G. (2017). Biosynthesis of silver nanoparticles using Myristica fragrans seed (nutmeg) extract and its antibacterial activity against multidrug-resistant (MDR) Salmonella enterica serovar Typhi isolates. *Environmental Science and Pollution Research International*, *24*(17), 14758–14769. doi:10.100711356-017-9065-7 PMID:28470497

Basavaraja, S., Balaji, S. D., Lagashetty, A., Rajasab, A. H., & Venkataraman, A. (2008). Extracellular biosynthesis of silver nanoparticles using the fungus Fusarium semitectum. *Materials Research Bulletin*, *43*(5), 1164–1170. doi:10.1016/j.materresbull.2007.06.020

Baser, K. H. C., & Buchbauer, G. (2015). *Handbook of essential oils: science, technology, and applications*. CRC Press. doi:10.1201/b19393

Bhattacharya, D., & Gupta, R. K. (2005). Nanotechnology and potential of microorganisms. *Critical Reviews in Biotechnology*, *25*(4), 199–204. doi:10.1080/07388550500361994 PMID:16419617

Bhawana, B. R., Buttar, H. S., Jain, V. K., & Jain, N. (2011). Curcumin nanoparticles: Preparation, characterization, and antimicrobial study. *Journal of Agricultural and Food Chemistry*, *59*(5), 2056–2061. doi:10.1021/jf104402t PMID:21322563

Binnig, G., Quate, C. F., & Gerber, Ch. (1986). Atomic force microscope. *Physical Review Letters*, *56*(9), 930–933. doi:10.1103/PhysRevLett.56.930 PMID:10033323

Blanco Andujar, C. (2014). *Sodium carbonate mediated synthesis of iron oxide nanoparticles to improve magnetic hyperthermia efficiency and induce apoptosis* (Doctoral dissertation). University College London.

Brar, S. K., & Verma, M. (2011). Measurement of nanoparticles by light-scattering techniques. *Trends in Analytical Chemistry*, *30*(1), 4–17. doi:10.1016/j.trac.2010.08.008

Brinck, T. (2014). *Introduction to green energetic materials*. Chichester, UK: John Wiley & Sons Ltd. doi:10.1002/9781118676448

Busó-Rogero, C., Brimaud, S., Solla-Gullon, J., Vidal-Iglesias, F. J., Herrero, E., Behm, R. J., & Feliu, J. M. (2016). Ethanol oxidation on shape-controlled platinum nanoparticles at different pHs: A combined in situ IR spectroscopy and online mass spectrometry study. *Journal of Electroanalytical Chemistry (Lausanne, Switzerland)*, *763*, 116–124. doi:10.1016/j.jelechem.2015.12.034

Castellano, J. J., Shafii, S. M., Ko, F., Donate, G., Wright, T. E., Mannari, R. J., ... Robson, M. C. (2007). Comparative evaluation of silver-containing antimicrobial dressings and drugs. *International Wound Journal*, *4*(2), 114–122. doi:10.1111/j.1742-481X.2007.00316.x PMID:17651227

Chainani-Wu, N. (2003). Safety and Anti-Inflammatory Activity of Curcumin: A Component of Tumeric (Curcuma longa). *Journal of Alternative and Complementary Medicine (New York, N.Y.)*, *9*(1), 161–168. doi:10.1089/107555303321223035 PMID:12676044

Chanda, N., Shukla, R., Zambre, A., Mekapothula, S., Kulkarni, R. R., Katti, K., ... Katti, K. V. (2010). An Effective Strategy for the Synthesis of Biocompatible Gold Nanoparticles Using Cinnamon Phytochemicals for Phantom CT Imaging and Photoacoustic Detection of Cancerous Cells. *Pharmaceutical Research*, *28*(2), 279–291. doi:10.100711095-010-0276-6 PMID:20872051

Chaudhry, N. M. A., & Tariq, P. (2006). Anti-microbial activity of Cinnamomum cassia against diverse microbial flora with its nutritional and medicinal impacts. *Pakistan Journal of Botany*, *38*(1), 169.

Chen, S., Zhang, X., Zhang, Q., & Tan, W. (2009). Trioctylphosphine as both solvent and stabilizer to synthesize CdS nanorods. *Nanoscale Research Letters*, *4*(10), 1159–1165. doi:10.100711671-009-9375-x PMID:20596487

Chryssanthi, D. G., Dedes, P. G., Karamanos, N. K., Cordopatis, P., & Lamari, F. N. (2011). Crocetin inhibits invasiveness of MDA-MB-231 breast cancer cells via downregulation of matrix metalloproteinases. *Planta Medica*, *77*(02), 146–151. doi:10.1055-0030-1250178 PMID:20803418

Crozier, A., Yokota, T., Jaganath, I. B., Marks, S. C., Saltmarsh, M., & Clifford, M. N. (2006). Secondary metabolites in fruits, vegetables, beverages and other plant based dietary components. *Plant secondary metabolites: Occurrence, structure and role in the human diet*, 208-302.

da Silva, A. C., de Freitas Santos, P. D., do Prado Silva, J. T., Leimann, F. V., Bracht, L., & Gonçalves, O. H. (2018). Impact of curcumin nanoformulation on its antimicrobial activity. *Trends in Food Science & Technology*, *72*, 74–82. doi:10.1016/j.tifs.2017.12.004

Das, S., Das, M. P., & Das, J. (2013). Fabrication of porous chitosan/silver nanocomposite film and its bactericidal efficacy against multi-drug resistant (MDR) clinical isolates. *Journal of Pharmacy Research*, *6*(1), 11–15. doi:10.1016/j.jopr.2012.11.006

Dhiman, J., Kundu, V., Kumar, S., Kumar, R., & Chakarvarti, S. K. (2014). *Eco-friendly Synthesis and Characterization of Silver Nanoparticles and Evaluation of Their Antibacterial Activity. American Journal of Materials Science and Technology*. doi:10.7726/ajmst.2014.1002

Dias, M. A., Lacerda, I. C. A., Pimentel, P. F., De Castro, H. F., & Rosa, C. A. (2002). Removal of heavy metals by an Aspergillus terreus strain immobilized in a polyurethane matrix. *Letters in Applied Microbiology*, *34*(1), 46–50. doi:10.1046/j.1472-765x.2002.01040.x PMID:11849492

Duarte, R. C., Fanaro, G. B., Koike, A. C. R., & Villavicencio, A. L. C. H. (2011). *Irradiation effect on antifungal potential myristica fragrans (nutmeg) essential oil, a preliminary study*. https://www.osti.gov/etdeweb/biblio/21517124

Duong, H. T., Chen, Y., Tawfik, S. A., Wen, S., Parviz, M., Shimoni, O., & Jin, D. (2018). Systematic investigation of functional ligands for colloidal stable upconversion nanoparticles. *RSC Advances*, *8*(9), 4842–4849. doi:10.1039/C7RA13765F

El-Batal, A. I., Al-Hazmi, N. E., Mosallam, F. M., & El-Sayyad, G. S. (2018). Biogenic synthesis of copper nanoparticles by natural polysaccharides and Pleurotus ostreatus fermented fenugreek using gamma rays with antioxidant and antimicrobial potential towards some wound pathogens. *Microbial Pathogenesis*, *118*, 159–169. doi:10.1016/j.micpath.2018.03.013 PMID:29530808

Engelbrekt, C., Jensen, P. S., Sørensen, K. H., Ulstrup, J., & Zhang, J. (2013). Complexity of gold nanoparticle formation disclosed by dynamics study. *The Journal of Physical Chemistry C*, *117*(22), 11818–11828. doi:10.1021/jp401883h

Eslami, M., Bayat, M., Nejad, A. S. M., Sabokbar, A., & Anvar, A. A. (2016). Effect of polymer/nanosilver composite packaging on long-term microbiological status of Iranian saffron (Crocus sativus L.). *Saudi Journal of Biological Sciences*, *23*(3), 341–347. doi:10.1016/j.sjbs.2015.07.004 PMID:27081358

Gade, A., Gaikwad, S., Tiwari, V., Yadav, A., Ingle, A., & Rai, M. (2010). Biofabrication of silver nanoparticles by Opuntia ficus-indica: In vitro antibacterial activity and study of the mechanism involved in the synthesis. *Current Nanoscience*, *6*(4), 370–375. doi:10.2174/157341310791659026

Ghodake, G. S., Deshpande, N. G., Lee, Y. P., & Jin, E. (2010). Pear fruit extract-assisted room-temperature biosynthesis of gold nanoplates. *Colloids and Surfaces. B, Biointerfaces*, *75*(2), 584–589. doi:10.1016/j.colsurfb.2009.09.040 PMID:19879738

Goldstein, J. I., Newbury, D. E., Michael, J. R., Ritchie, N. W., Scott, J. H. J., & Joy, D. C. (2017). *X-ray microanalysis*. Springer.

Gopalakrishnan, M. J. C. S., Narayanan, C. S., & Grenz, M. (1990). Nonsaponifiable lipid constituents of Cardamom. *Journal of Agricultural and Food Chemistry*, *38*(12), 2133–2136. doi:10.1021/jf00102a006

Haiss, W., Thanh, N. T., Aveyard, J., & Fernig, D. G. (2007). Determination of size and concentration of gold nanoparticles from UV– Vis spectra. *Analytical Chemistry*, *79*(11), 4215–4221. doi:10.1021/ac0702084 PMID:17458937

Harada, M., Saijo, K., & Sakamoto, N. (2009). Characterization of metal nanoparticles prepared by photoreduction in aqueous solutions of various surfactants using UV–vis, EXAFS and SAXS. *Colloids and Surfaces. A, Physicochemical and Engineering Aspects*, *349*(1-3), 176–188. doi:10.1016/j.colsurfa.2009.08.015

Hendel, T., Wuithschick, M., Kettemann, F., Birnbaum, A., Rademann, K., & Polte, J. (2014). In situ determination of colloidal gold concentrations with UV–Vis spectroscopy: Limitations and perspectives. *Analytical Chemistry*, *86*(22), 11115–11124. doi:10.1021/ac502053s PMID:25289517

Hill, L. E., Taylor, T. M., & Gomes, C. (2013). Antimicrobial Efficacy of Poly (DL-lactide-co-glycolide) (PLGA) Nanoparticles with Entrapped Cinnamon Bark Extract againstListeria monocytogenesandSalmonella typhimurium. *Journal of Food Science*, *78*(4), N626–N632. doi:10.1111/1750-3841.12069 PMID:23464835

Holmes, A. M., Lim, J., Studier, H., & Roberts, M. S. (2016). Varying the morphology of silver nanoparticles results in differential toxicity against micro-organisms, HaCaT keratinocytes and affects skin deposition. *Nanotoxicology*, *10*(10), 1503–1514. doi:10.1080/17435390.2016.1236993 PMID:27636544

Hoo, C. M., Starostin, N., West, P., & Mecartney, M. L. (2008). A comparison of atomic force microscopy (AFM) and dynamic light scattering (DLS) methods to characterize nanoparticle size distributions. *Journal of Nanoparticle Research*, *10*(1), 89–96. doi:10.100711051-008-9435-7

Huang, Y., Zhao, J., Zhou, L., Wang, J., Gong, Y., Chen, X., ... Jiang, W. (2010). Antifungal Activity of the Essential Oil of Illicium verum Fruit and Its Main Component trans-Anethole. *Molecules (Basel, Switzerland)*, *15*(11), 7558–7569. doi:10.3390/molecules15117558 PMID:21030909

Hubenthal, F., Blázquez Sánchez, D., & Träger, F. (2012). Determination of morphological parameters of supported gold nanoparticles: Comparison of AFM combined with optical spectroscopy and theoretical modeling versus TEM. *Applied Sciences (Basel, Switzerland)*, *2*(3), 566–583. doi:10.3390/app2030566

Iranshahy, M., & Iranshahi, M. (2011). Traditional uses, phytochemistry and pharmacology of asafoetida (Ferula assa-foetida oleo-gum-resin)—A review. *Journal of Ethnopharmacology*, *134*(1), 1–10. doi:10.1016/j.jep.2010.11.067 PMID:21130854

Iravani, S. (2011). Green synthesis of metal nanoparticles using plants. *Green Chemistry*, *13*(10), 2638–2650. doi:10.1039/c1gc15386b

Jain, D., Daima, H. K., Kachhwaha, S., & Kothari, S. L. (2009). Synthesis of plant-mediated silver nanoparticles using papaya fruit extract and evaluation of their anti microbial activities. *Digest Journal of Nanomaterials and Biostructures*, *4*(3), 557–563.

Jana, N. R., Wang, Z. L., Sau, T. K., & Pal, T. (2000). Seed-mediated growth method to prepare cubic copper nanoparticles. *CURRENT SCIENCE-BANGALORE*, *79*(9), 1367–1369.

Janaki, C., Sailatha, E., & Gunasekaran, S. (2015). Synthesis, characteristics and antimicrobial activity of ZnO nanoparticles. *Spectrochimica Acta. Part A: Molecular and Biomolecular Spectroscopy*, *144*, 17–22. doi:10.1016/j.saa.2015.02.041 PMID:25748589

Jayandran, M., Haneefa, M., & Balasubramanian, V. (2015). Green synthesis and characterization of Manganese nanoparticles using natural plant extracts and its evaluation of antimicrobial activity. *Journal of Applied Pharmaceutical Science*, 105–110. doi:10.7324/JAPS.2015.501218

Jha, A. K., & Prasad, K. (2008). Yeast mediated synthesis of silver nanoparticles. *International Journal of Nanoscience and Nanotechnology*, *4*(1), 17–22.

Jobitha, G., Annadurai, G., & Kannan, C. (2012). Green synthesis of silver nanoparticles using Elettaria cardamomom and assessment of its antimicrobial activity. *International Journal of Pharmaceutical Sciences and Research*, *3*, 323–330.

Jones, M. R., Macfarlane, R. J., Lee, B., Zhang, J., Young, K. L., Senesi, A. J., & Mirkin, C. A. (2010). DNA-nanoparticle superlattices formed from anisotropic building blocks. *Nature Materials*, *9*(11), 913–917. doi:10.1038/nmat2870 PMID:20890281

Kalishwaralal, K., Deepak, V., Ramkumarpandian, S., Nellaiah, H., & Sangiliyandi, G. (2008). Extracellular biosynthesis of silver nanoparticles by the culture supernatant of Bacillus licheniformis. *Materials Letters*, *62*(29), 4411–4413. doi:10.1016/j.matlet.2008.06.051

Kaur, H., Kaur, S., & Singh, M. (2013). Biosynthesis of silver nanoparticles by natural precursor from clove and their antimicrobial activity. *Biologia*, *68*(6). doi:10.247811756-013-0276-1

Kavoosi, G., Shakiba, A., Ghorbani, M., Dadfar, S. M. M., & Purfard, A. M. (2015). Antioxidant, antibacterial, water binding capacity and mechanical behavior of gelatin-ferula oil film as a wound dressing material. *Galen Medical Journal*, *4*(2), 103–114.

Kedia, A., Prakash, B., Mishra, P. K., & Dubey, N. K. (2014). Antifungal and antiaflatoxigenic properties of Cuminum cyminum (L.) seed essential oil and its efficacy as a preservative in stored commodities. *International Journal of Food Microbiology*, *168–169*, 1–7. doi:10.1016/j.ijfoodmicro.2013.10.008 PMID:24211773

Khameneh, B., Halimi, V., Jaafari, M. R., & Golmohammadzadeh, S. (2015). Safranal-loaded solid lipid nanoparticles: Evaluation of sunscreen and moisturizing potential for topical applications. *Iranian Journal of Basic Medical Sciences.*, *18*(1), 58. PMID:25810877

Khan, R., Zakir, M., Khanam, Z., Shakil, S., & Khan, A. U. (2010). Novel compound from Trachyspermum ammi (Ajowan caraway) seeds with antibiofilm and antiadherence activities against Streptococcus mutans: A potential chemotherapeutic agent against dental caries. *Journal of Applied Microbiology*, *109*(6), 2151–2159. doi:10.1111/j.1365-2672.2010.04847.x PMID:20846336

Kirschling, T. L., Golas, P. L., Unrine, J. M., Matyjaszewski, K., Gregory, K. B., Lowry, G. V., & Tilton, R. D. (2011). Microbial bioavailability of covalently bound polymer coatings on model engineered nanomaterials. *Environmental Science & Technology*, *45*(12), 5253–5259. doi:10.1021/es200770z PMID:21609011

Krausz, A. E., Adler, B. L., Cabral, V., Navati, M., Doerner, J., Charafeddine, R. A., ... Friedman, A. J. (2015). Curcumin-encapsulated nanoparticles as innovative antimicrobial and wound healing agent. *Nanomedicine; Nanotechnology, Biology, and Medicine*, *11*(1), 195–206. doi:10.1016/j.nano.2014.09.004 PMID:25240595

Kumar, G. S., Muthu, D., Karunakaran, G., Karthi, S., Girija, E. K., & Kuznetsov, D. (2018). Curcuma longa tuber extract mediated synthesis of hydroxyapatite nanorods using biowaste as a calcium source for the treatment of bone infections. *Journal of Sol-Gel Science and Technology*, *86*(3), 610–616. doi:10.100710971-018-4670-6

Kumar, P. B. A. N., Dushenkov, V., Motto, H., & Raskin, I. (1995). Phytoextraction: The Use of Plants To Remove Heavy Metals from Soils. *Environmental Science & Technology*, *29*(5), 1232–1238. doi:10.1021/es00005a014 PMID:22192016

Kumar, P. V., Pammi, S. V. N., Kollu, P., Satyanarayana, K. V. V., & Shameem, U. (2014). Green synthesis and characterization of silver nanoparticles using Boerhaavia diffusa plant extract and their anti bacterial activity. *Industrial Crops and Products*, *52*, 562–566. doi:10.1016/j.indcrop.2013.10.050

Laborda, F., Bolea, E., Cepriá, G., Gómez, M. T., Jiménez, M. S., Pérez-Arantegui, J., & Castillo, J. R. (2016). Detection, characterization and quantification of inorganic engineered nanomaterials: A review of techniques and methodological approaches for the analysis of complex samples. *Analytica Chimica Acta*, *904*, 10–32. doi:10.1016/j.aca.2015.11.008 PMID:26724760

Lapkin, A., Joyce, L., & Crittenden, B. (2004). Framework for evaluating the "greenness" of chemical processes: Case studies for a novel VOC recovery technology. *Environmental Science & Technology*, *38*(21), 5815–5823. doi:10.1021/es035414h PMID:15575305

Laxminarayan, R., & Chaudhury, R. R. (2016). Antibiotic Resistance in India: Drivers and Opportunities for Action. *PLoS Medicine*, *13*(3), e1001974. doi:10.1371/journal.pmed.1001974 PMID:26934098

Lazarides, A. A., Lance Kelly, K., Jensen, T. R., & Schatz, G. C. (2000). Optical properties of metal nanoparticles and nanoparticle aggregates important in biosensors. *Journal of Molecular Structure THEOCHEM*, *529*(1–3), 59–63. doi:10.1016/S0166-1280(00)00532-7

Lertsutthiwong & Rojsitthisak. (2011). *Chitosan-alginate nanocapsules for encapsulation of tumeric oil*. doi:10.1691/ph.2011.1068

Li, J., Zeng, H., Sun, S., Liu, J. P., & Wang, Z. L. (2004). Analyzing the Structure of CoFe– Fe3O4 Core– Shell Nanoparticles by Electron Imaging and Diffraction. *The Journal of Physical Chemistry B*, *108*(37), 14005–14008. doi:10.1021/jp047602f

Lu, W., Liu, G., Gao, S., Xing, S., & Wang, J. (2008). Tyrosine-assisted preparation of Ag/ZnO nanocomposites with enhanced photocatalytic performance and synergistic antibacterial activities. *Nanotechnology*, *19*(44), 445711. doi:10.1088/0957-4484/19/44/445711 PMID:21832753

Maggi, L., Carmona, M., Kelly, S. D., Marigheto, N., & Alonso, G. L. (2011). Geographical origin differentiation of saffron spice (Crocus sativus L. stigmas)–preliminary investigation using chemical and multi-element (H, C, N) stable isotope analysis. *Food Chemistry*, *128*(2), 543–548. doi:10.1016/j.foodchem.2011.03.063 PMID:25212167

Maliszewska, I., Szewczyk, K., & Waszak, K. (2009). Biological synthesis of silver nanoparticles. *Journal of Physics: Conference Series*, *146*(1), 012025. doi:10.1088/1742-6596/146/1/012025

Martin, R. C., Locatelli, E., Li, Y., Zhang, W., Li, S., Monaco, I., & Franchini, M. C. (2015). Gold nanorods and curcumin-loaded nanomicelles for efficient in vivo photothermal therapy of Barrett's esophagus. *Nanomedicine (London)*, *10*(11), 1723–1733. doi:10.2217/nnm.15.25 PMID:25706349

Mathew, S., Prakash, A., & Radhakrishnan, E. K. (2018). Sunlight mediated rapid synthesis of small size range silver nanoparticles using Zingiber officinale rhizome extract and its antibacterial activity analysis. *Inorganic and Nano-Metal Chemistry*, *48*(2), 139–145. doi:10.1080/24701556.2017.1373295

Meva, F. E. A., Segnou, M. L., Ebongue, C. O., Deli, V., Nyobe, J. C. N., & Mpondo, E. M. (2015). Synthesis, optimization and effect of condition reactions studies of seed kernel aqueous extract mediated silver nanoparticles from Ricinodendron heudelotii (*Baill*) Pierre Pax. Inter*national Journal of Biosciences, 7(4)*, 47–56. doi:10.12692/ijb/7.4.47-56

Milind, P., & Deepa, K. (2011). Pro-cholinergic, hypo-cholesterolemic and memory improving effects of clove. In*ternational Research Journal of Pharmacy,* 2(*4*), 119–126.

Montes, A., Bisson, M. A., Gardella, J. A. Jr, & Aga, D. S. (2017). Uptake and transformations of engineered nanomaterials: Critical responses observed in terrestrial plants and the model plant Arabidopsis thaliana. *The Science of the Total Environment*, *607*, 1497–1516. doi:10.1016/j.scitotenv.2017.06.190 PMID:28793406

Moritz, M., & Geszke-Moritz, M. (2013). The newest achievements in synthesis, immobilization and practical applications of antibacterial nanoparticles. *Chemical Engineering Journal*, *228*, 596–613. doi:10.1016/j.cej.2013.05.046

Muniyan, A., Ravi, K., Mohan, U., & Panchamoorthy, R. (2017). Characterization and in vitro antibacterial activity of saponin-conjugated silver nanoparticles against bacteria that cause burn wound infection. *World Journal of Microbiology & Biotechnology*, *33*(7), 147. doi:10.100711274-017-2309-3 PMID:28634713

Nadagouda, M. N., Hoag, G., Collins, J., & Varma, R. S. (2009). Green Synthesis of Au Nanostructures at Room Temperature Using Biodegradable Plant Surfactants. *Crystal Growth & Design*, *9*(11), 4979–4983. doi:10.1021/cg9007685

Naef, R., & Velluz, A. (2001). Volatile Constituents in Extracts of Mandarin and Tangerine Peel. *The Journal of Essential Oil Research*, *13*(3), 154–157. doi:10.1080/10412905.2001.9699647

Narayanan, K. B., & Sakthivel, N. (2008). Coriander leaf mediated biosynthesis of gold nanoparticles. *Materials Letters*, *62*(30), 4588–4590. doi:10.1016/j.matlet.2008.08.044

Oćwieja, M., Morga, M., & Adamczyk, Z. (2013). Self-assembled silver nanoparticles monolayers on mica-AFM, SEM, and electrokinetic characteristics. *Journal of Nanoparticle Research*, *15*(3), 1460. doi:10.100711051-013-1460-5 PMID:23519078

Panáček, A., Kvitek, L., Prucek, R., Kolář, M., Večeřová, R., Pizúrová, N., ... Zbořil, R. (2006). Silver colloid nanoparticles: Synthesis, characterization, and their antibacterial activity. *The Journal of Physical Chemistry B*, *110*(33), 16248–16253. doi:10.1021/jp063826h PMID:16913750

Paramelle, D., Sadovoy, A., Gorelik, S., Free, P., Hobley, J., & Fernig, D. G. (2014). A rapid method to estimate the concentration of citrate capped silver nanoparticles from UV-visible light spectra. *Analyst (London)*, *139*(19), 4855–4861. doi:10.1039/C4AN00978A PMID:25096538

Parashar, V., Parashar, R., Sharma, B., & Pandey, A. C. (2009). Parthenium leaf extract mediated synthesis of silver nanoparticles: A novel approach towards weed utilization. *Digest Journal of Nanomaterials and Biostructures*, *4*(1).

Patel, D., Perry, C., & Kennedy, S. (2007, February). Spectroscopic studies and AFM analysis of Ho3+ and Tm3+ doped yttrium oxide nanoparticles. In *Optical Components and Materials IV* (Vol. 6469). International Society for Optics and Photonics. doi:10.1117/12.701480

Pattanayak, M., & Nayak, P. L. (2013). Ecofriendly green synthesis of iron nanoparticles from various plants and spices extract. *International Journal of Plant. Animal and Environmental Sciences*, *3*(1), 68–78.

Perrault, S. D., & Chan, W. C. (2010). In vivo assembly of nanoparticle components to improve targeted cancer imaging. *Proceedings of the National Academy of Sciences of the United States of America*, *107*(25), 11194–11199. doi:10.1073/pnas.1001367107 PMID:20534561

Pitto-Barry, A., Perdigao, L. M., Walker, M., Lawrence, J., Costantini, G., Sadler, P. J., & Barry, N. P. (2015). Synthesis and controlled growth of osmium nanoparticles by electron irradiation. *Dalton Transactions (Cambridge, England)*, *44*(47), 20308–20311. doi:10.1039/C5DT03205A PMID:26418726

Press, C. R. C. (2002). *Handbook of Nutraceuticals and Functional Foods*. CRC Press.

Qiu, H., Gao, Y., Boott, C. E., Gould, O. E., Harniman, R. L., Miles, M. J., ... Manners, I. (2016). Uniform patchy and hollow rectangular platelet micelles from crystallizable polymer blends. *Science*, *352*(6286), 697–701. doi:10.1126cience.aad9521 PMID:27151866

Raghunandan, D., Bedre, M. D., Basavaraja, S., Sawle, B., Manjunath, S. Y., & Venkataraman, A. (2010). Rapid biosynthesis of irregular shaped gold nanoparticles from macerated aqueous extracellular dried clove buds (Syzygium aromaticum) solution. *Colloids and Surfaces. B, Biointerfaces*, *79*(1), 235–240. doi:10.1016/j.colsurfb.2010.04.003 PMID:20451362

Raghunandan, D., Borgaonkar, P. A., Bendegumble, B., Bedre, M. D., Bhagawanraju, M., Yalagatti, M. S., ... Abbaraju, V. (2011). Microwave-Assisted Rapid Extracellular Biosynthesis of Silver Nanoparticles Using Carom Seed (Trachyspermum copticum) Extract and in Vitro Studies. *American Journal of Analytical Chemistry*, *2*(4), 475–483. doi:10.4236/ajac.2011.24057

Raj, X. J., & Nishimura, T. (2014). Investigation of the Surface Potential on Iron Nanoparticles During the Corrosion by Atomic Force Microscopy (AFM) and Kelvin Probe Force Microscopy (KFM). *International Journal of Electrochemical Science*, *9*, 2090–2100.

Rajesh, K. M., Ajitha, B., Reddy, Y. A. K., Suneetha, Y., & Reddy, P. S. (2018). Assisted green synthesis of copper nanoparticles using Syzygium aromaticum bud extract: Physical, optical and antimicrobial properties. *Optik (Stuttgart)*, *154*, 593–600. doi:10.1016/j.ijleo.2017.10.074

Rane, A. V., Kanny, K., Abitha, V. K., & Thomas, S. (2018). Methods for synthesis of nanoparticles and fabrication of nanocomposites. In *Synthesis of inorganic nanomaterials* (pp. 121–139). Woodhead Publishing. doi:10.1016/B978-0-08-101975-7.00005-1

Reichert, J., Csáki, A., Köhler, J. M., & Fritzsche, W. (2000). Chip-Based Optical Detection of DNA Hybridization by Means of Nanobead Labeling. *Analytical Chemistry*, *72*(24), 6025–6029. doi:10.1021/ac000567y PMID:11140772

Rezvani, N., Sorooshzadeh, A., & Farhadi, N. (2012). Effect of nano-silver on growth of saffron in flooding stress. *World Academy of Science, Engineering and Technology*, *6*(1), 517–522.

Robert, M. (2015). Gold nanorods and curcumin-loaded nanomicelles for efficient in vivo photothermal therapy of Barrett's esophagus. *Nanomedicine (London)*, *10*(11), 1723–1733. doi:10.2217/nnm.15.25 PMID:25706349

Sahu, S., Rawat, D., & Singh, D. (2015). Antimicrobial activity of Trachyspermum ammi leaves mediated silver nanoparticles: Green approach. *International Journal of Research in Engineering and Technology*, *4*(9), 34–38. doi:10.15623/ijret.2015.0409006

Salam, H. A., Rajiv, P., Kamaraj, M., Jagadeeswaran, P., Gunalan, S., & Sivaraj, R. (2012). Plants: Green route for nanoparticle synthesis. *International Research Journal of Biological Sciences*, *1*(5), 85–90.

Sales, E. H., Sedeh, F. M., & Rajabifar, S. (2012). Effects of gamma irradiation and silver nano particles on microbiological characteristics of saffron, using hurdle technology. *Indian Journal of Microbiology*, *52*(1), 66–69. doi:10.100712088-011-0203-5 PMID:23449911

Sathyavathi, R., Krishna, M. B., Rao, S. V., Saritha, R., & Rao, D. N. (2010). Biosynthesis of silver nanoparticles using Coriandrum sativum leaf extract and their application in nonlinear optics. *Advanced Science Letters*, *3*(2), 138–143. doi:10.1166/asl.2010.1099

Senthil, B., Devasena, T., Prakash, B., & Rajasekar, A. (2017). Non-cytotoxic effect of green synthesized silver nanoparticles and its antibacterial activity. *Journal of Photochemistry and Photobiology. B, Biology*, *177*, 1–7. doi:10.1016/j.jphotobiol.2017.10.010 PMID:29028495

Seyed Mohammad, N., Dehpour, A. A., Ebrahimzadeh, M. A., & Seyed Fazel, N. (2009). Antioxidant activity of the methanol extract of Ferula assafoetida and its essential oil composition. *Grasas y Aceites*, *60*(4), 405–412. doi:10.3989/gya.010109

Shaban, M. A. E., Kandeel, K. M., Yacout, G. A., & Mehaseb, S. E. (1987). The chemical-composition of the volatile oil of elettaria cardamomum seeds. *Die Pharmazie*, *42*(3), 207–208.

Shalaby, T. I., Mahmoud, O. A., El Batouti, G. A., & Ibrahim, E. E. (2015). Green synthesis of silver nanoparticles: Synthesis, characterization and antibacterial activity. *Nanosci. Nanotechnol*, *5*(2), 23–29.

Shan, B., Cai, Y. Z., Brooks, J. D., & Corke, H. (2007). Antibacterial properties and major bioactive components of cinnamon stick (Cinnamomum burmannii): Activity against foodborne pathogenic bacteria. *Journal of Agricultural and Food Chemistry*, *55*(14), 5484–5490. doi:10.1021/jf070424d PMID:17567030

Shan, B., Cai, Y. Z., Sun, M., & Corke, H. (2005). Antioxidant capacity of 26 spice extracts and characterization of their phenolic constituents. *Journal of Agricultural and Food Chemistry*, *53*(20), 7749–7759. doi:10.1021/jf051513y PMID:16190627

Shankar, S. S., Ahmad, A., Pasricha, R., & Sastry, M. (2003). Bioreduction of chloroaurate ions by geranium leaves and its endophytic fungus yields gold nanoparticles of different shapes. *Journal of Materials Chemistry*, *13*(7), 1822–1826. doi:10.1039/b303808b

Sharma, G., Sharma, A. R., Kurian, M., Bhavesh, R., Nam, J. S., & Lee, S. S. (2014). Green synthesis of silver nanoparticle using myristica fragrans (nutmeg) seed extract and its biological activity. *Digest Journal of Nanomaterials and Biostructures*, *9*(1).

Sharma, V. K., Yngard, R. A., & Lin, Y. (2009). Silver nanoparticles: Green synthesis and their antimicrobial activities. *Advances in Colloid and Interface Science*, *145*(1–2), 83–96. doi:10.1016/j.cis.2008.09.002 PMID:18945421

Shevchenko, E. V., Talapin, D. V., Kotov, N. A., O'Brien, S., & Murray, C. B. (2006). Structural diversity in binary nanoparticle superlattices. *Nature, 439*(7072), 55–59. doi:10.1038/nature04414 PMID:16397494

Silva, A. C., da, Santos, P. D. de F., & Silva, J. T. (2018). Impact of curcumin nanoformulation on its antimicrobial activity. *Trends in Food Science & Technology, 72*, 74–82. doi:10.1016/j.tifs.2017.12.004

Singh, A. K., Talat, M., Singh, D. P., & Srivastava, O. N. (2010). Biosynthesis of gold and silver nanoparticles by natural precursor clove and their functionalization with amine group. *Journal of Nanoparticle Research, 12*(5), 1667–1675. doi:10.100711051-009-9835-3

Singh, D., Rathod, V., Ninganagouda, S., Herimath, J., & Kulkarni, P. (2013). Biosynthesis of silver nanoparticle by endophytic fungi Pencillium sp. isolated from Curcuma longa (turmeric) and its antibacterial activity against pathogenic gram negative bacteria. *Journal of Pharmacy Research, 7*(5), 448–453. doi:10.1016/j.jopr.2013.06.003

Singh, R. P., Magesh, S., & Rakkiyappan, C. (2011). Formation of fenugreek (Trigonella foenum-graecum) extract mediated Ag nanoparticles: Mechanism and applications. *Int J Bioeng Sci Technol, 2*(3), 64–73.

Singh, S. C., Zeng, H. B., Guo, C., & Cai, W. (Eds.). (2012). *Nanomaterials: processing and characterization with lasers*. John Wiley & Sons. doi:10.1002/9783527646821

Song, J. Y., Jang, H. K., & Kim, B. S. (2009). Biological synthesis of gold nanoparticles using Magnolia kobus and Diopyros kaki leaf extracts. *Process Biochemistry, 44*(10), 1133–1138. doi:10.1016/j.procbio.2009.06.005

Soshnikova, V., Kim, Y. J., Singh, P., Huo, Y., Markus, J., Ahn, S., ... Yang, D. C. (2017). Cardamom fruits as a green resource for facile synthesis of gold and silver nanoparticles and their biological applications. *Artificial Cells, Nanomedicine, and Biotechnology, 46*(1), 108–117. doi:10.1080/21691401.2017.1296849 PMID:28290213

Stokes, D. (2008). *Principles and practice of variable pressure/environmental scanning electron microscopy (VP-ESEM)*. John Wiley & Sons. doi:10.1002/9780470758731

Subhankari, I., & Nayak, P. L. (2013). Antimicrobial Activity of Copper Nanoparticles Synthesised by Ginger (Zingiber officinale) Extract. *World Journal of Nano Science & Technology, 2*(1), 10–13. doi:10.5829/idosi.wjnst.2013.2.1.21133

Sultanbawa, Y., & Sultanbawa, F. (2016). *Australian Native Plants: Cultivation and Uses in the Health and Food Industries*. CRC Press.

Thirumurugan, A., Jiflin, G. J., Rajagomathi, G., Tomy, N. A., Ramachandran, S., & Jaiganesh, R. (2010). Biotechnological synthesis of gold nanoparticles of Azadirachta indica leaf extract. *Internat J Biol Technol, 1*, 75–77.

Thomas, R., Nair, A. P., Soumya, K. R., Mathew, J., & Radhakrishnan, E. K. (2014). Antibacterial activity and synergistic effect of biosynthesized AgNPs with antibiotics against multidrug-resistant biofilm-forming coagulase-negative staphylococci isolated from clinical samples. *Applied Biochemistry and Biotechnology*, *173*(2), 449–460. doi:10.100712010-014-0852-z PMID:24699812

Tzitzios, V., Basina, G., Gjoka, M., Alexandrakis, V., Georgakilas, V., Niarchos, D., ... Petridis, D. (2006). Chemical synthesis and characterization of hcp Ni nanoparticles. *Nanotechnology*, *17*(15), 3750–3755. doi:10.1088/0957-4484/17/15/023

Valle Garcia-Rodriguez, M., Serrano-Diaz, J., Tarantilis, P. A., López-Córcoles, H., Carmona, M., & Alonso, G. L. (2014). Determination of saffron quality by high-performance liquid chromatography. *Journal of Agricultural and Food Chemistry*, *62*(32), 8068–8074. doi:10.1021/jf5019356 PMID:25075549

Velmurugan, P., Anbalagan, K., Manosathyadevan, M., Lee, K.-J., Cho, M., Lee, S.-M., ... Oh, B.-T. (2014). Green synthesis of silver and gold nanoparticles using Zingiber officinale root extract and antibacterial activity of silver nanoparticles against food pathogens. *Bioprocess and Biosystems Engineering*, *37*(10), 1935–1943. doi:10.100700449-014-1169-6 PMID:24668029

Verma, V. C., Kharwar, R. N., & Gange, A. C. (2010). Biosynthesis of antimicrobial silver nanoparticles by the endophytic fungus Aspergillus clavatus. *Nanomedicine (London)*, *5*(1), 33–40. doi:10.2217/nnm.09.77 PMID:20025462

Vidal-Vidal, J., Rivas, J., & López-Quintela, M. A. (2006). Synthesis of monodisperse maghemite nanoparticles by the microemulsion method. *Colloids and Surfaces. A, Physicochemical and Engineering Aspects*, *288*(1-3), 44–51. doi:10.1016/j.colsurfa.2006.04.027

Vijayakumar, R., Devi, V., Adavallan, K., & Saranya, D. (2011). Green synthesis and characterization of gold nanoparticles using extract of anti-tumor potent Crocus sativus. *Physica E, Low-Dimensional Systems and Nanostructures*, *44*(3), 665–671. doi:10.1016/j.physe.2011.11.002

Vilalta-Clemente, A., Gloystein, K., & Frangis, N. (2008). Principles of Atomic Force Microscopy (AFM). *Proceedings of Physics of Advanced Materials Winter School.*

Waidha, A. I., Pandiyarasan, V., Anusya, T., Waidha, K. M., Shah, A. H., & Pandiyarasan, V. (2015). Synthesis and characterization of silver nano rod like structures by green synthesis method using Curcumin longa. *International Journal of Chemtech Research*, *7*, 1504–1508.

Walkey, C. D., Olsen, J. B., Guo, H., Emili, A., & Chan, W. C. (2012). Nanoparticle size and surface chemistry determine serum protein adsorption and macrophage uptake. *Journal of the American Chemical Society*, *134*(4), 2139–2147. doi:10.1021/ja2084338 PMID:22191645

Wang, C., Kim, Y. J., Singh, P., Mathiyalagan, R., Jin, Y., & Yang, D. C. (2016). Green synthesis of silver nanoparticles by Bacillus methylotrophicus, and their antimicrobial activity. *Artificial Cells, Nanomedicine, and Biotechnology*, *44*(4), 1127–1132. PMID:25749281

Wei, D., Sun, W., Qian, W., Ye, Y., & Ma, X. (2009). The synthesis of chitosan-based silver nanoparticles and their antibacterial activity. *Carbohydrate Research*, *344*(17), 2375–2382. doi:10.1016/j.carres.2009.09.001 PMID:19800053

Wisam, J. A., & Haneen, A. J. (2018). A novel study of pH influence on Ag nanoparticles size with antibacterial and antifungal activity using green synthesis. *World Scientific News*, *97*, 139–152.

Yang, J.-F., Yang, C.-H., Chang, H.-W., Yang, C.-S., Wang, S.-M., Hsieh, M.-C., & Chuang, L.-Y. (2010). Chemical Composition and Antibacterial Activities of Illicium verum Against Antibiotic-Resistant Pathogens. *Journal of Medicinal Food*, *13*(5), 1254–1262. doi:10.1089/jmf.2010.1086 PMID:20828316

Yue, J., Feliciano, T. J., Li, W., Lee, A., & Odom, T. W. (2017). Gold nanoparticle size and shape effects on cellular uptake and intracellular distribution of siRNA nanoconstructs. *Bioconjugate Chemistry*, *28*(6), 1791–1800. doi:10.1021/acs.bioconjchem.7b00252 PMID:28574255

Zare, E., Pourseyedi, S., Khatami, M., & Darezereshki, E. (2017). Simple biosynthesis of zinc oxide nanoparticles using nature's source, and it's in vitro bio-activity. *Journal of Molecular Structure*, *1146*, 96–103. doi:10.1016/j.molstruc.2017.05.118

Zhang, M., Viennois, E., Prasad, M., Zhang, Y., Wang, L., Zhang, Z., ... Merlin, D. (2016). Edible ginger-derived nanoparticles: A novel therapeutic approach for the prevention and treatment of inflammatory bowel disease and colitis-associated cancer. *Biomaterials*, *101*, 321–340. doi:10.1016/j.biomaterials.2016.06.018 PMID:27318094

Zhaveh, S., Mohsenifar, A., Beiki, M., Khalili, S. T., Abdollahi, A., Rahmani-Cherati, T., & Tabatabaei, M. (2015). Encapsulation of Cuminum cyminum essential oils in chitosan-caffeic acid nanogel with enhanced antimicrobial activity against Aspergillus flavus. *Industrial Crops and Products*, *69*, 251–256. doi:10.1016/j.indcrop.2015.02.028

Zhuang, X., Deng, Z.-B., Mu, J., Zhang, L., Yan, J., Miller, D., ... Zhang, H.-G. (2015). Ginger-derived nanoparticles protect against alcohol-induced liver damage. *Journal of Extracellular Vesicles*, *4*(1), 28713. doi:10.3402/jcv.v4.28713 PMID:26610593

Zielinski, M. V. (2014). *Determination of thiamine in solution by UV-visible spectrophotometry: The effect of interactions with gold nanoparticles*. Academic Press.

Zomorodian, K., Saharkhiz, J., Pakshir, K., Immeripour, Z., & Sadatsharifi, A. (2018). The composition, antibiofilm and antimicrobial activities of essential oil of Ferula assa-foetida oleo-gum-resin. *Biocatalysis and Agricultural Biotechnology*, *14*, 300–304. doi:10.1016/j.bcab.2018.03.014

Chapter 17
Importance of Pest and Pathogen Control System With Special Emphasis on Coriander Crop on the Indian Subcontinent

Sunita Rao
Mody University of Science and Technology, India

Gajra Garg
MJRP University, Jaipur, India

ABSTRACT

India is a country known for its status as the largest producer and consumer for the crop Coriandrum sativum (L.). Improvement and alteration of cultivation techniques is highly required as the crop is highly susceptible to various diseases that are responsible for crop loss with small and marginal farmers every year. Proper guidance for soil preparation and nutritional fulfillment can result in a better yield of the spice crop. Integrated efforts for soil fertility with on-time pest management will enhance both productivity and profit. Therefore, a concise approach for pest-crop- pathogen management systems of coriander crops have been vividly presented in the present review chapter.

INTRODUCTION

Coriander of commerce is the dried ripe fruits of *Coriandrum sativum* (L.), also known as cilantro or Chinese parsley. It is one of the first spices to be used by humankind, having been identified as early as 5,000 B.C. The plant is an important member of the family Umbelliferae (Apiaceae) along with other 200 genera and 2900 species. The plant is indigenous to the Mediterranean region, extensively in India, Morocco, Russia, Hungary, Poland, Rumania, Czechoslovakia, Guatemala, Mexico, Turkey, and

DOI: 10.4018/978-1-7998-2524-1.ch017

Argentina (Coskuner and Karababa, 2007). It is a small aromatic annual herb, attaining a height of 0.3-1 meters. The lower leaves are broad with crenate-lobed Margins, and the upper one is finely cut with linear lobes. The flowers are white or pinkish arranged in compound terminal umbels (Burdock and Carabin, 2009). The fruit is a nearly globular, yellow-brown schizocarp. The plant requires a warm, dry summer with short, rainy winters and is cultivated as a cold-weather crop in northern India, mainly in Rajasthan, Uttar Pradesh, and Uttrakhand. The chemical composition of coriander seeds varies depending upon the country of its origin, agro-climatic, harvesting, and storage conditions. On average, seeds contain moisture (6.3%), protein (1.3%), fat (19.6%), carbohydrates (24%), mineral matter (5.3%), crude fiber (31.5%), and few traces of vitamin. Seeds are a good source of volatile and crude oil, tannins, saponins, cellulose, pentosans, and pigments. The seed oil is colorless or sometimes a pale yellow with a characteristic odor and taste. Indian coriander contains 45-70% coriander oil, which possesses a sweet and pleasant odor (Axel Diederichsen et al., 1996). The main components of the essential oil include linalool, linalyl acetate, geranial, camphor, limonene, geranyl acetate, γ-terpinene, etc. Linalool is the bioactive compound found to occur at high concentrations (70%) in the extract. It is used as an additive for processed foods, beverages, and as a fragrance ingredient in cosmetics and household detergent. It is the main compound responsible for its anti-microbial and anti-diabetic effects of cilantro seeds. As a medicinal plant, coriander has been used as an antifungal (Basilico and Basilico, 1999), antioxidant (Chithra and Leelamma, 1999), hypolipidemic (Chithra and Leelamma, 2000), antimicrobial (Singh, 2002), hypocholesterolemic (Chithra and Leelamma, 1997), and anticonvulsant substance (Hossein and Mohammad, 2000). In the traditional medicinal system, the leaves and fruits of the plant have been used to treat skin disease, and its paste is applied by mixing in water to wash the face and forehead. Also, it has been used as a carminative, stimulating, diuretic, tonic, stomachic agent by the people to get rid of the bad breath and mouth diseases. The leaves have been reported to treat convulsion, insomnia and anxiety and used to improve appetite (Heider, 1992) and much more, as shown in Figure 1.

The present review gives an overview of the better growth conditions required by plants so that it can be protected from pests and pathogensa. Pests belong to the phylum arthropods, which can harm the standing crop that has been listed here with preventive measures required, and the farmers must follow control strategies. In a nut-shell, the present review can be proven helpful for betterment for marginal and small farmers.

Diseases and Pests Affecting Coriander Crop Every Year

All developing nations are in high demand for better food and nutritional security. Still, there are few shortcomings, like numerous abiotic and biotic factors that are responsible for the fall in yield every year. Among the biotic factors, pathogens are highly accountable for the loss. These pathogens can get associated with the plants or crops since the very first day of sowing or can gain access to the produce after harvesting. During storage, these can be associated easily with the seeds externally or internally and extramurally or intramurally as a contaminant as well as related to inert matter. The most crucial step is to trace the exact location of the pathogen in the field or in storage for better management.

Coriander or cilantro has been affected by various pests and pathogens and a few are specifically attacking the crop, the rest of others are generalized pathogens, which have been summarized in Tables 1 and 2, respectively. According to Palamarja and Chotina (1953), fruits of coriander after harvesting will redistribute the bacteria among the healthy crop in the next sowing season. In 1995, Toben was able to describe biology, etiology, and the lifecycle of

Figure 1. Importance of Coriander sativum (L.) for the treatment of various diseases

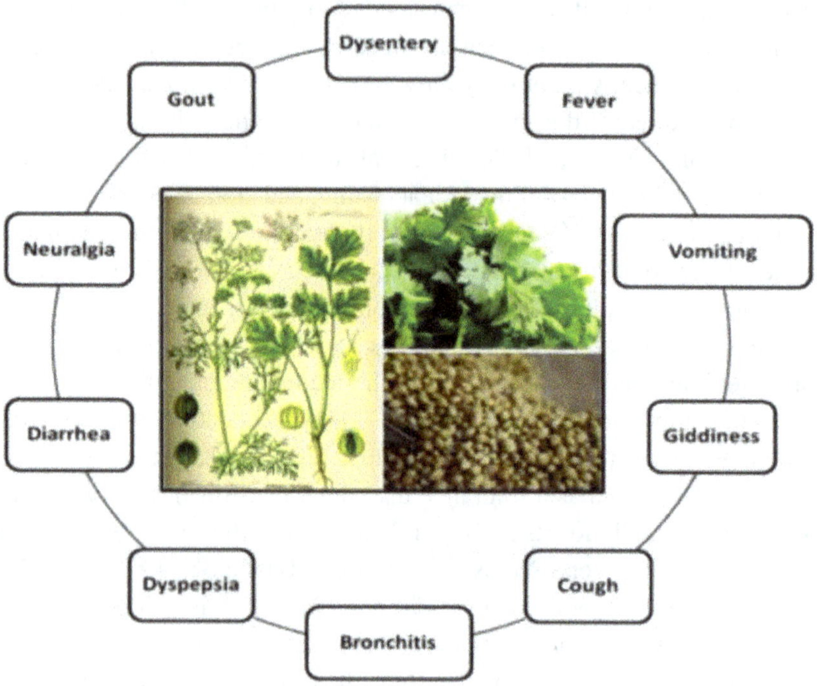

P. syringae pv. *Coriandricola,* associated with coriander. Two possibilities had been noted down for the spreading of the disease. First, in the process of pollination, these bacteria get adhered to the pollinating insects. They are transmitted to other plants, and later the same bacteria gets placed on the fruits and transferred to a long-distance during export and consumption. Secondly, the bacteria gets a room on the plant in the field, which is the same genus but is of different species or maybe with the aweeds. In the continuation, heat treatment has been proven a preventive measure for ripe fruits. Before sowing, these seeds must be treated with dry heat at approx. 65°C for at least six days so that infection can be effectively controlled and will not be transferred to the plants of the next-generation (Toben et al. 1994).

In extension to the previous work, Toben (1995) mentioned that other bacterial diseases affecting coriander crops are the *Erwinia* and *Xanthomonas* species along with several fungal infections. In Europe, *Ramularia coriandri* is of particular importance, and resistance breeding of this fungus has been carried out in the former Soviet Union. *Fusarium oxysporum* causes coriander wilt, and screenings of the resistant variety against this pathogen were done by Prakasam et al. (1987). Stem galls have been caused by *Protomyces macrosporus* (Das 1971), Grain mold diseases caused by *Helminthosporium* spp., *Fusarium* spp., *Curvularia* spp. and *Alternaria* spp. were studied by Rajan et al. (1990). Other fungal diseases are mildew (*Erisyphe polygoni*), rust, and leaf spots. The symptoms of several fungal diseases of the green plant are described by Palamarja and Chotina (1953). Fungicides for treatment of the seeds or application in the field do exist but had shown limited effects on the two viral diseases mentioned for coriander. The Alfalfa mosaic virus was isolated from coriander in Yemen (Alhubaishi et al. 1987). A specific insect adversely affecting the coriander is Systole coriandri (*Systole albipennis*), whose larva damages the fruits and survives for longer durations. Seeds of the affected fruits should be avoided for sowing. Jansen (1981) had described the severe losses of fruits caused by the chalcid fly *Systole albipen-*

Table 1. Microbial diseases affecting the production of coriander sativum (L.) crop

Disease/ pathogen	Symptoms	Favorable Conditions	Treatment
1. Powdery mildew *Erysiphe polygon* 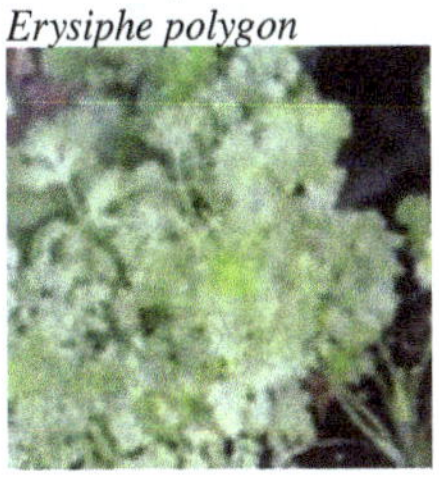	Visible small, white, powdery patches on young parts of stems, leaves. The occurrence of the premature sterility. Seed formation may not take place in affected plants.	The fungus can survive for the long term in the form of cleistothecia Capable of spreading by means of air. High humidity and cloudy weather are supportive of the disease. Most severe in the shad areas.	1.Pseudomonas fluorescent spray 10 g/kg 2.Wettable sulfur 1 kg/ha 3.Dinocap 250 ml/ha at the time of initial appearance of the disease and 2nd spray at ten days interval. 4.Neem seed kernel extracts 5 % by spraying on young plantlets
2. Wilt *Fusarium oxysporum sp. Coriander* 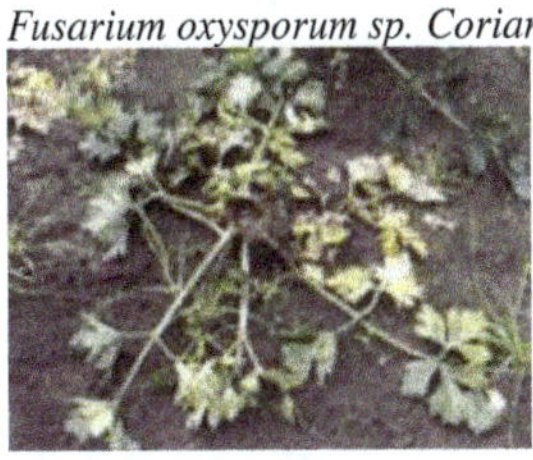	Drooping of the terminal portions, followed by withering and drying up of leaves. Discoloration of vascular system of the root is observed. Leaves become pinkish yellow to pale yellow.	The disease is soil borne. High soil moisture and temperature is responsible for the infection.	Treatment of Pseudomonas fluorescens (10g/kg) before sowing to seeds.
3. Stem gall *Protomyces macrospores Unger* 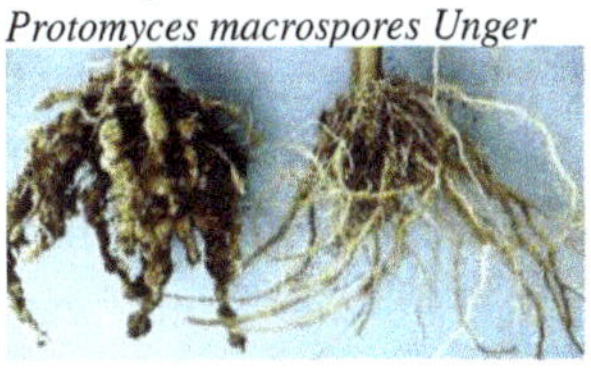	Swelling of leaf veins, stalks, peduncles, stems, as well as fruits. The infected leaf veins show a swollen hanging appearance to the leaves. Initially, the tumors are glossy in appearance, which ruptures later on and becomes rough.	High soil moisture and soil temperature is responsible for the infection.	1. Seeds treated with Thiram 4 g/kg and carbendazim2g/kg, before sowing. 2. A 0.1 % carbendazim at an interval of 20 days till the disease is incomplete controlled (Sharma et al. 2016)
4. Blight disease *Alternaria alternata* 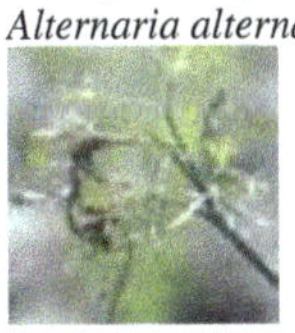	Dark brown spots appear on the stem and leaves of infected plants, emerging with no blooming flowers.	If soil is 70% moist and the weather is (12-25°C) An intermittent rain favors disease development.	1. A 0.2 % Mancozeb solution should be used to control the disease (Sharma et al. 2016)
5. Stem rot *Sclerotinia sclerotiorum* 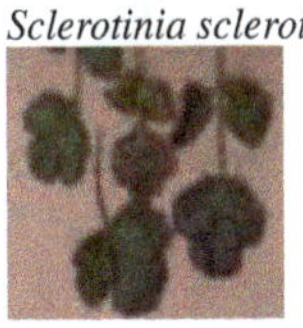	Infected seeds fail to germinate; rapid death of germinating seeds before emergence; water-soaked reddish lesions girdling the stem at the collar region results in the collapsing of emerged seedlings.	Fungus can spread by water, contaminated soil, or on equipment. Rainy season favors the development of the disease. Sclerotic infected plant parts or on the soil surface or with seed as a contaminant	

nis in Ethiopia, and reports the possibility of their biological control by the parasites *Tetrastichus* spp. and *Liondontomerus* spp. Singh and Baswana (1984) were successful in the screening of coriander for resistance to this specific pest in India. The aphids *Myzus persicae* (de Araujo, 1986) and *Hyadaphis coriandri* (Jain and Yadav 1988) have been mentioned for coriander. Other insect pests and methods to combat them, by sowing time or with pesticides, are described by Jain and Yadav (1989). One of them, the biscuit beetle (*Stegobium paniceum*) was also found in seed samples from genebanks. These insect pests can cause genetic erosion, and genebank curators need to ensure that the stored fruits are free of them. In India coriander has been screened several times for resistance to the nematodes *Meloidogyne incognita* (Midha and Trivedi 1988) and *Meloidogyne javanica* (Paruthi et al. 1987).

Apart from bacterial and fungal infections, few visible symptoms are commonly seen on the plant body as a result of the attack of the pests from the Arthropod phylum, which is the largest known phylum on earth and severely affects coriander crop has been listed in Table 2.

PROVEN REMEDIES FOR BETTER YIELD OF CROP

Enrichment of Soil

A most important step in coriander cultivation is the preparation of the soil bed, which is essential for nutrient and air supply as well as for getting rid of the existing pests and future outbreaks. Organic manure can be a good alternative for cultivation, as it can improve soil fertility, and in comparison to inorganic fertilizers, it can resist soft green growth, which is a good source of energy and food for pests.

Crop Rotation

Every year, growing the same crop in the same field can bring many unwanted pests and diseases, leading to various types of crop loss to the coriander crop. A possible reason is that pests and insects will become resistant after a few seasons due to the gain of resistance in the genome against the application of the same pesticide over some time. The plants can be grouped like onion and brinjal in which significant results have been obtained for the benefit of both the crops (Paul et al., 2015). Similarly, vegetables like carrots, celery, anise, coriander, dill, fennel, parsley should be kept on rotating in the same field over some time so that nutrient depletion can be controlled as well pests invading can be monitored easily.

Betterment of Growth Condition

A well-known and practiced fact is that the sowing season plays a vital role in the growth of the crop and to the disease-free condition as well. The period of October to December is appropriate for green leaves and the first fortnight of November is for the spice seed crop in India. The whole seed of coriander should not sow at once, it is advised to be divided into halves and grown. Spacing between the rows should be 20-30cm and plant to plant should be 20cm; this positioning and spacing condition is appropriate for better growth and yield.

Beneficial Organisms for the Crop

After sowing, weed removal is another important task that should be done at the proper time. Few crop-friendly insects can attract and eradicate pests such as ladybird, lacewings, frogs, toads, hedgehogs, and other domestic small birds.

Table 2. Infective pests affecting the coriander crop

Pathogen	Symptoms	Preventions	Control of disease
Aphids ***Cavariella aegopodii*** 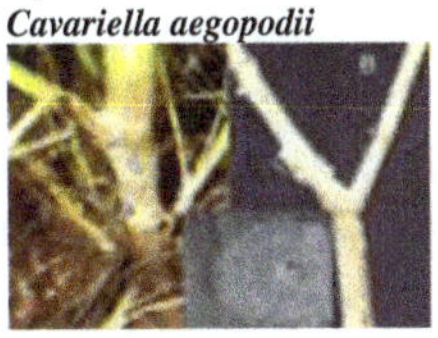	The pest causes the yellowing of the leaves with distorted and necrotic lesions on it and resulting in stunted growth of the plant. If there is a prolong period of stay on the stem, these start to secrete honeydew, which is sticky to touch results into the sooty mold on the plants.	Advisable to procure tolerant varieties of the crop. Silver colored plastic can prevent aphids from attacking and feeding on plants.	1. Spray of 1 % seed extract of neem (Azadirachata indica), karanj (Pongamia sp.), buken (Melia sp.) and pride of India (Lagerstroemia indica) 2. Spraying of Dimethoate 30 EC or Methyl demetone 25 EC 1 ltr / ha before flowering can control aphid population considerably.
Armyworm ***Pseudaletia unipuncta* Armyworm** 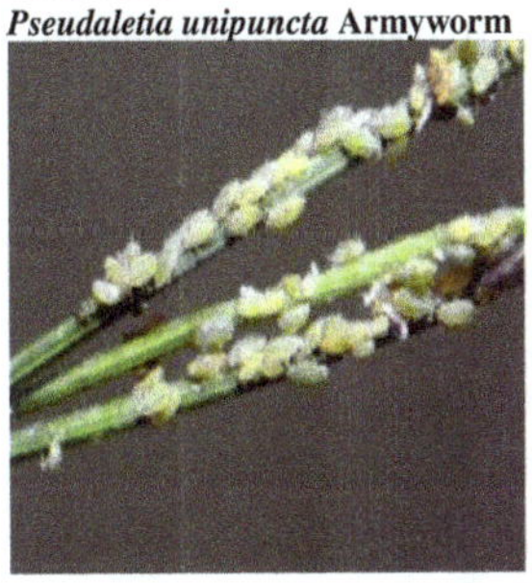	The appearance of single, adjacently grouped circular to irregularly shaped holes in leaves. Overfeeding by young larvae leads to skeletonized leaves, shallow, dry wounds on fruits. Egg clusters of 50-150 eggs may be present on the leaves, covered in a whitish scale that eventually destroys the stem.	1. Parasitize the larvae and the application of Bacillus thuringiensis of the worms. 2. Proper monitoring is required for better control.	
Cutworms ***Agrotis spp.*** 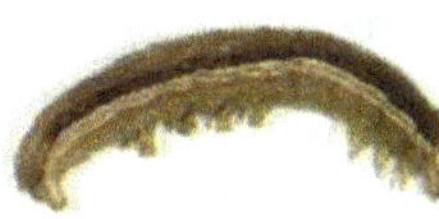	Infestation by worm occurs when the stem of young plantlet or seedlings touches at the soil line, irregular holes appear at the surface of fruits. The Larva becomes active at night and habitual to hide in the day time, at the base of the plants, or in plant debris of toppled plant. The larva is 2.5–5.0 cm long and may exhibit a variety of patterns and coloration but usually curl up into a C-shape when disturbed.	Cutworms have a wide host range and attack seasonal vegetables like asparagus, bean, cabbage corn, lettuce, pea, pepper, potato, and tomato.	1. Removal of the infected plant residue from the soil after harvest is necessary to step or at least two weeks before planting; this is especially important if the previous crop was another host such as alfalfa, beans or a leguminous cover crop 2. Plastic or foil collars fitted around plant stems a few centimeters above the soil line.
White Fly 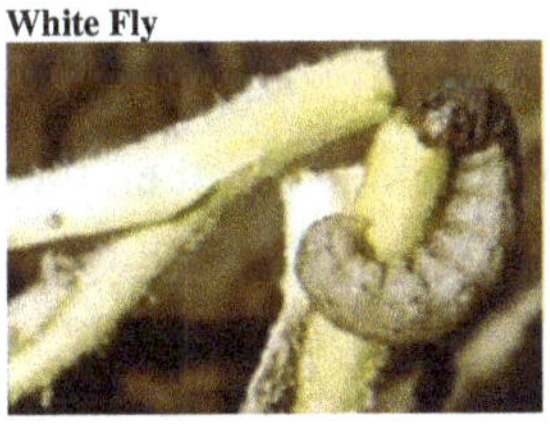	They remain underside the leaves and suck the sap. Continuous sucking the sap from the leaves results in chlorotic spots and later on leaves coalesce and become brittle and finally drop down from the plant prematurely	The honeydew secreted by the pest drop on the upper surface of the lower leaves and helps in the development of shooty molds which interferes with the photosynthesis of leaves (Kant et al. 2016).	Spraying of Dimethoate 30 EC or Methyl gemstone 25 EC one liter per ha before flowering can control aphid population considerably. This spray may be repeated in 10 days intervals. (Govt. of Raj. 2014)
Mite ***Petrobia lateens* (Muller)**	It remains active during winter with peak activity in March. It is a minute, no webbing and swift-moving mite and tends to dislodge from the plant which disturbed. The larva, nymphs, and adults feed on upper as well as the lower surface of leaves, leaf sheaths, and floral parts. Infested leaves started withering from the top downwards.	The plants become chlorotic due to loss of cell sap, resulting in poor seed formation. Heavily infested plants show sickly yellowish or bronzing appearance	

Field Free of Junk Material

Fields should be free of dumping yards, since old wood planks and dark and damp hides attract many night-dwellers like slugs and snails where they want to get shelter and later on at the same time will start uprooting the plants. Similarly, huge stones and old paving slabs also invite pests and predators of the crop. A junk free field is also important because it makes the hand removal of weeds a bit easier.

The Excessive Number of Plants in the Same Field

Seeds are required for the sowing and propagation of the crop. While sowing, initial growth after 48 hours is important because all the seeds come out of the soil as a seedling. This number is more than the actual requirement, although the seeds are the same, because its response to environmental conditions varies. So it is important to select only plants that seem to be healthier and taller in the whole slot on the soil bed. It can improve the chances of getting healthier plants and also helps in better utilization of resources.

Importance of Spacing In-Between the Plants

Spacing among plants and each row is a very important aspect for better yield. If the field is very crowded with nearly situated plants, then it makes the plants lack a proper supply of oxygen and also devoids them of required nutrients. If the condition persists for a longer duration, then rain or garden water will not evaporate easily, which leads to damping of the soil and supports the growth of molds and other fungus.

Selection of a Resistant Variety of the Crop

Re-emergence of the same pest or disease points towards selecting a better or more resistant variety for the upcoming season. The carrot fly is among one of the most prevalent pests all over the world known for damaging the crop. Still, no variety has been released that is resistant to this particular pest.

Field Free Of Seasonal Pests

During sowing season, if the forecast of weather is accurate, the emergence of pests is decidable and easily farmers can protect the crop from pests. If the farmer had all the information about weather, then planting of coriander early or late according to the time of the outbreak of aphids is possible. Similarly, if the forecast is proper, delaying in sowing will retard the plants growth. Thereby, flowering could be delayed, which will protect it from the moth, which is now incapable of egg-laying in the flower, hence the plant is preserved from the insect. Similar strategies could be planned which can protect the plants from seasonal pests.

Crop Management

There should be some preventive measures considered by farmers to protect the crop from infections. As per the advisory released by the local government and active scientists in the area, common cultural practices such as deep ploughing and soil solarizatuion have been suggested. Deep ploughing in fields during summer is used to control the nematode's population. Soil solarization is a technique in which soil beds are covered with 0.45 mm polythene sheets for 2-3 weeks before sowing, which will help in reducing the soil-borne pests and weeds. Castor plants can be grown as a trap crop which can manage spodopetra. Maize and sorghum can be proven alternatives for the management of whitefly, aphids, and mites. Crop rotation has also been proven to be effective against various pathogens. Application of

Trichoderma harzianum /viride and *Pseudomonas fluorescens* for treatment of seed/seedling/planting materials in the nurseries is also a proven method for better crop yield.

Removal of Weeds From The Field

There are a few weeds that intensively affect the crop yield; these are as follows: *Chenopodium album* L. (Chenopodiaceae); *Melilotus indica* L. (Fabaceae); *Asphodelus tenuifolius* Cav. (Liliaceae); *Anagallis arvensis* L. (Primulaceae); *Phalaris minor* Retz. (Poaceae); *Cynodon dactylon* L. (Pers.) (Poaceae) and *Cyperus rotundus* L. (Cyperaceae). These can lead to huge losses as they are able to dominate over the coriander crop and, if not removed on time, can lead to 100 percent yield loss. So, a weed control program is required along with the high inputs. For instance, hand weeding is one popular method across the world because the herbicide is not required, which has proven to be a danger to the earth in many ways but will not be a topic of discussion here. Hand weeding is not possible for those countries like Mexico and the U.S. because of labor cost, which is comparatively higher in these countries (Calvin et al. 2004; Martin 2007). Combinations of antigraminaceous herbicide Tiger platinum with soil-applied herbicides Tender, Silba Sharpen, Merlin flex, Smerch and Raft, and foliarly-applied herbicides Kalin flo, Eclipse, Sultan, Corrida and Lontrel does not reduce herbicide efficacy.

Deficiency of Nutrient

Macronutrients are essential for the growth of the coriander crop. The balanced supply of macronutrients is always required for the proper growth of plants (Amjad et al. 2014). Similarly, the role of micronutrients is not subjective to ignorance as these play an important role in chlorophyll functioning, nitrogen fixation, respiration, and various other metabolic processes as per the report of Sivaiah et al. 2013. Several other research groups had been exploring the effect of the micronutrient fertilizers on aromatic plants and successfully concluded that micronutrients appreciably improve the number of branches, umbel per plants, and seed yield (Nasiri et al. 2010; Joynul et al. 2012; Mazaheri et al. 2013). Nitrogen should be sprayed to the crops as a 1-2% foliar spray to the young plantlets to prevent the yellowing of the old leaves and to prevent stunted plant growth. Phosphorus is required through fertilizers at 4-5 kg/ acre or foliar spray of DAP at 2% for prevention of stunted growth and for prevention of the leaves changing color from purple to red (Kalidasu et al. 2008).

CONCLUSION

To conclude the article it is important to draw an inference about the requirement of better cultivation technology to prevent marginal and small farmers from huge losses because of weeds, pests, and pathogens. In India, traditional practices and tools are more practiced which has a poor working efficiency for coriander crops. Modern tools and technology are not only robust but also include suitable resistant varieties, weed eradication methods, and nutrient and pest management. These measures can surely help the farmers to get a better yield. The scene of "production equals consumption" could be changed shortly to meet the world's requirement exactly.

REFERENCES

Al-Shinawi, T. A. (1993). *Untersuchungen zur Anfälligkeit verschiedener Korianderherkünfte (Coriandrum sativum L.) für den Erreger der „Bakteriellen Doldenwelke" Pseudomonas syringae pv. coriandricola.* Magisterarbeit, Institut für Pflanzenpathologie und Pflanzenschutz, Universität Göttingen.

Alhubaishi, A. A., Walkey, D. G. A., Webb, M. J. W., Bolland, C. J., & Cook, A. A. (1987). A survey of horticultural plant virus diseases in the Yemen Arab Republic. *FAO Plant Protection Bulletin, 35*, 135–143.

Amjad, A., Sajida, P., Syed, N., Muhammad, S., Zengqiang, Z., Fazli, W., ... Abdul, M. (2014). Effect of foliar application of micronutrients on fruit quality of peach. *American Journal of Plant Sciences, 5*(09), 1258–1264. doi:10.4236/ajps.2014.59138

Araujo, C. Z. D. (1986). Occurrence of *Myzus persicae* (Sulzer, 1776) (*Homoptera, Aphididae*) on a crop of coriander *Coriandrum sativum* (Umbelliferae). *Anais da Sociedade Entomológica do Brasil, 15*, 173–174.

Avendan˜o & Schwentesius. (2004). The economics of food safety: the case of green onions and hepatitis A outbreaks. *USDA Economics Research Service*. http://www.ers.usda.gov/publications/vgs/nov04/ VGS30501/ VGS30501.pdf

Basilico, M. Z., & Basilico, J. C. (1999). Inhibitory effects of some spice essential oils on *Aspergillus ochraceus* NRRL 3174 growth and ochratoxin A production. *Letters in Applied Microbiology, 29*(4), 238–241. doi:10.1046/j.1365-2672.1999.00621.x PMID:10583751

Burdock, G. A., & Carabin, I. G. (2009). Safety assessment of coriander (*Coriandrum sativum* L.) essential oil as a food ingredient. *Food and Chemical Toxicology, 47*(1), 22–34. doi:10.1016/j.fct.2008.11.006 PMID:19032971

Chaudry, N. M. A., & Tariq, P. (2006). Bactericidal activity of black pepper, bay leaf, aniseed and coriander against oral isolates. *Pakistan Journal of Pharmaceutical Sciences, 19*, 214–218. PMID:16935829

Chithra, V., & Leelamma, S. (1999). *Coriandrum sativum* changes the levels of lipid peroxides and activity of antioxidant enzymes in experimental animals. *Indian Journal of Biochemistry & Biophysics, 36*(1), 59–61. PMID:10549163

Chithra, V., & Leelamma, S. (2000). *Coriandrum sativum*—Effect on lipid metabolism in 1,2-dimethyl hydrazine induced colon cancer. *Journal of Ethnopharmacology, 71*(3), 457–463. doi:10.1016/S0378-8741(00)00182-3 PMID:10940583

Coskuner, Y., & Karababa, E. (2007). Physical properties of coriander seeds (*Coriandrum sativum* L.). J. *Food Engineering, 80*(2), 408–416. doi:10.1016/j.jfoodeng.2006.02.042

Das, A. M. (1971). Studies on stem gall disease of coriander incited by *Protomyces macrosporus*. *Second International Symposium on Plant Pathology*.

Diederichsen, A. (1996). *Promoting the conservation and use of underutilized and neglected crops: Coriander (Coriandrum sativum L)* (1st ed.). International Plant Genetic Resources Institute IPGRI.

Heider, M. (1992). *Coriandrum sativum*: Applications of plants Prevention and Treatment of Illnesses. *Persian*, *1*, 247–252.

Jain, P. C., & Yadav, C. P. S. (1988). Relative susceptibility of coriander varieties to coriander aphid (*Hyadaphis coriandri* Das). *Indian Journal of Entomology*, *50*, 535–536.

Jain, P. C., & Yadav, C. P. S. (1989). Incidence of pests and their control on coriander. Indian Cocoa. *Arecanut and Spices J.*, *13*, 61–62.

Jansen, P. C. M. (1981). Coriandrum sativum L. condiments and medicinal plants in Ethiopia, their taxonomy and agricultural significance. College of Agriculture, Addis Ababa University, Ethiopia and The Agricultural University, Wageningen, The Netherlands.

Joynul, A. M., Nurul, A. M., Jamal, H. M., Nure, A. A., Kazi, M., & Faisal, H. (2012). Effect of micronutrients on growth and yield of onion under calcareous soil environment. *International Journal of Biosciences*, *2*, 95–101.

Kalidasu, G., Sarada, C., & Yellamanda, R. T. (2008). Influence of micronutrients on growth and yield of coriander (*Coriandrum sativum*) in rainfed vertisols. *Journal of Spices and Aromatic Crops*, *17*, 187–189.

Martin, P. (2007). Farm Labor Shortages: How Real, What Responses? ARE Update. *University of California, Davis*. http://www.agecon.ucdavis.edu/extension/update/articles/v10n5_3.pdf

Mazaheri, M., Fakheri, B., Piri, I., & Tavassoli, A. (2013). The effect of drought stress and micronutrient of Zn and Mn on yield and essential oil of (*Cuminum cyminum*). *Journal of Novel Applied Sciences*, *2*, 350–356.

Midha, R. L., & Trivedi, P. C. (1988). Evaluation of coriander varieties against *Meloidogyne incognita*. *Indian J. Nematol.*, *18*, 375.

Naga, S. K., Swain, S. K., Sandeep, V. V., & Raju, B. (2013). Effect of foliar application of micronutrients on growth parameters in tomato (*Lycopersicon esculentum* mill.). *Journal of Agriculture and Food Sciences*, *1*, 146–151.

Nasiri, Y., Saeid, Z.-S., Safar, N., Nosratollah, N., & Kazem, G. G. (2010). Effects of foliar application of micronutrients (Fe and Zn) on flower yield and essential oil of chamomile (*Matricaria chamomilla* L.). *Journal of Medicinal Plants Research*, *4*(17), 1733–1737.

Palamarja, N. S., & Chotina, A. A. (1953). Koriandr. Gosudarstvennoe izdatel'stvo sel'skochozjaistvennoj literatury, Moskva.

Paul, S. K., Mazumder, S., Mondal, S., Roy, S. K., & Kundu, S. (2015). Intercropping Coriander with Brinjal Forbrinjal Fruit and Shoot Borer Insect Suppression. *World Journal of Agricultural Sciences*, *11*(5), 303–306.

Pernice, R., Borriello, G., Ferracane, R., Borrelli, R. C., Cennamo, F., & Ritieni, A. (2009). Bergamot: A source of natural antioxidants for functionalized fruit juices. *Food Chemistry*, *112*(3), 545–550. doi:10.1016/j.foodchem.2008.06.004

Prakasam, V., Vedamuthu, P. G. B., Khader, M. A., & Jeyarajan, R. (1987). Screening coriander lines for wilt resistance. *South Indian Horticulture*, *35*, 258–259.

Rajan, F. S., Vedamuthu, P. G. B., Khader, M. K., & Jeyarajan, R. (1990). Screening coriander lines against grain mould disease. *South Indian Horticulture*, *38*, 168–169.

Schieber, A., Stintzing, F. C., & Carle, R. (2001). By-products of plant food processing as a source of functional compounds – recent developments. *Trends in Food Science & Technology*, *12*(11), 401–413. doi:10.1016/S0924-2244(02)00012-2

Singh, G., & Baswana, K. S. (1984). Screening of coriander germplasm against chalcid fly (*Systole albipennis*). *Ann. Appl. Biol. Supplement: Tests of Agrochemicals and Cultivars.*, *104*(5), 114–115.

Singh, G., Kapoor, I. P. S., Pandey, S. K., Singh, U. K., & Singh, R. K. (2002). Studies on essential oils: Part 10; antibacterial activity of volatile oils of some spices. *Phytotherapy Research*, *16*(7), 680–682. doi:10.1002/ptr.951 PMID:12410554

Singh, Y. N. (1986). Traditional medicine in Fiji: Some herbal folk cures used by Fiji Indians. *Journal of Ethnopharmacology*, *15*(1), 57–88. doi:10.1016/0378-8741(86)90104-2 PMID:3713228

Toben,, H.M., Meierzu, H., Beerentrup, K., Rudolph, H., &von der Schulenburg, G. (1994). Koriander als Petroselinsäurelieferant für die industrielle Verwendung. Stand der Züchtung und Bekämpfungsmöglichkeiten der „Bakteriellen Doldenwelke". Vortr. *Pflanzenzücht.*, *30*, 173–183.

Toben, H. M. (1995). *Die durch Pseudomonas syringae pv. coriandricola hervorgerufene Doldenwelke an Koriander, Charakterisierung des Erregers und Strategien zur Bekämpfung*. Göttingen: Cuvillier Verlag.

Chapter 18
Chili

Manas Kumar Pandit
Bidhan Chandra Krishi Viswavidyalaya, India

Ritoban Pandit
Hemvati Nandan Bahuguna Garhwal University, India

Sanjay Bairagi
Bidhan Chandra Krishi Viswavidyalaya, India

ABSTRACT

Chili is a unique and popular spice in the majority of the countries of the world and is well known for its hot, pungent flavor. Capsaicin is the bio-active compound that binds to pain receptors and causes an intense burning sensation. Capsanthin, a powerful antioxidant, is responsible for the red color of ripe fruits. Chili has its origin in Central America extending further south. This crop is of high commercial importance and huge genetic diversity exists. A systematic description of the crop with respect to its origin, distribution, botanical description, standard crop husbandry, and protection cum management of biotic stresses is given.

INTRODUCTION

Common hot chili (*Capsicum annuum* L., Solanaceae, 2n=2x=24) is one of the vegetables or spices known and used all over the world for its green fruits and pungency. Popularly called "capsicum", it is actually a non-pungent sweet pepper or *Simla Mirch* with a blocky fruit shape. The word capsicum has been derived from the Greek word *Kapsimo* meaning 'to burn'. Capsaicin ($C_{18}H_{27}NO_3$)is responsible for the pungency in chili, it is a condensation product of 3-hydroxy-4 methoxybenzylamine and decylenic acid. The red color of chili is due to the presence of Capsanthin, which is actually a mixture of esters of capsanthin, capsorubin, zeaxanthin, cryptoxanthin and other carotenoids (Sambamurty and Subrahmanyam, 1989). The chili fruit contains an essential oil Oleoresin that is used in pharmaceutical, food, and beverage industries for the preparation of value-added products.

DOI: 10.4018/978-1-7998-2524-1.ch018

Vernacular Names Of Chili

Bengali & Oriya – Lanka/ Lanka morich, **Kannad-**Mensana Kaya, **Tamil**- Mirapakaya, **Punjabi & Hindi**- Lalmirch,**Gujarati**- Marcha, **Malayalam**- Mulaku**Portuguese:** Pimento, **Spanish:** Chile dulce; pimiento; pimiento morron,**Myanmar:** Ngayok, **Netherlands:** SpaansePeper, **Sweden:** SpanskPeppar

ORIGIN AND SPREAD

Chilies have been reported to be in use since the infancy of agriculture. It is one of the oldest domesticated crops in the Western Hemisphere. Long before the arrival of Columbus in Americas, the local people already used peppers as food, as war artifacts and in religious rituals (Chiouet al., 2014).

Paleo-archeological findings suggest the antiquity of different chili peppers is 7000BC from caves excavated in Mexico and ancient burial grounds in Peru. Chilies originated in Mesoamerica, spreading from Central America to further South, and this is accepted as the primary center of origin for chili. The cultivated species *C. annuum* had been domesticated in the Tehuacan valley of Mexico during 5000 BC (Ettenberg, 2019), and it is now stated that the secondary centre is Guatemala. The globular, pea-sized fruits of the Wild Chili pepper (*C. annuum* var. *glabriusculum*), also called the "Mother Chili" the ancestor of domesticated *C. annuum,* are consumed and dispersed by frugivorous birds. The species spreads by seed and it has been transported through human and animal consumption as well as economic trade for hundreds of years (Basu and De, 2003).

Christopher Columbus brought chilies to Europe in 1493. In India, it was introduced by the Portuguese in the seventeenth century. Major chili growing states in India are Andhra Pradesh, Karnataka, Maharashtra, Orissa, Tamil Nadu, Madhya Pradesh, West Bengal and Rajasthan which accounts for more than 80% of the total area and production of the country. The North-Eastern states are bio-diversity hotspots for myriad variants of this crop. Chilies from India are exported mainly to Sri Lanka, USA, UK, Canada, Saudi Arabia, Malaysia, Singapore and Germany.

Biosystematics and Floral Biology

- Domain: Eukaryota
- Kingdom: Plantae
- Phylum: Spermatophyta
- Subphylum: Angiospermae
- Clade: Eudicots
- Class: Dicotyledonae
- Order: Solanales
- Family: Solanaceae
- Genus: Capsicum
- Species: annuum

There have been debates among taxonomists about the classification and species of chili since a long time ago, but presently about twenty-five to thirty wild and five domesticated species are recognized and accepted (Normah et al, 2013, Dewitt and Bosland, 1996; Arimbooret al., 2014).

Table 1. Five species under cultivation

Species	Conspicuous characters	Remarks
Capsicum annuum var. *annuum*	Anther blue with white corolla, calyx distinctly ridged with inconspicuous small teeth, solitary flowering or sometimes may bear 2-3 flowers	Major species grew on a large scale. Pungency is milder, but vitamin C content is more than that in *frutescens.* It includes bell peppers, wax, cayenne, jalapeños, chiltepin, and all forms of New Mexico chile.
*Capsicum baccatum*var. *pendulum*	Corolla white with yellow, green, tan or brown spots, calyx teeth present, anther yellow, flower/node1-2	Cultivation is restricted to central and south America. the South American ajipeppers
Capsicum pubescens	Both anther and corolla are purple, calyx teeth absent; flowering may be solitary or 2-3 per node. Seed color dark and rough	Cultivation is restricted to central and south America. The common one is rocoto peppers
Capsicum chinense	Corolla dull white or milky-greenish, calyx teeth absent, flower/node 2-3, seeds yellow and smooth	Widespread within Latin America. In India found in Kerala and north-eastern States. The types in it are Naga, habanero, Datil and Scotch bonnet
Capsicum frutescens	Corolla yellowish-white, sometimes yellowish blue or milky-greenish, anther blue, calyx teeth absent, flower/node 2-3, seeds yellow and smooth	Most of the small, highly pungent chilies (hot pepper) belong to this species, namely malagueta, tabasco and Thai peppers, piri and Malawian Kambuzi. It has a longer growing period than *annuum*.In India, this hot pepper is grown in coastal Kerala, Andhra Pradesh, Karnataka, Maharashtra and north-eastern states.

In *C. annuum*, there is the huge multiplicity of types; but no satisfactory classification of the variants is available. Recently Zhigila et al. (2014)provided a grouping on the basis of fruit morphology as described below.

- Abbreviatum; fruits ovate, wrinkled, 2-5 cm long. Also called wrinkled pepper;
- Acuminatum; fruits slender, curved, up to 11 cm long, mild to extremely pungent. Also called chili;
- Cerasiforme; fruits globose with firm flesh, up to 2.5 cm in diameter, mild to pungent, red, yellow or purple. Also called cherry pepper or bird's eye pepper;
- Conoides; fruits subconical, up to 3 cm long, very pungent. Also called cone pepper;
- Fasciculatum; fruits clustered, erect, up to 7.5 cm long, very pungent. Also called cluster pepper;
- Grossum: fruits large with basal depression, inflamed, red, orange, yellow, or purple, flesh thick and mild. Also called sweet pepper or paprika;
- Longum; fruits drooping, up to 30 cm long, mild or pungent, red, yellow or whitish. Also called long pepper.

C. annuum crosses both ways freely with *C. chinense* but with *frutescens* it crosses only as the male parent. The species name *annuum* suggests that it is of annual growth habit; sometimes, semi-perennial types are also found. Many of the wild relatives are perennial in nature. It is a hardy herb with erect growth and a strong taproot system; leaves are simple, variable in size, with flowers solitary, and the fruit is an indehiscent many-seeded berry. Anthesis takes place during the early morning at around 5 am, and the stigma remains receptive one day prior to anthesis to two days after anthesis. Pollens are best viable on the day of anthesis. Its fruit varies in size from 2-20 cm in length, from thin long to conical and thick fleshed blocky shapes.

Importance

§ Fruits are used as vegetables, spices, and pickles.

§ They are used in culinary dishes for adding flavor, color, and pungency.

§ Dry chilies are used to manufacture curry powder, curry paste and preparing sauces, soups, salads pickles etc.

§ Capsaicin is mainly present in the placenta of the central spongy tissue of fruits and also in seeds & ovary. It has good medicinal values, export potentialities and has physiological action potential to be used in many pharmaceutical preparations and ointments for cold, sore throat, asthma, chest congestion, headaches, arthritis etc.

§ Chilies are rich in vitamin A, C and E.

§ Capsanthin is responsible for red color in chili; it is a strong antioxidant and may fight cancer.

Varieties

§ NP 46 A (IARI): Suitable for green chili production, tolerant to thrips.

§ PusaJwala (IARI): Suitable for green chili production, pungency is high, fairly tolerant to thrips and aphids.

§ Bhaskar(X 235)(Agricultural Research Station,Lam,Guntur, Andhra Pradesh): Suitable for green chili production, flowers with yellow anthers, pungency is high, tolerant to thrips and mites, suitable for preparation of sauce.

§ Andhra Jyoti(G 5)(Agricultural Research Station, Lam, Guntur, Andhra Pradesh):suitable for salad purpose, cherry type fruits.

§ Bhagyalaxmi(G 4) (Agricultural Research Station, Lam, Guntur, Andhra Pradesh): Suitable for export as dry chilies, fairly tolerant to disease and pests.

§ Punjab Lal (PAU, Ludhiana): rich is capsaicin, suitable for export as dry chili, suitable for preparation of sauce, resistant to TMV, CMV and leaf curl viruses.

§ PusaSadabahar (IARI): Resistant to TMV, CMV and leaf curl viruses.

§ Pant C_1 (GBPUAT, Pantnagar): Tolerant to chili viruses, erect fruit bearing.

§ Pant C_2 (GBPUAT Pantnagar): Tolerant to chili viruses, pendant fruit bearing.

§ Suryamukhi and Bullet are two well-known landraces of West Bengal.

§ Bird's eye chili: Mainly grown in the North-Eastern Indian states of Mizoram, Manipur, Nagaland etc.; very pungent (50- 100 thousand Scoville Heat Units), perennial in growth habit, also found in Ethiopia.

§ **Bhutjolokia (ghost Chili): It** is an interspecific hybrid between *Capsicumchinense* and *C.frutescens*Chili pepper cultivated in Nepal as well as the Northeast Indian states of Arunachal Pradesh, Assam, Nagaland and Manipur. Extremely pungent (about 1million SHU); Bhutjolokia produces capsaicin in vesicles found in both the placenta around the seeds and throughout the fruit, rather than just the placenta(Bosland et al, 2015)

CROP IMPROVEMENT

Chili is diploid and basically self-pollinated. It has a huge genetic diversity that allows newer gene re-arrangements. The simplest and oldest breeding technique is mass selection, which is used to improve landraces and multiple traits. Other methods are pure line selection, pedigree method, single seed descent, backcrossing (used particularly for traits controlled by one or few genes), heterosis breeding, haploid diploidization and mutation.

Figure 1. Breeding goals in chili
(Source: Padilha and Barbieri, 2016)

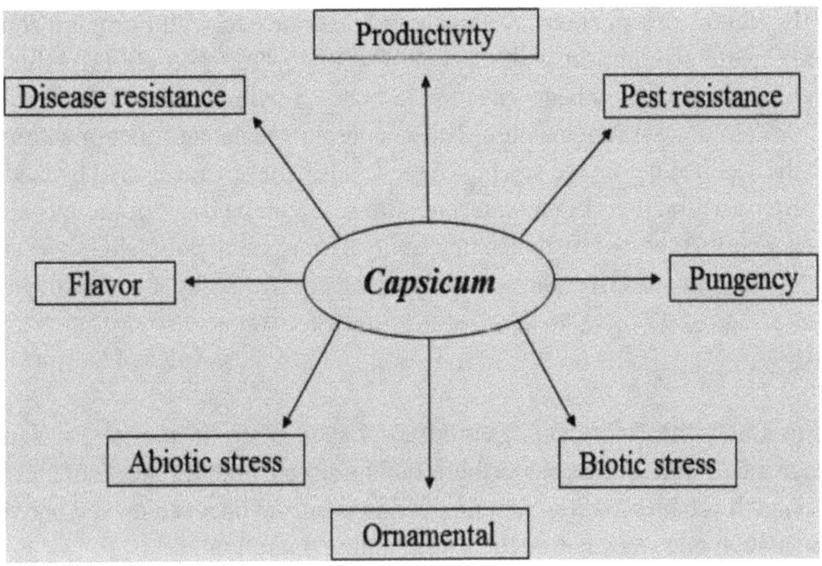

The choice of the best method or combination of them depends mainly on the type of inheritance (monogenic, oligogenic, or polygenic) from traits to be improved (Lee *et al.*, 2013). Use of molecular techniques and marker-assisted selection to improve fruit size, fruit production, pungency, abiotic stress tolerance, nutritional content, and disease resistance are presently done. Complete genome sequencing of chili is in need to cater the growing demand and volume of the commercial market worldwide.

Climate

Chili is a day-neutral crop making it fit for cultivating through the year in tropical and subtropical climates but it cannot withstand long frost. A temperature range of 15 -35^0 C is optimum for a satisfactory crop growth rate and yield. A little milder of a climate is required for sweet pepper. In chili, a soil temperature of 10^0 C or less, retards plant growth. Low temperature during fruit ripening delays color development. Temperatures beyond 40^{0}C results in a poor fruit set and in a severe flower and fruit drop. Chili requires 600-1200 mm rainfall. With chili an erratic temperature regime, insufficient water supply, excessive rainfall, and dry winds, particularly during the flowering stage, can cause bud, blossom and fruit drops, defoliation, and rotting of the plants.

Soil

Crops can grow in a wide range of soil, but well-aerated and well-drained loam soil rich in organic matter is found to be best, and the crop performs best at a soil pH of about 6.5. Vegetative growth and yields are higher in heavy textured soil, but the quality of fruits is better in lighter soil.

Nursery Management

About 1-2 kg of seeds of open-pollinated or improved cultivars and 250-400g of F_1hybrids, depending on the variety, are required to raise seedlings for one hectare of land. In sunny situations, 10-15 nursery beds of 3-4m x1 m or of convenient size are sufficient to obtain 50000-60000 seedlings for one hectare (Deshpande, 2001). Before sowing, nursery soli should be drenched with Formalin solution (1 part of Formaldehyde in 40 parts of water) or with Captan 0.3% (@ 5 litre solution/m^2). After drenching, the soil it should be covered with a polythene sheet for 48 hours. Sowing is done 7 days after the polythene sheet and 7-8 kg of FYM or cow dung manure, 100 g superphosphate, and 50 g of Muriate of potash/m^2 area is applied to the seedbed before the sowing of seed. It is better to cover seed beds with dry grasses/straw to ensure better germination. Light watering with rose can be done in the morning and evening according to the necessity. A temporary thatch made with a transparent polythene sheet at 3-3.5 feet high from the ground level is provided over the seedbed to protect it from direct sun, heavy rain, frost etc.

Transplanting

Prepare the land to a fine tilth, and seedlings are transplanted when they are 4-8 weeks old according to the season of sowing. Usual spacing in northern India is 45 cm and in south India 55 cm from row to row and plant to plant. It is better to transplant the seedlings during the evening and harden the seedlings by withholding irrigation one week before the transplanting operation.

Sowing Seasons

It is mainly grown during Kharif season (June-October) for dry red chilies and in other seasons for green chilies. South and central India: middle of May –mid July, Gangetic valley –June, Punjab and Rajasthan: April –May, West Bengal: May-June, Mid Sept-Mid November, Hilly areas: March –April, Under north India conditions sowing is done in June, transplanting in end of July, crops starts bearing by end of September, fruits start ripening by October, and this will give a continuous supply of fruits for three to four months.

Nutrient Management

For sowing one hectare of land, apply 20 ton FYM, 80 kg N, 60 kg P_2O_5 and 60 kg K_2O. Organic manure along with P_2O_5, K_2O, and one-third of the N should be mixed in the soil during land preparation. Remaining N is applied in two equal splits dose about 5 – 6 and 8 – 10 weeks after transplanting.

Water Management

In India, major areas under chili cultivation are rainfed. Irrigation depends on the season and soil type. Standard practice for irrigating chili is at an interval of 5-6 days in summer and 9-10 days in winter. Chili cannot withstand water stagnation and excess moisture. Maintenance of uniform soil moisture and proper drainage are required to prevent blossom and fruit drop. Water optimum moisture level should be maintained at the time of flowering, fruit set, and fruit development.

Cropping System

Garlic, soybean, and coriander as intercrops of chili in regions with black soil in southern parts of India are popular. Intercropping of groundnut and chili (3: 1) can give the maximum net return. Okra has been found to be the best intercrop for chili under semi-dry conditions. Incidence of thrips, mites, and nematodes is less if rotation with sorghum, maize, pulse, or groundnut is done. Through rotation with cereals and pulses, the incidence of fruit rot, bacterial disease, and mosaic are minimized in chili.

Use of Plant Growth Regulators

Unfavourable climatic conditions lead to poor fruit set and fruit drop in chili. Application of Planofix @ 10 ppm increased the number of branches. Branch number of chili is also increased with the application of CCC (500- 2000 ppm) and Ethrel (300-500 ppm). Fruit set in chili can be improved by the application of growth regulators like GA (10-100 ppm), NAA (20-200), and CCC (1000pm). Plant growth-promoting rhizobacteria (PGPR isolates)in chili rhizosphere can augment different direct plant growth promotion activities like ammonia production, phosphate solubilization, siderophore production, IAA production and indirect activities such as hydrocyanic acid (HCN) production, antagonistic effect on plant pathogenic bacteria (*Pseudomonas*, *Xanthomonas*) and *Fusarium* fungus (Datta et al, 2010).

Weed Management

Weed intensity is higher in *Kharif* season than in rabi or summer seasons. Two to three hand weedings are essential after transplanting. Herbicides like Triburalin and EPTC are generally applied as the pre-sowing soil incorporation. Diphenamid is extensively used as a pre-emergence herbicide. Pre-plant incorporation (10 DBT) of EPTC @ 3.75 kg/ha followed by application of either Nitrofen-1 @2kg a.i. /ha or Alachlor @ 2.5 kg a.i. /ha effectively controls *Cyperus rotundas* and annual weeds in chili crop.

Harvesting

Chilis, when used for vegetable purposes, are harvested when they are full-grown and still green, for pickles they are picked either green or ripe, and when used for drying are picked red or yellow when fully ripe. Qualities of green chili fruits are judged by size, color, and plumpness of the fruit. Normally green chilies are picked at frequent intervals, normally twice in a week.

Yield

Green chili: 7-10 t/ha for OP varieties and 12-15 t/ha for F_1hybrids. Dry chili: 0.5-1.0 t/ha 2(rainfed crop), 1.5-2.5 t/ha (irrigated crop).The yield of fresh green chilies is 3-4 times higher than fresh red ripe chilies and 6-10 times than dry Chilies, depending on quantity of seeds, pericarp, and inner wall thickness of the fruit(Deshpande,2001).

Post-harvest Handling

Damage and disease affected chilies are shorted out from the harvested lots, and as soon as possible, they are sent to the local market in gunny bags or in baskets. For dry red chilies fruits are harvested when they fully ripen and partially withered in the plant for better pungency and color retention. Keep harvested produce in heaps in shades for 2-3 days for uniform color development. Subsequently, fruits are dried in the sun by spreading them on cemented floor or on clean dry mats. Moisture in dried pods should be less than 10% to avoid microbial activity. Complete drying requires 15-20 days in sunlight. In the drier, they are kept at 55^0C for 2-3 days only. Later they are packed in gunny bags and sent to the local market. Modes of transport are head loads, carts, and trucks.

Storage

At room temperature, green chilies can be stored for 2-3 days. In cold storage they can be stored for 40 days at 0^0 C and 85-98% relative humidity. Dry chilies are stored in cool dry place, ensuring protection from dampness. They should preferably be exposed to sun periodically.

Seed Production

Basically chili is self-pollinated, but a good amount of outcrossing has been reported. That's why it is often a cross-pollinated crop and requires 200 and 400 m of isolation distance for certified and foundation seed production, respectively. Three rouging is required to remove off-types done before flowering, during flowering, and at pod maturity, respectively, on the basis of morphological, floral, and pod characters. Normal crop husbandry, along with plant protection measures, have to be followed.

PLANT PROTECTION (INSECT-PESTS)

Thrips (*Scirtothripsdorsalis*)

Thrips are common in almost all chili growing areas. It is a polyphagus pest. Besides chili, it also infests brinjal, mango, cotton, groundnut, citrus, castor, bottlegourd, guava, tea, sunflower and grapevine. It is more common on unirrigated chili crops than irrigated ones. A female adult inserts 40-48 white, minute eggs into veins. Both nymphs and adults lacerate the leaf tissues and suck the oozing sap, sometimes even the buds and flowers are attacked. Generally, they attack tender leaves and growing shoots. Rarely the older leaves are attacked. The insect is also responsible for transmitting a virus, causing leaf curl disease of chilies. The ETL level is three nymphs or adults per leaf.

- The infested leaves curl upward, crumble and shed
- Infested buds turn brittle with petiole becoming brown and drop down
- Affected fruits show light brown scars. Pest infestation is severe in dry weather. The damage ranges from 30-50%. In case of severe infestation, there is malformation of leaves, buds & fruits, which may damage half the crop. The attacked plants are stunted & may finally dry up.
- There are about 25 generations in a year with several overlapping generations. Reproduction in thrips is generally sexual, and parthenogenesis is also present. The adults are slender, yellowish-brown in color, having apically fringed pointed wings. They measure about 1 mm in length. The females possess long, narrow wings with the fore margin fringed with long hairs. The nymphs resemble the adults in shape & color but are wingless & smaller in size. There are three developmental stages viz. eggs, nymphs, and adults are found in its life cycle.

Management

- Seed treatment with Imidacloprid @ 3 -5 g/kg of seed.

Chili Mites (*Polyphagotarsonemuslatus*)

A minor pest emerged as a major pest in the recent past. The infestation starts in the nursery after 40 days of germination. Severe infestation is seen in the transplanted crops 2-3 months old. The tiny white transparent mites are found in large numbers on the undersurface of leaves under fine webs. Both nymphs and adults suck sap and devitalize the plant causing 'Murda' disease of chilies. Infestation results in:

- Downward curling of leaves.
- The affected leaves are becoming inverted boat-shaped.
- The leaves are rolling down along the margin with elongation of petioles.
- Affected leaves are turning dark green in certain cases.
- Younger leaves at the tip of branch clustering.

Management

- Foliar spraying of Dicofol 5ml/l or wettable sulphur 3g/l.
- Synthetic Pyrethroids were not used.
- If both thrips and mites are noticed, spraying Phosalone 3ml/l or Diafenthiuron 1.5 g /l or Chlorfenapyr 2 ml/l.

Chili Aphids (*Aphis gossypii, Myzuspersicae*)

They are polyphagous pests. Cloudy weather is very favorable for the multiplication of aphids. Heavy rains cause a reduction in their population. Adults are found in large numbers on the undersurface of leaves and growing shoots of plants. Both nymphs and adults suck sap and also excrete honeydew on which black sooty mold develops affecting photosynthetic activity thus causing:

- Retardation in growth and fruiting capacity of the plant.
- Sooty mold

Management

Foliar spray with methyl demeton 1 ml/l or acephate 1.5 g/l is effective.

Chili Pod Borers (*Spodopteralitura,S. exigua, Helicoverpaarmigera*, *Utetheisapulchella*)

Feeding by *S. litura*, *S. exigua* leads to irregular holes in the leaves and fruits. Affected pods turn whitish and dry up. In fruits, seeds are also eaten. Attack of *H.armigera* leads to round hole on fruits. In addition to these borers, sometimes *U. pulchella* also feeds on the pericarp leaving the seed intact. Ladder like marks are seen on chili pod due to *U.pulchella*. Their detailed history can be is given under pests of cotton and millets (*S. exigua*).

Management

1. Deep summer ploughing.
2. Monitoring with pheromone traps @ 4/acre
3. Raising trap crops like castor (*S. litura*), marigold (*H.armigera*).
4. Spraying with SNPV/HaNPV at 250LE/acre in the evening.
5. Spraying Novuluron 1.0 ml/l or Diflubenzuron 1.0 g/l controls just hatched larvae.
6. Foliar spraying of Thiodicarb 1.0 g/l or Acephate 1.5 g/l or Chlorpyriphos 2.5 ml/l or Spinosad 0.3ml/l or Qquinalphos 2 ml/l.
7. Poison baiting with rice bran 5 kg + Chlorpyriphos 500 ml or Carbaryl 500g + jaggery 500g with water in the form of small balls in the evening hours.

Root Grub (*Holotrichiaconsanguinea*)

It damages plants by eating the stem and roots. It initially survives on weed plants soon after planting chili and it attacks plants, which results in wilting and drying.

Management

- Application of well rotten Farm Yard Manure (FYM) will help in the prevention of root grubs
- Application of Carbofuram 3% granules @ 33 Kg per hectare or 10 kg Phorate 10% granules per hectare

Chili Blossom Midge (*Asphondyliacapsici*)

This fly is a dark reddish-brown mosquito-like midge that lays eggs in flower buds. The maggot is tiny pale, orange colored, and feeds on the floral parts leading to poor development of fruits. The ovary is distorted into gall like the structure of varied shape.

Management

Foliar spray with Triazophos 2 ml/l or Carbosulfan 2 ml/l followed by Chlorpyriphos 2.0 ml/L one week later, is found effective.

Stem Borer

Insects bore and enter into the main stem at 5-6 cm above ground level. Incidence of this pest is mainly during the early stages of the flowering stage. Due to stem damage, plant growth will be restricted, and plants will start slowly wilting. Damage by this insect leads to an inadequate supply of food and water, which results in the death of the plants.

Management

- Changing crop patterns, like not growing chili after brinjal, will help to some extent in prevention.
- Destroying the infected plants.
- Application of Choloropiriphos 2.5 ml or Thiodicarb 1 g by mixing in 1 litre of water.

Chili Whitefly (Bemisiatabaci)

Apart from chilies, this insect also feeds on cotton, cabbage, cauliflower, sarson, toria, melon, potato, brinjal, okra & some weeds. This pest is distributed throughout the northern & western regions of the Indian sub-continent & is also a very serious pest of American cotton, particularly in dry areas. It acts as a vector of various viral diseases including cotton leaf curl, tobacco leaf curl, vein clearing mosaic disease of okra & leaf curl of sesame.

Life-history: 3 developmental stages viz. are egg, nymph, and adult in its lifecycle. The total life cycle is completed in 14-22 days & almost 11 generations are completed in a year. In the winged stage, they are 1-1.5 mm long & their yellowish bodies are lightly dusted with a white waxy powder. They have 2 pairs of pure white wings & have prominent long hind wings.

Damage: The damage is caused by both the nymphs & adults by sucking the sap from the leaves. Insects exude honeydew, which attracts sooty mold. Therefore, in severe infestation, the plants not only become weak, but the mold interferes with the normal photosynthesis resulting in poor growth & yield. The ETL level is 20 nymphs or 8-10 adults/leaf or leaf stickiness due to the deposition of honeydew by insects in 50% of plants.

Management: Any one of the following insecticides can be used in 250 litres of water per ha. 750 ml of Formothion 25EC, or Oxydemeton methyl 25EC, 625 ml of Dimethoate 30EC, 100 ml of Imidacloprid 200SL,50 g of Acetamiprid 20SP, 100 g of Thiamethoxam 25WG.

DISEASES OF CHILI

Damping-off (*Pythiumaphanidermatum*)

Damping-off is a disease of nursery beds and young seedlings resulting in very high seedling mortality, reduced seed germination, and poor stand of seedlings. Infected areas turn brown and rot. Plants shrivel and collapse as a result of the softening of tissues at the collar region.

Management

- Raising nursery in light soil with proper drainage
- Avoid Excessive and frequent irrigation
- Rabbing – burning farm trash on the surface of the beds
- Sowing seed on raised beds of 6-8" high (15cm)
- Using the optimum seed rate of 650 g/cent
- Seed treatment with Thiram or Captan @ 2-3 g/kg.
- Soil drenching with Bordeaux mixture 1% or Copper oxychloride 0.3% or Metalaxyl (Ridomil) 0.2%
- Biocontrol with *Trichoderma viride* and *T. harzianum*
- Raising modern nurseries in portrays under controlled conditions in polyhouses

Die-back and Fruit Rot (*Colletotrichumcapsici*)

This disease is commonly known as Anthracnose and is more prevalent in the southern part of India, it is severe in Guntur and Krishna districts and some other states like Bihar, Uttar Pradesh, and Assam. The insect attacks young tender branches and flowers, resulting in flower drop. Branches start drying from the tips. Black spots appear on ripened fruits and lead to rotting of fruits. The pathogen is seed-borne.

Predisposing Factor-Relative Humudity-95-100%, temperature-28-32^0 C.

Symptoms: The pathogen shows two different types of symptoms at two different parts of the host.

A. **FRUIT ROT stage:** At the end and beginning of October, ripening fruits(turning red) show symptoms of small, dark, circular lesions. These lesions start to elongate along the axis, becoming sunken and elliptical in shape, which in the later stage diffuses. The central area turns black or straw-colored. Numerous fruiting bodies (*Acervulli*) in the form of black spots develop on the discolored areas arranged in concentric rings. One can see hyphae at the places on the lower surface of the fruit skin, in a cut-opened fruit. Seeds turn rusty in appearance as the seeds are covered with hyphae of the pathogen.

B. **DIE-BACK stage**: Prolonged deposition of dew on the leaves results in the occurrence of symptoms. Tender twigs and branches show necrosis beginning at the tip and advancing towards the base. Affected branches are water-soaked which later turns greyish-white. Finally, the twigs and branches wither.

Management

- Seed treatment with Captan or Thiram 3-4g/kg
- Collect seeds only form fruits without infection
- Avoid intercropping with susceptible turmeric cultivars
- Collect and destroy all infected plant parts
- Removal and destruction of Solanaceous weed hosts and infected plant debris
- Spray three times with Captan 1.5% or Mancozeb@0.25% just before flowering, at fruit formation stage and 15 days after the second spray
- 3-4 sprays of Blitox-50(0.5-1% concentration) and four sprays of Zineb(0.25% concentration) are effective in controlling both the stages of the disease.

Bacterial Leaf Spot (*Xanthomoascampestris***pv.** *vesicatoria*)

Leaves, fruits, and stems are affected, Lesions on the leaf begin as circular, water-soaked spots. Spots become necrotic with a brown center with chlorotic borders. Enlarged spots may develop straw colored centers. Lesions are slightly raised on the lower leaf surface, severely spotted leaves turn yellow and drop, raised brown lesions appear on fruits, and narrow, elongated lesions or streaks may develop on stems.

Management

- Seeds should be collected from healthy fruits
- Seed treatment with Copper oxychloride 2g/kg seed
- Field sanitation by removal and destruction of infected plant debris
- Add 1g Streptocycline or 2g Plantomycin to 10 litres of water and mix 3g of Copper oxychloride per litre of water and spray twice at 10 days interval

Cercospora Leaf Spot (*Cercosporacapsici*)

Circular spots with brown margins and grey centre appear on leaves. The spots enlarge and coalesce with others and the central portion of the spot becomes white and the leaves turn yellow and defoliate. Sometimes central portions of spot drops off. Spots also appear on stems and twigs as dark brown, irregular lesions with whitish centers. In severe cases die-back of twigs occur.

Management

- Seed treatment with Carbendazim @ 2g/Kg seed
- Spray Carbendazim 0.1% or Difolaton 0.15% @ 15 days interval

Choanephora Wet Rot (*Choanephoracucurbitarum*)

Plants from seedling to the early flowering stage are susceptible. Being a weak parasite, the fungus colonizes dead or dying tissues before it actively invades living tissues. Fruit infection is observed predominantly around calyx. Infected young fruits may abort.

Management

- Adopt recommended spacing to maintain adequate air circulation
- Field sanitation by destroying infected debris
- Select the seeds from healthy fruits and treat the seed with Captan or Thiram 3g/kg seed
- Spray Mancozeb 0.25% or Copper oxychloride 0.3%
  Spray wettable Sulphur 0.3% or Dinocap or Carbendazim or Tridemorph 0.1%.

Dry Root Rot (*Sclerotium* species / *Fusarium* Species)

Plants get infected by the fungus in the soil and dries

Management

- Crop rotation practices
- Application of Copper oxychloride at the plant base by mixing 3 g of Copper oxychloride in 1 litre water
- Application of 2 Kg of Trichoderma formulation in 90 Kg FYM and 10 Kg Neem seed powder

Powdery Mildew -*Leveillulataurica*

The disease is usually seen from December to February in cool and dry weather with high relative humidity.

The symptoms: A white powdery coating is seen on the lower surface of the leaf and occasionally yellow patches are seen on the upper surface. In case of severe infection, shedding of leaves occur. Sometimes powdery growth is also seen on branches and young fruits which do not grow further and drop-down prematurely.

Management

Spraying of wettable Sulphur 0.3% or Dinocap or Carbendazim or Tridemorph 0.1%.

VIRAL DISEASES

Leaf Curl (Gemini Virus)

It is transmitted by whiteflies. High humidity and rainy climatic conditions are favorable for whiteflies and help in the severe spread of the virus. Young leaves become small with upward curling. Leaves turn pale green and intermodal distance also decreases. Leaf curl virus symptoms resemble micronutrient deficiency symptoms. Whereas deficient plants can be observed in groups, virus-infected plants can spread all over the field here and there.

Cucumber Mosaic Virus

It is transmitted by aphids. The virus restricts the plant growth and black sooty mold can be observed on leaves and pods. The decrease in chlorophyll content of leaves leads to mosaic symptoms. Downward curling along the midribs is seen. Pods may be small or distorted. High humidity or persistent dew is conducive to the development of the disease.

Peanut bud Necrosis Virus

Virus develops on weeds, which grow on bunds like Parthenium, *Abutilon Indicum*, and are transmitted by thrips. The prolonged dry period after rains increases thrips incidences. Black spots occur on the stem and leaves that gradually transform into stripes. Necrotic spots occur on leaves resulting in leaves falling off.

CONCLUSION

Chili is not a staple food for millions but it can add taste and flavor to a bland meal. This is possibly the most prime cause of its rapid spread over the globe more so than potatoes or tomatoes. It is rich in loads of minerals and antioxidants, which can help the nutritional augmentation of marginal people. A consortium of growers, exporters, policy makers, and other stake holders are needed to ponder over and plan the improvement of the crop and enhancement of the quality of the spice. Market intelligence, supply chain management, and organic production standards have to be framed for better export trade.

REFERENCES

Arimboor, R., Natarajan, R. B., Menon, K. R., Chandrasekhar, L. P., & Moorkoth, V. (2014). Red pepper (*Capsicum annuum*) carotenoids as a source of natural food colors: Analysis and stability-a review. *Journal of Food Science and Technology*, *52*(3), 1258–1271. doi:10.100713197-014-1260-7 PMID:25745195

Basu, S. K., & De, A. K. (2003). Capsicum: historical and botanical perspectives. In A. K. De (Ed.), *Capsicum: The genus Capsicum* (pp. 1–15). London: Taylor and Francis.

Bosland, P., Coon, D., & Cooke, P. H. (2015). Novel Formation of Ectopic (Nonplacental) Capsaicinoid Secreting Vesicles on Fruit Walls Explains the Morphological Mechanism for Super-hot Chile Peppers. *Journal of the American Society for Horticultural Science*, *140*(3), 253–256. doi:10.21273/JASHS.140.3.253

Bosland, P. W. (1998). Capsicums: Innovative uses of an ancient crop". In J. Janick (Ed.), *Progress in New Crops* (pp. 479–487). Arlington, VA: ASHS Press.

Chiou, K. L., Hastorf, C. A., Bonavia, D., & Dillehay, T. D. (2014). Documenting cultural selection pressure changes on chile pepper (*Capsicum baccatum*L.) seed size through time in Coastal Peru (7,600 B.P. - Present). *Economic Botany*, *68*(2), 190–202. doi:10.100712231-014-9270-y

Datta, M., Sengupta, C., & Pandit, M. K. (2010). Isolation and characterization of bacterial isolates from chili (Capsicum annuum L.) rhizosphere as a potent plant growth promoter. *Journal of Crop and Weed*, *6*(2), 50–58.

Deshpande, A. A. (2001). Chili and capsicums. In S. Thamburaj & N. Singh (Eds.), *Textbook on vegetables, tuber crops and spices* (pp. 49–75). New Delhi: ICAR.

Dewitt, D., & Bosland, P. W. (1996). *Peppers of the World: An Identification Guide*. Berkeley, CA: Ten Speed Press.

Ettenberg, J. (2019). *A brief history of chili peppers*. https://www.legalnomads.com/history-Chili-peppers

Kuhn, Padilha. & LíaBarbieri. (2016). Plant breeding of Chili peppers (*Capsicum*, Solanaceae) – A review. *Australian Journal of Basic and Applied Sciences*, *10*(15), 148–154.

Lee, J. M., Jahn, M. M., & Yeam, I. (2013). Allelic relationships at the pvr1 locus in *Capsicum annuum*. *Euphytica*, *194*(3), 417–424. doi:10.100710681-013-0967-2

Normah, M. N., Chin, H. F., & Reed, B. M. (2013). *Conservation of tropical plant species*. Springer.

Sambamurty, A. V. S. S., & Subrahmanyam, N. S. (1989). Capsicums. In A textbook of economic botany. Wiley Eastern Ltd.

Zhigila, D. A., Abdul Rahaman, A. A., Kolawole, O. S., & Oladele, F. A. (2014). Fruit morphology as taxonomic features in five varieties of *Capsicum annuum* L. Solanaceae. *Journal of Botany*. http: //www. hindawi. Com /journals / jb / 2014/540868

Compilation of References

Abbai, R., Ramya Mathiyalagan, J. M., Kim, Y. J., Wang, C., Singh, P., Ahn, S., ... Yang, D. C. (2016). Green synthesis of multifunctional silver and gold nanoparticles from the oriental herbal adaptogen: Siberian ginseng. *International Journal of Nanomedicine*, *11*, 3131–3143. doi:10.2147/IJN.S108549 PMID:27468232

Abbas, K., & Tahere, R. (2012). Composition and insecticidal activity of essential oil from *Coriandrum sativum* seeds against tribolium confusum and callosobruchus maculatus. ISRN Pharmaceutics, 5.

Abbaszadegan, A., Gholami, A., Ghahramani, Y., Ghareghan, R., Ghareghan, M., Kazemi, A., ... Ghasemi, Y. (2016). Antimicrobial and cytotoxic activity of Cuminum cyminum as an intracanal medicament compared to chlorhexidine gel. *Iranian Endodontic Journal*, *11*(1), 44. PMID:26843877

Abderrahmane, A., Soumia, Z., Zafar, H., & Badiaam, I. L. (2011). Hypoglycemic and hypolipidemic effects of *Coriandrum sativum* L. in *Merionesshawi* rats. *Journal of Ethnopharmacology*, *137*(1), 652–661. doi:10.1016/j.jep.2011.06.019 PMID:21718774

Abu-zaid, A. A., Alopidi, M. A., & El-Sehrawy, M. H. (2013). *In vitro* antibacterial, anticancer and antioxidant properties of some oil plant extract. *The Journal of American Science*, *9*(11), 83–94.

Abu-Zaiton, A. S. (2010). Anti-Diabetic Activity of Ferula assafoetida Extract in Normal and Alloxan-Induced Diabetic Rats. *Pakistan Journal of Biological Sciences*, *13*(2), 97–100. doi:10.3923/pjbs.2010.97.100 PMID:20415145

Acharya, S. N., Thomas, J. E., & Basu, S. K. (2008). Fenugreek, an alternative crop for semiarid regions of North America. *Crop Science*, *48*(3), 841–853. doi:10.2135/cropsci2007.09.0519

Adel, S. P. R., & Prakash, J. (2010). Chemical composition and antioxidant properties of ginger root (Zingiber officinale). *Journal of Medicinal Plants Research*, *4*(24), 2674–2679. doi:10.5897/JMPR09.464

Adeyemi, M. M. H. (2011). A review of secondary metabolites from plant materials for post-harvesting. *IJPAS*, *6*, 94–102.

Adisakwattana, S., Lerdsuwankij, O., Poputtachai, U., Minipun, A., & Suparpprom, C. (2011). Inhibitory activity of cinnamon bark species and their combination effect with acarbose against intestinal α-glucosidase and pancreatic α-amylase. *Plant Foods for Human Nutrition (Dordrecht, Netherlands)*, *66*(2), 143–148. doi:10.100711130-011-0226-4 PMID:21538147

Aggarwal, B. B., Kumar, A., & Aggarwal, M. S. (2005). Curcumin derived from turmeric (Curcuma longa): a spice for all seasons. In P. D. Debases Bagchi & H. G. Preuss (Eds.), *Phytochemicals in Cancer Chemoprevention* (pp. 349–387). New York: CRC Press.

Agrawal, P., Kotagiri, D., & Kolluru, V. C. (2018). Comparative analysis of antimicrobial activity of herbal extracts against pathogenic microbes. *Current Trends in Biomedical Engineering & Biosciences*, *16*, 1–7.

Agu, C. S., Igwe, J. E., Amanze, N. N., & Oduma, O. (2016). Effect of oven drying on proximate composition of ginger. *American Journal of Engineering Research*, *5*(8), 58–61.

Ahmad, A., Alghamdi, S. S., Mahmood, K., & Afzal, M. (2016). Fenugreek a multipurpose crop: Potentialities and improvements. *Saudi Journal of Biological Sciences*, *23*(2), 300–310. doi:10.1016/j.sjbs.2015.09.015 PMID:27307778

Ahmed, M. A., Ibrahim, O. M., & Elham, A. B. (2010). Effect of bio and mineral phosphorus fertilizer on the growth, productivity and nutritional value of fenugreek (*Trigonellafoenumgraecum* L.) in newly cultivated land. *Research Journal of Agriculture and Biological Sciences*, *6*(3), 339–348.

Ahmed, T., & Gilani, A. H. (2009). Inhibitory effect of curcuminoids on acetylcholinesterase activity and attenuation of scopolamine-induced amnesia have medicinal use of turmeric in Alzheimer's disease. *Pharmacology, Biochemistry, and Behavior*, *91*(4), 554–559. doi:10.1016/j.pbb.2008.09.010 PMID:18930076

Ahn, T., Kim, J. H., Yang, H. M., Lee, J. W., & Kim, J. D. (2012). Formation pathways of magnetite nanoparticles by coprecipitation method. *The Journal of Physical Chemistry C*, *116*(10), 6069–6076. doi:10.1021/jp211843g

Ahui, M. L., Champy, P., Ramadan, A., Pham Van, L., Araujo, L., Brou André, K., ... Herbelin, A. (2008). Ginger prevents Th2-mediated immune responses in a mouse model of airway inflammation. *International Immunopharmacology*, *8*(12), 1626–1632. doi:10.1016/j.intimp.2008.07.009 PubMed

Aissaoui, A., El-Hilaly, J., Israili, Z. H., & Lyoussi, B. (2008). Acute diuretic effect of continuous intravenous infusion of an aqueous extract of *Coriandrum sativum* L. in anesthetized rats. *Journal of Ethnopharmacology*, *115*(1), 89–95. doi:10.1016/j.jep.2007.09.007

Ajayi, O. B., Akomolafe, S. F., & Akinyemi, F. T. (2013). Food value of two varieties of ginger (Zingiber officinale) commonly consumed in Nigeria. *ISRN Nutrition*. doi:10.5402/2013/359727

Akbari, B., Tavandashti, M. P., & Zandrahimi, M. (2011). Particle size characterization of nanoparticles–a practicalapproach. *Iranian Journal of Materials Science and Engineering*, *8*(2), 48–56.

Akhani, S. P., Vishwakarma, S. L., & Goyal, R. K. (2004). Anti-diabetic activity of Zingiber officinale in streptozotocin-induced type I diabetic rats. *The Journal of Pharmacy and Pharmacology*, *56*(1), 101–105. doi:10.1211/0022357022403 PubMed

Akimoto, M., Iizuka, M., Kanematsu, R., Yoshida, M., & Takenaga, K. (2015). Anticancer effect of ginger extract against pancreatic cancer cells mainly through reactive oxygen species-mediated autotic cell death. *PLoS One*, *10*(5). doi:10.1371/journal.pone.0126605

Al Jasass, F. M., & Al Jasser, M. S. (2012). Chemical composition and fatty acid content of some spices and herbs under Saudi Arabia conditions. *TheScientificWorldJournal*, *2012*, 1–5. doi:10.1100/2012/859892 PMID:23319888

Alam, K., Goher, Z., & Anderson, R. A. (2009). Bay leaves improves glucose and lipid profile of people with type 2 diabetes. *Journal of Clinical Biochemistry and Nutrition*, *44*(1), 52–56. doi:10.3164/jcbn.08-188 PMID:19177188

Alfonso, A. A., Altarejos, J., & Salido, S. (2017). Phytochemicals and Biological Activities of Laurel Tree (Laurus nobilis). *Natural Product Communications*, *12*(5), 743–757. PMID:30496684

Al-Hadi, L. M. (2011). The antibacterial activity of aqueous extract of peppermint and bay leaf against Staphylococcus aureus. *Journal of Baghdad College of Dentistry*, *23*(2), 146–150.

al-Hashimi, A. G., & Mahmood, S. A. (2016). The nutritional value and antioxidant activity of bay leaves (*laurusn obilis L.*). *Magallat al-Basrat Li-l-Abhat al-Baytariyyat*, *15*(4), 10–23.

Al-Hashimi, A. G., & Mahmood, S. A. (2016). The nutritional value and antioxidant activity of bay leaves (Laurus nobilis L.). *Magallat al-Basrat Li-l-Abhat al-Baytariyyat, 15*(2), 246–259. doi:10.33762/bvetr.2016.124310

Alhubaishi, A. A., Walkey, D. G. A., Webb, M. J. W., Bolland, C. J., & Cook, A. A. (1987). A survey of horticultural plant virus diseases in the Yemen Arab Republic. *FAO Plant Protection Bulletin, 35*, 135–143.

Ali, B. H., Blunden, G., Tanira, M. O., & Nemmar, A. (2008). Some phytochemical, pharmacological and toxicological properties of ginger (Zingiber officinale Roscoe): A review of recent research. *Food and Chemical Toxicology, 46*(2), 409–420. doi:10.1016/j.fct.2007.09.085 PubMed

Aligita, W., Susilawati, E., Sukmawati, I.K., Holidayanti, L. & Riswanti, J. (2018). Article. *The Indonesian Biomedical Journal, 10*(2), 165. DOI: 20 doi:10.18585/inabj.v10i2.405

Alison, M. G., & Peter, R. F. (1999). Insulin-releasing and insulin-like activity of the traditional anti-diabetic plant *Coriandrum sativum* (coriander). *British Journal of Nutrition, 81*(3), 203–209. doi:10.1017/S0007114599000392

Al-Qattan, K., Thomson, M. and Ali, M., (2008). Garlic (Allium sativum) and ginger (Zingiberofficinale) attenuate structural nephropathy progression in streptozotocin-induced diabetic rats. *Eur E J Clin NutrMetab, 3*, e62-e71.

Al-Said, M. S., Al-Khamis, K. I., Islam, M. W., Parmar, N. S., Tariq, M., & Ageel, A. M. (1987). Post-coital antifertility activity of the seeds of *Coriandrum sativum* in rats. *Journal of Ethnopharmacology, 21*(2), 165–173. doi:10.1016/0378-8741(87)90126-7

AlSalhi, M., Devanesan, S., Alfuraydi, A., Vishnubalaji, R., Munusamy, M. A., Murugan, K., ... Benelli, G. (2016). Green synthesis of silver nanoparticles using <em>Pimpinella anisum</em> seeds: Antimicrobial activity and cytotoxicity on human neonatal skin stromal cells and colon cancer cells. *International Journal of Nanomedicine, 11*, 4439–4449. doi:10.2147/IJN.S113193 PMID:27660438

Alsammarraie, F. K., Wang, W., Zhou, P., Mustapha, A., & Lin, M. (2018). Green synthesis of silver nanoparticles using turmeric extracts and investigation of their antibacterial activities. *Colloids and Surfaces. B, Biointerfaces, 171*, 398–405. doi:10.1016/j.colsurfb.2018.07.059 PMID:30071481

Al-Shinawi, T. A. (1993). *Untersuchungen zur Anfälligkeit verschiedener Korianderherkünfte (Coriandrum sativum L.) für den Erreger der „Bakteriellen Doldenwelke" Pseudomonas syringae pv. coriandricola.* Magisterarbeit, Institut für Pflanzenpathologie und Pflanzenschutz, Universität Göttingen.

Al-Snafi, A. E. (2016). The pharmacological activities of Cuminumcyminum - A review. *IOSR Journal of Pharmacy., 6*(6), 46–65.

Altuntas, E., Ozgoz, E., & Taser, O. F. (2005). Some physical properties of fenugreek (*Trigonellafoenumgraecum* L. seeds. *Journal of Food Engineering, 71*(1), 37–43. doi:10.1016/j.jfoodeng.2004.10.015

Alu'datt, M. H., Rababah, T., Alhamad, M. N., Gammoh, S., Ereifej, K., Johargy, A., ... Rawashdeh, M. (2016). Optimization of Phenolic Content, Antioxidant, and Inhibitory Activities of α-Glucosidase and Angiotensin Converting (AC) Enzymes from *Zingiber Officinale* Z. *International Journal of Food Properties, 19*(6), 1303–1316. doi:10.1080/10942912.2015.1063066

Al-Yasiry, K., Kathum, W., & Al-Ganimi, Y. (2014). Evaluation of antidiabetic effect of cinnamon in patients with diabetes mellitus type Ii in Kerbala City. *Journal of Natural Sciences Research, 4*(4), 43–45.

Alzoreky, N. S., & Nakahara, K. (2003). Antibacterial activity of extracts from some edible plants commonly consumed in Asia. *International Journal of Food Microbiology, 80*(3), 223–230. doi:10.1016/S0168-1605(02)00169-1 PMID:12423924

Amin, A., Alkaabi, A., & Al-Falasi, S. (2005). Chemopreventive activities of *Trigonellafoenumgraecum* (Fenugreek) against breast cancer. *Cell Biology International*, *29*(8), 687–694. doi:10.1016/j.cellbi.2005.04.004 PMID:15936223

Amjad, A., Sajida, P., Syed, N., Muhammad, S., Zengqiang, Z., Fazli, W., ... Abdul, M. (2014). Effect of foliar application of micronutrients on fruit quality of peach. *American Journal of Plant Sciences*, *5*(09), 1258–1264. doi:10.4236/ajps.2014.59138

Ammon, H. P., & Wahl, M. A. (1991). Pharmacology of Curcuma longa. *Planta Medica*, *57*(01), 1–7. doi:10.1055-2006-960004 PMID:2062949

Amran, A. Z., Jantan, I., Dianita, R., & Buang, F. (2015). Protective effects of the standardized extract of Zingiber officinale on myocardium against isoproterenol-induced biochemical and histopathological alterations in rats. *Pharmaceutical Biology*, *53*(12), 1795–1802. doi:10.3109/13880209.2015.1008147 PubMed

Anandakumar, P., Kamaraj, S., Jagan, S., Ramakrishnan, G., Vinodjkumar, R., & Devaki, T. (2008). Capsaicin modulates pulmonary antioxidant defense system during benzo(a)pyrene-induced lung cancer in swiss albino mice. *Phytotherapy Research*, *22*(4), 529–533. doi:10.1002/ptr.2393 PMID:18338764

Anastas, P. T., & Warner, J. C. (1998). Green chemistry: Theory and practice. Oxford University Press.

Anderson, R. A., Broadhurst, C. L., Polansky, M. M., Schmidt, W. F., Khan, A., Flanagan, V. P., ... Graves, D. J. (2004). Isolation and characterization of polyphenol type-A polymers from cinnamon with insulin-like biological activity. *Journal of Agricultural and Food Chemistry*, *52*(1), 65–70. doi:10.1021/jf034916b PMID:14709014

Anderson, R. A., Zhan, Z., Luo, R., Guo, X., Guo, Q., Zhou, J., ... Stoecker, B. A. (2016). Cinnamon extract lowers glucose, insulin and cholesterol in people with elevated serum glucose. *Journal of Traditional and Complementary Medicine*, *6*(4), 332–336. doi:10.1016/j.jtcme.2015.03.005 PMID:27774415

Andronikashvili, M., & Reichmuth, C. H. (2003), Repellency and toxicity of essential oils from Ocimum gratissimum (Lamiaceae) and Laurus nobilis (Lauraceae) from Georgia against the rust-red flour beetle Tribolium castaneum (Herbst.) (Coleoptera: Tenebrionidae). *Proceedings of the 8th International Working Conference of Stored Product Protection*, 749-762.

An, K., Zhao, D., Wang, Z., Wua, J., Xu, Y., & Xiao, G. (2016). Comparison of different drying methods on Chinese ginger (Zingiber officinale Roscoe): Changes in volatiles, chemical profile, antioxidant properties, and microstructure. *Food Chemistry*, *197*, 1292–1300. doi:10.1016/j.foodchem.2015.11.033 PubMed

Ankamwar, B., Damle, C., Ahmad, A., & Sastry, M. (2005). Biosynthesis of gold and silver nanoparticles using Emblica officinalis fruit extract, their phase transfer and transmetallation in an organic solution. *Journal of Nanoscience and Nanotechnology*, *5*(10), 1665–1671. doi:10.1166/jnn.2005.184 PMID:16245525

Anon. (1992). Les agentsantioxygenes. *Pour la Science*, *179*, 10–12.

Anuradha, M., Pragyandip, D., Murthy, P. N., Siddique, H. H., & Poonam, K. (2012). A classical review on Rajika (Brassica juncea). *Res Rev J Biol Sci*, *1*(1), 18–23.

Aranda, P., Fernandes, F. M., Wicklein, B., Ruiz-Hitzky, E., Hill, J. P., & Ariga, K. (2012). *Bioinspired materials chemistry I: organic–inorganic nanocom-posites. In Bioinspiration and biomimicry in chemistry: reverse-engineering nature* (1st ed., pp. 121–138). Hoboken, NJ: John Wiley & Sons. doi:10.1002/9781118310083.ch5

Araujo, C. Z. D. (1986). Occurrence of *Myzus persicae* (Sulzer, 1776) (*Homoptera, Aphididae*) on a crop of coriander *Coriandrum sativum* (Umbelliferae). *Anais da Sociedade Entomológica do Brasil*, *15*, 173–174.

Arends, J. (2010). Metabolism in cancer patients. *Anticancer Research*, *30*, 1863–1868. PMID:20592393

Arias, B. A., & Ramon-Laca, L. (2005). Pharmacological properties of citrus and their ancient and medieval uses in the Mediterranean region. *Journal of Ethnopharmacology*, *97*(1), 89–95. doi:10.1016/j.jep.2004.10.019 PMID:15652281

Arimboor, R., Natarajan, R. B., Menon, K. R., Chandrasekhar, L. P., & Moorkoth, V. (2014). Red pepper (*Capsicum annuum*) carotenoids as a source of natural food colors: Analysis and stability-a review. *Journal of Food Science and Technology*, *52*(3), 1258–1271. doi:10.100713197-014-1260-7 PMID:25745195

Arshadi, S., Azarbayjani, M.A., & Hajaghaalipor, F. (2015). Evaluation of *Trigonellafoenum-graecum* extract in combination with swimming exercise compared to glibenclamide consumption on type 2 diabetic rodents. *Food Nutr. Res.*, *59*.doi: .v59.29717 doi:10.3402/fnr

Arulselvan, P., Ghofar, H. A. A., Karthivashan, G., Halim, M. F. A., Ghafar, M. S. A., & Fakurazi, S. (2014). Antidiabetic therapeutics from natural source: A systematic review. *Biomedicine & Preventive Nutrition*, *4*(4), 607–617. doi:10.1016/j.bionut.2014.07.009

Asfaw, D., (2019) Review on Use of Bioactive Compounds in Some Spices in Food Preservation. *Food Sci and Quality Manag., 87.*

Ashokkumar, K., Arjun, P., Murugan, M., Dhanya, M. K., Sathyan, T., Sivakumar, P., & Surya, R. (2018a). Simple and rapid extraction method for determination of carotenoids in the edible parts of Vitis vinifera, Vaccinum sect. cyanococcus, Ipomoea batatas and Capsicum annum. Advances in Research, 17(4), 1–8. doi:10.9734/AIR/2018/45132

Ashokkumar, K., Murugan, M., Dhanya, M. K., Surya, R., & Kamaraj, D. (2019b). Phytochemical variations among four distinct varieties of Indian cardamom Elettaria cardamomum (L.) Maton. Natural Product Research, 1–4. doi:10.1080/14786419.2018.1561687

Ashokkumar, K., Pandian, A., Murugan, M., Dhanya, M. K., Sathyan, T., Sivakumar, P., . . . Warkentin, T. D. (2019). Profiling bioactive flavonoids and carotenoids in select south Indian spices and nuts. Natural Product Research, 1–5. doi:10.1080/14786419.2018.1557179

Ashokkumar, K., Diapari, M., Jha, A. B., Tar'an, B., Arganosa, G., & Warkentin, T. D. (2015). Genetic diversity of nutritionally important carotenoids in 94 pea and 121 chickpea accessions. *Journal of Food Composition and Analysis*, *43*, 49–60. doi:10.1016/j.jfca.2015.04.014

Ashokkumar, K., Elayabalan, S., Shobana, V. G., Sivakumar, P., & Pandiyan, M. (2018b). Nutritional value of cultivars of Banana (Musa spp.) and its future prospects. *Journal of Pharmacognosy and Phytochemistry*, *7*(3), 2972–2977.

Ashokkumar, K., Kumarakurubaran, S., & Saradha Devi, S. M. (2013). Reverse phase-high performance liquid chromatography-diode array detector (RP-HPLC-DAD) analysis of flavonoids profile from curry leaf (Murraya koenigii L). *Journal of Medicinal Plants Research*, *7*, 3393–3399. doi:10.5897/JMPR2013.5150

Ashokkumar, K., Murugan, M., Dhanya, M. K., & Warkentin, T. D. (2020). Botany, traditional uses, phytochemistry and biological activities of cardamom [Elettaria cardamomum (L.) Maton] - A critical review. *Journal of Ethnopharmacology*, *246*, 112244. doi:10.1016/j.jep.2019.112244 PubMed

Ashokkumar, K., & Shunmugam, A. S. K. (2016). Curry leaf (Muraya koenji L. Spreng): its phytochemistry and pharmacological properties - A review. Medicinal Plants: Phytochemistry. *Pharmacology & Therapeutics*, *4*, 375–390.

Ashokkumar, K., Sivakumar, P., & Saradha Devi, M. (2018). Identification and determination of naturally occurring folates in grains of rice (Oryza sativa L.) by UPLC-MS/MS analysis. *Natural Product Research*, *32*(14), 1733–1737. doi:10.1080/14786419.2017.1392957 PubMed

Ashokkumar, K., Tar'an, B., Diapari, M., Arganosa, G., & Warkentin, T. D. (2014). Effect of cultivar and environment on carotenoid profile of pea and chickpea. *Crop Science*, *54*(5), 2225–2235. doi:10.2135/cropsci2013.12.0827

Ashok, P. K., & Upadhyaya, K. (2012). Tannins are asrigent. *Journal of Pharmacognosy and Phytochemistry*, *1*, 45–50.

Ashraf, R., Aamir, K., Shaikh, R. A., & Ahmed, T. (2005). Effects of garlic on dyslipidemia in patients with type 2 diabetes mellitus. *Journal of Ayub Medical College*, *17*(3), 60–64. PMID:16320801

Atawodi, S. E., Atawodi, J. C., Idakwo, G. A., Pfundstein, B., Haubner, R., & Wurtel, G. (2011). Spiegelhalder & Owen, R.W. (2011). *Journal of Medicinal Food*, *12*(6), 1316. doi:10.1089/jmf.2008.0211 PMID:20041787

Auta, K. I., Galadima, J. U., Olowoniyi, O. D., Moses, O. O., & Yako, A. B. (2011). Antimicrobial properties of the ethanolic extracts of Zingiber officinale (Ginger) on Escherichia coli and Pseudomonas aeruginosa. *Research Journal of Biological Sciences*, *6*(1), 37–39. doi:10.3923/rjbsci.2011.37.39

Avendan˜o & Schwentesius. (2004). The economics of food safety: the case of green onions and hepatitis A outbreaks. *USDA Economics Research Service*. http://www.ers.usda.gov/publications/vgs/nov04/VGS30501/ VGS30501.pdf

Ayodhya, S., Kusum, S., & Anjali, S. (2010). Hypoglycaemic activity of different extracts of various herbal plants. *International Journal of Research in Ayurveda and Pharmacy*, *1*(1), 212–224.

Azizi, S., Mohamad, R., Rahim, R. A., Moghaddam, A. B., Moniri, M., Ariff, A., ... Namvab, F. (2016). ZnO-Ag core shell nanocomposite formed by green method using essential oil of wild ginger and their bactericidal and cytotoxic effects. *Applied Surface Science*, *384*, 517–524. doi:10.1016/j.apsusc.2016.05.052

Aziz, W., & Jassim, H. A. (2018). A novel study of pH influence on Ag nanoparticles size with antibacterial and antifungal activity using green synthesis. *World Sci News*, *97*, 139–152.

Bag, A., & Chattopadhyay, R. R. (2015). Evaluation of synergistic antibacterial and antioxidant efficacy of essential oils of spices and herbs in combination. *PLoS One*, *10*(7), 1–17. doi:10.1371/journal.pone.0131321 PMID:26132146

Bagherzade, G., Tavakoli, M. M., & Namaei, M. H. (2017). Green synthesis of silver nanoparticles using aqueous extract of saffron (Crocus sativus L.) wastages and its antibacterial activity against six bacteria. *Asian Pacific Journal of Tropical Biomedicine*, *7*(3), 227–233. doi:10.1016/j.apjtb.2016.12.014

Balakrishnan, K. V. (2007). Postharvest technology and processing of turmeric. In P. N. Ravindran, K. Nirmal Babu, & K. Sivaraman (Eds.), *Turmeric: The Genus Curcuma* (pp. 193–256). Boca Raton, FL: CRC Press.

Balakrishnan, S., Sivaji, I., Kandasamy, S., Duraisamy, S., Kumar, N. S., & Gurusubramanian, G. (2017). Biosynthesis of silver nanoparticles using Myristica fragrans seed (nutmeg) extract and its antibacterial activity against multidrug-resistant (MDR) Salmonella enterica serovar Typhi isolates. *Environmental Science and Pollution Research International*, *24*(17), 14758–14769. doi:10.100711356-017-9065-7 PMID:28470497

Balch, P. A. (2003). Prescription for dietary wellness (2nd ed.). Penguin Group.

Baliga, M. S., Haniadka, R., Pereira, M. M., D'Souza, J. J., Pallaty, P. L., Bhat, H. P., & Popuri, S. (2011). Update on the chemopreventive effects of ginger and its phytochemicals. *Critical Reviews in Food Science and Nutrition*, *51*(6), 499–523. doi:10.1080/10408391003698669 PubMed

Banerjee, S. K., Mukherjee, P. K., & Maulik, S. K. (2003). Garlic as an antioxidant: The good, the bad and the ugly. *Phytotherapy Research*, *17*(2), 97–106. doi:10.1002/ptr.1281 PMID:12601669

Bang, Lee, Kim, Sung, & Jeong. (2016). Metabolic engineering of *Escherichia coli* for the production of cinnamaldehyde. *Microbial Cell Factories*, *15*(1), 16.

Ban, J. O., Oh, J. H., Kim, T. M., Kim, D. J., Jeong, J. S., Han, S. B., & Hong, J. T. (2009). Anti-inflammatory and arthritic effects of thiacremonone, a novel sulfur compound isolated from garlic via inhibition of NF-κB. *Arthritis Research & Therapy*, *11*(5), R145. doi:10.1186/ar2819 PMID:19788760

Basavaraja, S., Balaji, S. D., Lagashetty, A., Rajasab, A. H., & Venkataraman, A. (2008). Extracellular biosynthesis of silver nanoparticles using the fungus Fusarium semitectum. *Materials Research Bulletin*, *43*(5), 1164–1170. doi:10.1016/j.materresbull.2007.06.020

Basch, E., Ulbricht, C., & Kuo, G. (2003). Therapeutic applications of fenugreek. *Alternative Medicine Review*, *8*(1), 20–27. PMID:12611558

Baser, K. H. C., & Buchbauer, G. (2015). *Handbook of essential oils: science, technology, and applications*. CRC Press. doi:10.1201/b19393

Basha, S. K., Sudarshanam, G., & Prveen, D. (2011). Plant sources for the treatment of jaundice in the Sugali tribes of Yerramalais forest of Eastern Ghats, Andhra Pradesh, India. *Life Sciences Leaflets*, *14*, 449–457.

Basilico, M. Z., & Basilico, J. C. (1999). Inhibitory effects of some spice essential oils on *Aspergillus ochraceus* NRRL 3174 growth and ochratoxin A production. *Letters in Applied Microbiology*, *29*(4), 238–241. doi:10.1046/j.1365-2672.1999.00621.x PMID:10583751

Basu, S. K., Acharya, S. N., & Thomas, J. E. (2008). Application of phosphate fertilizer and harvest management for important fenugreek (Trigonellafoenum-graecumL.) seed and forage yield in a dark brown soil zone of Canada. *KMITL Sci Tech J*, *8*(1), 1–7.

Basu, S. K., & De, A. K. (2003). Capsicum: historical and botanical perspectives. In A. K. De (Ed.), *Capsicum: The genus Capsicum* (pp. 1–15). London: Taylor and Francis.

Begum, S. S., Jayalakshmi, H. K., & Vidyavathi, H. G. (2016). A novel extract of fenugreek husk (FenuSMARTTM) alleviates postmenopausal symptoms and helps to establish the hormonal balance: A randomized, double-blind, Placebo-Controlled Study. *Phytotherapy Research*, *30*(11), 1775–1784. doi:10.1002/ptr.5680 PMID:27406028

Beinvogl, B., Burch, E., Snyder, J., Schechter, N., Hale, A., Okazaki, Y., ... Nurko, S. (2018). Multidisciplinary treatment of pediatric functional gastrointestinal disorders results in improved pain and functioning. *Clinical Gastroenterology and Hepatology*.

Bellik, Y. (2014). Total antioxidant activity and antimicrobial potency of the essential oil and oleoresin of Zingiber officinale Roscoe. *Asian Pacific Journal of Tropical Disease*, *4*(1), 40–44. doi:10.1016/S2222-1808(14)60311-X

Benavides, G. A., Squadrito, G. L., Mills, R. W., Patel, H. D., Isbell, T. S., Patel, R. P., ... Kraus, D. W. (2007). Hydrogen sulfide mediates the vasoactivity of garlic. *Proceedings of the National Academy of Sciences of the United States of America*, *104*(46), 17977–17982. doi:10.1073/pnas.0705710104 PMID:17951430

Bendahou, M., Muselli, A., Grignon-Dubois, M., Benyoucef, M., Desjobert, J. M., Bernardini, A. F., & Costa, J. (2008). Antimicrobial activity and chemical composition of OriganumglandulosumDesf. Essential oil and extract obtained by microwave extraction. Comparison with hydro distillation. *Food Chemistry*, *106*(1), 132–139. doi:10.1016/j.foodchem.2007.05.050

Bernard, G. T., Esteban, P., & Christopher, J. S. (1982). Turmerones: Isolation from turmeric and their structure determination. *Chemical Communications*, *6*, 363.

Besong, E. E., Balogun, M. E., Djobissie, S. F. A., Mbamalu, O. S., & Obimma, J. N. (2016). A review of *Piper guineense*(African Black Pepper). *Inter J of Pharm and Pharma Res*, *6*, 368–384.

Betty, R. (2008). *The many healing virtues of fenugreek.* Spice India.

Bhandari, U., Kanojia, R., & Pillai, K. K. (2005). Effect of ethanolic extract of Zingiber officinale on dyslipidaemia in diabetic rats. *Journal of Ethnopharmacology, 97*(2), 227–230. doi:10.1016/j.jep.2004.11.011 PubMed

Bhattacharya, D., & Gupta, R. K. (2005). Nanotechnology and potential of microorganisms. *Critical Reviews in Biotechnology, 25*(4), 199–204. doi:10.1080/07388550500361994 PMID:16419617

Bhawana, B. R., Buttar, H. S., Jain, V. K., & Jain, N. (2011). Curcumin nanoparticles: Preparation, characterization, and antimicrobial study. *Journal of Agricultural and Food Chemistry, 59*(5), 2056–2061. doi:10.1021/jf104402t PMID:21322563

Bhowmik, D., & Jayakar, B. (2008). Turmeric. Herbal and traditional medicine. *Archives of Applied Science Research, 1*(2), 86–108.

Bhuiyan, N. I., Begum, J., & Sultana, M. (2009). Chemical composition of leaf and seed essential oil of Coriandrum sativumL. from Bangladesh. *Bangladesh Journal of Pharmacology, 4*(2), 150–153. doi:10.3329/bjp.v4i2.2800

Billman, G. E. (2013). The effects of omega-3 polyunsaturated fatty acids on cardiac rhythm: A critical assessment. *Pharmacology & Therapeutics, 140*(1), 53–80. doi:10.1016/j.pharmthera.2013.05.011 PMID:23735203

Binnig, G., Quate, C. F., & Gerber, Ch. (1986). Atomic force microscope. *Physical Review Letters, 56*(9), 930–933. doi:10.1103/PhysRevLett.56.930 PMID:10033323

Bi, X., Lim, J., & Henry, C. J. (2017). Spices in the management of diabetes mellitus. *Food Chemistry, 217*, 281–293. doi:10.1016/j.foodchem.2016.08.111 PMID:27664636

Blanco Andujar, C. (2014). *Sodium carbonate mediated synthesis of iron oxide nanoparticles to improve magnetic hyperthermia efficiency and induce apoptosis* (Doctoral dissertation). University College London.

Blumenthal, M., Goldberg, A., & Brinckmann, J. (2000). Herbal Medicine: Expanded Commission E Monographs. American Botanical Council, Integrative Medicine Communications.

Blumenthal, M. (1998). *The complete German Commission E monographs: therapeutic guide to herbal medicines.* Austin, TX: American Botanical Council.

Bode, A. M., & Dong, Z. (2004). Ginger. In L. Packer, C. N. Ong, & B. Halliwell (Eds.), Herbal and traditional medicine: molecular aspects of health (pp. 131–156). New York: Marcel Dekker; doi:10.1201/9780203025901.ch8.

Bolhasani, A., Bathaie, S. Z., Yavari, I., Moosavi-Movahedi, A. A., & Ghaffari, M. (2005). Separation and purification of some components of Iranian saffron. *Chemistry, an Asian Journal, 17*, 725–729.

Bone, M. E., Wilkinson, D. J., Young, J. R., McNeil, J., & Charlton, S. (1990). Ginger root, a new antiemetic. The effect of ginger root on postoperative nausea and vomiting after major gynaecological surgery. *Anaesthesia, 45*(8), 669–671. doi:10.1111/j.1365-2044.1990.tb14395.x PubMed

Bordia, A., Verma, S. K., & Srivastava, K. C. (1997). Effect of ginger and fenugreek on blood lipids, blood sugar and platelet aggregation in patients with coronary disease Prostaglandins, Leukotrienes and Essential Fatty Acids. *Pharmacological Research, 36*, 379–384.

Boroushaki, M. T., Mofidpour, H., & Sadeghnia, H. (2007). Protective effect of safranal against hexachlorobutadiene-induced nephrotoxicity in rat. *Iranian Journal of Medical Sciences, 32*, 173–176.

Borrelli, F., Capasso, R., Aviello, G., Pittler, M. H., & Izzo, A. A. (2005). Effectiveness and safety of ginger in the treatment of pregnancy induced Nausea and vomiting. *Obstetrics and Gynecology, 105*(4), 849–856. doi:10.1097/01.AOG.0000154890.47642.23 PubMed

Bosland, P. W. (1998). Capsicums: Innovative uses of an ancient crop". In J. Janick (Ed.), *Progress in New Crops* (pp. 479–487). Arlington, VA: ASHS Press.

Bosland, P., Coon, D., & Cooke, P. H. (2015). Novel Formation of Ectopic (Nonplacental) Capsaicinoid Secreting Vesicles on Fruit Walls Explains the Morphological Mechanism for Super-hot Chile Peppers. *Journal of the American Society for Horticultural Science*, *140*(3), 253–256. doi:10.21273/JASHS.140.3.253

Brar, S. K., & Verma, M. (2011). Measurement of nanoparticles by light-scattering techniques. *Trends in Analytical Chemistry*, *30*(1), 4–17. doi:10.1016/j.trac.2010.08.008

Brewer, M.S. (2011) Natural Antioxidants: Sources, Compounds, Mechanisms of Action, and Potential Applications. *Inst food technol, 10*, 221-247.

Brinck, T. (2014). *Introduction to green energetic materials*. Chichester, UK: John Wiley & Sons Ltd. doi:10.1002/9781118676448

Broca, C., Breil, V., Cruciani-Guglielmacci, C., Manteghetti, M., Rouault, C., Derouet, M., ... Taouis, M. (2004). The insulinotrophic agent 1D1101(4-hydroxyisoleucine) activates insulin signaling in rat. *American Journal of Physiology. Endocrinology and Metabolism*, *287*(3), E463–E471. doi:10.1152/ajpendo.00163.2003 PMID:15082420

Broek, H., Robbins, K., & Randall, J. (2004). Rosemary extract: Taking freshness back to basics. In: Fats and oils-their role in food and health. In *Proceedings of the biennial conference*. Australian Section of the American Oil Chemists Society.

Brummer, Y., Cui, W., & Wang, Q. (2003). Extraction, purification and physicochemical characterization of fenugreek gum. *Food Hydrocolloids*, *3*(3), 229–236. doi:10.1016/S0268-005X(02)00054-1

Bukhari, S. B., Bhanger, M. I., & Memon, S. (2008). Antioxidative activity of extracts from fenugreek. *Pakistan Journal of Analytical & Environmental Chemistry*, *9*(2), 78–83.

Burdock, G. A., & Carabin, I. G. (2009). Safety assessment of coriander (*Coriandrum sativum* L.) essential oil as a food ingredient. *Food and Chemical Toxicology*, *47*(1), 22–34. doi:10.1016/j.fct.2008.11.006 PMID:19032971

Busó-Rogero, C., Brimaud, S., Solla-Gullon, J., Vidal-Iglesias, F. J., Herrero, E., Behm, R. J., & Feliu, J. M. (2016). Ethanol oxidation on shape-controlled platinum nanoparticles at different pHs: A combined in situ IR spectroscopy and online mass spectrometry study. *Journal of Electroanalytical Chemistry (Lausanne, Switzerland)*, *763*, 116–124. doi:10.1016/j.jelechem.2015.12.034

Butt, M. S., & Sultan, M. T. (2011). Ginger and its health claims: Molecular aspects. *Critical Reviews in Food Science and Nutrition*, *51*(5), 383–393. doi:10.1080/10408391003624848 PubMed

Butt, M. S., Sultan, M. T., Butt, M. S., & Iqbal, J. (2009). Garlic: Nature's Protection Against Physiological Threats. *Critical Reviews in Food Science and Nutrition*, *49*(6), 538–551. doi:10.1080/10408390802145344 PMID:19484634

Caballero-Ortega, H., Pereda-Miranda, R., & Abdullaev, F. I. (2007). HPLC quantification of major active components from 11 different saffron (*Crocus sativus* L.) sources. *Food Chemistry*, *100*(3), 1126–1131. doi:10.1016/j.foodchem.2005.11.020

Cabello, C. M., Bair, W. B. III, Lamore, S. D., Ley, S., Bause, A. S., Azimian, S., & Wondrak, G. T. (2009). The cinnamon-derived Michael acceptor cinnamic aldehyde impairs melanoma cell proliferation, invasiveness, and tumor growth. *Free Radical Biology & Medicine*, *46*(2), 220–231. doi:10.1016/j.freeradbiomed.2008.10.025 PMID:19000754

Cao, H., Urban, J. F. Jr, & Anderson, R. A. (2008). Cinnamon Polyphenol Extract Affects Immune Responses by Regulating Anti- and Proinflammatory and Glucose Transporter Gene Expression in Mouse Macrophages. *The Journal of Nutrition*, *138*(5), 833–840. doi:10.1093/jn/138.5.833 PMID:18424588

Cao, J., Liu, Y., Jia, L., Jiang, L. P., Geng, C. Y., Yao, X. F., ... Zhong, L. F. (2008). Curcumin attenuates acrylamide-induced cytotoxicity and genotoxicity in HepG2 cells by ROS scavenging. *Journal of Agricultural and Food Chemistry*, *56*(24), 12059–12063. doi:10.1021/jf8026827 PMID:19012407

Castellano, J. J., Shafii, S. M., Ko, F., Donate, G., Wright, T. E., Mannari, R. J., ... Robson, M. C. (2007). Comparative evaluation of silver-containing antimicrobial dressings and drugs. *International Wound Journal*, *4*(2), 114–122. doi:10.1111/j.1742-481X.2007.00316.x PMID:17651227

Chahal, K. K., Bansal, R., & Kaur, R. (2016). Chemistry and insecticidal potential of bay leaf essential oil against stored grain pest of wheat. *Journal of Applied and Natural Science*, *8*(4), 2049–2054. doi:10.31018/jans.v8i4.1085

Chahal, K. K., Singh, R., Kumar, A., & Bhardwaj, U. (2017). Chemical composition and biological activity of *Coriandrum sativum* Lin [review]. *Indian Journal of Natural Products and Resources*, *8*(3), 193–203.

Chainani-Wu, N. (2003). Safety and Anti-Inflammatory Activity of Curcumin: A Component of Tumeric (Curcuma longa). *Journal of Alternative and Complementary Medicine (New York, N.Y.)*, *9*(1), 161–168. doi:10.1089/107555303321223035 PMID:12676044

Chaiyasit, K., Khovidhunkit, W., & Wittayalertpanya, S. (2009). Relationships between Free Radical Scavenging and Antioxidant Activity in Foods. *Journal of the Medical Association of Thailand*, *92*, 108–113. PMID:19260251

Chaiyata, P., Puttadechakum, S., & Komindr, S. (2003). Bioactives from spices and herbs. *Journal of the Medical Association of Thailand*, *86*, 854–860.

Chakraborty, B., Nath, A., Saikia, H., & Sengupta, M. (2014). Bactericidal activity of selected medicinal plants against multidrug resistant bacterial strains from clinical isolates. *Asian Pacific Journal of Tropical Medicine*, *7*, S435–S441. doi:10.1016/S1995-7645(14)60271-6 PubMed

Chanda, N., Shukla, R., Zambre, A., Mekapothula, S., Kulkarni, R. R., Katti, K., ... Katti, K. V. (2010). An Effective Strategy for the Synthesis of Biocompatible Gold Nanoparticles Using Cinnamon Phytochemicals for Phantom CT Imaging and Photoacoustic Detection of Cancerous Cells. *Pharmaceutical Research*, *28*(2), 279–291. doi:10.100711095-010-0276-6 PMID:20872051

Chandra, D., & Gupta, S. S. (1972). Anti-inflammatory and antiarthritic activity of volatile oil of Curcuma longa. *The Indian Journal of Medical Research*, *60*, 138–142. PMID:5029117

Chang, K. S., & Ahn, Y. J. (2002). Fumigant activity of (E)-anethole identified in Illiciumverum fruit against Blattellagermanica. *Journal of Pest Management Science*, *58*(2), 161–166. doi:10.1002/ps.435 PMID:11852640

Chatterjee, S., Variyar, P. S., & Sharma, A. (2010). Bioactive lipid constituents of fenugreek. *Food Chemistry*, *1*(1), 349–353. doi:10.1016/j.foodchem.2009.05.076

Chaudhry, N. M. A., & Tariq, P. (2006). Anti-microbial activity of Cinnamomum cassia against diverse microbial flora with its nutritional and medicinal impacts. *Pakistan Journal of Botany*, *38*(1), 169.

Chaudhry, N. M., & Tariq, P. (2006). Bactericidal activity of black pepper, bay leaf, aniseed and coriander against oral isolates. *Pakistan Journal of Pharmaceutical Sciences*, *19*(3), 214–218.

Chauhan, G., Sharma, M., & Varma, A. (2010). Phytochemical analysis and anti-inflammatory potential of fenugreek, Medicinal plants. *Int. J. Phytomedicine. Rel. Ind*, *2*(1), 39–44.

Chelladurai, P. K., & Ramalingam, R. (2017). *Myristica malabarica*: A comprehensive review. *Journal of Pharmacognosy and Phytochemistry*, *6*, 255–258.

Chen, N., Chang, C. C., Ng, C. C., Wang, C. Y., Shyu, Y. T., & Chang, T. I. (2008). Antioxidant and antimicrobial activity of Zingiberaceae plants in Taiwan. *Plant Foods for Human Nutrition (Dordrecht, Netherlands)*, *63*(1), 15–20. doi:10.100711130-007-0063-7 PMID:18157743

Chen, S., Zhang, X., Zhang, Q., & Tan, W. (2009). Trioctylphosphine as both solvent and stabilizer to synthesize CdS nanorods. *Nanoscale Research Letters*, *4*(10), 1159–1165. doi:10.100711671-009-9375-x PMID:20596487

Chiou, K. L., Hastorf, C. A., Bonavia, D., & Dillehay, T. D. (2014). Documenting cultural selection pressure changes on chile pepper (*Capsicum baccatum*L.) seed size through time in Coastal Peru (7,600 B.P. - Present). *Economic Botany*, *68*(2), 190–202. doi:10.100712231-014-9270-y

Chithra, V., & Leelamma, S. (1999). *Coriandrum sativum* changes the levels of lipid peroxides and activity of antioxidant enzymes in experimental animals. *Indian Journal of Biochemistry & Biophysics*, *36*(1), 59–61. PMID:10549163

Chithra, V., & Leelamma, S. (2000). *Coriandrum sativum*—Effect on lipid metabolism in 1,2-dimethyl hydrazine induced colon cancer. *Journal of Ethnopharmacology*, *71*(3), 457–463. doi:10.1016/S0378 8741(00)00182-3 PMID:10940583

Chitra, V., Dharani, P. P., Pavan, K. K., & Alla, N. R. (2009). Wound healing activity of alcoholic extract of Buchanania lanzan in Albino rats. *International Journal of Chemtech Research*, *1*(4), 1026–1031.

Chiwendu, S., Ejike, E. N., Ejeke, B. U., Oti, W., & Uwachukwu, I. (2016). Phytochemical properties of Uziza leave (*Piper guineesnse*). *J of Pure and App Chem*, *3*, 12–15.

Choudhary, D., Kala, S. P., Todaria, N. P., Dasgupta, S., Kinhal, G., & Kollmair, M. (2013). Essential oil from bay leaves in India and Nepal: An analysis for quality oriented value chain development. *International Journal of Medicinal and Aromatic Plants*, *3*(1), 11–17.

Choudhury, D., Das, A., Bhattacharya, A., & Chakrabarti, G. (2010). Aqueous extract of ginger shows antiproliferative activity through disruption of microtubule network of cancer cells. *Food and Chemical Toxicology*, *48*(10), 2872–2880. doi:10.1016/j.fct.2010.07.020 PubMed

Chryssanthi, D. G., Dedes, P. G., Karamanos, N. K., Cordopatis, P., & Lamari, F. N. (2011). Crocetin inhibits invasiveness of MDA MB 231 breast cancer cells via downregulation of matrix metalloproteinases. *Planta Medica*, *77*(02), 146–151. doi:10.1055-0030-1250178 PMID:20803418

Cook, N. C., & Samman, S. (1996). Flavonoids- chemistry, metabolism, cardioprotective effects, and dietary sources. *Nutritional Biochemistry*, *7*(2), 66–76. doi:10.1016/0955-2863(95)00168-9

Coon, J. S. T., & Ernst, E. (2003). Herbs for serum cholesterol reduction: A systematic view. *The Journal of Family Practice*, *52*, 468–478. PMID:12791229

Coriander (cilantro) leaves, raw. (n.d.). Retrieved from https://www.nutritionvalue.org/Coriander_(cilantro)_leaves,_raw_nutritional_value.html

Coriandrum sativum (coriander). (n.d.). Retrieved from https://www.cabi.org/isc/datasheet/15300

Coskuner, Y., & Karababa, E. (2007). Physical properties of coriander seeds (*Coriandrum sativum L.*). *Journal of Food Engineering*, *80*(2), 408–416. doi:10.1016/j.jfoodeng.2006.02.042

Craig, W. J. (1999). Health-promoting properties of common herbs. *The American Journal of Clinical Nutrition*, *70*(3), 491–499. doi:10.1093/ajcn/70.3.491s PMID:10479221

Cristian, D., Liliana, G., Petru, A., & Stefan, D. (2013). Encapsulation of coriander essential oil in alginate and alginate/chitosan microspheres by emulsification of external gelation method. *Inside Food Symposium*, 9-12.

Crozier, A., Yokota, T., Jaganath, I. B., Marks, S. C., Saltmarsh, M., & Clifford, M. N. (2006). Secondary metabolites in fruits, vegetables, beverages and other plant based dietary components. *Plant secondary metabolites: Occurrence, structure and role in the human diet*, 208-302.

Crozier, A., Jaganath, I. B., & Clifford, M. N. (2009). Dietary phenolics chemistry, bioavailability and effect on health. *Natural Product Reports*, *26*(8), 1001–1043. doi:10.1039/b802662a PMID:19636448

Cusi, K., & DeFronzo, R. (2000). Recombinant human insulin-like growth factor I treatment for 1 week improves metabolic control in type 2 diabetes by ameliorating hepatic and muscle insulin resistance. *The Journal of Clinical Endocrinology and Metabolism*, *85*, 3077–3084. PMID:10999789

Czygan, F. C. D., Frohne, C., Holtzel, A., Nagell, & Pfander, H. J. (2001). Norman Grainger Bisset and max Wichtl. Herbal Drugs and Phytopharmaceuticals. In A Handbook for practices on a scientific basics with reference to German commission and Monographs (2nd ed.). Medpharm Scientific Publishers.

D'Alessandro, A. M., Mancini, A., Lizzi, A. R., Simone, A. D., Marroccella, C. E., Gravina, G. L., ... Festuccia, C. (2013). Crocus sativus stigma extract and its major constituent crocin possess significant antiproliferative properties against human prostate cancer. *Nutrition and Cancer*, *65*(6), 930–942. doi:10.1080/01635581.2013.767368 PMID:23909737

da Silva, A. C., de Freitas Santos, P. D., do Prado Silva, J. T., Leimann, F. V., Bracht, L., & Gonçalves, O. H. (2018). Impact of curcumin nanoformulation on its antimicrobial activity. *Trends in Food Science & Technology*, *72*, 74–82. doi:10.1016/j.tifs.2017.12.004

Damanik, R., Wahlqvist, M. L., & Wattanapenpaiboon, N. (2004). The use of a putative lactogogue plant on breast milk production in Simalungun, North Sumatra, Indonesia. *Asia Pacific Journal of Clinical Nutrition*, *13*, S118.

Darughe, F., Barzegar, M., & Sahari, M. A. (2012). Antioxidant and antifungal activity of coriander (*Coriandrum sativum* L.) essential oil in cake. *International Food Research*, *19*(3), 1253–1260.

Das, A. M. (1971). Studies on stem gall disease of coriander incited by *Protomyces macrosporus*. *Second International Symposium on Plant Pathology*.

Das, S., Das, M. P., & Das, J. (2013). Fabrication of porous chitosan/silver nanocomposite film and its bactericidal efficacy against multi-drug resistant (MDR) clinical isolates. *Journal of Pharmacy Research*, *6*(1), 11–15. doi:10.1016/j.jopr.2012.11.006

Datta, M., Sengupta, C., & Pandit, M. K. (2010). Isolation and characterization of bacterial isolates from chili (Capsicum annuum L.) rhizosphere as a potent plant growth promoter. *Journal of Crop and Weed*, *6*(2), 50–58.

De Figueiredo, R. O., Marques, M. O. M., Nakagawa, J., & Ming, L. C. (2004). Composition of coriander essential oil from Brazil. *Acta Horticulturae*, (62): 135–137. doi:10.17660/ActaHortic.2004.629.18

De Milto, L., & Frey, R. J. (2005). Nutmeg. In Gale Encyclopedia of Alternative Medicine (2nd ed. vol. 3). Detroit, MI: Thomson Gale.

Debatin, K. M. (1999). Activation of apoptosis pathways by anticancer drugs. *Advances in Experimental Medicine and Biology*, *457*, 237–244. doi:10.1007/978-1-4615-4811-9_25 PMID:10500798

Debbarma, J., Kishore, P., Nayak, B. B., Kannuchamy, N., & Gudipati, V. (2013). Antibacterial activity of ginger, eucalyptus and sweet orange peel essential oils on fish-borne bacteria. *Journal of Food Processing and Preservation*, *37*(5), 1022–1030. doi:10.1111/j.1745-4549.2012.00753.x

Deepa, G., Ayesha, S., Nishtha, K., & Thankamani, M. (2013). Comparative evaluation of various total antioxidant capacity assays applied to phytochemical compounds of Indian culinary spices. *International Food Research Journal*, *20*(4), 1711–1716.

Dehghani, I., Mostajeran, A., & Asghari, G. (2011). In vitro and in vivo production of gingerols and zingiberene in ginger plant (Zingiber officinale Roscoe). *Indian Journal of Pharmaceutical Sciences*, *7*, 129–133.

Delecroix, B., Abaïdia, A. E., Leduc, C., Dawson, B., & Dupont, G. (2017). Article. *Journal of Sports Science & Medicine*, *16*, 147–153. PMID:28344463

Delisle, J., Amiot, J., Goulet, G., Simard, C., Brisson, G. J., & Jones, J. D. (1984). Nutritive value of protein fractions extracted from soybean, rapeseed and wheat flours in the rat. *Plant Foods for Human Nutrition (Dordrecht, Netherlands)*, *34*(4), 243–251. doi:10.1007/BF01126553

De, M., De, A. K., Sen, P., & Banerjee, A. B. (2002). Antimicrobial properties of star anise (Illiciumverum Hook f). *Journal of Phytotherapy Research*, *16*(1), 94–95. doi:10.1002/ptr.989 PMID:11807977

Derwich, E., Benziane, Z., & Chabir, R. (2011). *Aromatic and medicinal plants of Morocco: Chemical composition of essential oils of Rosmarinus officinalis and Juniperus Phoenicea*. Academic Press.

Desai, U. (2005). *The Ayurvedic cookbook: A personalized guide to good nutrition and health*. New Delhi: Motilal-Banarsidass.

Deshpande, A. A. (2001). Chili and capsicums. In S. Thamburaj & N. Singh (Eds.), *Textbook on vegetables, tuber crops and spices* (pp. 49–75). New Delhi: ICAR.

Devaki, T., Venmahdi, S., & Govindaraju, P. (1992). Alterations in protein metabolism in ethanol-ingested rats treated with garlic. *Medical Science Research*, *20*, 725–727.

Devi, B. A., Kamalakkannan, N., & Prince, P. S. (2003). Supplementation of fenugreek leaves to diabetic rats-Effect on carbohydrate metabolic enzymes in diabetic liver and kidney. *Phytotherapy Research*, *17*(10), 1231 1233. doi:10.1002/ptr.1357 PMID:14669264

Dewitt, D., & Bosland, P. W. (1996). *Peppers of the World: An Identification Guide*. Berkeley, CA: Ten Speed Press.

Dhanapakiam, P., & Joseph, J., Mini, Ramaswamy, V. K. M., Moorthi, & Senthil Kumar, A. (2008). The cholesterol lowering property of coriander seeds (Coriandrumsativum): Mechanism of action. *Journal of Environmental Biology*, *29*(1), 53–56. PMID:18831331

Dhanapakiam, P., Mini Joseph, J., Ramaswamy, V. K., Moorthi, M., & Senthil Kumar, A. (2008). The cholesterol lowering property of coriander seeds (Coriandrum sativum): Mechanism of action. *Journal of Environmental Biology*, *29*(1), 53–56. PMID:18831331

Dhiman, J., Kundu, V., Kumar, S., Kumar, R., & Chakarvarti, S. K. (2014). *Eco-friendly Synthesis and Characterization of Silver Nanoparticles and Evaluation of Their Antibacterial Activity*. American Journal of Materials Science and Technology. doi:10.7726/ajmst.2014.1002

Dhingra, D., & Sharma, A. (2006). Antidepressant-like activity of n-hexane extract of nutmeg (Myristica fragrans) seeds in mice. *Journal of Medicinal Food*, *9*(1), 84–89. doi:10.1089/jmf.2006.9.84 PMID:16579733

Dhuley, J. N. (1999). Anti-oxidant effects of cinnamon (Cinnamomum verum) bark and greater cardamon (Amomum subulatum) seeds in rats fed high fat diet. *Indian Journal of Experimental Biology*, *37*(3), 238–242. PMID:10641152

Dias, L. S., Luzia, D. M. M., & Jorge, N. (2013). Physicochemical and bioactive properties of *Hymenaea courbaril* L. pulp and seed lipid fraction. *Industrial Crops and Products*, *49*, 610–618. doi:10.1016/j.indcrop.2013.06.005

Dias, M. A., Lacerda, I. C. A., Pimentel, P. F., De Castro, H. F., & Rosa, C. A. (2002). Removal of heavy metals by an Aspergillus terreus strain immobilized in a polyurethane matrix. *Letters in Applied Microbiology*, *34*(1), 46–50. doi:10.1046/j.1472-765x.2002.01040.x PMID:11849492

Diederichsen, A. (1996). *An ecogeographical study of promoting the conservation and use of underutilized and neglected crops: Coriander*. International Plant Genetic Resources Institute.

Diederichsen, A. (1996). *Promoting the conservation and use of underutilized and neglected crops:Coriander (Coriandrum sativum L)* (1st ed.). International Plant Genetic Resources Institute IPGRI.

Dighe, V. V., Gursale, A. A., Sane, R. T., Menon, S., & Patel, P. H. (2005). Quantitative determination of eugenol from Cinnamomum tamala nees and eberm: Leaf powder and polyherbal formulation using reverse phase liquid chromatography. *Chromatographia*, *61*(9-10), 443–446. doi:10.136510337-005-0527-6

Dixit, P., Ghaskadbi, S., Mohan, H., & Devasagayam, T. P. A. (2005). Antioxidant properties of germinated fenugreek seeds. *Phytotherapy Research*, *19*(11), 977–983. doi:10.1002/ptr.1769 PMID:16317656

Duan, L., Tao, H. W., Hao, X. J., Gu, Q. Q., & Zhu, W. M. (2009). Cytotoxic and antioxidative phenolic compounds from the traditional Chinese medicinal plant, *Myristica fragrans. Planta Medica*, *75*(11), 1241–1245. doi:10.1055-0029-1185506 PMID:19326328

Duarte, R. C., Fanaro, G. B., Koike, A. C. R., & Villavicencio, A. L. C. H. (2011). *Irradiation effect on antifungal potential myristica fragrans (nutmeg) essential oil, a preliminary study*. https://www.osti.gov/etdeweb/biblio/21517124

Duarte, A., Ferreira, S., Silva, F. C., & Domingues, F. C. (2012). Synergistic activity of coriander oil and conventional antibiotics against Acinetobacter baumannii. *Phytomedicine*, *19*(3–4), 236–238. doi:10.1016/j.phymed.2011.11.010

Dubie, J., Stancik, A., Morra, M., & Nindo, C. (2013). Antioxidant extraction from mustard (Brassica juncea) seed meal using high-intensity ultrasound. *Journal of Food Science*, *78*(4), 542–548. doi:10.1111/1750-3841.12085 PMID:23488824

Dugasani, S., Pichika, M. R., Nadarajah, V. D., Balijepalli, M. K., Tandra, S., & Korlakunta, J. N. (2010). Comparative antioxidant and anti-inflammatory effects of [6]-gingerol, [8]-gingerol, [10]-gingerol and [6]-shogaol. *Journal of Ethnopharmacology*, *127*(2), 515–520. doi:10.1016/j.jep.2009.10.004 PubMed

Dugoua, J. J., Seely, D., Perri, D., Cooley, K., Forelli, T., Mills, E., & Koren, G. (2007). From type 2 diabetes to antioxidant activity: A systematic review of the safety and efficacy of common and cassia cinnamon bark. *Canadian Journal of Physiology and Pharmacology*, *85*(9), 837–847. doi:10.1139/Y07-080 PMID:18066129

Duke, J. A., Bogenschutz-Godwin, M. J., deCellier, J., & Duke, P. K. (2003). Elettaria cardamomum Maton (Zingiberaceae) Cardamon, Malabar or Mysore cardamon. CRC Handbook of Medicinal Spices, 120-138.

Duke, J. A. (2002). *Handbook of Medicinal Herbs* (2nd ed.). Boca Raton, FL: CRC Press LLC. doi:10.1201/9781420040463

Duke, J. A., Bogenschutz-Godwin, M. J., deCellier, J., & Duke, P. K. (2003). *Syzygiumaromaticum(L.)Merr.and L. M. Perry (Myrtaceae) Clavos, Clove, Clovetree. In CRC Handbook of Medicinal Spices* (p. 281). Washington, DC: CRC Press.

Dumbre, R. K., Kamble, M. B., & Patil, V. R. (2014). Inhibitory effects by ayurvedic plants on prostate enlargement induced in rats. *Pharmacognosy Research*, *6*(2), 127. doi:10.4103/0974-8490.129031 PMID:24761116

Duong, H. T., Chen, Y., Tawfik, S. A., Wen, S., Parviz, M., Shimoni, O., & Jin, D. (2018). Systematic investigation of functional ligands for colloidal stable upconversion nanoparticles. *RSC Advances*, *8*(9), 4842–4849. doi:10.1039/C7RA13765F

Dzoyem, J. P., McGaw, L.J., Kuete, V., & Bakowsky, U. (2017). *Medicinal Spices and Vegetables from Africa*. Academic Press.

Eguale, T., Tilahun, G., Debella, A., Feleke, A., & Makonnen, E. (2007). In vitro and in vivo anthelmintic activity of crude extracts of Coriandrum sativum against Haemonchuscontortus. *Journal of Ethnopharmacology*, *110*(3), 428–433. doi:10.1016/j.jep.2006.10.003 PMID:17113738

Eidi, A., Eidi, M., & Esmaeili, E. (2006). Antidiabetic effect of garlic (Allium sativum L.) in normal and streptozotocin-induced diabetic rats. *Phytomedicine*, *13*(9-10), 624–629. doi:10.1016/j.phymed.2005.09.010 PMID:17085291

Ekanem, A. P., Udoh, V. F., & Oku, E. E. (2010). Effects of ethanol extract of *Piper guineense* seeds (Schum and Thonn) on the conception of mice (MuaMusculus). *African Journal of Pharmacy and Pharmacology*, *4*, 362–367.

El Nasri, N. A., & El Tinay, A. (2007). Functional properties of Fenugreek (*Trigonellafoenumgraecum*) protein concentrate. *Food Chemistry*, *2*(2), 582–589. doi:10.1016/j.foodchem.2006.09.003

El-Alfy, A., Wilson, L., ElSohly, M. A., & Abourashed, E. A. (2009). Towards a better understanding of the psychopharmacology of nutmeg: Activities in the mouse tetrad assay. *Journal of Ethnopharmacology*, *126*(2), 280–286. doi:10.1016/j.jep.2009.08.026 PMID:19703539

El-Baroty, G. S., El-Baky, H. H. A., Farag, R. S., & Saleh, M. A. (2010). Characterization of antioxidant and antimicrobial compounds of cinnamon and ginger essential oils. *African Journal of Biochemistry Research*, *6*, 167–174.

El-Batal, A. I., Al-Hazmi, N. E., Mosallam, F. M., & El-Sayyad, G. S. (2018). Biogenic synthesis of copper nanoparticles by natural polysaccharides and Pleurotus ostreatus fermented fenugreek using gamma rays with antioxidant and antimicrobial potential towards some wound pathogens. *Microbial Pathogenesis*, *118*, 159–169. doi:10.1016/j.micpath.2018.03.013 PMID:29530808

El, S. N., Karagozlu, N., Karakaya, S., & Sahın, S. (2014). Antioxidant and antimicrobial activities of essential oils extracted from Laurus nobilis L. leaves by using solvent-free microwave and hydrodistillation. *Food and Nutrition Sciences*, *5*(02), 97–106. doi:10.4236/fns.2014.52013

El-Sawi, S. A., Ibrahim, M. E., & Ali, A. M. (2009). In vitro cytotoxic, antioxidant and antimicrobial activities of essential oil of leaves of Lauras nobilis L. grown in Egypt and its chemical composition. *Medicinal and Aromatic Plant Science and Biotechnology*, *3*(1), 16–23.

Elvin-Lewis, M. (2001). Should we be concerned about herbal remedies? *Journal of Ethnopharmacology*, *75*(2-3), 141–164. doi:10.1016/S0378-8741(00)00394-9 PMID:11297844

Enaydede, A., Meloa, J. M., Filhob, N. B., Guerrac, E. G., & Heidari-Hamedani. (2006). *Sedative-hypnotic activity of extracts and essential oil of coriander seeds*. Academic Press.

Enaydede, A. (2005). Characterization of antioxidant compounds in aqueous coriander extract (*Coriandrum sativum* L.). *Lebensmittel-Wissenschaft + Technologie*, *38*(1), 15–19. doi:10.1016/j.lwt.2004.03.011

Engelbrekt, C., Jensen, P. S., Sørensen, K. H., Ulstrup, J., & Zhang, J. (2013). Complexity of gold nanoparticle formation disclosed by dynamics study. *The Journal of Physical Chemistry C*, *117*(22), 11818–11828. doi:10.1021/jp401883h

Erturk, O. (2006). Antibacterial and antifungal activity of ethanolic extracts from eleven spice plants. *Section Cellular and Molecular Biology*, *61*(3), 275–278. doi:10.247811756-006-0050-8

Eshrat, H., & Hussain, M. A. (2002). Hypoglycemic, hypolipidemic and antioxidant properties of combination of curcumin from Curcuma longa Linn. and partially purified product from Abromaaugusta Linn. in streptozotocin induced diabetes. *Indian Journal of Clinical Biochemistry*, *17*(2), 33–43. doi:10.1007/BF02867969 PMID:23105348

Eslami, M., Bayat, M., Nejad, A. S. M., Sabokbar, A., & Anvar, A. A. (2016). Effect of polymer/nanosilver composite packaging on long-term microbiological status of Iranian saffron (Crocus sativus L.). *Saudi Journal of Biological Sciences*, *23*(3), 341–347. doi:10.1016/j.sjbs.2015.07.004 PMID:27081358

Ettenberg, J. (2019). *A brief history of chili peppers*. https://www.legalnomads.com/history-Chili-peppers

Everett, T. H. (1981). *Myristica. In Illustrated Encyclopaedia of Horticulture*. New York: Garland Publishing Inc.

Fabio, A., Cermelli, C., Fabio, G., Nicoletti, P., & Quaglio, P. (2007). Screening of the antibacterial effects of a variety of essential oils on microorganisms responsible for respiratory infections. *Phytotherapy Research*, *21*(4), 374–377. doi:10.1002/ptr.1968 PMID:17326042

Fang, S. H., Rao, Y. K., & Tzeng, Y. M. (2004). Cytotoxic effect of trans-cinnamaldehyde from cinnamomum osmophloeum leaves on Human cancer cell lines. *International Journal of Applied Science and Engineering*, *2*(2), 136–147.

Fang, X. D., Yang, F., Zhu, L., Shen, Y. L., Wang, L. L., & Cheng, Y. Y. (2009). Curcumin ameliorates high glucose-induced acute vascular endothelial dysfunction in rat thoracic aorta. *Clinical and Experimental Pharmacology & Physiology*, *36*(12), 1177–1182. doi:10.1111/j.1440-1681.2009.05210.x PMID:19473193

Farag, M. F. S. (2013). Evaluation of radioprotective effects of coriander (Coriandrum sativum L.) in male rats. *Arab Journal of Nuclear Science and Applications*, *46*(1), 240–249.

Farooqi, A. A., Sreeramu, B. S., & Srinivasappa, K. N. (2005). Cultivation of spice crops. Hyderabad: Universities Press (India) Private Limited.

Ferreira, E. B., Neves, F. E. A., da Costa, M. E. D., do Prado, W. A., Ferri, L. A., & … . (2006). Comparative effects of Stevia rebaudiana leaves and stevioside on glycaemia and hepatic gluconeogenesis. *Planta Medica*, *72*(08), 691–696. doi:10.1055-2006-931586 PMID:16732523

Filomena, S., & Fernanda, C. D. (2017). Antimicrobial activity of coriander oil and its effectiveness as a food preservative. *Critical Reviews in Food Science and Nutrition*, *57*(1), 35–47. doi:10.1080/10408398.2013.847818

Filomena, S., & Susana, F. (2011). Antifungal activity of *Coriandrum sativum* essential oil, its mode of action against Candida species and potential synergism with amphotericin B. *Phytomedicine*, *19*(1), 42–47. doi:10.1016/j.phymed.2011.06.033

Filomena, S., Susana, F., & Joao, A. (2011). Essential oil: Its antibacterial activity and mode of action evaluated by flow cytometry. *Journal of Medical Microbiology*, *60*(10), 1479–1486. doi:10.1099/jmm.0.034157-0

Flammang, A., Cifone, M., Erexson, G., & Stankowski, L. F. Jr. (2004). Genotoxicity testing of a fenugreek extract. *Food and Chemical Toxicology*, *11*(11), 1769–1775. doi:10.1016/j.fct.2004.07.003 PMID:15350674

Flückinger, F. A. (1879). *Pharmacographia: A History of the Principal Drugs of Vegetable Origin, Met with in Great Britain and British India*. London: Macmillan.

Forrester, M. B. (2005). Nutmeg intoxication in Texas, 1998-2004. *Human and Experimental Toxicology*, *24*(11), 563–566. doi:10.1191/0960327105ht567oa PMID:16323572

Freires, I. D. A., Murata, R. M., Furletti, V. F., Sartoratto, A., De Alencar, S. M. D., & Figueira, G. M. (2019). *Coriandrum sativum* L. (Coriander) essential oil: Antifungal activity and mode of action on Candida spp. and molecular targets affected in human whole-genome expression. *PLoS One*, *9*(6), e99086. doi:10.1371/journal.pone.0099086

Fuhrman, B., Rosenblat, M., Hayek, T., Coleman, R., & Aviram, M. (2000). Ginger extract consumption reduces plasma cholesterol, inhibits LDL oxidation and attenuates development of atherosclerosis in atherosclerotic, apolipoprotein E-deficient mice. *The Journal of Nutrition*, *130*(5), 1124–1131. doi:10.1093/jn/130.5.1124 PubMed

Gade, A., Gaikwad, S., Tiwari, V., Yadav, A., Ingle, A., & Rai, M. (2010). Biofabrication of silver nanoparticles by Opuntia ficus-indica: In vitro antibacterial activity and study of the mechanism involved in the synthesis. *Current Nanoscience*, *6*(4), 370–375. doi:10.2174/157341310791659026

Garcia-Olmo, D. C., Riese, H. H., Escribano, J., Ontanon, J., Fernandez, J. A., Atienzar, M., & Garcia-Olmo, D. (1999). Effects of long-term treatment of colon adenocarcinoma with crocin, a carotenoid from saffron (Crocussativus L.): An experimental study in the rat. *Nutrition and Cancer*, *35*(2), 120–126. doi:10.1207/S15327914NC352_4 PMID:10693164

Garg, S. N., Siddiqui, M. S., & Agarwal, S. K. (1992). New fatty acid esters and hydroxyl ketones from fruits of Laurus nobilis. *Journal of Natural Products*, *55*(9), 1315–1319. doi:10.1021/np50087a023

Geeta, G. S., & Reddy, T. K. R. (1990). Aspergillus flavus link and its occurrence in relation to other mycoflora on stored spices. *Journal of Stored Products Research*, *26*(4), 211–213. doi:10.1016/0022-474X(90)90024-M

Gende, L. B., Floris, I., Fritz, R., & Eguaras, M. J. (2008). Antimicrobial activity of cinnamon (*Cinnamomum zeylanicum*) essential oil and its main components against paenibacillus larvae from argentine. *Bulletin of Insectology*, *61*(1), 1–4.

Ghadermazi, R., Keramat, J., & Goli, S. A. H. (2017). Antioxidant activity of clove (Eugenia caryophyllataThunb), oregano (Oringanumvulgare L) and sage (Salvia officinalis L) essential oils in various modelsystems. *International Food Research Journal*, *24*(4), 1628–1635.

Ghayur, M. N., Gilani, A. H., Afridi, M. B., & Houghton, P. J. (2005). Cardiovascular effects of ginger aqueous extract and its phenolic constituents are mediated through multiple pathways. *Vascular Pharmaco, 43*(4), 234-241.

Ghedira, K., Goetz, P. L. J. R., & Le Juene, R. (2010). Fenugrec: *Trigonellafoenumgraecum* L. (Fabaceae ex. Leguminosae). *Phytothérapie*, *8*(3), 180–184. doi:10.100710298-010-0551-z

Ghodake, G. S., Deshpande, N. G., Lee, Y. P., & Jin, E. (2010). Pear fruit extract-assisted room-temperature biosynthesis of gold nanoplates. *Colloids and Surfaces. B, Biointerfaces*, *75*(2), 584–589. doi:10.1016/j.colsurfb.2009.09.040 PMID:19879738

Giacosa, A., Morazzoni, P., Bombardelli, E., Riva, A., Bianchi, P. G., & Rondanelli, M. (2015). Can nausea and vomiting be treated with ginger extract? *European Review for Medical and Pharmacological Sciences*, *19*, 1291–1296. PMID:25912592

Gilani, A. H., Bashir, S., & Khan, A. U. (2007). Pharmacological basis for the use of *Borago officinalis* in gastrointestinal, respiratory and cardiovascular disorders. *Journal of Ethnopharmacology*, *114*(3), 393–399. doi:10.1016/j.jep.2007.08.032 PMID:17900837

Goldstein, J. I., Newbury, D. E., Michael, J. R., Ritchie, N. W., Scott, J. H. J., & Joy, D. C. (2017). *X-ray microanalysis*. Springer.

Goodman, P. S. (2005). *Star Rises in Fight Against Bird Flu. Demand for a Chinese Fruit 2Skyrockets.* Washington Post Foreign Service.

Gopalakrishnan, M. J. C. S., Narayanan, C. S., & Grenz, M. (1990). Nonsaponifiable lipid constituents of Cardamom. *Journal of Agricultural and Food Chemistry*, *38*(12), 2133–2136. doi:10.1021/jf00102a006

Gopalan, C., Ramasastri, B.V., & Balasubramaniyam, S.C. (1989). *Nutritive value of Indian food.* National Institute of Nutrition, ICMR Hydrabad.

Goud, V. K., Polasa, K., & Krishnaswamy, K. (1993). Effect of turmeric on xenobiotic metabolising enzymes. *Plant Foods for Human Nutrition (Dordrecht, Netherlands)*, *44*(1), 87–92. doi:10.1007/BF01088486 PMID:8332589

Governa, P., Baini, G., Borgonetti, V., Cettolin, G., Giachetti, D., Magnano, A. R., ... Biagi, M. (2018). Phytotherapy in the management of diabetes: A review. *Molecules (Basel, Switzerland)*, *23*(1), 1–22. doi:10.3390/molecules23010105 PMID:29300317

Goyal, R. K., & Kadnur, S. V. (2006). Beneðcial effects of *Zingiber officinale* on gold thioglucose induced obesity. *Fitoterapia*, *77*(3), 160–163. doi:10.1016/j.fitote.2006.01.005 PMID:16513292

Grigoleit, H. G., & Grigoleit, P. (2005). Gastrointestinal clinical pharmacology of peppermint oil. *Phytomedicine*, *12*(8), 607–611. doi:10.1016/j.phymed.2004.10.006 PMID:16121522

Grontved, A., Brask, T., Kambskard, J., & Hentzer, E. (1988). Ginger root against seasickness: A controlled trial on the open sea. *Acta Oto-Laryngologica*, *105*(1-2), 45–49. doi:10.3109/00016488809119444 PubMed

Grover, J. K., Rathi, S. S., & Vats, V. (2002). Amelioration of experimental diabetic neuropathy and gastropathy in rats following oral administration of plant (Eugenia jambolana, Mucunapruriens and Tinosporacordifolia) extracts. *Indian Journal of Experimental Biology*, *40*, 273–276. PMID:12635695

Grover, J. K., Yadav, S. P., & Vats, V. (2003). Effect of feeding murrayakoeingii and brassica juncea diet on [correction] kidney functions and glucose levels in streptozotocin-diabetic mice. *Journal of Ethnopharmacology*, *85*(1), 1–5. doi:10.1016/S0378-8741(02)00355-0 PMID:12576195

Grzanna, R., Phan, P., Polotsky, A., Lindmark, L., & Fondoza, C. G. (2004). Ginger Extract Inhibits β-Amyloid Peptide–Induced Cytokine and Chemokine Expression in Cultured THP-1 Monocytes. *Journal of Alternative and Complementary Medicine (New York, N.Y.)*, *10*(6), 1009–1013. doi:10.1089/acm.2004.10.1009 PMID:15673995

Guldiken, B., Özkan, G., Catalkaya, G., Ceylan, F.D., Yalçınkaya, İ. E., & Capanoglu, E. (2018). Phytochemicals of herbs and spices: Health versus toxicological effects. *Food and Chemical Toxicology*. doi:10.1016/j.fct.2018.05.050 PMID:29802945

Gunasekar, M., Geemon, K., & Mariwala, S. J. (2012). Health benefits of bioactive molecules from spices and aromatic plants. *JOSAC21*, 87–101.

Guo, J. B., Fan, Y., Zhang, W. J., Wu, H., Du, L. M., & Chang, Y. X. (2017). Extraction of gingerols and shogaols from ginger (Zingiber officinale Roscoe) through microwave technique using ionic liquids. *Journal of Food Composition and Analysis*, *62*, 35–42. doi:10.1016/j.jfca.2017.04.014

Gupta, A. D., & Rajpurohit, D. (2011). Antioxidant and Antimicrobial Activity of Nutmeg (Myristica fragrans). In V. R. Preedy, R. R. Watson, & V. B. Patel (Eds.), Nuts & Seeds in Health and Disease Prevention (pp. 831-839). London, UK: Academic Press is an imprint of Elsevier.

Gupta, A. D., Bansal, V. K., Babu, V., & Maithil, N. (2013). Chemistry, antioxidant and antimicrobial potential of nutmeg (*Myristica fragrans* Houtt). *Journal of Genetic Engineering and Biotechnology*, *11*(1), 25–31. doi:10.1016/j.jgeb.2012.12.001

Gupta, A., Gupta, R., & Lal, B. (2001). Effect of *Trigonellafoenum- graecum*(fenugreek) seeds on glycaemic control and insulin resistance in type 2 diabetes mellitus: A double blind placebo controlled study. *The Journal of the Association of Physicians of India*, *49*, 1057–1061. PMID:11868855

Gupta, A., Gupta, R., & Lal, B. (2001). Effect of Trigonellafoenum-graecum (fenugreek) seeds on glycemic control and insulin resistance in type-2 diabetes mellitus: A double blind placebo controlled study. *J Assoc Physi Ind*, *49*, 1057–1061. PMID:11868855

Gupta, M. (2010). Pharmacological Properties and Traditional Therapeutic Uses of Important Indian Spices: A Review. *International Journal of Food Properties*, *13*(5), 1092–1116. doi:10.1080/10942910902963271

Gupta, R. K., & Watal, G. (2005). Hypoglycemic effects of Murrayakoenigii on normal and alloxan-diabetic rabbits. *Journal of Ethnopharmacology*, *97*(2), 247–251. doi:10.1016/j.jep.2004.11.006 PMID:15707761

Gupta, V. B., Indi, S. S., & Rao, K. S. (2009). Garlic extract exhibits antiamyloidogenic activity on amyloid-beta fibrillogenesis: Relevance to Alzheimer's disease. *Phytotherapy Research*, *23*(1), 111–115. doi:10.1002/ptr.2574 PMID:18844255

Gupta, V. B., & Rao, K. S. (2007). Anti-amyloidogenic activity of S-allyl-L-cysteine and its activity to destabilize Alzheimer's beta-amyloid fibrils in vitro. *Neuroscience Letters*, *429*, 75–80.

Gurib-Fakim, A., Maudarbaccus, N., Leach, D., Doimo, L., & Wohlmuth, H. (2002). Essential oil composition of zingiberaceae species from Mauritius. *The Journal of Essential Oil Research*, *14*(4), 271–273. doi:10.1080/10412905.2002.9699850

Gutierrez, J., Barry-Ryan, C., & Bourke, P. (2008). The antimicrobial efficacy of plant essential oil combinations and interactions with food ingredients. *International Journal of Food Microbiology*, *124*(1), 91–97. doi:10.1016/j.ijfoodmicro.2008.02.028 PMID:18378032

Gutierrez, J., Barry-Ryan, C., & Bourke, P. (2009). Antimicrobial activity of plant essential oils using food model media: Efficacy, synergistic potential and interactions with food components. *Food Microbiology*, *26*(2), 142–150. doi:10.1016/j.fm.2008.10.008 PMID:19171255

Guynot, M. E., Marin, S., Setu, L., Sanchis, V., & Ramos, A. J. (2005). Screening for antifungal activity of some essential oils against common spoilage fungi of bakery products. *Food Science & Technology International*, *11*(1), 25–32. doi:10.1177/1082013205050901

Guynot, M. E., Ramos, A. J., Seto, L., Purroy, P., Sanchis, V., & Marin, S. (2003). Antifungal activity of volatile compounds generated by essential oils against fungi commonly causing deterioration of bakery products. *Journal of Applied Microbiology*, *94*(5), 893–899. doi:10.1046/j.1365-2672.2003.01927.x PMID:12694455

Haiss, W., Thanh, N. T., Aveyard, J., & Fernig, D. G. (2007). Determination of size and concentration of gold nanoparticles from UV– Vis spectra. *Analytical Chemistry*, *79*(11), 4215–4221. doi:10.1021/ac0702084 PMID:17458937

Hamden, K., Jaouadi, B., Carreau, S., Aouidet, A., El-Fazaa, S., Gharbi, N., & Elfeki, A. (2010). Potential protective effect on key steroidogenesis and metabolic enzymes and sperm abnormalities by fenugreek steroids in testis and epididymis of surviving diabetic rats. *Archives of Physiology and Biochemistry*, *116*(3), 146–155. doi:10.3109/13813455.2010.486405 PMID:20507258

Hannan, J. M. A., Ali, L., Rokeya, B., Khaleque, J., Akhter, M., Flatt, P. R., & Abdel-Wahab, Y. H. A. (2007). Soluble dietary fibre fraction of *Trigonellafoenum-graecum*(fenugreek) seed improves glucose homeostasis in animal models of type 1and type 2 diabetes by delaying carbohydrate digestion and absorption and enhancing insulin action. *British Journal of Nutrition*, *97*(3), 514–521. doi:10.1017/S0007114507657869 PMID:17313713

Hannan, J. M., Rokeya, B., Faruque, O., Nahar, N., Mosihuzzaman, M., Azad Khan, A. K., & Ali, L. (2003). Effect of soluble dietary fibre fraction of Trigonellafoenum-graecum on glycemic, insulenimic, lipidemic and platelet aggregation status of Type II diabetic model rats. *Journal of Ethnopharmacology*, *88*(1), 73–77. doi:10.1016/S0378-8741(03)00190-9 PMID:12902054

Haouala, R., Hawala, S., El-Ayeb, A., Khanfir, R., & Boughanmi, N. (2008). Aqueous and organic extracts of *Trigonellafoenumgraecum* L. inhibit the mycelia growth of fungi. *Journal of Environmental Sciences (China)*, *20*(12), 1453–1457. doi:10.1016/S1001-0742(08)62548-6 PMID:19209631

Harada, M., Saijo, K., & Sakamoto, N. (2009). Characterization of metal nanoparticles prepared by photoreduction in aqueous solutions of various surfactants using UV–vis, EXAFS and SAXS. *Colloids and Surfaces. A, Physicochemical and Engineering Aspects*, *349*(1-3), 176–188. doi:10.1016/j.colsurfa.2009.08.015

Harliyansyahm, H., Murad, N. A., & Wan Ngah, W. Z. (2007). Antiproliferative, antioxidant and apoptosis effects of Zingiber officinale and 6-gingerol on HepG2 cells. *Asian Journal of Biochemistry*, *2*(6), 421–426. doi:10.3923/ajb.2007.421.426

Harsha, S. N., & Anila, K. K. R. (2012). Effects of *Coriandrum sativum* extract on exploratory behavior pattern and locomotor activity in mice: An experimental study. *IJGB*, *6*(2), 157–162.

Hassiotis, C. N. (2010). Evaluation of essential oil antifungal activity against mycorrhizal fungi: The case of Laurus nobilis essential oil. *Israel Journal of Ecology & Evolution*, *56*(1), 35–54. doi:10.1560/IJEE.56.1.35

Heider, M. (1992). *Coriandrum sativum*: Applications of plants Prevention and Treatment of Illnesses. *Persian*, *1*, 247–252.

Heikens, H., Fliers, E., Endert, E., Acknermans, M., & van Montfrans, G. (1995). Linquorice-induced hypertension—A new understanding of an old disease. *Journal of Medicinal Chemistry*, *5*, 230–234.

Heitzman, M. E., Neto, C. C., Winiarz, E., Vaisberg, A. J., & Hammond, G. B. (2005). Ethnobotany, phytochemistry and pharmacology of Uncaria (Rubiaceae). *Phytochemistry*, *66*(1), 5–29. doi:10.1016/j.phytochem.2004.10.022 PMID:15649507

Helle, W. (2004). Antioxidant activity in extracts from coriander. *Food Chemistry*, *88*(2), 293–297. doi:10.1016/j.foodchem.2004.01.047

Hendel, T., Wuithschick, M., Kettemann, F., Birnbaum, A., Rademann, K., & Polte, J. (2014). In situ determination of colloidal gold concentrations with UV–Vis spectroscopy: Limitations and perspectives. *Analytical Chemistry*, *86*(22), 11115–11124. doi:10.1021/ac502053s PMID:25289517

Héritier, V. N. V., Arthur, D. N., Augustin, M. M., Nadège, N. K., & Roger, K. V., Eric et, S. Z. L. P., & Jude-Thaddée, M. N. (2018). Article. *J. Pharmacogn.Phytochem.*, *7*(1), 643–648.

Hibasami, H., Moteki, H., & Ishikawa, H. (2003). Protodioscin isolated from fenugreek (*Trigonellafoenumgraecum*) induces cell death and morphological change indicative of apoptosis in leukemic cell line H-60 but not in gastric cancer line KATO III. *International Journal of Molecular Medicine*, *11*, 23–26. PMID:12469212

Hill, L. E., Taylor, T. M., & Gomes, C. (2013). Antimicrobial Efficacy of Poly (DL-lactide-co-glycolide) (PLGA) Nanoparticles with Entrapped Cinnamon Bark Extract againstListeria monocytogenesandSalmonella typhimurium. *Journal of Food Science*, *78*(4), N626–N632. doi:10.1111/1750-3841.12069 PMID:23464835

Hiserodt, R. D., Franzblau, S. G., & Rosen, R. T. (1998). Isolation of 6-, 8-, and 10-gingerol from ginger rhizome by HPLC and preliminary evaluation of inhibition of Mycobacterium avium and Mycobacterium tuberculosis. *Journal of Agricultural and Food Chemistry*, *46*(7), 2504–2508. doi:10.1021/jf9709481

Hitokoto, H., Morozumi, S., Wauke, T., Sakai, S., & Kurata, H. (1980). Inhibitory effects of spices on growth and toxin production of toxigenic fungi. *Applied and Environmental Microbiology*, *39*(4), 818–822. doi:10.1128/AEM.39.4.818-822.1980 PMID:6769391

Hlebowicz, J., Wickenberg, J., & Ingemansson, S. L. (2007). Effects of Curcuma longa (turmeric) on postprandial plasma glucose and insulin in healthy subjects. *Nutrition Journal*, *9*, 43. PMID:20937162

Holmes, A. M., Lim, J., Studier, H., & Roberts, M. S. (2016). Varying the morphology of silver nanoparticles results in differential toxicity against micro-organisms, HaCaT keratinocytes and affects skin deposition. *Nanotoxicology*, *10*(10), 1503–1514. doi:10.1080/17435390.2016.1236993 PMID:27636544

Hong, J. W., Yang, G. E., Kim, Y. B., Eom, S. H., Lew, J. H., & Kang, H. (2012). Anti-inflammatory activity of cinnamon water extract in vivo and in vitro LPS-induced models. *BMC Complementary and Alternative Medicine*, *12*(1), 237. doi:10.1186/1472-6882-12-237 PMID:23190501

Hoo, C. M., Starostin, N., West, P., & Mecartney, M. L. (2008). A comparison of atomic force microscopy (AFM) and dynamic light scattering (DLS) methods to characterize nanoparticle size distributions. *Journal of Nanoparticle Research*, *10*(1), 89–96. doi:10.100711051-008-9435-7

Ho, S. H., Ma, Y., Goh, P. M., & Sim, K. Y. (1995). Star anise, Illiciumverum Hook f. as a potential grain protectant against Ttiboliumcastaneum (Herbst) and Sitophilus zeamaisMotsch. *Postharvest Biology and Technology*, *6*(3-4), 341–347. doi:10.1016/0925-5214(95)00015-X

Hosseinzadeh, H., & Talebzadeh, F. (2005). Anticonvulsant evaluation of safranal and crocin from *Crocus sativus* in mice. *Fitoterapia*, *76*(7–8), 722–724. doi:10.1016/j.fitote.2005.07.008 PMID:16253437

Hosseinzadeh, H., Ziaee, T., & Sadeghi, A. (2008). The effect of saffron, Crocus sativus stigma, extract and its constituents, safranal, and crocin on sexual behaviors in normal male rats. *Phytomedicine*, *15*(6-7), 491–495. doi:10.1016/j.phymed.2007.09.020 PMID:17962007

Hsu, M. H., Kuo, S. C., Chen, C. J., Chung, J. G., Lai, Y. Y., & Huang, L. J. (2005). 1-(3,4-Dimethoxyphenyl 3,5-dodecenedione (I6) induces G1 arrest and apoptosis in human promyelocytic leukemia HL-60 cells. *Leukemia Research*, *29*(12), 1399–1406. doi:10.1016/j.leukres.2005.04.014 PubMed

Huang, E. S., Shook, M., Jin, L., Chin, M. H., & Meltzer, D. O.ADA. (2006). The impact of patient preferences on the cost-effectiveness of intensive glucose control in older patients with new-onset diabetes. *Diabetes Care*, *29*(2), 259–264. doi:10.2337/diacare.29.02.06.dc05-1443 PMID:16443870

Huang, Y., Zhao, J., Zhou, L., Wang, J., Gong, Y., Chen, X., ... Jiang, W. (2010). Antifungal Activity of the Essential Oil of Illicium verum Fruit and Its Main Component trans-Anethole. *Molecules (Basel, Switzerland)*, *15*(11), 7558–7569. doi:10.3390/molecules15117558 PMID:21030909

Hubenthal, F., Blázquez Sánchez, D., & Träger, F. (2012). Determination of morphological parameters of supported gold nanoparticles: Comparison of AFM combined with optical spectroscopy and theoretical modeling versus TEM. *Applied Sciences (Basel, Switzerland)*, *2*(3), 566–583. doi:10.3390/app2030566

Hu, Q., Pan, R., Wang, L., Peng, B., Tang, J., & Liu, X. (2010). Platycodongrandiflorum induces apoptosis in SKOV3 human ovarian cancer cells through mitochondrial-dependent pathway. *The American Journal of Chinese Medicine*, *38*(02), 373–386. doi:10.1142/S0192415X10007919 PMID:20387232

Hussain, F., Sher, H., & Ibrar, M. (2004). Ethnobotanical profile of some plants of District Swat, Pakistan. *Pak J Pl Sci*, *10*, 85–104.

Hussain, Z., Swindle, J., & Hauptman, P. J. (2006). Digoxin useand digoxin toxicity in the post-DIG trial era. *Journal of Cardiac Failure*, *12*(5), 343–346. doi:10.1016/j.cardfail.2006.02.005 PMID:16762795

Hussein, K. A., & Joo, J. H. (2018). Antifungal activity and chemical composition of ginger essential oil against ginseng pathogenic fungi. Current Research in Environmental & Applied Mycology, 8(2), 194–203. doi:10.5943/cream/8/2/4

Hussien, J., Teshale, C., & Mohammed, J. (2011). Assessment of the antimicrobial effects of some Ethiopian aromatic spice and herb hydrosols. *International Journal of Pharmacology*, *7*(5), 635–640. doi:10.3923/ijp.2011.635.640

Hwa, J. S., Jin, Y. C., Lee, Y. S., Ko, Y. S., Kim, Y. M., Shi, L. Y., ... Chang, K. C. (2012). 2- Methoxycinnamaldehyde from Cinnamomum cassia reduces rat myocardial ischemia and reperfusion injury in vivo due to HO-1 induction. *Journal of Ethnopharmacology*, *139*(2), 605–615. doi:10.1016/j.jep.2011.12.001 PMID:22179023

Hwang, E., Lee, D. G., Park, S. H., Oh, M. S., & Kim, S. Y. (2014). Coriander leaf extract exerts antioxidant activity and protects against UVB-induced photoaging of skin by regulation of procollagen type I and MMP-1 expression. *Journal of Medicinal Food*, *17*(9), 985–995. doi:10.1089/jmf.2013.2999

IJpma, I., Renken, R. J., Ter Horst, G. J., & Reyners, A. K. (2015). Metallic taste in cancer patients treated withchemotherapy. *Cancer Treatment Reviews*, *41*(2), 179–186. doi:10.1016/j.ctrv.2014.11.006 PMID:25499998

Indrianingsih, A., Tachibana, S., & Itoh, K. (2015). In vitro evaluation of antioxidant and α-glucosidase inhibitory assay of several tropical and subtropical plants. *Procedia Environmental Sciences*, *28*, 639–648. doi:10.1016/j.proenv.2015.07.075

Iqbal, M., Akhtar, N., Zafar, S., & Ali, I. (2008). Genotypic responses for yield and seed oil quality of two Brassica species under semi-arid environmental conditions. *South African Journal of Botany*, *74*(4), 567–571. doi:10.1016/j.sajb.2008.02.003

Iranshahy, M., & Iranshahi, M. (2011). Traditional uses, phytochemistry and pharmacology of asafoetida (Ferula assa-foetida oleo-gum-resin)—A review. *Journal of Ethnopharmacology*, *134*(1), 1–10. doi:10.1016/j.jep.2010.11.067 PMID:21130854

Iravani, S. (2011). Green synthesis of metal nanoparticles using plants. *Green Chemistry*, *13*(10), 2638–2650. doi:10.1039/c1gc15386b

Irfan, U., & Ali, S. (2016). The antibacterial effect of curry leaves (*Murraya Koenigii*). *Euro J. Pharma. and Medi Resea.*

Iriti, M., Vitalini, S., Fico, G., & Faoro, F. (2010). Neuroprotective Herbs and Foods from Different Traditional Medicines and Diets. *Molecules (Basel, Switzerland)*, *15*(5), 3517–3555. doi:10.3390/molecules15053517 PMID:20657497

Isao, Kubo, & Fujita, Kubo,& Nihei. (2004). Antibacterial activity of coriander volatile compounds against Salmonella choleraesuis. *Journal of Agricultural and Food Chemistry.*

Islam, M. S., & Choi, H. (2008). Comparative effects of dietary ginger (Zingiberofficinale) and garlic (Allium sativum) investigated in a type2 diabetes model of rats. *Journal of Medicinal Food*, *11*(1), 152–159. doi:10.1089/jmf.2007.634 PMID:18361751

Itoigawa, M., Ito, C., Tokuda, H., Enjo, F., Nishino, H., & Furukawa, H. (2004). Cancer chemopreventive activity of phenylpropanoids and phytoquinoids from *Illicium plants. Cancer Letters*, *214*(2), 165–169. doi:10.1016/j.canlet.2004.05.005 PMID:15363542

Ivanovic, J., Misic, D., Ristic, M., Pesic, O., & Zizovic, I. (2010). Supercritical carbon dioxide extract and essential oil of bay (Laurus nobilis L.): Chemical composition and antibacterial activity. *Journal of the Serbian Chemical Society*, *75*(3), 395–404. doi:10.2298/JSC090303003I

Iweala, E. E. J., Liu, F. F., Cheng, R. R., Li, Y., Ononhinmin, C. A., & Zhand, Y. J. (2015). Anticancer and free radical scavenging acivity of some Nigerian food plants *in vitro. International Journal of Cancer Research*, *11*(1), 41–51. doi:10.3923/ijcr.2015.41.51

Iwu, M. M. (2014). *Handbook of African medicinal plants*. Boca Raton, FL: Francis & Taylorn Group. doi:10.1201/b16292

Iyengar, M. A. (1997). *Pharmacognosy of powdered crude drugs*. Manipal, Karnataka: Manipal Power Press.

Iyengar, M. A. (2004). *Study of crude drugs*. Manipal, Karnataka: Manipal Power Press.

Iyengar, M. A., & Nayak, S. G. K. (1991). *Anatomy of crude drugs*. Manipal, Karnataka: Manipal Power Press.

Jafri, M. A., Farah, Javed, K., & Singh, S. (2001). Evaluation of the gastric antiulcerogenic effect of large cardamom (fruits of AmomumsubulatumRoxb). *Journal of Ethnopharmacology*, *75*(2-3), 89–94. doi:10.1016/S0378-8741(00)00398-6 PMID:11297839

Jain, D., Daima, H. K., Kachhwaha, S., & Kothari, S. L. (2009). Synthesis of plant-mediated silver nanoparticles using papaya fruit extract and evaluation of their anti microbial activities. *Digest Journal of Nanomaterials and Biostructures*, *4*(3), 557–563.

Jain, P. C., & Yadav, C. P. S. (1988). Relative susceptibility of coriander varieties to coriander aphid (*Hyadaphis coriandri* Das). *Indian Journal of Entomology*, *50*, 535–536.

Jain, P. C., & Yadav, C. P. S. (1989). Incidence of pests and their control on coriander. Indian Cocoa. *Arecanut and Spices J.*, *13*, 61–62.

Jain, R. C., & Vyas, C. R. (1974). Hypoglycemic action of onion on rabbits. *British Medical Journal*, *2*(5921), 730. doi:10.1136/bmj.2.5921.730-b PMID:4852817

Jain, S. C., Purohit, M., & Jain, R. (1992). Pharmacological evaluation of Cuminumcyminum. *Fitoterapia*, *63*(4), 291–294.

Jakhetia, V., Patel, R., Khatri, P., Pahuja, N., Garg, S., Pandey, A., & Sharma, S. (2010). Cinnamon: A pharmacological review. *International Journal of Advances in Scientific Research*, *1*(2), 19–23.

Janaki, C., Sailatha, E., & Gunasekaran, S. (2015). Synthesis, characteristics and antimicrobial activity of ZnO nanoparticles. *Spectrochimica Acta. Part A: Molecular and Biomolecular Spectroscopy*, *144*, 17–22. doi:10.1016/j.saa.2015.02.041 PMID:25748589

Jana, N. R., Wang, Z. L., Sau, T. K., & Pal, T. (2000). Seed-mediated growth method to prepare cubic copper nanoparticles. *CURRENT SCIENCE-BANGALORE*, *79*(9), 1367–1369.

Jani, R., Udipi, S., & Ghugre, P. (2009). Mineral content of complementary foods. *Indian Journal of Pediatrics*, *1*(1), 37–44. doi:10.100712098-009-0027-z PMID:19391001

Jansen, P. C. M. (1981). Coriandrum sativum L. condiments and medicinal plants in Ethiopia, their taxonomy and agricultural significance. College of Agriculture, Addis Ababa University, Ethiopia and The Agricultural University, Wageningen, The Netherlands.

Janssens, P. L., Hursel, R., & Westerterp-Plantenga, M. S. (2014). Capsaicin increases sensation of fullness in energy balance, and decreases desire to eat after dinner in negative energy balance. *Appetite*, *77*, 44–49. doi:10.1016/j.appet.2014.02.018 PMID:24630935

Jari, Ä. (2007). An ethnobotanical study on the usage of wild medicinal herbs from Kopaonik Mountain (Central Serbia). *Journal of Ethnopharmacology*, *111*(1), 160–175. doi:10.1016/j.jep.2006.11.007 PMID:17145148

Jayandran, M., Haneefa, M., & Balasubramanian, V. (2015). Green synthesis and characterization of Manganese nanoparticles using natural plant extracts and its evaluation of antimicrobial activity. *Journal of Applied Pharmaceutical Science*, 105–110. doi:10.7324/JAPS.2015.501218

Jelodar, G. A., Maleki, M., Motadayen, M. H., & Sirus, S. (2005). Effect of fenugreek, onion and garlic on blood glucose and histopathology of pancreas of alloxan induced diabetic rats. *Indian Journal of Medical Sciences*, *59*(2), 64–69. doi:10.4103/0019-5359.13905 PMID:15738612

Jemaa, J. M. B., Tersim, N., & Khouja, M. L. (2011). Composition and repellent efficacy of essential oil from Laurus nobilis against adults of the cigarette beetle Lasioderma serricorne (Coleoptera: Anobiidae). *Tunisian Journal of Plant Protection*, *6*(1), 29–42.

Jemaa, J. M. B., Tersim, N., Toudert, K. T., & Khouja, M. L. (2012). Insecticidal activities of essential oils from leaves of Laurus nobilis L. from Tunisia, Algeria and Morocco and comparative chemical composition. *Journal of Stored Products Research*, *48*, 97–104. doi:10.1016/j.jspr.2011.10.003

Jessie Suneetha, W., & Krishnakantha, T. P. (2008). Antiplatelet activity of coriander and curry leaf spices. *Pharmaceutical Biology*, *43*(3), 230–233. doi:10.1080/13880200590928807

Jha, A. B., Ashokkumar, K., Diapari, M., Ambrose, S. J., Zhang, H., Tar'an, B., ... Purves, R. W. (2015). Genetic diversity of folates profiles in seeds of common bean, lentil, chickpea, and pea. *Journal of Food Composition and Analysis*, *42*, 134–140. doi:10.1016/j.jfca.2015.03.006

Jha, A. K., & Prasad, K. (2008). Yeast mediated synthesis of silver nanoparticles. *International Journal of Nanoscience and Nanotechnology*, *4*(1), 17–22.

Jiang, S., Han, J., Li, T., Xin, Z., Ma, Z., Di, W., & Wang, D. (2017). 880 Curcumin as a potential protective compound against cardiac diseases. *Pharmacological Research*, *119*, 373–383. doi:10.1016/j.phrs.2017.03.001 PMID:28274852

Jiang, T. A. (2019). Health Benefits of Culinary Herbs and Spices. *Journal of AOAC International*, *102*(2), 395–411. doi:10.5740/jaoacint.18-0418 PMID:30651162

Jiang, Y., Wu, N., Fu, Y. J., Wang, W., Luo, M., Zhao, C. J., ... Liu, X. L. (2011). Chemical composition and antimicrobial activity of the essential oil of rosemary. *Environmental Toxicology and Pharmacology*, *32*(1), 63–68. doi:10.1016/j.etap.2011.03.011 PMID:21787731

Jin, D. Q., Lim, C. S., Hwang, J. K., Ha, I., & Han, J. S. (2005). Anti-oxidant and anti-inflammatory activities of macelignan in murine hippocampal cell line and primary culture of rat microglial cells. *Biochemical and Biophysical Research Communications*, *331*(4), 1264–1269. doi:10.1016/j.bbrc.2005.04.036 PMID:15883012

Jobitha, G., Annadurai, G., & Kannan, C. (2012). Green synthesis of silver nanoparticles using Elettaria cardamomom and assessment of its antimicrobial activity. *International Journal of Pharmaceutical Sciences and Research*, *3*, 323–330.

John, A. A., & Soba, N. (2011). Hepatoprotective activity of Brassica juncea (L) Czernagainst carbon tertrachloride induced hepatotoxicity in albino rats. *Pharmacologyonline*, *3*, 609–621.

Jones, M. R., Macfarlane, R. J., Lee, B., Zhang, J., Young, K. L., Senesi, A. J., & Mirkin, C. A. (2010). DNA-nanoparticle superlattices formed from anisotropic building blocks. *Nature Materials*, *9*(11), 913–917. doi:10.1038/nmat2870 PMID:20890281

Jorge, A. P., Aristides, R., & Victor, F. (1990). Composition of the seed oil of *Coriandrum sativum* L. from Cuba. *The Journal of Essential Oil Research*, *8*, 97–98.

Joukar, S., & Dehesh, M. M. (2015). The safety assessment of saffron (*Crocus sativus* L.) on sympathovagal balance and heart rate variability; a comparison with amiodarone. *Autonomic & Autacoid Pharmacology*, *35*(4), 46–50. doi:10.1111/aap.12040 PMID:27329172

Joynul, A. M., Nurul, A. M., Jamal, H. M., Nure, A. A., Kazi, M., & Faisal, H. (2012). Effect of micronutrients on growth and yield of onion under calcareous soil environment. *International Journal of Biosciences*, *2*, 95–101.

Junheon, K., Sun-Mi, S., Sang-Gil, L., & Sang-Chul, S., & Il-Kwon, P. (2008). Nematicidal activity of plant essential oils and components from coriander (Coriandrum sativum), oriental sweetgum (Liquidambar orientalis), and valerian (Valeriana wallichii) essential oils against pinewood nematode (Bursaphelenchus xylophilus). *Journal of Agricultural and Food Chemistry*.

Kadhim, M., & Ibrahim, R. K. (2013). Abd-Sahib Antibacterial Activity of Nutmeg (*Myristica fragrans*) Seed Extracts Against Some Pathogenic Bacteria. *Journal of Al-Nahrain University*, *16*(2), 188–192. doi:10.22401/JNUS.16.2.29

Kaefer, C. M., & Milner, J. A. (2011). Herbs and Spices in Cancer Prevention and Treatment. In Source Herbal Medicine: Biomolecular and Clinical Aspects (2nd ed.). CRC Press/Taylor & Francis. doi:10.1201/b10787-18

Kakani, R.K., Anwer, M.M., & Meena, S.S. (2009). Advance production technology of fenugreek. *NRCSS Tech. Release*, 1-24.

Kalidasu, G., Sarada, C., & Yellamanda, R. T. (2008). Influence of micronutrients on growth and yield of coriander (*Coriandrum sativum*) in rainfed vertisols. *Journal of Spices and Aromatic Crops*, *17*, 187–189.

Kalishwaralal, K., Deepak, V., Ramkumarpandian, S., Nellaiah, H., & Sangiliyandi, G. (2008). Extracellular biosynthesis of silver nanoparticles by the culture supernatant of Bacillus licheniformis. *Materials Letters*, *62*(29), 4411–4413. doi:10.1016/j.matlet.2008.06.051

Kanari, M., Tomoda, M., Gonda, R., Shimizu, N., Kimura, M., Kawaguchi, M., & Kawabe, C. (1989). A reticuloendothelial system-activating arabinoxylan from the bark of Cinnamomum cassia. *Chemical & Pharmaceutical Bulletin*, *37*(12), 3191–3194. doi:10.1248/cpb.37.3191 PMID:2632069

Kandaswami, C., Lee, L. T., Lee, P. P., Hwang, J. J., Ke, F. C., Huang, Y. T., & Lee, M. T. (2005) The antitumor activities of flavonoids. In Vivo, 19(5), 895-909.

Kandhare, A. D., Bodhankar, S. L., Mohan, V., & Thakurdesai, P. A. (2015). Acute and repeated doses (28 days) oral toxicity study of glycosides based standardized fenugreek seed extract in laboratory mice. *Regulatory Toxicology and Pharmacology*, *72*(2), 323–334. doi:10.1016/j.yrtph.2015.05.003 PMID:25979642

Kang, J. H., Tsuyoshi, G., Han, I. S., Kawada, T., Kim, Y. M., & Yu, R. (2010). Dietary capsaicin reduces obesity induced insulin resistance and hepatic steatosis in obese mice fed a high fat diet. *Obesity (Silver Spring, Md.)*, *18*(4), 780–787. doi:10.1038/oby.2009.301 PMID:19798065

Kapoor, I. P., Singh, B., Singh, G., De-Heuluan, C. S., De Lampasona, M. P., & Catalan, C. A. N. (2009). Chemistry and in Vitro Antioxidant Activity of Volatile Oil and Oleoresins of Black Pepper (*Piper nigrum*). *Journal of Agricultural and Food Chemistry*, *57*(12), 5358–5364. doi:10.1021/jf900642x PMID:19456163

Kapoor, L. D. (1990). *Handbook of Ayurvedic Medicinal Plants*. Boca Raton, FL: CRC Press.

Kara, S., Gencer, B., Karaca, T., Tufan, H., Arikan, S., Ersan, I., … Volkan, H. (2019). *Protective Effect of Hesperetin and Naringenin against Apoptosis in Ischemia/Reperfusion-Induced Retinal Injury in Rats*. Academic Press.

Karampour, N. S., Arzi, A., Rezaie, A., Pashmforoosh, M., & Kordi, F. (2019). Gastro protective effect of zingerone on ethanol-induced gastric ulcers in rats. Medicina, 55(3), 64. doi:10.3390/medicina55030064

Karimi, E., Oskoueian, E., Hendra, R., & Jaafar, H. Z.Stigma Phenolic and Flavonoid Compounds and Its Antioxidant Activity. (2010). Evaluation of Crocus sativus L.stigma phenolic and flavonoid compounds and its antioxidant activity. *Molecules (Basel, Switzerland)*, *15*(9), 6244–6256. doi:10.3390/molecules15096244 PMID:20877220

Karlsson, F. H., Tremaroli, V., Nookaew, I., Bergström, G., Behre, C. J., Fagerberg, B., ... Bäckhed, F. (2013). Gut metagenome in European women with normal, impaired and diabetic glucose control. *Nature*, *498*(7452), 99–103. doi:10.1038/nature12198 PMID:23719380

Karnick, C. R. (1991). A clinical trial of a composite herbal drug in the treatment of diabetes mellitus. *Aryavaidyan.*, *5*, 36–46.

Karuppiah, P., & Rajaram, S. (2012). Antibacterial effect of Allium sativum, cloves and Zingiber officinale rhizomes against multiple-drug resistant clinical pathogens. *Asian Pacific Journal of Tropical Biomedicine*, *8*(8), 597–601. doi:10.1016/S2221-1691(12)60104-X PubMed

Kasuga, S., Ushijima, M., Morihara, N., Itakura, Y., & Nakata, Y. (1999). Effect of aged garlic extract (AGE) on hyperglycemia induced by immobilization stress in mice. *Nippon Yakurigaku Zasshi*, *114*(3), 191–197. doi:10.1254/fpj.114.191 PMID:10553583

Katiyar, S. K., Agarwal, R., & Mukhtar, H. (1996). Inhibition of tumor promotion in SENCARmouse skin by ethanol extract of Zingiber officinale rhizome. *Cancer Research*, *56*(5), 1023–1030. PubMed

Kato, S., Yuzawa, Y., Tsuboi, N., Maruyama, S., Morita, Y., Matsuguchi, T., & Matsuo, S. (2004). Endotoxin-induced chemokine expression in murine peritoneal mesothelial cells: The role of toll-like receptor 4. *Journal of the American Society of Nephrology*, *5*, 1289–1299. PMID:15100369

Kaur, G., Athar, M., & Alam, M. S. (2010). Eugenol precludes cutaneous chemical carcinogenesis in mouse by preventing oxidative stress and inflammation and by inducing apoptosis. *Molecular Carcinogenesis*, *49*(3), 290–301. PMID:20043298

Kaur, H., Kaur, S., & Singh, M. (2013). Biosynthesis of silver nanoparticles by natural precursor from clove and their antimicrobial activity. *Biologia*, *68*(6). doi:10.247811756-013-0276-1

Kaurinovic, B., Popovic, M., & Vlaisavljevic, S. (2010). In vitro and in vivo effects of Laurus nobilis L. leaf extracts. *Molecules (Basel, Switzerland)*, *15*(5), 3378–3390. doi:10.3390/molecules15053378 PMID:20657487

Kaviarasan, S., Naik, G., Gangabhagirathi, R., Anuradha, C. V., & Priyadarsini, K. I. (2007). In vitro studies on antiradical and antioxidant activities of fenugreek (*Trigonellafoenumgraecum*) seeds. *Food Chemistry*, *103*(1), 31–37. doi:10.1016/j.foodchem.2006.05.064

Kavoosi, G., Shakiba, A., Ghorbani, M., Dadfar, S. M. M., & Purfard, A. M. (2015). Antioxidant, antibacterial, water binding capacity and mechanical behavior of gelatin-ferula oil film as a wound dressing material. *Galen Medical Journal*, *4*(2), 103–114.

Kawabata, F., Inoue, N., Yazawa, S., Kawada, T., Inoue, K., & Fushiki, T. (2006). Effects of CH-19 Sweet, a Non-Pungent Cultivar of Red Pepper, in Decreasing the Body Weight and Suppressing Body Fat Accumulation by Sympathetic Nerve Activation in Humans. *Bioscience, Biotechnology, and Biochemistry*, *70*(12), 2824–2835. doi:10.1271/bbb.60206 PMID:17151481

Kayaardi, S., Durak, F., Kayacier, A., & Kayaardi, M. (2005). Chemical characteristics of kavurma with selected condiments. *International Journal of Food Properties*, *8*(3), 513–520. doi:10.1080/10942910500269568

Kedia, A., Prakash, B., Mishra, P. K., & Dubey, N. K. (2014). Antifungal and antiaflatoxigenic properties of Cuminum cyminum (L.) seed essential oil and its efficacy as a preservative in stored commodities. *International Journal of Food Microbiology*, *168–169*, 1–7. doi:10.1016/j.ijfoodmicro.2013.10.008 PMID:24211773

Keskin, D., & Toroglu, S. (2011). Studies on antimicrobial activities of solvent extracts of different spices. *Journal of Environmental Biology*, *32*(2), 251–256. PMID:21882663

Khajehdehi, P. (2012). Turmeric: Reemerging of a neglected Asian traditional remedy. *Journal of Nephropathology*, *1*(1), 17–22. doi:10.5812/jnp.5 PMID:24475382

Khaki, A., & Fathiazad, F. (2012). Diabetic nephropathy-using herbals in diabetic nephropathy prevention and treatment - the role of ginger (Zingiber officinale) and onion (Allium cepa) in diabetics' nephropathy. In A. Bhattacharya (Ed.), A Compendium of Essays on Alternative Therapy (pp. 207–232). Rijeka, Croatia: InTech Publisher; doi:10.5772/34953.

Khameneh, B., Halimi, V., Jaafari, M. R., & Golmohammadzadeh, S. (2015). Safranal-loaded solid lipid nanoparticles: Evaluation of sunscreen and moisturizing potential for topical applications. *Iranian Journal of Basic Medical Sciences.*, *18*(1), 58. PMID:25810877

Khan, A., Safdar, M., Ali Khan, M.M., Khattak, K.N. & Anderson, R.A. (2003). Cinnamon improves glucose and lipids of people with type 2. *Diabetics Care, 26*, 3215-3218.

Khan, A., Safdar, M., Ali Khan, M. M., Khattak, K. N., & Anderson, R. A. (2003). Cinnamon improves glucose and lipids of people with type-2 diabetes. *Diabetes Care*, *26*(12), 3215–3218. doi:10.2337/diacare.26.12.3215 PMID:14633804

Khan, I., Pandotra, P., Gupta, A. P., Sharma, R., Gupta, B. D., Dhar, J. K., ... Gupta, S. (2010). RP-thin layer chromatographic method for the quantification of three gingerol homologs of ultrasonic-assisted fresh rhizome extracts of Zingiber officinale collected from North Western Himalayas. *Journal of Separation Science*, *33*(4-5), 558–563. doi:10.1002/jssc.200900629 PubMed

Khan, R., Zakir, M., Khanam, Z., Shakil, S., & Khan, A. U. (2010). Novel compound from Trachyspermum ammi (Ajowan caraway) seeds with antibiofilm and antiadherence activities against Streptococcus mutans: A potential chemotherapeutic agent against dental caries. *Journal of Applied Microbiology*, *109*(6), 2151–2159. doi:10.1111/j.1365-2672.2010.04847.x PMID:20846336

Khatoon, N., Gupta, R. K., & Tyagi, Y. K. (2015). Nutraceutical potential and phytochemical screening of Buchanania lanzan, an underutilized exotic Indian nut and its use as a source of functional food. *Journal of Pharmacognosy and Phytochemistry*, *4*(1).

Khattab, R. Y., & Arntfield, S. D. (2009). Functional properties of raw and processed canola meal. *Lebensmittel-Wissenschaft + Technologie*, *42*(6), 1119–1124. doi:10.1016/j.lwt.2009.02.009

Khonche, A., Biglaria, O., Panahi, Y., Valizadegan, G., Soflaei, S. S., Ghamarchehreh, M. E., ... Sahebkar, A. (2016). Adjunctive Therapy with Curcumin for Peptic Ulcer: A Randomized Controlled Trial. *Drug Research (Stuttgart)*, *66*(08), 444–448. doi:10.1055-0042-109394 PMID:27351245

Kianbakht, S., & Hajiaghaee, R. (2011). Anti-hyperglycemic effects of saffron and its active constituents, crocin and safranal, in alloxan-induced diabetic rats. *Faslnamah-i Giyahan-i Daruyi*, *3*(39), 82–89.

Kianbakht, S., & Hashem, D. F. (2015). Anti-obesity and anorectic effects of saffron and itsconstituent crocin in obese Wistar rat. *Faslnamah-i Giyahan-i Daruyi*, *1*(53), 25–33.

Kikusaki, H., & Nakatani, N. (1993). Antioxidant effect of some ginger constituents. *Journal of Food Science*, *58*(6), 1407–1410. doi:10.1111/j.1365-2621.1993.tb06194.x

Kim, D. H., Kim, C. H., Kim, M. S., Kim, J. Y., Chung, J. H., Lee, J. W., ... Chung, H. Y. (2007). Suppression of age-related inflammatory NF-κB activation by cinnamaldehyde. *Biogerontology*, *8*(5), 545–554. doi:10.100710522-007-9098-2 PMID:17486422

Kim, M. J., Park, H. J., Hong, M. S., Kim, M. S., Leem, K. H., Kim, J. B., ... Kim, H. K. (2005). Citrus Reticulatablanco induces apoptosis in human gastric cancer cells SNU-668. *Nutrition and Cancer*, *51*(1), 78–82. doi:10.120715327914nc5101_11 PMID:15749633

Kim, S. H., Hyun, S. H., & Choung, S. Y. (2006). Anti-diabetic effect of cinnamon extract on blood glucose in db/db mice. *Journal of Ethnopharmacology*, *104*(1-2), 119–123. doi:10.1016/j.jep.2005.08.059 PMID:16213119

Kim, S. H., & Lee, Y. C. (2009). Piperine inhibits eosinophil infiltration and airway hyperresponsiveness by suppressing T cell activity and Th2 cytokine production in the ovalbumin-induced asthma model. *The Journal of Pharmacy and Pharmacology*, *61*(3), 353–359. doi:10.1211/jpp.61.03.0010 PMID:19222908

Kim, T., Davis, J., Zhang, A. J., He, X., & Matthews, S. T. (2009). Curcumin activates AMPK and suppresses gluconeogenic gene expression in hepatoma cells. *Biochemical and Biophysical Research Communications*, *388*(2), 377–382. doi:10.1016/j.bbrc.2009.08.018 PMID:19665995

Kiran, C. R., Chakka, A. K., Padmakumari Amma, K. P., Menon, A. N., Sree Kumar, M. M., & Venugopalan, V. V. (2013). Essential oil composition of fresh ginger cultivars from North-East India. *The Journal of Essential Oil Research*, *25*(5), 380–387. doi:10.1080/10412905.2013.796496

Kirschling, T. L., Golas, P. L., Unrine, J. M., Matyjaszewski, K., Gregory, K. B., Lowry, G. V., & Tilton, R. D. (2011). Microbial bioavailability of covalently bound polymer coatings on model engineered nanomaterials. *Environmental Science & Technology*, *45*(12), 5253–5259. doi:10.1021/es200770z PMID:21609011

Kirtikar, K.R. (1935). *Indian medicinal plants: Lalit mohan basu*. Allahabad, India: Academic Press.

Kirtikar, K. R., Basu, B. D., Blatter, E., Caius, J. F., & Mhaskar, K. S. (1993). *Indian Medicinal Plants* (2nd ed., Vol. 2). Allahabad, India: Lalit Mohan Basu.

Kiuchi, F., Shibuya, M., & Sankawa, U. (1982). Inhibitors of prostaglandin biosynthesis from ginger. *Chemical & Pharmaceutical Bulletin*, *30*(2), 754–757. doi:10.1248/cpb.30.754 PubMed

Kodati, D., Pareta, S., & Patra, K. C. (2010). Antiulcer activity of ethanolic extract of B. lanzan Spreng roots. *Annals of Biological Research*, *1*(4), 234–239.

Kokate, C. K., & Gokhlae. (2007). *Text book of Pharmacognosy*. New Delhi: Nirali Prakashan.

Kokate, C. K., Purohit, A. P., & Gokhale, S B. (2010). Text Book of Pharmacognosy. *Nirali prakashan, 46*(1-2), 80.

Kong, J.-Q. (2015). Phenylalanine ammonia-lyase, a key component used for phenylpropanoids production by metabolic engineering. *RSC Advances*, *5*(77), 62587–62603. doi:10.1039/C5RA08196C

Kothari, S. K., Bhattacharya, A. K., & Ramesh, S. (2004). Essential oil yield and quality of methyl eugenol rich Ocimumtenuiflorum L. f. (syn. O. sanctum L.) grown in South India as influenced by method of harvest. *Journal of Chromatography. A*, *1054*(1-2), 67–72. doi:10.1016/j.chroma.2004.03.019 PMID:15553132

Krausz, A. E., Adler, B. L., Cabral, V., Navati, M., Doerner, J., Charafeddine, R. A., ... Friedman, A. J. (2015). Curcumin-encapsulated nanoparticles as innovative antimicrobial and wound healing agent. *Nanomedicine; Nanotechnology, Biology, and Medicine*, *11*(1), 195–206. doi:10.1016/j.nano.2014.09.004 PMID:25240595

Krishnamoorthy, B., & Rema, J. (2001). Nutmeg and mace. In K. V. Peter (Ed.), *Hand Book of Herbs and Spices* (pp. 239–248). Cambridge, UK: Woodhead Publishing Limited.

Kubra, I. R., & Rao, L. J. M. (2012). An impression on current developments in the technology, chemistry, and biological activities of Ginger (Zingiber officinale Roscoe). *Critical Reviews in Food Science and Nutrition*, *52*, 651–688.

Kuhn, Padilha. & LíaBarbieri. (2016). Plant breeding of Chili peppers (*Capsicum*, Solanaceae) – A review. *Australian Journal of Basic and Applied Sciences*, *10*(15), 148–154.

Kumar, G. S., Muthu, D., Karunakaran, G., Karthi, S., Girija, E. K., & Kuznetsov, D. (2018). Curcuma longa tuber extract mediated synthesis of hydroxyapatite nanorods using biowaste as a calcium source for the treatment of bone infections. *Journal of Sol-Gel Science and Technology*, *86*(3), 610–616. doi:10.100710971-018-4670-6

Kumar, J., Vengaiah, P. C., Srivastava, P. P., & Bhowmick, P. K. (2012). Chironji nut (Buchanania lanzan) processing, present practise and scope. *Indian Journal of Traditional Knowledge*, *11*(1), 202–204.

Kumar, P. B. A. N., Dushenkov, V., Motto, H., & Raskin, I. (1995). Phytoextraction: The Use of Plants To Remove Heavy Metals from Soils. *Environmental Science & Technology*, *29*(5), 1232–1238. doi:10.1021/es00005a014 PMID:22192016

Kumar, P. V., Pammi, S. V. N., Kollu, P., Satyanarayana, K. V. V., & Shameem, U. (2014). Green synthesis and characterization of silver nanoparticles using Boerhaavia diffusa plant extract and their anti bacterial activity. *Industrial Crops and Products*, *52*, 562–566. doi:10.1016/j.indcrop.2013.10.050

Kumar, S., & Mukkadan, J. (2013). Anti diabetic effect of oral administration of cinnamon in Wistar Albino Rats. *Bali Medical Journal*, *2*(3), 97–99.

Kumar, V., Thakur, A. K., Barothia, N. D., & Chatterjee, S. S. (2011). Therapeutic potentials of Brassica juncea: An overview. *Tang*, *1*(1), 2–1. doi:10.5667/tang.2011.0005

Kumpulainen, J. T., & Salonen, J. T. (1999). *Natural Antioxidants and Anticarcinogens in Nutrition. In Health and Disease* (pp. 178–187). The Royal Society of Chemistry. doi:10.1533/9781845698409

Kuriyama, T., Schmidt, T. J., Okuyama, E., & Ozoe, Y. (2002). Structure–activity relationships of secoprezizaaneterpenoids in gamma-aminobutyric acid receptors of houseflies and rats. *Bioorganic & Medicinal Chemistry*, *10*(6), 1873–1881. doi:10.1016/S0968-0896(02)00011-1 PMID:11937345

Kwon, H. K., Hwang, J. S., So, J. S., Lee, C. G., Sahoo, A., Ryu, J. H., ... Park, Z. Y. (2010). Cinnamon extract induces tumor cell death through inhibition of NFκB and AP1. *BMC Cancer*, *10*(1), 392. doi:10.1186/1471-2407-10-392 PMID.20653974

Laborda, F., Bolea, E., Cepriá, G., Gómez, M. T., Jiménez, M. S., Pérez-Arantegui, J., & Castillo, J. R. (2016). Detection, characterization and quantification of inorganic engineered nanomaterials: A review of techniques and methodological approaches for the analysis of complex samples. *Analytica Chimica Acta*, *904*, 10–32. doi:10.1016/j.aca.2015.11.008 PMID:26724760

Lai, M., Yao, W., Yang, M., Huang, P., Liu, B., & Zheng, X. (1997). Studies on the pharmacognosy of Cortex Illicii and its adulterants. *Zhong Yao Cai*, *20*(12), 601–604. PMID:12572500

Lai, P. K., & Roy, J. (2004). Antimicrobial and Chemopreventive Properties of Herbs and Spices. *Current Medicinal Chemistry*, *11*(11), 1451–1460. doi:10.2174/0929867043365107 PMID:15180577

Lao, C. D., Ruffin, M. T. IV, Normolle, D., Heath, D. D., Murray, S. I., Bailey, J. M., ... Brenner, D. E. (2006). Ruffin4th M. T, Normolle D. Dose escalation of a curcuminoid formulation. *BMC Complementary and Alternative Medicine*, *6*(1), 10–13. doi:10.1186/1472-6882-6-10 PMID:16545122

Lapkin, A., Joyce, L., & Crittenden, B. (2004). Framework for evaluating the "greenness" of chemical processes: Case studies for a novel VOC recovery technology. *Environmental Science & Technology*, *38*(21), 5815–5823. doi:10.1021/es035414h PMID:15575305

Laribi, B., Kouki, K., M'Hamdi, M., & Bettaieb, T. (2015). Coriander (*Coriandrum sativum* L.) and its bioactive constituents. *Fitoterapia, 103*, 9–26. doi:10.1016/j.fitote.2015.03.012

Laroubi, A., Touhami, M., Farouk, L., Zrara, I., Aboufatima, R., Benharref, A., & Chait, A. (2007). Prophylaxis effect of *Trigonellafoenumgraecum* L. seeds on renal stone formation in rats. *Phytotherapy Research, 21*(10), 921–925. doi:10.1002/ptr.2190 PMID:17582593

Latha, K., Rammohan, B., Sunanda, B. P., Maheswari, M. S., & Mohan, S. K. (2015). Evaluation of anxiolytic activity of aqueous extract of *Coriandrum sativum* Linn in mice: A preliminary experimental study. *Pharmacognosy Research,* 7(5Suppl 1), S47–S51. doi:10.4103/0974-8490.157996

Latha, P. G., Sindhu, P. G., Suja, S. R., Geetha, B. S., Pushpangadan, P., & Rajasekharan, S. (2005). Pharmacology and chemistry of *Myristica fragrans* Houtt. a review. *Journal of Spices and Aromatic Crops, 14*, 94–101.

Latona, D. F., Oyeleke, G. O., & Olayiwola, O. A. (2012). Chemical analysis of ginger root. IOSR Journal of Applied Chemistry, 1(1), 47–49. doi:10.9790/5736-0114749

Laxminarayan, R., & Chaudhury, R. R. (2016). Antibiotic Resistance in India: Drivers and Opportunities for Action. *PLoS Medicine, 13*(3), e1001974. doi:10.1371/journal.pmed.1001974 PMID:26934098

Lazarides, A. A., Lance Kelly, K., Jensen, T. R., & Schatz, G. C. (2000). Optical properties of metal nanoparticles and nanoparticle aggregates important in biosensors. *Journal of Molecular Structure THEOCHEM, 529*(1–3), 59–63. doi:10.1016/S0166-1280(00)00532-7

Lee, D.H., Park, K.I., Park, H.S., Kang, S.R., Nagappan, A., Kim, J.A., … Kim, G.S. (2012b). Flavonoids isolated from Korea Citrus aurantium L. induce G2/M phase arrest and apoptosis in human gastric cancer AGS Cells. *Evid.-Based Complement.Altern Med: eCAM*, 515901.

Lee, H. S., & Ahn, Y. J. (1998). Growth-inhibiting effects of Cinnamomum cassia bark-derived materials on human intestinal bacteria. *Journal of Agricultural and Food Chemistry, 46*(1), 8–12. doi:10.1021/jf970548y PMID:10554188

Lee, H. S., Seo, E. Y., Kang, N. E., & Kim, W. K. (2008). [6]-Gingerol inhibits metastasis of MDS-MB-231 human breast cancer cells. *The Journal of Nutritional Biochemistry, 19*(5), 313–319. doi:10.1016/j.jnutbio.2007.05.008 PubMed

Lee, J. M., Jahn, M. M., & Yeam, I. (2013). Allelic relationships at the pvr1 locus in *Capsicum annuum. Euphytica, 194*(3), 417–424. doi:10.100710681-013-0967-2

Lee, J. Y., & Park, W. (2011). Anti-inflammatory effect of myristicin on RAW 264.7 macrophages stimulated with polyinosinic-polycytidylic acid. *Molecules (Basel, Switzerland), 16*(8), 7132–7142. doi:10.3390/molecules16087132 PMID:21991618

Lee, K. H., Abas, F., Alitheen, M., Banu, N., Shaari, K., Lajis, N. H., & Syahida, A. (2015). Chemopreventive effects of a curcuminlike diarylpentanoid [2,6-bis (2, 5-dimethoxybenzylidene) cyclohexanone] in cellular targetsof rheumatoid arthritis in vitro. *International Journal of Rheumatic Diseases, 18*(6), 616–627. doi:10.1111/1756-185X.12341 PMID:24832356

Leela, N., & Shafeekh, K. (2008). *Fenugreek. Chemistry of Spices*. Pondicherry, India: CAB. International.

Lee, S. J., Umano, K., Shibamoto, T., & Lee, K.-G. (2005). Identification of volatile components in basil (*Ocimum-basilicum* L.) and thyme leaves (*Thymus vulgaris* L.) and their antioxidant properties. *Food Chemistry, 1*(1), 131–137. doi:10.1016/j.foodchem.2004.05.056

Lee, S. W., Li, G., Lee, K. S., Jung, J. S., Xu, M. L., Seo, C. S., ... Son, J. K. (2003). Preventive agents against sepsis and new phenylpropanoid glucosides from the fruits of *Illiciumverum. Planta Medica, 69*(9), 861–864. doi:10.1055-2003-43210 PMID:14598217

Lee, S. W., Li, G., Lee, K. S., Song, D.-K., & Son, J.-K. (2003). A new phenylpropanoid glucoside from the fruits ofIllicium verum. *Archives of Pharmacal Research*, *26*(8), 591–593. doi:10.1007/BF02976705 PMID:12967191

Lee, Y. M., Gweon, O. C., Seo, Y. J., Im, J., Kang, M. J., Kim, M. J., & Kim, J. I. (2009). Antioxidant effect of garlic and aged black garlic in animal model of type 2 diabetes mellitus. *Nutrition Research and Practice*, *3*(2), 156–161. doi:10.4162/nrp.2009.3.2.156 PMID:20016716

Lejeune, M. P., Kovacs, E. M., & Westerterp-Plantenga, M. S. (2003). Effect of capsaicin on substrate oxidation and weight maintenance after modest body-weight loss in human subjects. *British Journal of Nutrition*, *90*(3), 651–659. doi:10.1079/BJN2003938 PMID:13129472

Lertsutthiwong & Rojsitthisak. (2011). *Chitosan-alginate nanocapsules for encapsulation of tumeric oil*. doi:10.1691/ph.2011.1068

Lewis, Y. (1984). *Spices and herbs for the food industry*. Food Trade Press Ltd.

Li, S., Wan, C., Wang, M., Li, W., Matsumoto, K., & Tang, Y. (n.d.). *Antidepressant like effects of piperine in chronic mild stress treated mice and its possible mechanisms*. Academic Press.

Li, J., Zeng, H., Sun, S., Liu, J. P., & Wang, Z. L. (2004). Analyzing the Structure of CoFe– Fe3O4 Core– Shell Nanoparticles by Electron Imaging and Diffraction. *The Journal of Physical Chemistry B*, *108*(37), 14005–14008. doi:10.1021/jp047602f

Lin, C.-C., Wu, S.-J., Chang, C.-H., & Ng, L.-T. (2003). Antioxidant activity of *Cinnamomum cassia*. *Phytotherapy Research*, *17*(7), 726–730. doi:10.1002/ptr.1190 PMID:12916067

Ling, J., Wei, B., Lv, G., Ji, H., & Li, S. (2012). Antihyperlipidaemic and antioxidant effects of turmeric oil in hyperlipidaemic rats. *Food Chemistry*, *130*(2), 229–235. doi:10.1016/j.foodchem.2011.07.039

Li, Q., Cui, Y., Jin, R., Lang, H., Yu, H., Sun, F., ... Zhu, Z. (2017). Enjoyment of Spicy Flavor Enhances Central Salty-Taste Perception and Reduces Salt Intake and Blood Pressure. *Hypertension*, *70*(6), 1291–1299. doi:10.1161/HYPERTENSIONAHA.117.09950 PMID:29089370

Li, R., & Jiang, Z. (2004). Chemical composition of the essential oil of Cuminumcyminum L. from China. *Flavour and Fragrance Journal*, *19*(4), 311–313. doi:10.1002/ffj.1302

Li, R., Liang, T., Xu, L., Li, Y., Zhang, S., & Duan, X. (2013). Protective Effect of Cinnamon Polyphenols against STZ-diabetic Mice Fed High-Sugar, High-Fat Diet and Its Underlying Mechanism. *Food and Chemical Toxicology*, *51*, 419–425. doi:10.1016/j.fct.2012.10.024 PMID:23127600

Li, T. Y., Brennan, A. M., Wedick, N. M., Petersen, J. M., Stonehouse, O. W., Jerling, J. C., ... White, Z. (2006). Antioxidant rich spice added to hamburger meat during cooking results in reduced meat, plasma, and urine malondialdehyde concentrations. *The American Journal of Clinical Nutrition*, *84*, 95–135.

Liu, C. T., Wong, P. L., Lii, C. K., Hse, H., & Sheen, L. Y. (2006). Antidiabetic effect of garlic oil but not diallyl disulfide in rats with streptozotocin-induced diabetes. *Food and Chemical Toxicology*, *44*(8), 1377–1384. doi:10.1016/j.fct.2005.07.013 PMID:16690190

Liu, R. H. (2003). Health benefits of fruit and vegetables are from additive and synergistic combinations of phytochemicals. *The American Journal of Clinical Nutrition*, *78*(3), 517S–520S. doi:10.1093/ajcn/78.3.517S PMID:12936943

Lobo, V., Patil, A., Phatak, A., & Chandra, N. (2010). Free radicals, antioxidants and functional foods: Impact on human health. *Pharmacognosy Reviews*, *4*(8), 118–126. doi:10.4103/0973-7847.70902 PMID:22228951

Loizzo, M. R., Saab, A. M., Tundis, R., Statti, G. A., Menichini, F., Lampronti, I., ... Doerr, H. W. (2008). Phytochemical analysis and in vitro antiviral activities of the essential oils of seven Lebanon species. *Chemistry & Biodiversity*, *5*(3), 461–470. doi:10.1002/cbdv.200890045 PMID:18357554

Lucky, E., Igbinosa, O. E., & Jonahan, I. (2017). Antimicrobial activity of Zingiber officinale against multidrug resistant microbial isolates. *Health Science Research*, *4*, 76–81.

Lu, W., Liu, G., Gao, S., Xing, S., & Wang, J. (2008). Tyrosine-assisted preparation of Ag/ZnO nanocomposites with enhanced photocatalytic performance and synergistic antibacterial activities. *Nanotechnology*, *19*(44), 445711. doi:10.1088/0957-4484/19/44/445711 PMID:21832753

Lu, X., Rasco, B. A., Jabal, J. M. F., Aston, D. E., Lin, M., & Kondel, M. E. (2011). Investigating antibacterial effects of garlic (*Allium sativum*) concentrate and garlic-derived organosulfur compounds on *Campylobacter jejuni* by using fourier transform infrared spectroscopy, raman spectroscopy, and electron microscopy. *Applied and Environmental Microbiology*, *77*(15), 5257–5269. doi:10.1128/AEM.02845-10 PMID:21642409

Machado, D. G., Bettio, L. E., Cunha, M. P., Capra, J. C., Dalmarco, J. B., Pizzolatti, M. G., & Rodrigues, A. L. S. (2009). Antidepressant-like effect of the extract of Rosmarinus officinalis in mice: Involvement of the monoaminergic system. *Progress in Neuro-Psychopharmacology & Biological Psychiatry*, *33*(4), 642–650. doi:10.1016/j.pnpbp.2009.03.004 PMID:19286446

Mackeen, M. M., Ali, A. M., El-Sharkawy, S. H., Manap, M. Y., Salleh, K. M., Lajis, N. H., & Kawazu, K. (1997). Antimicrobial and cytotoxic properties of some Malaysian vegetables (Ulam). *International Journal of Pharmacognosy*, *35*(3), 174–178. doi:10.1076/phbi.35.3.174.13294

Madreseh-Ghahfarokhi, S., Pirali, Y., Dehghani-Samani, A., & Dehghani-Samani, A. (2018). The insecticidal and repellent activity of ginger (Zingiber officinale) and eucalyptus (Eucalyptus globulus) essential oils against Culex theileri Theobald, 1903 (Diptera: Culicidae. *Annals of Parasitology*, *64*(4), 351–360. PubMed

Mae, T., Nishiyama, T., Kishida, H., Takagaki, R., & Yamamoto, M. (2007). *Agent for preventing/ ameliorating life style related diseases containing turmeric essential oil component*. European Patent Application, Intl Nat Pub No. WO 2005/115366, EP1752144A1, 1–12. Spices and aromatic plants–health benefits 100.

Maggi, L., Carmona, M., Kelly, S. D., Marigheto, N., & Alonso, G. L. (2011). Geographical origin differentiation of saffron spice (Crocus sativus L. stigmas)–preliminary investigation using chemical and multi-element (H, C, N) stable isotope analysis. *Food Chemistry*, *128*(2), 543–548. doi:10.1016/j.foodchem.2011.03.063 PMID:25212167

Maghtader & Salari. (2012). Comparative survey on the essential oil composition from the leaves and flowers of Laurus nobilis L. from Kerman province. *Journal of Ecology and the Natural Environment*, *4*(6), 150–153.

Mahady, G. B., Pendland, S. L., Yun, G. S., Lu, Z. Z., & Stoia, A. (2003). Ginger (Zingiber officinale Roscoe) and the gingerols inhibit the growth of Cag A+ strains of helicobacter pylori. *Anticancer Research*, *23*, 3699–3702. PubMed

Mahendra, P., & Bisht, S. (2011). Anti-anxiety activity of *Coriandrum sativum* assessed using different experimental anxiety models. *Indian Journal of Pharmacology*, *43*(5), 574–577. doi:10.4103/0253-7613.84975

Mahendra, P., & Bisht, S. (2011). Coriandrum sativum: A daily use spice with great medicinal effect department of pharmacology. *Pharmacognosy Journal*, *3*(21), 84–88. doi:10.5530/pj.2011.21.16

Maheshwari, A., Verma, N., Swaroop, A., Bagchi, M., Preuss, H. G., Tiwari, K., & Bagchi, D. (2017). Efficacy of Furosap™, a novel *Trigonella foenum-graecum* seed extract, in Enhancing Testosterone Level and Improving Sperm Profile in Male Volunteers. *International Journal of Medical Sciences*, *14*(1), 58–66. doi:10.7150/ijms.17256 PMID:28138310

Mahindru, S. N. (1982). *Spices in Indian Life*. New Delhi: Sultanchand and Sons.

Maitre, S., Neher, J., & Safranek, S. (2011). FPIN's clinical inquiries: Ginger for the treatment of nausea and vomiting in pregnancy. *American Family Physician*, *84*, 1–2. PubMed

Ma, J., Hwang, Y. K., Cho, W. H., Han, S. H., Hwang, J. K., & Han, J. S. (2009). Macelignan attenuates activations of mitogen-activated protein kinases and nuclear factor kappa B induced by lipopolysaccharide in microglial cells. *Biological & Pharmaceutical Bulletin*, *32*(6), 1085–1090. doi:10.1248/bpb.32.1085 PMID:19483320

Majeed, M. (1995). *Curcuminoids: Antioxidant Phytonutrient*. NutriScience Publishers Inc.

Malan, R., Walia, A., Saini, V., & Gupta, S. (2011). Comparison of different extracts leaf of Brassica juncea Linn on wound healing activity. *European Journal of Experimental Biology*, *1*(2), 33–40.

Maliszewska, I., Szewczyk, K., & Waszak, K. (2009). Biological synthesis of silver nanoparticles. *Journal of Physics: Conference Series*, *146*(1), 012025. doi:10.1088/1742-6596/146/1/012025

Mancini-Filho, J., van-Koiij, A., Mancini, D. A. P., Cozzolino, F. F., & Torres, R. P. (1998). Antioxidant activity of cinnamon (Cinnamomum zeylanicum, breyne) extracts. *Bollettino Chimico Farmaceutico*, *137*(11), 443–447. PMID:10077878

Mandal, S., & Mandal, M. (2015). Coriander (Coriandrum sativum L.) essential oil. *Chemistry and Biological Activity*, *5*(6), 421–428.

Manohar, R. P., Pushpan, R., & Rohini, S. (2009). Mustard and its uses in Ayurveda. *Indian Journal of Traditional Knowledge*, *8*, 400–404.

Mansour, S. M., Bahgat, A. K., El-Khatib, A. S., & Khayyal, M. T. (2011). Ginkgo biloba extract (EGb 761) normalizes hypertensionin 2K, 1C hypertensive rats: Role ofantioxidant mechanisms, ACE inhibiting activityand improvement of endothelial dysfunction. *Phytomedicine*, *18*(8-9), 641–647. doi:10.1016/j.phymed.2011.01.014 PMID:21353510

Martin, P. (2007). Farm Labor Shortages: How Real, What Responses? ARE Update. *University of California, Davis*. http://www.agecon.ucdavis.edu/extension/update/articles/v10n5_3.pdf

Martin, R. C., Locatelli, E., Li, Y., Zhang, W., Li, S., Monaco, I., & Franchini, M. C. (2015). Gold nanorods and curcumin-loaded nanomicelles for efficient in vivo photothermal therapy of Barrett's esophagus. *Nanomedicine (London)*, *10*(11), 1723–1733. doi:10.2217/nnm.15.25 PMID:25706349

Marzouki, H., Piras, A., Marongiu, B., Rosa, A., & Dessì, M. A. (2008). Extraction and separation of volatile and fixed oils from berries of *laurus nobilis* l. by supercritical co_2. *Molecules (Basel, Switzerland)*, *13*(8), 1702–1711. doi:10.3390/molecules13081702 PMID:18794780

Masuda, Y., Kikuzaki, H., Hisamoto, M., & Nakatani, N. (2004). Antioxidant properties of gingerol related compounds from ginger. *BioFactors (Oxford, England)*, *21*(1-4), 293–296. doi:10.1002/biof.552210157 PubMed

Matan, N., Rimkeeree, H., Mawson, A. J., Chompreeda, P., Haruthaithanasan, V., & Parker, M. (2006). Antimicrobial activity of cinnamon and clove oils under modified atmosphere conditions. *International Journal of Food Microbiology*, *107*(2), 180–185. doi:10.1016/j.ijfoodmicro.2005.07.007 PMID:16266767

Mathew, S., & Abraham, T. E. (2006). Studies on the antioxidant activities of cinnamon (*Cinnamomum verum*) bark extracts, through various in vitro models. *Food Chemistry*, *94*(4), 520–528. doi:10.1016/j.foodchem.2004.11.043

Mathew, S., Prakash, A., & Radhakrishnan, E. K. (2018). Sunlight mediated rapid synthesis of small size range silver nanoparticles using Zingiber officinale rhizome extract and its antibacterial activity analysis. *Inorganic and Nano-Metal Chemistry*, *48*(2), 139–145. doi:10.1080/24701556.2017.1373295

Matsuda, D., Ohte, S., Ohshiro, T., Jiang, W., Rudel, L., Hong, B., ... Tomoda, H. (2008). Ectomycorrhizal fungal community of naturally regenerated *Pinus thunbergii* seedlings in a coastal pine forest. *Biological & Pharmaceutical Bulletin, 31*, 1063–1066. doi:10.1248/bpb.31.1063 PMID:18520030

Mazaheri, M., Fakheri, B., Piri, I., & Tavassoli, A. (2013). The effect of drought stress and micronutrient of Zn and Mn on yield and essential oil of (*Cuminum cyminum*). *Journal of Novel Applied Sciences, 2*, 350–356.

McCaffrey, R., Thomas, D. J., & Kinzelman, A. O. (2009). The effects of lavender and rosemary essential oils on test-taking anxiety among graduate nursing students. *Holistic Nursing Practice, 23*(2), 88–93. doi:10.1097/HNP.0b013e3181a110aa PMID:19258850

McCormick. (2017). *The History of Spices*. Available online: https://www.mccormickscienceinstitute.com/resources/history-of-spices

Medagama, B. (2015). The glycaemic outcomes of Cinnamon, a review of the experimental evidence and clinical trials. *Nutrition Journal, 14*(108), 2015. doi:10.118612937-015-0098-9 PMID:26475130

Meghwal, M., & Goswami, T. K. (2012). A review on the functional properties, nutritional content, medicinal utilization and potential application of fenugreek. *Journal of Food Processing & Technology, 3*(09). doi:10.4172/2157-7110.1000181

Mehdizadeh, R., Parizadeh, M. R., Khooei, A. R., Mehri, S., & Hosseinzadeh, H. (2013). Cardioprotective Effect of Saffron Extract and Safranal in Isoproterenol-Induced Myocardial Infarction in Wistar Rats. *Iranian Journal of Basic Medical Sciences., 16*(1), 56–63. PMID:23638293

Mehrafarin, A., Rezazahdeh, S. H., & Naghdi, B. H. (2011). A review on biology, cultivation and biotechnology of fenugreek (*Trigonellafoenumgraecum* L.) as a valuable medicinal plant and multipurpose. *Faslnamah-i Giyahan-i Daruyi, 10*, 6–24.

Mehta, K. S., Nayeem, N., & Bains, N. (2011). Adaptogenic activity of methanol extract of B. Lanzanleaves an experimental study in rat model. *Der Pharmacia Sinica, 2*(3), 107–112.

Meisner, W. (1818). Beitragzur Geschichte des Chrom. *Annalen der Physik, 60*(12), 366–394. doi:10.1002/andp.18180601204

Menon, V. P., & Sudheer, A. R. (2007). Antioxidant and anti-inflammatory properties of Curcumin. *Advances in Experimental Medicine and Biology, 595*, 105–125. doi:10.1007/978-0-387-46401-5_3 PMID:17569207

Merah, O. (2015). Genetic Variability in Glucosinolates in Seed of Brassica juncea: Interest in mustard condiment. *Journal of Chemistry*.

Mercan, N., Guvensen, A., Celik, A., & Katircioglu, H. (2007). Antimicrobial activity and pollen composition of honey samples collected from different provinces in Turkey. *Natural Product Research, 21*(3), 187–195. doi:10.1080/14786410600906277 PMID:17365707

Mesomo, M. C., Corazza, M. L., Ndiaye, P. M., Santa, O. R. D., Cardozo, L., & Scheer, A. P. (2013). Supercritical CO2 extracts and essential oil of ginger (Zingiber officinale R.): Chemical composition and antibacterial activity. *The Journal of Supercritical Fluids, 80*, 44–49. doi:10.1016/j.supflu.2013.03.031

Meva, F. E. A., Segnou, M. L., Ebongue, C. O., Deli, V., Nyobe, J. C. N., & Mpondo, E. M. (2015). Synthesis, optimization and effect of condition reactions studies of seed kernel aqueous extract mediated silver nanoparticles from Ricinodendron heudelotii (*Baill*) Pierre Pax. Inter*national Journal of Biosciences, 7(4)*, 47–56. doi:10.12692/ijb/7.4.47-56

Mhemdi, H., Rodier, E., Kechaou, N., & Fages, J. (2011). A supercritical tuneable process for the selective extraction of fats and essential oil from coriander seeds. Jour*nal of Food Engineering, 105(4)*, 609–616. doi:10.1016/j.jfoodeng.2011.03.030

Midha, R. L., & Trivedi, P. C. (1988). Evaluation of coriander varieties against Meloidogyne incognita. *Indian J. Nematol., 18, 375.*

Milind, P., & Deepa, K. (2011). Pro-cholinergic, hypo-cholesterolemic and memory improving effects of clove. *International Research Journal of Pharmacy,* 2(4), 119–126.

Min, B. S., Cuong, T. D., Hung, T. M., Min, B. K., Shin, B. S., & Woo, M. H. (2011). Inhibitory Effect of Lignans from *Myristica fragrans* on LPS-induced NO Production in RAW264.7 Cells. *Bulletin of the Korean Chemical Society, 32*(11), 4059–4062. doi:10.5012/bkcs.2011.32.11.4059

Minpei, K., Yoshihiro, M., Tozo, N., Tatsumasa, M., Hideyuki, K., Misuzu, T., ... Mikio, K. (2005). Hypoglycemic effects of turmeric (Curcuma longa L.) rhizomes on genetically diabetic KK-Ay mice. *Biological & Pharmaceutical Bulletin, 28*(5), 937–939. doi:10.1248/bpb.28.937 PMID:15863912

Minu, V., Harsh, V., Ravikant, T., Paridhi, J., & Noopur, S. (2012). Medicinal plants of chhattisgarh with anti-snake venom property. *International Journal of Current Pharmaceutical Research*, *3*(2), 1–10.

Mitchell, R., & Fleetwood-Walker, S. (2015). *TRP Channels As Therapeutic Targets.* Academic Press.

Modaghegh, M. H., Shahabian, M., Esmaeili, H. A., Rajbai, O., & Hosseinzadeh, H. (2008). Safety evaluation of saffron (Crocus sativus) tablets in healthy volunteers. *Phytomedicine, 15*(12), 1032–1037. doi:10.1016/j.phymed.2008.06.003 PMID:18693099

Mohajeri, D., & Amouoghli, T. B. (2008). Mousavi Gh, Mesgari M. Antidiabetic activity of Crocus sativus L. (saffron) stigma ethanolic extract in alloxan-induced diabetic rats. *Research Journal of Biological Sciences*, *3*(9), 1102–1108.

Mohamed, W. S., Mostafa, A. M., Mohamed, K. M., & Serwah, A. H. (2015). Effects of fenugreek, Nigella, and termis seeds in nonalcoholic fatty liver in obese diabetic albino rats. *Arab Journal of Gastroenterology*, *16*(1), 1–9. doi:10.1016/j.ajg.2014.12.003 PMID:25670619

Montes, A., Bisson, M. A., Gardella, J. A. Jr, & Aga, D. S. (2017). Uptake and transformations of engineered nanomaterials: Critical responses observed in terrestrial plants and the model plant Arabidopsis thaliana. *The Science of the Total Environment*, *607*, 1497–1516. doi:10.1016/j.scitotenv.2017.06.190 PMID:28793406

Montgomery, J. (2009). *The potential of Fenugreek (Trigonellafoenumgraecum) as a forage for dairy herds in central Alberta*. University of Alberta.

Moradi, K. N., & Moradi, K. (2013). Physiological and pharmaceutical effects of fenugreek (*Trigonellafoenumgraecum* L.) as multipurpose and valuable medicinal plant. *Global J. Med. Plant Res.*, *1*, 199-206.

Morita, T., Jinno, K., Kawagishi, H., Arimoto, Y., Suganuma, H., Inakuma, T., & Sugiyama, K. (2003, March). Hepatoprotective effect of myristicin from nutmeg (Myristica fragrans) on lipopolysaccharide/d-galactosamine-induced liver injury. *Journal of Agricultural and Food Chemistry*, *51*(6), 1560–1565. doi:10.1021/jf020946n PMID:12617584

Moritz, M., & Geszke-Moritz, M. (2013). The newest achievements in synthesis, immobilization and practical applications of antibacterial nanoparticles. *Chemical Engineering Journal*, *228*, 596–613. doi:10.1016/j.cej.2013.05.046

Moselhy, S. S., & Ali, H. K. (2009). Hepatoprotective effect of cinnamon extracts against carbon tetrachloride induced oxidative stress and liver injury in rats. *Biological Research*, *42*(1), 93–98. doi:10.4067/S0716-97602009000100009 PMID:19621136

Mowla, A., Alauddin, M., & Rahman, M. A. (2009). Antihyperglycemic effect of *TrigonellaFoenum-Graecum* (Fenugreek) seed extract in alloxan-induced diabetic rats and its use in diabetes mellitus: A brief qualitative phytochemical and acute toxicity test on the extract. *AJTCAM*, *6*(3), 255–261. PMID:20448850

Muchuweti, M., Kativu, E., Mupure, C. H., Chidewe, C., Ndhlala, A. R., & Benhura, M. A. N. (2007). Phenolic composition and antioxidant properties of some spices. *American Journal of Food Technology*, *2*, 414–420. doi:10.3923/ajft.2007.414.420

Mueller, M., & Jungbauer, A. (2009). Culinary plants, herbs and spices – A rich source of PPARγ ligands. *Food Chemistry*, *117*(4), 660–667. doi:10.1016/j.foodchem.2009.04.063

Mughal, M. H. (2019). Spices; a mechanistic anticancer treatise. *J Nutr Food Technol.*, *2*(1), 14–19. doi:10.30881/jnfrt.00016

Muniyan, A., Ravi, K., Mohan, U., & Panchamoorthy, R. (2017). Characterization and in vitro antibacterial activity of saponin-conjugated silver nanoparticles against bacteria that cause burn wound infection. *World Journal of Microbiology & Biotechnology*, *33*(7), 147. doi:10.100711274-017-2309-3 PMID:28634713

Muthukrishnan, S. D., Ashokkumar, K., & Annapoorani, S. (2014). Identification and determination of flavonoids, carotenoids and chlorophyll concentration in Cynodon dactylon (L.) by HPLC analysis. *Natural Product Research*, *29*(8), 785–790. doi:10.1080/14786419.2014.986125 PubMed

Nabavi, S. F., Di Lorenzo, A., Izadi, M., Sobarzo-Sánchez, E., Daglia, M., & Nabavi, S. M. (2015). Antibacterial effects of cinnamon: From farm to food, cosmetic and pharmaceutical industries. *Nutrients*, *7*(9), 7729–7748. doi:10.3390/nu7095359 PMID:26378575

Nadagouda, M. N., Hoag, G., Collins, J., & Varma, R. S. (2009). Green Synthesis of Au Nanostructures at Room Temperature Using Biodegradable Plant Surfactants. *Crystal Growth & Design*, *9*(11), 4979–4983. doi:10.1021/cg9007685

Nadeem, M., Anjum, F. M., Khan, M. I., Tehseen, S., El-Ghorab, A., & Sultan, J. I. (2013). Nutritional and medicinal aspects of coriander (*Coriandrum sativum* L.)-a review. *British Food Journal*, *115*(5), 743–755. doi:10.1108/00070701311331526

Naef, R., & Velluz, A. (2001). Volatile Constituents in Extracts of Mandarin and Tangerine Peel. *The Journal of Essential Oil Research*, *13*(3), 154–157. doi:10.1080/10412905.2001.9699647

Naga, S. K., Swain, S. K., Sandeep, V. V., & Raju, B. (2013). Effect of foliar application of micronutrients on growth parameters in tomato (*Lycopersicon esculentum* mill.). *Journal of Agriculture and Food Sciences*, *1*, 146–151.

Naidu, M. M., Shyamala, B., & Naik, J. P. (2011). Chemical composition and antioxidant activity of the husk and endosperm of fenugreek seeds. *Lebensmittel-Wissenschaft + Technologie*, *2*(2), 451–456. doi:10.1016/j.lwt.2010.08.013

Naikodi, M. A. R., Waheed, M. A., Shareef, M. A., Ahmad, M., & Nagaiah, K. (2011). Standardization of the Unani drug, *Myristica fragrans* Houtt. (Javetri) with modern analytical techniques. *Pharmaceutical Methods*, *2*(2), 76–82. doi:10.4103/2229-4708.84438 PMID:23781434

Nanjundaiah, S. M., Annaiah, H. N. M., & Dharmesh, S. M. (2011). Gastroprotective Effect of Ginger Rhizome (Zingiber officinale) Extract: Role of Gallic Acid and Cinnamic Acid in H+, K+-ATPase/H. pylori Inhibition and Anti-Oxidative Mechanism. *Evidence-Based Complementary and Alternative Medicine*. doi:10.1093/ecam/nep060

Nanjundan, P., Arunachalam, A., & Thakur, R. (2009). Antinociceptive property of *Trigonellafoenumgraecum*(fenugreek seeds) in high fat diet-fed/low dose streptozotocin-induced diabetic neuropathy in rats. *Pharmacology*, 24–36.

Narasimhamurthy, K., Vishwanatha, S., & Ramesh, B. S. (1999). Acute and subchronic toxicity assessment of debitterized fenugreek powder in the mouse and rat. *Food and Chemical Toxicology*, *37*(8), 831–838. doi:10.1016/S0278-6915(99)00076-9 PMID:10506006

Narayanan, K. B., & Sakthivel, N. (2008). Coriander leaf mediated biosynthesis of gold nanoparticles. *Materials Letters*, *62*(30), 4588–4590. doi:10.1016/j.matlet.2008.08.044

Narender, T., Puri, A., Shweta, A., Khaliq, T., Saxena, R., Bhatia, G., & Chandra, R. (2006). 4-hydroxyisoleucine an unusual amino acid as antidyslipidemic and antihyperglycemic agent. *Bioorganic & Medicinal Chemistry Letters*, *16*(2), 293–296. doi:10.1016/j.bmcl.2005.10.003 PMID:16246556

Nasiri, Y., Saeid, Z.-S., Safar, N., Nosratollah, N., & Kazem, G. G. (2010). Effects of foliar application of micronutrients (Fe and Zn) on flower yield and essential oil of chamomile (*Matricaria chamomilla* L.). *Journal of Medicinal Plants Research*, *4*(17), 1733–1737.

Natta, L. K., & Orapin, N., Krittika, & Pantip, B. (2008). Essential oil from five Zingiberaceae for anti-food-borne bacteria. *International Food Research Journal*, *15*, 337–346.

Nazrul Islam, B., Jaripa, B., & Mahbuba, S. (2009). Chemical composition of leaf and seed essential oil of *Coriandrum sativum* L. from Bangladesh. *Bangladesh Journal of Pharmacology*, *4*, 150–153.

Neelkanthan, N., Narayanan, M., & de Souza, R. J. (2014). Effect of fenugreek (*Trigonellafoenum-graecum*L.) intake on glycemia: A meta-analysis of clinical trials. *Nutrition Journal*, *13*(1), 7. doi:10.1186/1475-2891-13-7 PMID:24438170

Neveu, V., Perez-Jiménez, J., Vos, F., Crespy, V., & du Chaffaut, L. (2010). *Database*. doi:/bap024 doi:10.1093/database

Newman, D. J., & Cragg, G. M. (2012). Natural Products as Sources of New Drugs over the 30 Years from 1981 to 2010. *Journal of Natural Products*, *75*(3), 311–335. doi:10.1021/np200906s PMID:22316239

Ngubane, P. S., Masola, B., & Musabayane, C. T. (2011). The effects of Syzygiumaromaticum-derived oleanolic acid on glycogenic enzymes in streptozotocin-induced diabetic rats. *Renal Failure*, *33*(4), 434–439. doi:10.3109/0886022X.2011.568147 PMID:21529273

Nguyen, P. H., Le, T. V., Kang, H. W., Chae, J., Kim, S. K., Kwon, K. I., ... Oh, W. K. (2010). AMP-activated protein kinase (AMPK) activators from *Myristica fragrans* (nutmeg) and their anti-obesity effect. *Bioorganic & Medicinal Chemistry Letters*, *20*(14), 4128–4131. doi:10.1016/j.bmcl.2010.05.067 PMID:20541406

Nishizono, S., Hayami, T., Ikeda, I., & Imaizumi, K. (2000). Protection against diabetogenic effect of feeding tert-butylhydroxyquinone to rats prior to the administration of streptozotocin. *Bioscience, Biotechnology, and Biochemistry*, *64*(6), 1153–1158. doi:10.1271/bbb.64.1153 PMID:10923784

Nomura, T., Shinoda, S., Yamori, T., Sawaki, S., Nagata, I., Ryoyama, K., & Fuke, Y. (2005). Selective sensitivity to wasabi-derived 6-(methylsulfinyl)hexyl isothiocyanate of human breast cancer and melanoma cell lines studied *in vitro*. *Cancer Detection and Prevention*, *29*(2), 155–160. doi:10.1016/j.cdp.2004.07.010 PMID:15829375

Normah, M. N., Chin, H. F., & Reed, B. M. (2013). *Conservation of tropical plant species*. Springer.

O'Mahony, R., Al-khtheeri, H., & Weerasekera, D. (2005). Bactericidal and antiadhesive properties of culinary and medicinal plants against *Helicobactor pylori*. *World Journal of Gastroenterology*, *11*(47), 7499–7507. doi:10.3748/wjg.v11.i47.7499 PMID:16437723

Oboh, G., Agunloye, O. M., Adefegha, S. A., Akinyemi, A. J., & Ademiluyi, A. O. (2015). Caffeic and chlorogenic acids inhibit key enzymes linked to type 2 diabetes (in vitro): A comparative study. *Journal of Basic and Clinical Physiology and Pharmacology*, *26*(2), 165–170. doi:10.1515/jbcpp-2013-0141 PMID:24825096

Oćwieja, M., Morga, M., & Adamczyk, Z. (2013). Self-assembled silver nanoparticles monolayers on mica-AFM, SEM, and electrokinetic characteristics. *Journal of Nanoparticle Research*, *15*(3), 1460. doi:10.100711051-013-1460-5 PMID:23519078

Odebunmi, E. O., Oluwaniyi, O. O., & Bashiru, M. O. (2010). Comparative proximate analysis of some food condiments. *Journal of Applied Sciences Research*, *6*(3), 272–274.

Ogbuewu, I. P., Jiwuba, P. D., Ezeokeke, C. T., Uchegbu, M. C., Okoli, I. C., & Iloeje, M. U. (2014). Evaluation of phytochemical and nutritional composition of ginger rhizome powder. *International Journal of Agriculture & Rural Development*, *17*(1), 1663–1670.

Ogbunugafor, H. A., Ugochukwu, C. J., & Kyrian-Ogbonna, A. E. (2017). The role of spices in nutrition and health: a review of three popular spices used in Southern Nigeria. *J Food QualSaf*, *1*, 171–185.

Ogbunugafor, H. A. (2011). Physico-chemical and antioxidant properties of *Moringaoleifera*seed oil. *Pakistan Journal of Nutrition*, *10*(5), 409–414. doi:10.3923/pjn.2011.409.414

Ohshiro, M., Kuroyanag, M., & Keno, A. (1990). Structures of sesquiterpenes from Curcuma longa. *Phytochemistry*, *29*(7), 2201–2205. doi:10.1016/0031-9422(90)83038-3

Ojewole, J. A. O. (2006). Analgesic, antiinflammatory and hypoglycaemic effects of ethanol extract of Zingiber officinale (Roscoe) rhizomes (Zingiberaceae) in mice and rats. *Phytotherapy Research*, *20*(9), 764–772. doi:10.1002/ptr.1952 PubMed

Okamoto, M., Irii, H., Tahara, Y., Ishii, H., Hirao, A., Udagawa, H., ... Shimizu, I. (2011). Synthesis of a new [6]- gingerol analogue and its protective effect with respect to the development of metabolic syndrome in mice fed a high-fat diet. *Journal of Medicinal Chemistry*, *54*(18), 6295–6304. doi:10.1021/jm200662c PubMed

Okoye, E. I., & Ebeledike, A. O. O. (2013). *Phytochemical constituents of Piperngguineense(Uziza) and their health implications on some microorganisms*. Academic Press.

Olajide, O. A., Makinde, J. M., & Awe, S. O. (2000). Evaluation of the pharmacological properties of nutmeg oil in rats and mice. *Pharmaceutical Biology*, *38*(5), 385–390. doi:10.1076/phbi.38.5.385.5976

Omidi, A., Riahinia, N., Montazer, T. M., & Behdani, M. (2014). Hepatoprotective effect of Crocus sativus (saffron) petals extract against acetaminophen toxicity in male Wistar rats. *Avicenna Journal of Phytomedicine*, *4*(5), 330–336. PMID:25386395

Omotayo, O. A., Adepoju, O., Thomas, K., & Oluremi, O. (2013). Evaluation of micronutrient potentials of seven commonly consumed indigenous spices from Nigeria. *American Journal of Food and Nutrition*, *3*(3), 122–126. doi:10.5251/ajfn.2013.3.3.122.126

Onimawo, I. A., Esekheigbe, A., & Okoh, J. E. (2019). Determination of Proximate and Mineral Composition of Three Traditional Spices. *Acta Scientific Nutritional Health*, *3*, 111–114.

Onyenekwe, P. C., & Hashimoto, S. (1999). The composition of the essential oil of dried Nigerian ginger (Zingiber officinale Roscoe). *European Food Research and Technology*, *209*(6), 407–410. doi:10.1007/s002170050517

Opara, E. I., & Chohan, M. (2014). Culinary Herbs and Spices: Their Bioactive Properties the Contribution of Polyphenols and the Challenges in Deducing Their True Health Benefits. *International Journal of Molecular Sciences*, *15*(10), 19183–19202. doi:10.3390/ijms151019183 PMID:25340982

Otunola, G. A., Oloyede, O. B., Oladiji, A. T., & Afolayan, A. J. (2010). Comparative analysis of the chemical composition of three spices - Allium sativum L. Zingiber officinale Rosc.andCapsicum frutescens L. commonly consumed in Nigeria. *African Journal of Biotechnology*, *9*(41), 6927–6931.

Ouibrahim, A., Tlili-Ait-kaki, Y., Bennadja, S., Amrouni, S., Djahoudi, A. G., & Djebarl, M. R. (2013). Evaluation of antibacterial activity of Laurus nobilis L, Rosmarinus officinalis L. and Ocimum basilicum L. from Northeast of Algeria. *African Journal of Microbiological Research*, *7*(42), 4968–4973. doi:10.5897/AJMR2012.2390

Ozcan, B., Esen, M., Sangun, M. K., Coleri, A., & Caliskan, M. (2010). Effective antibacterial and antioxidant properties of methanolic extract of Laurus nobilis seed oil. *Journal of Environmental Biology*, *31*(5), 637–641. PMID:21387914

Padmashree, A., Roopa, N., Semwal, A. D., Sharma, G. K., Agathian, G., & Bawa, A. S. (2007). Star-anise (*Illicium verum*) and black caraway (*Carumnigrum*) as natural antioxidants. *Food Chemistry*, *104*(1), 59–66. doi:10.1016/j.foodchem.2006.10.074

Palamarja, N. S., & Chotina, A. A. (1953). Koriandr. Gosudarstvennoe izdatel'stvo sel'skochozjaistvennoj literatury, Moskva.

Pal, D., & Verma, P. (2013). Flavonoids: A powerful and abundant source of antioxidants. *Interl J of Pharm and Pharmaceu Sci*, *5*, 97–106.

Pal, M., Srivastava, M., Soni, D. K., Kumar, A., & Tewari, S. K. (2011). Composition and anti-microbial activity of essential oil of *Myristica fragrans* from Andaman Nicobar Island. *International Journal of Pharmacy and Life Sciences*, *2*, 1115–1117.

Panáček, A., Kvitek, L., Prucek, R., Kolář, M., Večeřová, R., Pizúrová, N., ... Zbořil, R. (2006). Silver colloid nanoparticles: Synthesis, characterization, and their antibacterial activity. *The Journal of Physical Chemistry B*, *110*(33), 16248–16253. doi:10.1021/jp063826h PMID:16913750

Panda, S., Tahiliani, P., & Kar, A. (1999). Inhibition of Triiodothyronine production by fenugreek seeds extract in mice and rats. *Pharmacological Research*, *40*(5), 405–409. doi:10.1006/phrs.1999.0510 PMID:10527654

Paramelle, D., Sadovoy, A., Gorelik, S., Free, P., Hobley, J., & Fernig, D. G. (2014). A rapid method to estimate the concentration of citrate capped silver nanoparticles from UV-visible light spectra. *Analyst (London)*, *139*(19), 4855–4861. doi:10.1039/C4AN00978A PMID:25096538

Parashar, V., Parashar, R., Sharma, B., & Pandey, A. C. (2009). Parthenium leaf extract mediated synthesis of silver nanoparticles: A novel approach towards weed utilization. *Digest Journal of Nanomaterials and Biostructures*, *4*(1).

Park, G., Kim, H. G., Kim, Y. O., Park, S. H., Kim, S. Y., & Oh, M. S. (2012). *Coriandrum sativum* L. protects human keratinocytes from oxidative stress by regulating oxidative defense systems. *Skin Pharmacology and Physiology*, *25*(2), 93–99. doi:10.1159/000335257

Park, G., Kim, H. G., Lim, S., Lee, W., Sim, Y., & Oh, M. S. (2014). Coriander alleviates 2,4-dinitrochlorobenzene-induced contact dermatitis-like skin lesions in mice. *Journal of Medicinal Food*, *17*(8), 862–868. doi:10.1089/jmf.2013.2910

Park, M., Bae, J., & Lee, D. S. (2008). Antibacterial activity of [10]-gingerol and [12]-gingerol isolated from ginger rhizome against periodontal bacteria. *Phytotherapy Research*, *22*(11), 1446–1449. doi:10.1002/ptr.2473 PubMed

Park, S. H., Ryu, S. N., Bu, Y., Kim, H., Simon, J. E., & Kim, K. S. (2010). Antioxidant components as potential neuroprotective agent in sesame (Sesamumindicum L.) food rev. *Int.*, *26*, 103–121.

Patel, D., Perry, C., & Kennedy, S. (2007, February). Spectroscopic studies and AFM analysis of Ho3+ and Tm3+ doped yttrium oxide nanoparticles. In *Optical Components and Materials IV* (Vol. 6469). International Society for Optics and Photonics. doi:10.1117/12.701480

Patil, R. N., & Rothe, S. P. (2017). Buchanania lanzan: An enormous medicinal value. *International Journal of Advance Research and Innovative Ideas in Education*, *3*(1), 2395–4396.

Patra, K. C., Pareta, S. K., Harwansh, R. K., & Kumar, J. (2011). Antioxidant activity of B. lanzan spreng. *Pharmacologyonline*, *1*, 733–739.

Patsnaik, A. K., Kodati, D., Pareta, S. K., Patra, K. C., & Harwansh, R. K. (2011). Analgesic and anti-inflammatory activities of BuchananialanzanSpreg. roots. *Research Journal of Pharmaceutical, Biological and Chemical Sciences*, *2*(1), 419–425.

Pattanayak, M., & Nayak, P. L. (2013). Ecofriendly green synthesis of iron nanoparticles from various plants and spices extract. *International Journal of Plant. Animal and Environmental Sciences*, *3*(1), 68–78.

Pattnaik, A., Sarkar, R., Sharma, A., Yadav, K. K., Kumar, A., Roy, P., ... Sen, T. (2013). Pharmacological studies on Buchanania lanzan Spreng.-A focus on wound healing with particular reference to anti-biofilm properties. *Asian Pacific Journal of Tropical Biomedicine*, *3*(12), 967–974. doi:10.1016/S2221-1691(13)60187-2 PMID:24093788

Paul, S. K., Mazumder, S., Mondal, S., Roy, S. K., & Kundu, S. (2015). Intercropping Coriander with Brinjal Forbrinjal Fruit and Shoot Borer Insect Suppression. *World Journal of Agricultural Sciences*, *11*(5), 303–306.

Pawar, S. (2012). Plant based folk recipes for treatment of hepatic disorders in Jalgaon district (ms) India. *International. Journal of Basic and Applied Sciences*, *1*, 109–114.

Pérez-Jiménez, J., Neveu, V., Vos, F., & Scalbert, A. (2010). Identification of the 100 richest dietary sources of polyphenols: An application of the phenol-explorer database. *European Journal of Clinical Nutrition*, *64*(3), 112–120. doi:10.1038/ejcn.2010.221 PMID:21045839

Pernice, R., Borriello, G., Ferracane, R., Borrelli, R. C., Cennamo, F., & Ritieni, A. (2009). Bergamot: A source of natural antioxidants for functionalized fruit juices. *Food Chemistry*, *112*(3), 545–550. doi:10.1016/j.foodchem.2008.06.004

Perrault, S. D., & Chan, W. C. (2010). In vivo assembly of nanoparticle components to improve targeted cancer imaging. *Proceedings of the National Academy of Sciences of the United States of America*, *107*(25), 11194–11199. doi:10.1073/pnas.1001367107 PMID:20534561

Persson, I. A., Persson, K., Hägg, S., & Andersson, R. G. (2011). Effects of cocoa extract and dark chocolate on angiotensin-converting enzyme and nitric oxide in human endothelial cells and healthy volunteersanutrigenomics perspective. *Journal of Cardiovascular Pharmacology*, *57*(1), 44–50. doi:10.1097/FJC.0b013e3181fe62e3 PMID:20966764

Peter, K. V. (2004). Handbook of herbs and spices. Cambridge: Woodhead Publishing Ltd.

Petit, P., Sauvaire, Y., Ponsin, G., Manteghetti, M., Fave, A., & Ribes, G. (1993). Effects of a fenugreek seed extract on feeding behavior in the rat: Metabolic endocrine correlates. *Pharmacology, Biochemistry, and Behavior*, *2*(2), 369–374. doi:10.1016/0091-3057(93)90253-P PMID:8327543

Petropoulos, G. A. (2002). *Fenugreek, The genus Trigonella*. London: Taylor and Francis. doi:10.4324/9780203217474

Piaru, S. P., Mahmud, R., Abdul Majid, A. M., Ismail, S., & Man, C. N. (2012). Chemical composition, antioxidant and cytotoxicity activities of the essential oils of *Myristica fragrans* and *Morinda citrifolia*. *Journal of the Science of Food and Agriculture*, *92*(3), 593–597. doi:10.1002/jsfa.4613 PMID:25520982

Pimentel, M., Bonorris, G. G., Chow, E. J., & Lin, H. C. (2001). Peppermint oil improves the manometric findings in diffuse esophageal spasm. *Journal of Clinical Gastroenterology*, *33*(1), 27–31. doi:10.1097/00004836-200107000-00007 PMID:11418786

Ping, H., Zhang, G., & Ren, G. (2010). Antidiabetic Effects of Cinnamon Oil in Diabetic KK-Ay Mice. *Food and Chemical Toxicology*, *48*(8), 2344–2349. doi:10.1016/j.fct.2010.05.069 PMID:20561948

Pino, J. A., Marbot, R., Rosado, A., & Batista, A. (2004). Chemical composition of the essential oil of Zingiber officinale Roscoe L. from Cuba. *The Journal of Essential Oil Research*, *16*(3), 186–188. doi:10.1080/10412905.2004.9698692

Pitsikas, N., Boultadakis, A., Gergiadou, G., Tarantilis, P. A., & Sakellaridis, N. (2008). Effects of the active constituents of Crocus sativus L. in an animal model of anxiety. *Phytomedicine*, *15*, 1135.

Pitto-Barry, A., Perdigao, L. M., Walker, M., Lawrence, J., Costantini, G., Sadler, P. J., & Barry, N. P. (2015). Synthesis and controlled growth of osmium nanoparticles by electron irradiation. *Dalton Transactions (Cambridge, England), 44*(47), 20308–20311. doi:10.1039/C5DT03205A PMID:26418726

Platel, K., & Srinivasan, K. (2004). Article. *The Indian Journal of Medical Research, 119*, 167–179. PMID:15218978

Poma, A., Fontecchio, G., Carlucci, G., & Chichiricco, G. (2012). Anti-Inflammatory Properties of Drugs from saffron crocus. *Anti-Inflammatory & Anti-Allergy Agents in Medicinal Chemistry, 11*(1), 37–51. doi:10.2174/187152312803476282 PMID:22934747

Portincasa, P., Bonfrate, L., de Bari, O., Lembo, A., & Ballou, S. (2017). Irritable bowel syndrome and diet. *Gastroenterology Report, 5*(1), 11–19. doi:10.1093/gastro/gow047 PMID:28110300

Prakasam, V., Vedamuthu, P. G. B., Khader, M. A., & Jeyarajan, R. (1987). Screening coriander lines for wilt resistance. *South Indian Horticulture, 35*, 258–259.

Prasad, S., & Tyagi, A. K. (2015). Ginger and Its Constituents: Role in Prevention and Treatment of Gastrointestinal Cancer. Gastroenterology Research and Practice. doi:10.1155/2015/142979

Prasad, R. C., Herzog, B., Boone, B., Sims, L., & Waltner-Law, M. (2005). An extract of Syzygiumaromaticum represses genes encoding hepatic gluconeogenic enzymes. *Journal of Ethnopharmacology, 96*(1-2), 295–301. doi:10.1016/j.jep.2004.09.024 PMID:15588682

Prasad, S., Gupta, S. C., Tyagi, A. K., & Aggarwal, B. B. (2014). Curcumin, acomponent of golden spice: From bedside to bench and back. *Biotechnology Advances, 32*(6), 1053–1064. doi:10.1016/j.biotechadv.2014.04.004 PMID:24793420

Press, C. R. C. (2002). *Handbook of Nutraceuticals and Functional Foods*. CRC Press.

Preuss, H. G., Echard, B., Polansky, M. M., & Anderson, R. (2006). Whole Cinnamon and Aqueous Extracts Ameliorate Sucrose-Induced Blood Pressure Elevations in Spontaneously Hypertensive Rats. *Journal of the American College of Nutrition, 25*(2), 144–150. doi:10.1080/07315724.2006.10719525 PMID:16582031

Qaiser, J. (2009). Coriander fruit exhibits gut modulatory, blood pressure lowering, and diuretic activities. *Journal of Ethnopharmacology, 122*(1), 123–130. doi:10.1016/j.jep.2008.12.016

Qin, B., Polansky, M. M., Sato, Y., Adeli, K., & Anderson, R. A. (2010). Cinnamon extract inhibits the postprandial overproduction of apolipoprotein B48-containing lipoproteins in fructose-fed animals. *The Journal of Nutritional Biochemistry, 20*(11), 901–908. doi:10.1016/j.jnutbio.2008.08.005 PMID:18993048

Qin, F., & Xu, H. (2008). Active compounds in gingers and their therapeutic uses in complimentary medication. *Medicinal and Aromatic Plant Science and Biotechnology, 2*(2), 72–78.

Qiu, H., Gao, Y., Boott, C. E., Gould, O. E., Harniman, R. L., Miles, M. J., ... Manners, I. (2016). Uniform patchy and hollow rectangular platelet micelles from crystallizable polymer blends. *Science, 352*(6286), 697–701. doi:10.1126cience.aad9521 PMID:27151866

Qiu, P., Dong, P., Guan, H., Li, S., Ho, C. T., Pan, M. H., ... Xiao, H. (2010). Inhibitory effects of 5-hydroxy polymethoxyflavones on colon cancer cells. *Molecular Nutrition & Food Research, 54*(S2), S244–S252. doi:10.1002/mnfr.200900605 PMID:20397199

Qiu, Q., Zhang, G., Sun, X., & Liu, X. (2004). Study on chemical constituents of the essential oil from *Myristica fragrans* Houtt. by supercritical fluid extraction and steam distillation. *Zhong Yao Cai, 27*, 823–826. PMID:15810588

Qureshi, A. A., Qureshi, N., Wright, J. J., Shen, Z., Kramer, G., Gapor, A., ... Peterson, D. M. (1991). Lowering of serum cholesterol in hypercholesterolemic humans by tocotrienols (palmvitee). *The American Journal of Clinical Nutrition*, *53*(4), 1021S–1026S. doi:10.1093/ajcn/53.4.1021S PMID:2012010

R'ıos, J. L., Recio, M. C., Ginger, R. M., & M'a˜nez, S. (1996). An updated review of saffron and its active constituents. *Phytotherapy Research*, *10*(3), 189–193. doi:10.1002/(SICI)1099-1573(199605)10:3<189::AID-PTR754>3.0.CO;2-C

Rababah, T. M., Ereifej, K. I., Esoh, R. B., Al-u'datt, M. H., Alrababah, M. A., & Yang, W. (2011). Antioxidant activities, total phenolics and HPLC analyses of the phenolic compounds of extracts from common Mediterrarean plants. *Natural Product Research*, *6*(6), 596–605. doi:10.1080/14786419.2010.488232 PMID:21409721

Radojčić Redovniković, I., Glivetic, T., Delonga, K., & Vorkapić-Furač, J. (2008). Glucosinolates and their potential role in plant. *Periodicum Biologorum*, *110*(4), 297–309.

Raghunandan, D., Bedre, M. D., Basavaraja, S., Sawle, B., Manjunath, S. Y., & Venkataraman, A. (2010). Rapid biosynthesis of irregular shaped gold nanoparticles from macerated aqueous extracellular dried clove buds (Syzygium aromaticum) solution. *Colloids and Surfaces. B, Biointerfaces*, *79*(1), 235–240. doi:10.1016/j.colsurfb.2010.04.003 PMID:20451362

Raghunandan, D., Borgaonkar, P. A., Bendegumble, B., Bedre, M. D., Bhagawanraju, M., Yalagatti, M. S., ... Abbaraju, V. (2011). Microwave-Assisted Rapid Extracellular Biosynthesis of Silver Nanoparticles Using Carom Seed (Trachyspermum copticum) Extract and in Vitro Studies. *American Journal of Analytical Chemistry*, *2*(4), 475–483. doi:10.4236/ajac.2011.24057

Rahmani, S., Asgary, S., Askar, G., Keshvari, M., Hataminpour, M., Feizi, A., & Sahebkar, A. (2016). Treatment of Non-alcoholic Fatty Liver Disease with Curcumin: A Randomized Placebo-controlled Trial. *Phytotherapy Research*, *30*(9), 1540–1548. doi:10.1002/ptr.5659 PMID:27270872

Raina, V. K., Kumar, A., & Aggarwal, K. K. (2005). Essential oil composition of ginger (Zingiber officinale Roscoe) rhizomes from different place in india. *Journal of Essential Oil-Bearing Plants*, *8*(2), 187–191. doi:10.1080/0972060X.2005.10643442

Rajan, F. S., Vedamuthu, P. G. B., Khader, M. K., & Jeyarajan, R. (1990). Screening coriander lines against grain mould disease. *South Indian Horticulture*, *38*, 168–169.

Rajesh, K. M., Ajitha, B., Reddy, Y. A. K., Suneetha, Y., & Reddy, P. S. (2018). Assisted green synthesis of copper nanoparticles using Syzygium aromaticum bud extract: Physical, optical and antimicrobial properties. *Optik (Stuttgart)*, *154*, 593–600. doi:10.1016/j.ijleo.2017.10.074

Raju, J., Gupta, D., Rao, A. R., Yadava, P. K., & Baquer, N. Z. (2001). *Trigonellafoenumgraecum* (Fenugreek) seed powder improves glucose homeostasis in alloxan diabetic rat tissues by reversing the altered glycolytic, gluconeogenic and lipogenic enzymes. *Molecular and Cellular Biochemistry*, *224*(1/2), 45–51. doi:10.1023/A:1011974630828 PMID:11693199

Raju, J., Patlolla, J. M., Swamy, M. V., & Rao, C. V. (2004). Diosgenin, a steroid saponin of *Trigonellafoenum graecum* (Fenugreek), inhibits azoxymethane-induced aberrant crypt foci formation in F344 rats and induces apoptosis in HT-29 human colon cancer cells. *Cancer Epidemiology, Biomarkers & Prevention*, *13*, 1392–1398. PMID:15298963

Raj, X. J., & Nishimura, T. (2014). Investigation of the Surface Potential on Iron Nanoparticles During the Corrosion by Atomic Force Microscopy (AFM) and Kelvin Probe Force Microscopy (KFM). *International Journal of Electrochemical Science*, *9*, 2090–2100.

Ram, A., Lauria, P., Gupta, R., & Sharma, V. N. (1996). Hypolipidaemic effect of *Myristica fragrans* fruit extract in rabbits. *Journal of Ethnopharmacology*, *55*(1), 49–53. doi:10.1016/S0378-8741(96)01473-0 PMID:9121167

Ramadan, M. F.&Morsel, J. T. (2002). Oil composition of coriander (Coriandrum sativum L.) fruit seeds. *European Food Research and Technology, 215*, 204-209.

Ramadan, G., Al-Kahtani, M. A., & El-Sayed, W. M. (2011). Anti-inflammatory and anti-oxidant properties of Curcuma longa (turmeric) versus Zingiber officinale (ginger) rhizomes in rat adjuvant-induced arthritis. *Inflammation, 34*(4), 291–301. doi:10.1007/s10753-010-9278-0 PubMed

Ramadan, M. M., & Abd Algader, N. N. E. (2013). Chemopreventive effect of Coriandrum sativum fruits on hepatic toxicity in male rats. *World Journal of Medical Sciences*, *8*(4), 322–333.

Ramasamy, R. (2007). Aroma characterization of coriander (*Coriandrum sativum* L.) oil samples. *European Food Research and Technology*, *225*(3-4), 367–374. doi:10.100700217-006-0425-7

Ramos-Tovar, E. (2019). Dietary Interventions in Liver Disease. *Foods, Nutrients, and Dietary Supplements*, 101-121.

Randhir, R., Lin, Y. T., & Shetty, K. (2004). Phenolics, their antioxidant and antimicrobial activity in dark germinated fenugreek sprouts in response to peptide and phytochemical elicitors. *Asia Pacific Journal of Clinical Nutrition, 13*, 295–307. PMID:15331344

Randhir, R., & Shetty, K. (2007). Improved alpha-amylase and *Helicobactor pylori* inhibition by fenugreek extracts derived via solid-state bioconversion using *Rhizopusoligosporous. Asia Pacific Journal of Clinical Nutrition, 16*, 382–392. PMID:17704018

Rane, A. V., Kanny, K., Abitha, V. K., & Thomas, S. (2018). Methods for synthesis of nanoparticles and fabrication of nanocomposites. In *Synthesis of inorganic nanomaterials* (pp. 121–139). Woodhead Publishing. doi:10.1016/B978-0-08-101975-7.00005-1

Rao, A., Steels, E., Beccaria, G., Inder, W. J., & Vitetta, L. (2015). Influence of a Specialized Trigonella foenum-graecum Seed Extract (Libifem), on Testosterone, Estradiol and Sexual Function in Healthy Menstruating Women, a Randomised Placebo Controlled Study. *Phytotherapy Research*, *29*(8), 1123–1130. doi:10.1002/ptr.5355 PMID:25914334

Rao, A., Steels, E., Inder, W. J., Abraham, S., & Vitetta, L. (2016). Testofen, a specialised Trigonella foenum-graecum seed extract reduces age-related symptoms of androgen decrease, increases testosterone levels and improves sexual function in healthy aging males in a double-blind randomised clinical study. *The Aging Male*, *19*(2), 134–142. doi:10.3109/13685538.2015.1135323 PMID:26791805

Rao, P. V., & Gan, S. H. (2014). Cinnamon: A multifaceted medicinal plant. *Evidence-Based Complementary and Alternative Medicine*. PMID:24817901

Rathi, S. S., Grover, J. K., Vats, V., & Biswas, N. R. (2002). Prevention of experimental diabetic cataract by Indian Ayurvedic plant extracts. *Phytotherapy Research*, *16*(8), 774–777. doi:10.1002/ptr.1064 PMID:12458487

Rathore, B., Jaggi, K., Thakur, S. K., Mathur, A., & Mahdi, F. (2015). Anti-inflammatory activity of Crocus sativus extracts in experimental arthritis. *International Journal of Pharmaceutical Sciences and Research*, *6*(4), 1473–1478.

Ravindran, P. N., Nirmal Babu, K., & Shiva, K. N. (2005). Botany and crop improvement of ginger. In P. N. Ravindran & K. Nirmal Babu (Eds.), *Ginger: The Genus Zingiber* (Vol. 41, pp. 15–85). Boca Raton, FL: Medicinal and Aromatic Plants-Industrial Profiles.

Ravindran, P., Shylaja, M., Nirmal Babu, K., & Krishnamoorthy, B. (2004). Botany and crop improvement of cinnamon and cassia. In P. N. Ravindran & K. N. Babu (Eds.), *Cinnamon and Cassia—The Genus Cinnamomum*. CRC Press.

Regnault-Roger, C., & Hamraoui, A. (1995). Fumigant toxic activity and reproductive inhibition induced by monoterpenes on acanthoscelides obtectus (Say) (coleoptera), a bruchid of kidney bean (phaseolus vulgaris L.). *Journal of Stored Products Research*, *31*(4), 291–299. doi:10.1016/0022-474X(95)00025-3

Reichert, J., Csáki, A., Köhler, J. M., & Fritzsche, W. (2000). Chip-Based Optical Detection of DNA Hybridization by Means of Nanobead Labeling. *Analytical Chemistry*, *72*(24), 6025–6029. doi:10.1021/ac000567y PMID:11140772

Reid, I. R., Ames, R. W., Evans, M. C., Gamble, G. D., & Sharpe, S. J. (1993). Effect of calcium supplementation on bone loss in postmenopausal women. *The New England Journal of Medicine*, *328*(7), 460–464. doi:10.1056/NEJM199302183280702 PMID:8421475

Rezvani, N., Sorooshzadeh, A., & Farhadi, N. (2012). Effect of nano-silver on growth of saffron in flooding stress. *World Academy of Science, Engineering and Technology*, *6*(1), 517–522.

Riaz, H., Begum, A., Raza, S. A., Khan, Z. M.-U.-D., Yousaf, H., & Tariq, A. (2015). Antimicrobial property and phytochemical study of ginger found in local area of Punjab, Pakistan. International Current Pharmaceutical Journal, 4(7), 405–409. doi:10.3329/icpj.v4i7.23591

Ried, K., Travica, N., & Sali, A. (2016). The effect of aged garlic extract on bloodpressure and other cardiovascular risk factors in uncontrolled hypertensives: The AGE at Heart trial. *Integrated Blood Pressure Control*, *9*, 9. doi:10.2147/IBPC.S93335 PMID:26869811

Rizvi, S. S. H., Benado, A. L., Zollweg, J. A., & Daniels, J. A. (1986). Supercritical fluid extraction operating principles and food applications. *Food Technology (Chicago)*, *40*(7), 57–64.

Roberts, K. T. (2011). The potential of fenugreek (*Trigonellafoenumgraecum)* as a functional food and nutraceutical and its effects on glycemia and lipidemia. *Journal of Medicinal Food*, *14*(12), 1485–1489. doi:10.1089/jmf.2011.0002 PMID:21861724

Rodriguez, L., Ramirez, M., Badillo, M., León-Buitimea, A., & Reyes-Esparza, J. (2006). Toxicological evaluation of *Coriandrum sativum* (cilantro) using in vivo and in vitro models. *The FASEB Journal*, *20*, A645.

Rohit, R. P., Kavindra, R. J., & Chintan, K. M. (2011, April). Image morphological operation-based quality analysis of coriander seed (Coriandrum sativum L.). In *Emerging Trends in Networks and Computer Communications (ETNCC) International Conference on* (pp. 22-24). Academic Press.

Rosello, J., Sampere, F., Sans-Berzosa, I., Amparo, C. A., & Santamarina, J. M. P. (2015). Antifungal activity and potential use of essential oils against Fusarium culmorum and Fusarium verticillioides. *Journal of Essential Oil-Bearing Plants*, *18*(2), 359–367. doi:10.1080/0972060X.2015.1010601

Rosti, L., & Gastaldi, G. (2005). Chronic Salmonellosis and Cinnamon. *Pediatrics*, *116*(4), 1057. doi:10.1542/peds.2005-1521 PMID:16199729

Roussel, A. M., Hininger, I., Benaraba, R., Ziegenfuss, T. N., & Anderson, R. A. (2009). Antioxidant Effects of a Cinnamon Extract in People with Impaired Fasting Glucose That Are Overweight or Obese. *Journal of the American College of Nutrition*, *28*(1), 16–21. doi:10.1080/07315724.2009.10719756 PMID:19571155

Rubió, L., Motilva, M. J., & Romero, M. P. (2013). Recent advances in biologically active compounds in herbs and spices: A review of the most effective antioxidant and anti-inflammatory active principles. *Critical Reviews in Food Science and Nutrition*, *53*(9), 943–953. doi:10.1080/10408398.2011.574802 PMID:23768186

Rubio-Moraga, A., Trapero, A., Ahrazem, O., & Gomez-Gomez, L. (2010). Crocins transport in Crocus sativus: The long road from a senescent stigma to a new born corm. *Phytochemistry*, *71*, 1506–1513.

Ruby, A. J., Kuttan, G., Babu, K. D., Rajasekharan, K. N., & Kuttan, R. (1995). Anti-tumour and antioxidant activity of natural curcuminoids. *Cancer Letters*, *94*(1), 79–83. doi:10.1016/0304-3835(95)03827-J PMID:7621448

Ruby, B., Gaskill, S., Slivka, D., & Harger, S. G. (2005). The addition of fenugreek extract (*Trigonellafoenum- graecum)* to glucose feeding increases muscle glycogen resynthesis after exercise. *Amino Acids*, *1*(1), 71–76. doi:10.100700726-004-0143-z PMID:15719265

Rudzki, E., & Grzywa, Z. (1976). Sensitizing and irritating properties of star anise oil. *Contact Dermatitis*, *2*(6), 305–308. doi:10.1111/j.1600-0536.1976.tb03065.x PMID:1032123

Sachan, A.K., Rao, C.V., & Sachan, N.K. (2016). Ethnobotanicalsurvey of indigenous medicines practiced in Chambal valley of Uttar Pradesh. *Bharatiya Vaigyanik Evam Audyogik Anusandhan Patrika, 23*(2), 132-135.

Sachan, A. K. R., Kumar, S., Kumari, K., & Singh, D. (2018). Medicinal uses of spices used in our traditional culture world wide. *JMPS*, *6*, 116–122.

Sachan, A. K., Das, D. R., & Kumar, M. (2016). Carum carvi- An important medicinal plant. *Journal of Chemical and Pharmaceutical Research*, *8*, 529–533.

Sachan, P. L., Singh, M., Patel, M. L., & Sachan, R. A. (2018). Study on cervical cancer screening using pap smear test and clinical correlation. *Asia-Pacific Journal of Oncology Nursing*, *5*(3), 337–341. doi:10.4103/apjon.apjon_15_18 PMID:29963597

Saeed, F., Nadeem, M., Ahmad, R. S., Nadeem, M. T., Arshad, M. S., & Ullah, A. (2016). Studying the impact of nutritional immunology underlying the modulation of immune responses by nutritional compounds – A review. *Food and Agricultural Immunology*, *27*(2), 205–229. doi:10.1080/09540105.2015.1079600

Safia, Z. (2010). Essential oil composition of *Coriandrum sativum* seed cultivated in Algeria as food grains protectant. *Food Chemistry*, *122*(4), 1226–1228. doi:10.1016/j.foodchem.2010.03.119

Sahib, S. (2016). Anti-diabetic and antioxidant effect of cinnamon in poorly controlled type-2 diabetic Iraqi patients: A randomized, placebocontrolled clinical trial. *Journal of Intercultural Ethnopharmacology*, *5*(2), 108–113. doi:10.5455/jice.20160217044511 PMID:27104030

Sahu, S., Rawat, D., & Singh, D. (2015). Antimicrobial activity of Trachyspermum ammi leaves mediated silver nanoparticles: Green approach. *International Journal of Research in Engineering and Technology*, *4*(9), 34–38. doi:10.15623/ijret.2015.0409006

Said, C. M., & Hussein, K. (2014). Determination of the chemical and genetic differences of Laurus collected from three different geographic and climatic areas in Lebanon. *European Scientific Journal*, *2*, 412–419.

Salam, H. A., Rajiv, P., Kamaraj, M., Jagadeeswaran, P., Gunalan, S., & Sivaraj, R. (2012). Plants: Green route for nanoparticle synthesis. *International Research Journal of Biological Sciences*, *1*(5), 85–90.

Sales, E. H., Sedeh, F. M., & Rajabifar, S. (2012). Effects of gamma irradiation and silver nano particles on microbiological characteristics of saffron, using hurdle technology. *Indian Journal of Microbiology*, *52*(1), 66–69. doi:10.100712088-011-0203-5 PMID:23449911

Sambamurty, A. V. S. S., & Subrahmanyam, N. S. (1989). Capsicums. In A textbook of economic botany. Wiley Eastern Ltd.

Samejima, K., Kanazawa, K., Ashida, H., & Danno, G. (1998). Bay laurel contains antimutagenic kaempferyl coumarate acting against the dietary carcinogen 3-amino-1-methyl-5h-pyrido [4, 3- b]indole. *Journal of Agricultural and Food Chemistry*, *46*(12), 4864–4868. doi:10.1021/jf980714h

Sandasi, M., Leonard, C. M., & Viljoen, A. M. (2008). The effect of five common essential oil components on Listeria monocytogenes biofilms. *Food Control, 19*(11), 1070–1075. doi:10.1016/j.foodcont.2007.11.006

Sangal, A. (2011). Role of cinnamon as beneficial antidiabetic food adjunct: A review. *Advances in Applied Science Research, 2*(4), 440450.

Sangal, A. (2011). Role of cinnamon as beneficial antidiabetic food adjunct: A review. *Advances in Applied Science Research, 2*(4), 440–450.

Sa-Nguanpuag, K., Kanlayanarat, S., Srilaong, V., Tanprasert, K., & Techavuthiporn, C. (2011). Ginger (Zingiber officinale) oil as an antimicrobial agent for minimally processed produce: A case study in shredded green papaya. *International Journal of Agriculture and Biology, 13*, 895–901.

Saputri, F. C., & Jantan, I. (2011). Effects of selected medicinal plants on human low-density lipoprotein oxidation, 2,2-diphenyl-1-picrylhydra-zyl (DPPH) radicals and human platelet aggregation. *Journal of Medicinal Plants Research, 5*, 6182–6199.

Sarris, J. (2007). Herbal medicines in the treatment of psychiatric disorders: A systematic review. *Phytotherapy Research, 21*(8), 703–706. doi:10.1002/ptr.2187 PMID:17562566

Sasidharan, I., & Menon, A. N. (2010). Comparative chemical composition and antimicrobial activity fresh & dry ginger oils (Zingiber officinale Roscoe). *International Journal of Current Pharmaceutical Research, 2*, 40–43.

Sathyavathi, R., Krishna, M. B., Rao, S. V., Saritha, R., & Rao, D. N. (2010). Biosynthesis of silver nanoparticles using Coriandrum sativum leaf extract and their application in nonlinear optics. *Advanced Science Letters, 3*(2), 138–143. doi:10.1166/asl.2010.1099

Satyanarayana, M. N. (2006). Capsaicin and Gastric Ulcers. *Critical Reviews in Food Science and Nutrition, 46*(4), 275–328. doi:10.1080/1040-830491379236 PMID:16621751

Sauvaire, Y., Petit, P., Broca, C., Manteghetti, M., Baissac, Y., Fernandez-Alvarez, J., ... Ribes, G. (1998). 4-Hydroxyisoleucine: A novel amino acid potentiator of insulin secretion. *Diabetes, 47*(2), 206–210. doi:10.2337/diab.47.2.206 PMID:9519714

Sauvare, Y., Pett, P., & Baissao, Y. (2000). Chemistry and pharmacology of fenugreek. In G. Mazza & B. D. Oomah (Eds.), *Herbs, Botanicals and Teas* (pp. 107–129). Technomic Publishing Company Inc.

Saxena, R., & Patil, P. (2012). Phytochemical Studies on Myristica fragrance Essential Oil, Biological Forum –. *International Journal (Toronto, Ont.), 4*, 62–64.

Sayyah, M., Valizadeh, J., & Kamalinejad, M. (2002). Anticonvulsant activity of the leaf essential oil of Laurus nobilis against pentylenetetrazole and maximal electroshock–induced seizures. *Phytomedicine, 9*(3), 212–216. doi:10.1078/0944-7113-00113 PMID:12046861

Schieber, A., Stintzing, F. C., & Carle, R. (2001). By-products of plant food processing as a source of functional compounds – recent developments. *Trends in Food Science & Technology, 12*(11), 401–413. doi:10.1016/S0924-2244(02)00012-2

Schwingshackl, L., Missbach, B., & Hoffmann, G. (2016). An umbrella review of garlic intake and risk of cardiovascular disease. *Phytomedicine, 23*(11), 1127–1133. doi:10.1016/j.phymed.2015.10.015 PMID:26656227

Selvam, R., Subramanian, L., Gayathri, R., & Angayarkanni, N. (1995). The anti-oxidant activity of turmeric (Curcuma longa). *Journal of Ethnopharmacology, 47*(2), 59–67. doi:10.1016/0378-8741(95)01250-H PMID:7500637

Semwal, R. B., Semwal, D. K., Combrinck, S., & Viljoen, A. M. (2015). Gingerols and shogaols: Important nutraceutical principles from ginger. *Phytochemistry*, *117*, 554–568. doi:10.1016/j.phytochem.2015.07.012 PubMed

Senthil, B., Devasena, T., Prakash, B., & Rajasekar, A. (2017). Non-cytotoxic effect of green synthesized silver nanoparticles and its antibacterial activity. *Journal of Photochemistry and Photobiology. B, Biology*, *177*, 1–7. doi:10.1016/j.jphotobiol.2017.10.010 PMID:29028495

Seyed Mohammad, N., Dehpour, A. A., Ebrahimzadeh, M. A., & Seyed Fazel, N. (2009). Antioxidant activity of the methanol extract of Ferula assafoetida and its essential oil composition. *Grasas y Aceites*, *60*(4), 405–412. doi:10.3989/gya.010109

Shaban, M. A. E., Kandeel, K. M., Yacout, G. A., & Mehaseb, S. E. (1987). The chemical-composition of the volatile oil of elettaria cardamomum seeds. *Die Pharmazie*, *42*(3), 207–208.

Shabbeer, S., Sobolewski, M., Anchoori, R. K., Kachhap, S., Hidalgo, M., Jimeno, A., ... Khan, S. R. (2009). Fenugreek: A naturally occurring edible spice as an anticancer agent. *Cancer Biology & Therapy*, *8*(3), 2720–278. doi:10.4161/cbt.8.3.7443 PMID:19197146

Shah, G. M., Hussain, M., & Abbasi, A. M. (2015). *Medicinal Plants Used to Treat Respiratory Tract Illness in Kaghan Valley*. Himalayan Region-Pakistan.

Shahid, M., & Hussain, F. (2012). Chemical composition and mineral contents of Zingiber officinale and Alpinia allughas (Zingiberaceae) rhizomes. *International Journal of Chemical and Biochemical Science*, *2*, 101–104.

Shalaby, T. I., Mahmoud, O. A., El Batouti, G. A., & Ibrahim, E. E. (2015). Green synthesis of silver nanoparticles: Synthesis, characterization and antibacterial activity. *Nanosci. Nanotechnol*, *5*(2), 23–29.

Shammari, A. M. N. A. (2018). Protective effect of ginger (Zingiber officinale) consumption against kidney damage in rats. *Life Science Journal*, *15*(1), 80–85.

Shan, B., Cai, Y. Z., Brooks, J. D., & Corke, H. (2007). Antibacterial properties and major bioactive components of cinnamon stick (Cinnamomum burmannii): Activity against foodborne pathogenic bacteria. *Journal of Agricultural and Food Chemistry*, *55*(14), 5484–5490. doi:10.1021/jf070424d PMID:17567030

Shan, B., Cai, Y. Z., Sun, M., & Corke, H. (2005). Antioxidant capacity of 26 spice extracts and characterization of their phenolic constituents. *Journal of Agricultural and Food Chemistry*, *53*(20), 7749–7759.

Shankar, S. S., Ahmad, A., Pasricha, R., & Sastry, M. (2003). Bioreduction of chloroaurate ions by geranium leaves and its endophytic fungus yields gold nanoparticles of different shapes. *Journal of Materials Chemistry*, *13*(7), 1822–1826. doi:10.1039/b303808b

Sharma, A., Mathur, R., & Dixit, V. P. (1995). Prevention of hypercholesterolemia and atherosclerosis in rabbits after supplementation of *Myristica fragrans* seed extract. *Indian Journal of Physiology and Pharmacology*, *39*, 407–410. PMID:8582756

Sharma, G., Sharma, A. R., Kurian, M., Bhavesh, R., Nam, J. S., & Lee, S. S. (2014). Green synthesis of silver nanoparticle using myristica fragrans (nutmeg) seed extract and its biological activity. *Digest Journal of Nanomaterials and Biostructures*, *9*(1).

Sharma, N., Sharma, P., Jasuja, N. D., & Joshi, C. (2013). Hypocholesterolemic and Antioxidant Potentials of Some plants and herbs: A review. *Journal of Zoological Sciences, RRJZS*, *1*(2), 26–42.

Sharma, N., Tiwari, R., & Srivastava, M. P. (2013). Zingiberofficinale Roscoe. Oil: A preservative of stored commodities against storage Mycoflora. *International Journal of Current Microbiology and Applied Sciences*, *2*, 123–134.

Sharma, P. K., Singh, V., & Ali, M. (2016). Chemical composition and antimicrobial activity of fresh rhizome essential oil of Zingiber officinale Roscoe. *Pharmacognosy Journal*, *8*(3), 185–190. doi:10.5530/pj.2016.3.3

Sharma, R. D., Raghuram, T. C., & Rao, N. S. (1990). Effect of fenugreek seeds on blood glucose and serum lipids in type I diabetes. *European Journal of Clinical Nutrition*, *44*(4), 301–306. PMID:2194788

Sharma, V. K., Yngard, R. A., & Lin, Y. (2009). Silver nanoparticles: Green synthesis and their antimicrobial activities. *Advances in Colloid and Interface Science*, *145*(1–2), 83–96. doi:10.1016/j.cis.2008.09.002 PMID:18945421

Sheela, C. G., Kumud, K., & Augusti, K. T. (1995). Antidiabetic effect of onion and garlic sulfoxide amino acids in rats. *Planta Medica*, *61*(04), 356–357. doi:10.1055-2006-958099 PMID:7480182

Shelef, L. A. (2003). Herbs: Herbs of the Umbelliferae. In *Encyclopedia of Food Sciences and Nutrition*. Retrieved from https://www.sciencedirect.com/topics/agricultural-and-biological-sciences/coriandrum-sativum

Sheng, L., & Zhu, M. J. (2014). Inhibitory effect of Cinnamomum cassia oil on non-O157 Shiga toxin-producing Escherichia coli. *Food Control*, *46*, 374–381. doi:10.1016/j.foodcont.2014.05.050

Shevchenko, E. V., Talapin, D. V., Kotov, N. A., O'Brien, S., & Murray, C. B. (2006). Structural diversity in binary nanoparticle superlattices. *Nature*, *439*(7072), 55–59. doi:10.1038/nature04414 PMID:16397494

Shin, D. Y., Kim, G. Y., Li, W., Choi, B. T., Kim, N. D., Kang, H. S., & Choi, Y. H. (2009). Implication of intracellular ROS formation, caspase-3 activation and Egr-1 induction in platycodon D-induced apoptosis of U937 human leukemia cells. *Biomedicine and Pharmacotherapy*, *63*(2), 86–94. doi:10.1016/j.biopha.2008.08.001 PMID:18804340

Shishu, N. A. (2011). A Review of Recent Investigations on Medicinal Herbs Possessing Anti-Diabetic Properties. *Journal of Nutritional Disorders & Therapy*, *1*(102), 2.

Shobana, S., & Naidu, K. A. (2000). Antioxidant activity of selected Indian spices. *Prostaglandins, Leukotrienes, and Essential Fatty Acids*, *62*(2), 107–110. doi:10.1054/plef.1999.0128 PubMed

Shokoohinia, Y., Yegdaneh, A., Amin, G., & Ghannadi, A. (2014). Seasonal variations of Laurus nobilis L. leaves volatile oil components in Isfahan, Iran. *Research Journal of Pharmacognosy*, *1*(3), 1–6.

Shukla, Y., & Singh, M. (2007). Cancer preventive properties of ginger: A brief review. *Food and Chemical Toxicology*, *45*(5), 683–690. doi:10.1016/j.fct.2006.11.002 PubMed

Siddiqui, M. J., Saleh, M. S., Basharuddin, S. N. B., Zamri, S. H. B., Mohd Najib, M. H., Che Ibrahim, M. Z., ... Khatib, A. (2018). Saffron (Crocus sativus L.): As an antidepressant. *Journal of Pharmacy & Bioallied Sciences*, *10*(4), 173. doi:10.4103/JPBS.JPBS_83_18 PMID:30568374

Sigiura, M., Saito, H., & Abe, K. (1995). Ethanol extract of Crocus sativus L.antagonizes the inhibitory action of ethanol on hippocampal long-term potentiation in vivo. *Phytotherapy Research*, *9*(2), 100–104. doi:10.1002/ptr.2650090204

Silalahi, J. (2002). Anticancer and health protective properties of citrus fruit components. *Asia Pacific Journal of Clinical Nutrition*, *11*(1), 79–84. doi:10.1046/j.1440-6047.2002.00271.x PMID:11890643

Singh, R. H., Sankat, C. K., & Mujaffar. (2003). *The nutmeg and spice industry in grenada: innovations and competitiveness- A Case Study*. Workshop on the Role of Science, Technology and Innovation in Increasing Competitiveness in the Productive Sector, Organized by The Office of Science and Technology (OS&T) of the Organization of American States (OAS) and the Secretariat of Science, Technology and Productive Innovation (SeCYT).

Singh, A. K., Talat, M., Singh, D. P., & Srivastava, O. N. (2010). Biosynthesis of gold and silver nanoparticles by natural precursor clove and their functionalization with amine group. *Journal of Nanoparticle Research*, *12*(5), 1667–1675. doi:10.100711051-009-9835-3

Singh, D., Rathod, V., Ninganagouda, S., Herimath, J., & Kulkarni, P. (2013). Biosynthesis of silver nanoparticle by endophytic fungi Pencillium sp. isolated from Curcuma longa (turmeric) and its antibacterial activity against pathogenic gram negative bacteria. *Journal of Pharmacy Research*, *7*(5), 448–453. doi:10.1016/j.jopr.2013.06.003

Singh, G., & Baswana, K. S. (1984). Screening of coriander germplasm against chalcid fly (*Systole albipennis*). *Ann. Appl. Biol. Supplement: Tests of Agrochemicals and Cultivars.*, *104*(5), 114–115.

Singh, G., Kapoor, I. P. S., Pandey, S. K., Singh, U. K., & Singh, R. K. (2002). Studies on essential oils: Part 10; antibacterial activity of volatile oils of some spices. *Phytotherapy Research*, *16*(7), 680–682. doi:10.1002/ptr.951 PMID:12410554

Singh, G., Kapoor, I. P. S., Singh, P., De Heluani, C. S., De Lampasona, M. P., & Catalan, C. A. N. (2008). Chemistry, antioxidant and antimicrobial investigations on essential oil and oleoresins of Zingiber officinale. *Food and Chemical Toxicology*, *46*(10), 3295–3302. doi:10.1016/j.fct.2008.07.017 PubMed

Singh, G., Maurya, S., & Catalan, C. A. (2007). A comparison of chemical, antioxidant and antimicrobial studies of cinnamon leaf and bark volatile oils, oleoresins and their constituents. *Food and Chemical Toxicology*, *45*(9), 1650–1661. doi:10.1016/j.fct.2007.02.031 PMID:17408833

Singh, G., Maurya, S., De Lampasona, M. P., & Catalan, C. A. N. (2006). Studies on the essential oils part41: Chemical composition, antifungal, antioxidant, and sprout suppressant activities of coriander (Coriandrum sativum L.) essential oil and its oleoresin. *Flavour and Fragrance Journal*, *21*(3), 472–479. doi:10.1002/ffj.1608

Singh, G., Maurya, S., Marimuthu, P., Murali, H. S., & Bawa, A. S. (2007). Antioxidant and Antibacterial investigations on essential oils and acetone extracts of some spices. *Journal of Natural Product Radiance*, *6*(2), 114–121.

Singh, M. P., & Panda, H. (2005). *Medicinal herbs with their formulations*. New Delhi: Daya Publishing House.

Singh, R. B., Gupta, D., Kumar, S., Singh, K., & Tiwari, C. (2018). Buchanania lanzan spreng (Chironji): A vulnerable multipurpose tree species in Vindhyam region. *Journal of Pharmacognosy and Phytochemistry*, *7*(5), 833–836.

Singh, R. P., Magesh, S., & Rakkiyappan, C. (2011). Formation of fenugreek (Trigonella foenum-graecum) extract mediated Ag nanoparticles: Mechanism and applications. *Int J Bioeng Sci Technol*, *2*(3), 64–73.

Singh, R., Singh, N., Saini, B. S., & Rao, H. S. (2008). In vitro antioxidant activity of pet ether extract of black pepper. *International Journal of Pharmacology*, *40*, 147–151. PMID:20040947

Singh, R., Singh, S., Parihar, P., Mishra, R. K., Tripathi, D. K., Singh, V. P., ... Prasad, S. M. (2016). Reactive Oxygen Species (ROS): Beneficial Companions of Plants' Developmental Processes. *Front Plant Sci*, *7*, 1299. doi:10.3389/fpls.2016.01299 PMID:27729914

Singh, S. C., Zeng, H. B., Guo, C., & Cai, W. (Eds.). (2012). *Nanomaterials: processing and characterization with lasers*. John Wiley & Sons. doi:10.1002/9783527646821

Singh, Y. N. (1986). Traditional medicine in Fiji: Some herbal folk cures used by Fiji Indians. *Journal of Ethnopharmacology*, *15*(1), 57–88. doi:10.1016/0378-8741(86)90104-2 PMID:3713228

Sinha, R., Rauniar, G. P., & Panday, D. R. (2015). Fenugreek: Pharmacological actions. *World Journal of Pharmacy and Pharmaceutical Sciences*, *5*(1), 1481–1489.

Slim, H. B., Black, H. R., & Thompson, P. D. (2011). Older bloodpressure medications-do they still have a place? *The American Journal of Cardiology*, *108*(2), 308–316. doi:10.1016/j.amjcard.2011.03.041 PMID:21550576

Smith, C., Crowther, C., Willson, K., Hotham, N., & McMillian, V. (2004). A randomized controlled trial of ginger to treat nausea and vomiting in pregnancy. *Obstetrics and Gynecology*, *103*(4), 639–645. doi:10.1097/01.AOG.0000118307.19798.ec PMID:15051552

Snitker, S., Fujishima, Y., Shen, H., Ott, S., Pi-Sunyer, X., Furuhata, Y., ... Takahashi, M. (2009). Effects of novel capsinoid treatment on fatness and energy metabolism in humans: Possible pharmacogenetic implications. *The American Journal of Clinical Nutrition*, *89*(1), 45–50. doi:10.3945/ajcn.2008.26561 PMID:19056576

Sofowora, A. (1982). *Medicinal plant and traditional medicine in Africa*. New York: John Wiley and Sons.

Sogara, P. P. U. (2014). Pengaruh ekstrak etanol buah ketumbar (coriandrum sativum l.) Terhadap penurunan kadar gula darah tikus putih yang diinduksi aloksan. *Pharmacon, 3*(3).

Somani, R. S., & Singhai, A. K. (2008). Hypoglycemic and antidiabetic activities of seeds of Myristica fragrans in normoglycemic and alloxan-induced diabetic rats. *Asian Journal of Experimental Sciences*, *22*, 95–102.

Song, F., Li, H., Sun, J., & Wang, S. (2013). Protective effects of cinnamic acid and cinnamic aldehyde on isoproterenol-induced acute myocardial ischemia in rats. *Journal of Ethnopharmacology*, *150*(1), 125–130. doi:10.1016/j.jep.2013.08.019 PMID:24001892

Song, J. Y., Jang, H. K., & Kim, B. S. (2009). Biological synthesis of gold nanoparticles using Magnolia kobus and Diopyros kaki leaf extracts. *Process Biochemistry*, *44*(10), 1133–1138. doi:10.1016/j.procbio.2009.06.005

Soshnikova, V., Kim, Y. J., Singh, P., Huo, Y., Markus, J., Ahn, S., ... Yang, D. C. (2017). Cardamom fruits as a green resource for facile synthesis of gold and silver nanoparticles and their biological applications. *Artificial Cells, Nanomedicine, and Biotechnology*, *46*(1), 108–117. doi:10.1080/21691401.2017.1296849 PMID:28290213

Soureshjan, E. H., & Heidari, M. (2014). In vitro variation in antibacterial activity plant extracts on Glaucium elegansand saffron (Crocus sativus). *Bangladesh Journal of Pharmacology*, *9*, 275–278.

Sowmya, P., & Rajyalakshmi, P. (1999). Hypocholesterolemic effect of germinated fenugreek seeds in human subjects. *Plant Foods for Human Nutrition (Dordrecht, Netherlands)*, *4*(4), 359–365. doi:10.1023/A:1008021618733 PMID:10540988

Spiller, F., Alves, M. K., Vieira, S. M., Carvalho, T. A., Leite, C. E., Lunardelli, A., ... de Oliviera, J. R. (2008). Anti-inflammatory effects of red pepper (Capsicum baccatum) on carrageenan- and antigen-induced inflammation. *The Journal of Pharmacy and Pharmacology*, *60*, 473–478.

Sreejayan, N., & Rao, M. N. A. (1994). Curcuminoids as potent inhibitors of lipid peroxidation. *The Journal of Pharmacy and Pharmacology*, *46*(12), 1013–1016. doi:10.1111/j.2042-7158.1994.tb03258.x PMID:7714712

Srichamroen, A., Field, C. J., Thomson, A. B., & Basu, T. K. (2008). The Modifying Effects of Galactomannan from Canadian-Grown Fenugreek (*Trigonella foenum-graecum L.*) on the Glycemic and Lipidemic Status in Rats. *Journal of Clinical Biochemistry and Nutrition*, *43*(3), 167–174. doi:10.3164/jcbn.2008060 PMID:19015751

Srinivasan, K. (2005). Role of Spices Beyond Food Flavoring: Nutraceuticals with Multiple Health Effects. *Food Reviews International*, *21*(2), 167–188. doi:10.1081/FRI-200051872

Srinivasan, K. (2005). Spices as influencers of body metabolism: An overview of three decades of research. *Food Research International*, *38*(1), 77–86. doi:10.1016/j.foodres.2004.09.001

Srinivasan, K. (2006). Fenugreek (*Trigonellafoenumgraecum* L.): A review of health beneficial physiological effects. *Food Reviews International*, *2*, 2013–2224.

Srinivasan, K. (2007). Black Pepper and its Pungent Principle-Piperine: A Review of Diverse Physiological Effects. *Critical Reviews in Food Science and Nutrition*, *47*(8), 735–748. doi:10.1080/10408390601062054 PMID:17987447

Srinivasan, K. (2014). Antioxidant potential of spices and their active constituents. *Critical Reviews in Food Science and Nutrition*, *54*(3), 352–372. doi:10.1080/10408398.2011.585525 PMID:24188307

Srivastava, G., & Mehta, J. L. (2009). Currying the Heart: Curcumin and Cardioprotection. *Journal of Cardiovascular Pharmacology and Therapeutics*, *14*(1), 22–27. doi:10.1177/1074248408329608 PMID:19153099

Srivastava, K. C., & Mustafa, T. (1989). Spices: Antiplatelet activity and prostanoid metabolism. *Prostaglandins, Leukotrienes, and Essential Fatty Acids*, *38*(4), 255–266. doi:10.1016/0952-3278(89)90129-4 PubMed

Srivastava, R., Ahmed, H., Dixit, R. K., Dharamveer, & Saraf, S. A. (2010). Crocus sativus L: A comprehensive review. *Pharmacognosy Reviews*, *4*(8), 200. doi:10.4103/0973-7847.70919 PMID:22228962

Stangl, V., Lorenz, M., & Stangl, K. (2006). The role of tea and tea flavonoids in cardiovascular health. *Molecular Nutrition & Food Research*, *50*(2), 218–228. doi:10.1002/mnfr.200500118 PMID:16404706

Stein, U., Greyer, H., & Hentschel, H. (2001). Nutmeg (myristicin) poisoning— Report on a fatal case and a series of cases recorded by a poison information centre. *Forensic Science International*, *118*(1), 87–90. doi:10.1016/S0379-0738(00)00369-8 PMID:11343860

Stoilova, I., Krastanv, A., Stoyanova, A., Denev, P., & Gargova, S. (2007). Antioxidant activity of a ginger extract (Zingiber officinale). *Food Chemistry*, *102*(3), 764–770. doi:10.1016/j.foodchem.2006.06.023

Stokes, D. (2008). *Principles and practice of variable pressure/environmental scanning electron microscopy (VP-ESEM)*. John Wiley & Sons. doi:10.1002/9780470758731

Stoyanova, A., Konakchiev, A., Damyanova, S., Stoilova, I., & Suu, P. T. (2006). Composition and antimicrobial activity of ginger essential oil from Vietnam. *Journal of Essential Oil-Bearing Plants*, *9*(1), 93–98. doi:10.1080/0972060X.2006.10643478

Subash Babu, P., Prabuseenivasan, S., & Ignacimuthu, S. (2007). Cinnamaldehyde--a potential antidiabetic agent. *Phytomedicine*, *14*(1), 15–22. doi:10.1016/j.phymed.2006.11.005 PMID:17140783

Subhankari, I., & Nayak, P. L. (2013). Antimicrobial Activity of Copper Nanoparticles Synthesised by Ginger (Zingiber officinale) Extract. *World Journal of Nano Science & Technology*, *2*(1), 10–13. doi:10.5829/idosi.wjnst.2013.2.1.21133

Subramoniam. (2016). *Plants with Anti-Diabetes Mellitus Properties*. . doi:10.1201/978131537148

Sultanbawa, Y., & Sultanbawa, F. (2016). *Australian Native Plants: Cultivation and Uses in the Health and Food Industries*. CRC Press.

Sultan, M., Bhatti, H. N., & Iqbal, Z. (2005). Chemical analysis of essential oil of ginger (Zingiber officinale). *Pakistan Journal of Biological Sciences*, *8*(11), 1576–1578. doi:10.3923/pjbs.2005.1576.1578

Suresh, K. G., Shetty, A. K., & Salimath, P. V. (2005). Modulatory effect of fenugreek seed mucilage and spent turmeric on intestinal and renal disaccharidases in streptozotocin induced diabetic rats. *Plant Foods for Human Nutrition (Dordrecht, Netherlands)*, *60*(2), 87–91. doi:10.100711130-005-5104-5 PMID:16021836

Sureshkumar, D., Begum, S., Johannah, N. M., Maliakel, B., & Krishnakumar, I. M. (2018). Toxicological evaluation of a saponin-rich standardized extract of fenugreek seeds (FenuSMART): Acute, sub-chronic and genotoxicity studies. *Toxicology Reports*, *5*, 1060–1068. doi:10.1016/j.toxrep.2018.10.008 PMID:30416976

Surh, Y. J., Park, K. K., Chun, K. S., Lee, L. J., Lee, E., & Lee, S. S. (1999). Anti-tumor-promoting activities of selected pungent phenolic substances present in ginger. *Journal of Environmental Pathology, Toxicology and Oncology*, *18*, 131–139. PubMed

Sushma, N., Smitha, P. V., Gopal, Y. V., Vinay, R., Reddy, N. S., Mohan, M., & Raju, B. (2013). Antidiabetic, antihyperlipidaemic, antioxidant activities of Buchanania lanzan Spreng methanol leaf extract in streptozotocin induced Types I & II diabetic rats. *Tropical Journal of Pharmaceutical Research*, *12*(2), 221–226.

Švarc-Gajić, J., Cvetanović, A., Segura-Carretero, A., Linares, I. B., & Maškovic, P. (2017). Characterization of ginger extracts obtained by subcritical water. *The Journal of Supercritical Fluids*, *123*, 92–100. doi:10.1016/j.supflu.2016.12.019

Tahiliani, P., & Kar, A. (2003). Mitigation of thyroxine induced hyperglycaemia by two plant extracts. *Phytotherapy Research*, *17*(3), 294–296. doi:10.1002/ptr.1121 PMID:12672166

Tahir, A. A., Abdul Sani, N. F., Morad, N. A., Makpol, S., Ngah, W. Z., & Yusof, Y. A. (2015). Combined ginger extract and gelam honey modulate Ras/ERK and P13/AKT pathway genes in colon cancer HT29 cells. *Nutrition Journal*, *14*(1), 31. doi:10.1186/s12937-015-0015-2 PubMed

Tamaddonfard, E., Farshid, A. A., Eghdami, K., Samadi, F., & Erfanparast, A. (2013). Comparison of the effects of crocin, safranal and diclofenac on local inflammation andinflammatory pain responses induced by carrageenan in rats. *Pharmacological Reports*, *65*(5), 1272–1280. doi:10.1016/S1734-1140(13)71485-3 PMID:24399723

Tanwar, V., Sachdeva, J., Golechha, M., Kumari, S., & Arya, D. S. (2010). Curcumin protects rat myocardium against isoproterenol-induced ischemic injury: Attenuation of ventricular dysfunction through increased expression of hsp27alongwith strengthening antioxidant defense system. *Journal of Cardiovascular Pharmacology*, *55*(4), 377–384. doi:10.1097/FJC.0b013e3181d3da01 PMID:20125031

Tapsell, L. C., Hemphill, I., Cobiac, L., Patch, C. S., Sullivan, D. R., Fenech, M., ... Inge, K. (2006). Health benefits of herbs and spices: The past, the present, the future. *The Medical Journal of Australia*, *185*(S4), S1–S24. doi:10.5694/j.1326-5377.2006.tb00548.x PMID:17022438

Tayoub, G., Odeh, A., & Ghanem, I. (2014). Chemical composition and fumigation toxicity of Laurus nobilis L. and Salvia officinalis L. Essential oils on larvae of khapra beetle (Trogoderma granarium Everts). *Herba Polonica*, *58*(2), 26–37.

Tchombé, N. L., Louajri, A., & Benajiba, M. H. (2012). Therapeutic effects of ginger (Zingiber officinale). *ISESCO Journal of Science and Technology*, *8*, 64–69.

Thanekar, D., Dhodi, J., & Juvekar, A. (2013). Evaluation of in vitro cytotoxic activity of petroleum ether, methanol and aqueous extracts of Indian bay leaf, Cinnamomum tamala (Buch. -ham) T. Nees and eberm on cancer cells. *World Journal of Pharmacy and Pharmaceutical Sciences*, *3*(1), 519–533.

Thatte, U. M., & Dahanukar, S. A. (1986). Ayurveda and contemporary scientific thought. *Trends in Pharmacological Sciences*, *7*, 247–251. doi:10.1016/0165-6147(86)90336-6

The Chemistry of Coriander. (2014). Retrieved from https://www.compoundchem.com

The Columbia Encyclopedia. (2001-2005). (6th ed.). New York: Columbia University Press.

The wealth of India: A dictionary of Indian raw materials and industrial products. (2000). New Delhi: National Institute of Science Communication.

Thirumalai, T., Therasa, S. V., Elumalai, E., & David, E. (2011). Hypoglycemic effect of Brassica juncea (seeds) on streptozotocin induced diabetic male albino rat. *Asian Pacific Journal of Tropical Biomedicine*, *1*(4), 323–325. doi:10.1016/S2221-1691(11)60052-X PMID:23569784

Thirumurugan, A., Jiflin, G. J., Rajagomathi, G., Tomy, N. A., Ramachandran, S., & Jaiganesh, R. (2010). Biotechnological synthesis of gold nanoparticles of Azadirachta indica leaf extract. *Internat J Biol Technol*, *1*, 75–77.

Thiyagrajan, M., & Sharma, S. S. (2004, January 9). Neuroprotective effect of curcumin in middle cerebral artery occlusion induced focal cerebral ischemia in rats. *Life Sciences*, *74*(8), 969–985. doi:10.1016/j.lfs.2003.06.042 PMID:14672754

Thomas, R., Nair, A. P., Soumya, K. R., Mathew, J., & Radhakrishnan, E. K. (2014). Antibacterial activity and synergistic effect of biosynthesized AgNPs with antibiotics against multidrug-resistant biofilm-forming coagulase-negative staphylococci isolated from clinical samples. *Applied Biochemistry and Biotechnology*, *173*(2), 449–460. doi:10.100712010-014-0852-z PMID:24699812

Thomson, M., Al-Qattan, K. K., Al-Sawan, S. M., Alnaqeeb, M. A., Khan, I., & Ali, M. (2002). The use of ginger (Zingiber officinale Rosc.) as a potential anti-inflammatory and antithrombotic agent. *Prostaglandins, Leukotrienes, and Essential Fatty Acids*, *67*(6), 475–478. doi:10.1054/plef.2002.0441 PubMed

Thongson, C., Davidson, P. M., Mahakarnchanakul, W., & Vibulsresth, P. (2005). Antimicrobial effect of Thai spices against Listeria monocytogenes and Salmonella Typhimurium DT104. *Journal of Food Protection*, *68*(10), 2054–2058. doi:10.4315/0362-028X-68.10.2054 PubMed

Toader, O. R. (2014). Study of the effects of Zingiber officinale (ginger) on spermatogenesis in mice. *Annals of West University of Timisoara. Series of Biology*, *17*, 145–152.

Toben,, H.M., Meierzu, H., Beerentrup, K., Rudolph, H., &von der Schulenburg, G. (1994). Koriander als Petroselinsäurelieferant für die industrielle Verwendung. Stand der Züchtung und Bekämpfungsmöglichkeiten der „Bakteriellen Doldenwelke". Vortr. *Pflanzenzücht.*, *30*, 173–183.

Toben, H. M. (1995). *Die durch Pseudomonas syringae pv. coriandricola hervorgerufene Doldenwelke an Koriander, Charakterisierung des Erregers und Strategien zur Bekämpfung*. Göttingen: Cuvillier Verlag.

Toda, S., Miyase, T., & Arich, H. (1985). Natural Antioxidants. III. Antioxidative components isolated from rhizomes of Curcuma longa L. *Chemical & Pharmaceutical Bulletin*, *33*(4), 1725–1728. doi:10.1248/cpb.33.1725 PMID:4042250

Townsend, E. A., Siviski, M. E., Zhang, Y., Xu, C., Hoonjan, B., & Emala, C. W. (2013). Effects of ginger and its constituents on airway smooth muscle relaxation and calcium regulation. *American Journal of Respiratory Cell and Molecular Biology*, *48*(2), 157–163. doi:10.1165/rcmb.2012-0231OC PubMed

Trease, G. E., & Evans, M. C. (2002). Textbook of Pharmacognosy (15th ed.). London: Academic Press.

Trease, G. E., & Evans, W. C. (1989). *Pharmacognosy* (13th ed.). Bailliere Tindall Ltd.

Tung, Y.-T., Chua, M.-T., Wang, S.-Y., & Chang, S.-T. (2008). Anti-inflammation activities of essential oil and its constituents from indigenous cinnamon (*Cinnamomum osmophloeum*) twigs. *Bioresource Technology*, *99*(9), 3908–3913. doi:10.1016/j.biortech.2007.07.050 PMID:17826984

Tzeng, T. F., & Liu, I. M. (2013). 6-Gingerol prevents adipogenesis and the accumulation of cytoplasmic lipid droplets in 3T3-L1 cells. *Phytomedicine*, *20*(6), 481–487. doi:10.1016/j.phymed.2012.12.006 PubMed

Tzitzios, V., Basina, G., Gjoka, M., Alexandrakis, V., Georgakilas, V., Niarchos, D., ... Petridis, D. (2006). Chemical synthesis and characterization of hcp Ni nanoparticles. *Nanotechnology*, *17*(15), 3750–3755. doi:10.1088/0957-4484/17/15/023

Uhl. (2000). Effects of mustard sprouts and allylisothiocyanate. *Ensuring global food safety. Exploring global harmonization.*

Uma, B., Prabhakar, K., Rajendran, S., Sarayu, Y., & Lakshmi. (2009). Antimicrobial activity and phytochemical analysis of *Coriander sativum* against infectious diarrhoea. *Ethnobotanical Leaflets*, 5.

USDA/ERS. (2011). Food availability (Per Capita) Data System. *United States Department of Agriculture Economic Research Service*. Available at: http://www.ers.usda.gov/Data/ FoodConsumption/

USDA-ARS. (2009). Germplasm Resources Information Network (GRIN). Online Database. Beltsville, MD: National Germplasm Resources Laboratory. https://npgsweb.ars-grin.gov/gringlobal/taxon/taxonomysearch.aspx

Vahidi, H., Kamalinejad, M., & Sedaghati, N. (2002). Antimicrobial Properties of Crocus sativus L. *Iranian Journal of Pharmaceutical Research*, *1*, 33–35.

Vajragupta, O., Boonchoong, P., Watanabe, H., Tohda, M., Kummasud, N., & Sumanont, Y. (2003). Manganese complexes of curcumin and its derivatives: Evaluation for the radical scavenging ability and neuroprotective activity. *Free Radical Biology & Medicine*, *35*(12), 1632–1644. doi:10.1016/j.freeradbiomed.2003.09.011 PMID:14680686

Valle Garcia-Rodriguez, M., Serrano-Diaz, J., Tarantilis, P. A., López-Córcoles, H., Carmona, M., & Alonso, G. L. (2014). Determination of saffron quality by high-performance liquid chromatography. *Journal of Agricultural and Food Chemistry*, *62*(32), 8068–8074. doi:10.1021/jf5019356 PMID:25075549

Vangalapati, M., Satya, N. S., Prakash, S. D. V., & Avanigadda, S. (2012). A review on pharmacological activities and clinical effects of cinnamon species. *Research Journal of Pharmaceutical, Biological and Chemical Sciences*, *3*(1), 653–663.

Vardapetyan, H., Tiratsuyan, S., & Hovhannisyan, A. (2014). Antioxidant and antibacterial activities of selected armenian medicinal plants. *Journal of Experimental Biology and Agricultural Sciences*, *2*(3), 300–330.

Varni, J. W., Bendo, C. B., Nurko, S., Shulman, R. J., Self, M. M., Franciosi, J. P., ... Pohl, J. F. (2015). Pediatric Quality of Life Inventory (PedsQL) Gastrointestinal Symptoms Module Testing Study Consortium Health-related quality of life in pediatric patients with functional and organic gastrointestinal diseases. *The Journal of Pediatrics*, *166*(1), 85–90. doi:10.1016/j.jpeds.2014.08.022 PMID:25241177

Vasala, P. A. (2004). Ginger. In K. V. Peter (Ed.), *Handbook of Herbs and Spices* (Vol. 1, pp. 195–206). Cambridge, UK: Woodhead.

Vasudevan, M., & Milind, P. (2009). Memory enhancing activity of Coriandrum sativum in rats. *Pharmacologyonline*, 2, 827–839.

Vekaria, R. H., Patel, M. N., Bhalodiya, P. N., Patel, V., Desai, T. R., & Tirgar, P. R. (2012). Evaluation of the neuroprotective effect of *Coriandrum sativum* Linn. against ischemic-reperfusion on insulin in the brain. *International Journal of Phytopharmacology*, *3*(2), 86–193.

Velaga, M. K., Yallapragada, P. R., Williams, D., Rajanna, S., & Bettaiya, R. (2014). Hydroalcoholic seed extract of *Coriandrum sativum* (coriander) alleviates lead-induced oxidative stress in different regions of rat brain. *Biological Trace Element Research*, *159*(1-3), 351–363. doi:10.100712011-014-9989-4

Velmurugan, P., Anbalagan, K., Manosathyadevan, M., Lee, K.-J., Cho, M., Lee, S.-M., ... Oh, B.-T. (2014). Green synthesis of silver and gold nanoparticles using Zingiber officinale root extract and antibacterial activity of silver nanoparticles against food pathogens. *Bioprocess and Biosystems Engineering*, *37*(10), 1935–1943. doi:10.100700449-014-1169-6 PMID:24668029

Verma, S. K., Singh, S. K., & Mathur, A. (2010). In vitro cytotoxicity of Calotropisprocera and *Trigonellafoenum-graecum* against human cancer cell lines. *Journal of Chemical and Pharmaceutical Research*, 2, 861–865.

Verma, V. C., Kharwar, R. N., & Gange, A. C. (2010). Biosynthesis of antimicrobial silver nanoparticles by the endophytic fungus Aspergillus clavatus. *Nanomedicine (London)*, *5*(1), 33–40. doi:10.2217/nnm.09.77 PMID:20025462

Vidal-Vidal, J., Rivas, J., & López-Quintela, M. A. (2006). Synthesis of monodisperse maghemite nanoparticles by the microemulsion method. *Colloids and Surfaces. A, Physicochemical and Engineering Aspects*, *288*(1-3), 44–51. doi:10.1016/j.colsurfa.2006.04.027

Vijayakumar, A., Duraipandiyan, V., Jeyaraj, B., Agastian, P., Raj, M. K., & Ignacimuthu, S. (2012). Phytochemical analysis and in vitro antimicrobial activity of Illicium griffithii Hook. f. & Thoms extracts. *Asian Pacific Journal of Tropical Disease*, *2*(3), 190–199. doi:10.1016/S2222-1808(12)60045-0

Vijayakumar, M. V., & Bhat, M. K. (2008). Hypoglycemic effect of a novel dialysed feungreek seeds extract is sustainable and is mediated, in part, by the activation of hepatic enzymes. *Phytotherapy Research*, *22*(4), 500–505. doi:10.1002/ptr.2351 PMID:18338783

Vijayakumar, R., Devi, V., Adavallan, K., & Saranya, D. (2011). Green synthesis and characterization of gold nanoparticles using extract of anti-tumor potent Crocus sativus. *Physica E, Low-Dimensional Systems and Nanostructures*, *44*(3), 665–671. doi:10.1016/j.physe.2011.11.002

Vijaykumar, M. V., Singh, S., & Chhipa, R. R. (2005). The hypoglycaemic activity of fenugreek seed extract is mediated through the stimulation of an insulin signaling pathway. *British Journal of Pharmacology*, *146*(1), 41–48. doi:10.1038j.bjp.0706312 PMID:15980869

Vilalta-Clemente, A., Gloystein, K., & Frangis, N. (2008). Principles of Atomic Force Microscopy (AFM). *Proceedings of Physics of Advanced Materials Winter School.*

Wahab, A., Ul Haq, R., Ahmed, A., Khan, R. A., & Raza, M. (2009). Anticonvulsant activities of nutmeg oil of *Myristica fragrans. Phytotherapy Research*, *23*(2), 153–158. doi:10.1002/ptr.2548 PMID:19067329

Waidha, A. I., Pandiyarasan, V., Anusya, T., Waidha, K. M., Shah, A. H., & Pandiyarasan, V. (2015). Synthesis and characterization of silver nano rod like structures by green synthesis method using Curcumin longa. *International Journal of Chemtech Research*, *7*, 1504–1508.

Walkey, C. D., Olsen, J. B., Guo, H., Emili, A., & Chan, W. C. (2012). Nanoparticle size and surface chemistry determine serum protein adsorption and macrophage uptake. *Journal of the American Chemical Society*, *134*(4), 2139–2147. doi:10.1021/ja2084338 PMID:22191645

Wang, C., Kim, Y. J., Singh, P., Mathiyalagan, R., Jin, Y., & Yang, D. C. (2016). Green synthesis of silver nanoparticles by Bacillus methylotrophicus, and their antimicrobial activity. *Artificial Cells, Nanomedicine, and Biotechnology*, *44*(4), 1127–1132. PMID:25749281

Wang, S. L., Li, Y., Wen, Y., Chen, Y. F., Na, L. X., Li, S. T., & Sun, C. H. (2009). Curcumin, a potential inhibitor of up-regulation of TNF-alpha and IL-6 induced by palmitate in 3T3-L1 adipocytes through NF-kappaB and JNK pathway. *Biomedical and Environmental Sciences*, *22*(1), 32–39. doi:10.1016/S0895-3988(09)60019-2 PMID:19462685

Warokar, A. S., Ghante, M. H., Duragkar, N. J., & Bhusari, K. P. (2010). Anti-inflammatory and antioxidant activities of methanolic extract of Buchananialanzan Kernel. *Indian Journal of Pharmaceutical Education*, *44*(4), 363–368.

Wei1a, L., Hua, R., Lilc, M., Huan, Y., Lile, S., He1f, Y., & Shen, Z. (2014). Chemical composition and biological activity of star anise *Illiciumverum*extracts against maize weevil, *Sitophilus zeamais*adults. *Journal of Insect Science*, *14*.

Wei, D., Sun, W., Qian, W., Ye, Y., & Ma, X. (2009). The synthesis of chitosan-based silver nanoparticles and their antibacterial activity. *Carbohydrate Research*, *344*(17), 2375–2382. doi:10.1016/j.carres.2009.09.001 PMID:19800053

Wei, Q. Y., Ma, J. P., Cai, Y. J., Yang, L., & Liu, Z. L. (2005). Cytotoxic and apoptotic activities of diarylheptanoids and gingerol-related compounds from the rhizome of Chinese ginger. *Journal of Ethnopharmacology*, *102*(2), 177–184. doi:10.1016/j.jep.2005.05.043 PubMed

WHO. (1991). *Traditional medicine and modern health care: progress report by the director general document A 44(10)*. World Health Organization.

WHO. (2001). *The World health report: Mental health: new understanding*. Geneva: New Hope.

Wikipedia. (2009). *Mustard seed.* Available http://en.wikipedia.org/wiki/mustard_seed

Willatgamuva, S. A., Platel, K., Sarawathi, G., & Srinivasan, K. (1998). Antidiabetic influence of dietary cumin seeds (Cuminumcyminum) in streptozotocin induced diabetic rats. *Nutrition Research (New York, N.Y.)*, *18*(1), 131–142. doi:10.1016/S0271-5317(97)00207-8

Williams, S. R. (1973). *Nutrition and diet therapy*. Jones & Bartlett Publishers.

Wisam, J. A., & Haneen, A. J. (2018). A novel study of pH influence on Ag nanoparticles size with antibacterial and antifungal activity using green synthesis. *World Scientific News*, *97*, 139–152.

Wohlmuth, H., Leach, D. N., Smith, M. K., & Myers, S. P. (2005). Gingerol content of diploid and tetraploid clones of ginger (Zingiber officinale Roscoe). *Journal of Agricultural and Food Chemistry*, *53*(14), 5772–5778. doi:10.1021/jf050435b PubMed

Wong, Y. C., Ahmad-Mudzaqqirand, M. Y., & Wan-Nurdiyana, W. A. (2014). Extraction of Essential Oil from Cinnamon (*Cinnamomum zeylanicum*). *Oriental Journal of Chemistry*, *30*(1), 37–47. doi:10.13005/ojc/300105

World Health Organization. (2016). *Global report on diabetes*. World Health Organization.

Xiao, H., Yang, C. S., Li, S., Jin, H., Ho, C. T., & Patel, T. (2009). Monodemethylatedpolymethoxyflavones from sweet orange (Citrus sinensis) peel inhibit growth of human lung cancer cells by apoptosis. *Molecular Nutrition & Food Research*, *53*(3), 398–406. doi:10.1002/mnfr.200800057 PMID:19065586

Xie, J. T., Chang, W. T., Wang, C. Z., Mehendale, S. R., Li, J., Ambihaipahar, R., & Yuan, C. S. (2006). Curry leaf (MurrayakoenigiiSpreng.) reduces blood cholesterol and glucose levels in ob/ob mice. *The American Journal of Chinese Medicine*, *34*(02), 279–284. doi:10.1142/S0192415X06003825 PMID:16552838

Yadav, R., Kaushik, R., & Gupta, D. (2011). The health benefits of *Trigonellafoenum- graecum*: A review. *Int. J. Engineering Research and Applications*, *1*(1), 32-35.

Yadava, D. K., Giri, S. C., Vignesh, M., Vasudev, S., Yadav, A. K., Dass, B., ... Prabhu, K. V. (2011). Genetic variability and trait association studies in Indian mustard (Brassica juncea). *Indian Journal of Agricultural Sciences*, *81*(8), 712–716.

Yadav, S. K., Yadava, D. K., Vasudev, S., Yadav, S., Kumar, P. R., & Nigam, R. (2013). Assessment of seed quality and oil content in different branches of Indian mustard (Brassica juncea) cultivars at different storage intervals. *Indian Journal of Agricultural Sciences*, *83*(2), 227–233.

Yadav, S., Sharma, P. K., & Alam, M. A. (2016). Ginger medicinal uses and benefits. *European Journal Pharmaceutical and Medical Research*, *3*, 127–135.

Yamada, K., Takada, S., Nakamura, S., & Hirata, S. (1965). The structure of noranisatin, an oxidation product of anisatin. *Tetrahedron Letters*, *52*(52), 4785–4794. doi:10.1016/S0040-4039(01)89035-3

Yamamoto-Ribeiro, M. M. G., Grespan, R., Kohiyama, C. Y., Dias, F., Galerani, S. A., Leite, E., ... Machinski, M. (2013). Effect of Zingiber officinale essential oil on Fusarium verticillioides and Fumonisin production. *Food Chemistry*, *141*(3), 3147–3152. doi:10.1016/j.foodchem.2013.05.144 PubMed

Yang, C. H., Chang, F. R., Chang, H. W., Wang, S. M., Hsieh, M. C., & Chuang, L. Y. (2011). Investigation of the anti-oxidant activity of *Illiciumverum* extracts. *Journal of Medicinal Plants Research*, *6*(2), 314–324.

Yang, J.-F., Yang, C.-H., Chang, H.-W., Yang, C.-S., Wang, S.-M., Hsieh, M.-C., & Chuang, L.-Y. (2010). Chemical Composition and Antibacterial Activities of Illicium verum Against Antibiotic-Resistant Pathogens. *Journal of Medicinal Food*, *13*(5), 1254–1262. doi:10.1089/jmf.2010.1086 PMID:20828316

Yang, X. W., Huang, X., & Ahmat, M. (2008). New neolignan from the seed of *Myristica fragrans*. *Zhongguo Zhongyao Zazhi*, *33*, 397–402. PMID:18533495

Yan, J. H., Xiao, X. X., & Huang, K. L. (2002). Component analysis of volatile oil from Illicium Verum Hook. f. *Journal of Central South University of Technology*, *9*(3), 173–176. doi:10.100711771-002-0021-3

Yan, Y.-M., Fang, P., Yang, M.-T., Li, N., Lu, Q., & Cheng, Y.-X. (2015). Anti-Diabetic Nephropathy Compounds from Cinnamomum Cassia. *Journal of Ethnopharmacology*, *165*, 141–147. doi:10.1016/j.jep.2015.01.049 PMID:25725434

Yazdani, D., Rezazadeh, S., Amin, G., Zainal Abidin, M.A., Shahnazi, S., & Jamalifar, H. (2009). Antifungal Activity of Dried Extracts of Anise (*PimpinellaanisumL.*) and Star anise (*IlliciumverumHook.* f.) Against Dermatophyte and Saprophyte Fungi. *Journal of Medicinal Plans*, *8*(S5).

Yeh, G. Y., Eisenberg, D. M., Kaptchuk, T. M., & Phillips, R. S. (2003). Systematic review of herbs and dietary supplements for glycemic control in diabetes. *Diabetes Care*, *26*(4), 1277–1294. doi:10.2337/diacare.26.4.1277 PMID:12663610

Yeh, H. F., Luo, C. Y., Lin, C. Y., Cheng, S. S., Hsu, Y. R., & Chang, S. T. (2013). Methods for thermal stability enhancement of leaf essential oils and their main constituents from indigenous cinnamon (*Cinnamomumosmophloeum*). *Journal of Agricultural and Food Chemistry*, *61*(26), 6293–6298. doi:10.1021/jf401536y PMID:23738884

Yiming, Li., Tran, V. H., Duke, C. C., & Roufogalis, B. D. (2012). Preventive and protective properties of Zingiberofficinale (ginger) in diabetes mellitus, diabetic complications, and associated lipid and other metabolic disorders: A brief review. *Evidence-Based Complementary and Alternative Medicine*.

Yoo, M. J., Kim, Y. S., & Shin, D. H. (2006). Antibacterial effects of natural essential oils from ginger and mustard against Vibrio species inoculated on sliced raw flatfish. *Food Science and Biotechnology*, *15*, 462–465.

Youn, H. S., Lee, J. K., Choi, Y. J., Saitoh, S. I., Miyake, K., Hwang, D. H., & Lee, J. Y. (2008). Cinnamaldehyde suppresses toll-like receptor 4 activation mediated through the inhibition of receptor oligomerization. *Biochemical Pharmacology*, *75*(2), 494–502. doi:10.1016/j.bcp.2007.08.033 PMID:17920563

Yue, J., Feliciano, T. J., Li, W., Lee, A., & Odom, T. W. (2017). Gold nanoparticle size and shape effects on cellular uptake and intracellular distribution of siRNA nanoconstructs. *Bioconjugate Chemistry*, *28*(6), 1791–1800. doi:10.1021/acs.bioconjchem.7b00252 PMID:28574255

Yu, J. S., & Kim, A. K. (2010). Platycodin D induces apoptosis in MCF-7 human breast cancer cells. *Journal of Medicinal Food*, *13*(2), 298–305. doi:10.1089/jmf.2009.1226 PMID:20412017

Yuki, M., Komazawa, Y., Kobayashi, Y., Kusunoki, M., Takahashi, Y., Nakashima, S., ... Kinoshita, Y. (2015). Effects of Daikenchuto on abdominal bloating accompanied by chronic constipation:A prospective, single-center randomized open trial. *Current Therapeutic Research, Clinical and Experimental*, *77*, 58–62. doi:10.1016/j.curtheres.2015.04.002 PMID:27069528

Yu, S. M., Wu, T. S., & Teng, C. M. (1994). Pharmacological characterization of cinnamophilin, a novel dual inhibitor of thromboxane synthase and thromboxane A2 receptor. *British Journal of Pharmacology*, *111*(3), 906–912. doi:10.1111/j.1476-5381.1994.tb14824.x PMID:8019768

Yusof, Y. A. M., Ahmad, N., & Das, S. (2009). Chemopreventive efficacy of ginger (Zingiber officinale) in ethionine induced rat hepatocarcinogenesis. *African Journal of Traditional, Complementary, and Alternative Medicines*, *6*, 87–93. PubMed

Zandi, P., Basu, S.K., & Khatibani, L.B. (2015). Fenugreek (*Trigonellafoenum-graecum* L.) seed: a review of physiological and biochemical properties and their genetic improvement. *Acta. Physiol. Plant.*, *37*, 1714. DOI 10.1007/s11738-014-1714-6

Zarate, R., & Yeoman, M. M. (1996). Changes in the amounts of [6]-gingerol and derivatives during a culture cycle of ginger, Zingiber officinale. *Plant Science*, *121*(1), 115–122. doi:10.1016/S0168-9452(96)04512-8

Zare, E., Pourseyedi, S., Khatami, M., & Darezereshki, E. (2017). Simple biosynthesis of zinc oxide nanoparticles using nature's source, and it's in vitro bio-activity. *Journal of Molecular Structure*, *1146*, 96–103. doi:10.1016/j.molstruc.2017.05.118

Zhang, M., Viennois, E., Prasad, M., Zhang, Y., Wang, L., Zhang, Z., ... Merlin, D. (2016). Edible ginger-derived nanoparticles: A novel therapeutic approach for the prevention and treatment of inflammatory bowel disease and colitis-associated cancer. *Biomaterials*, *101*, 321–340. doi:10.1016/j.biomaterials.2016.06.018 PMID:27318094

Zhang, Y., Shoyama, Y., Sugiura, M., & Saito, H. (1994). Effect of Crocus sativus L. On the ethanol-induced impairment of passive avoidance performances in mice. *Biological & Pharmaceutical Bulletin*, *17*, 217–221.

Zhaveh, S., Mohsenifar, A., Beiki, M., Khalili, S. T., Abdollahi, A., Rahmani-Cherati, T., & Tabatabaei, M. (2015). Encapsulation of Cuminum cyminum essential oils in chitosan-caffeic acid nanogel with enhanced antimicrobial activity against Aspergillus flavus. *Industrial Crops and Products*, *69*, 251–256. doi:10.1016/j.indcrop.2015.02.028

Zheng, G., Kenney, P. M., & Lam, L. K. (1992). Myristicin: A potential cancer chemopreventive agent from parsley leaf oil. *Journal of Agricultural and Food Chemistry*, *40*(1), 107–110. doi:10.1021/jf00013a020

Zheng, Q., Hirose, Y., Yoshimi, N., Murakami, A., Koshimizu, K., Ohigashi, H., ... Mori, H. (2002). Further investigation of the modifying effect of various chemopreventive agents on apoptosis and cell proliferation in human colon cancer cells. *Journal of Cancer Research and Clinical Oncology*, *128*(10), 539–546. doi:10.100700432-002-0373-y PMID:12384797

Zheng, W., & Wang, S. Y. (2001). Antioxidant activity and phenolic compounds in selected herbs. *Journal of Agricultural and Food Chemistry*, *49*(11), 5165–5170. doi:10.1021/jf010697n PMID:11714298

Zhigila, D. A., Abdul Rahaman, A. A., Kolawole, O. S., & Oladele, F. A. (2014). Fruit morphology as taxonomic features in five varieties of *Capsicum annuum* L. Solanaceae. *Journal of Botany*. http: //www. hindawi. Com /journals / jb / 2014/540868

Zhuang, X., Deng, Z.-B., Mu, J., Zhang, L., Yan, J., Miller, D., ... Zhang, H.-G. (2015). Ginger-derived nanoparticles protect against alcohol-induced liver damage. *Journal of Extracellular Vesicles*, *4*(1), 28713. doi:10.3402/jev.v4.28713 PMID:26610593

Zia, T., Hasnain, S. N., & Hasan, S. K. (2001). Evaluation of the oral hypoglycaemic effect of *Trigonellafoenumgraecum* L.(methi) in normal mice. *Journal of Ethnopharmacology*, *75*(2-3), 191–195. doi:10.1016/S0378-8741(01)00186-6 PMID:11297850

Zielinski, M. V. (2014). *Determination of thiamine in solution by UV-visible spectrophotometry: The effect of interactions with gold nanoparticles*. Academic Press.

Zomorodian, K., Saharkhiz, J., Pakshir, K., Immeripour, Z., & Sadatsharifi, A. (2018). The composition, antibiofilm and antimicrobial activities of essential oil of Ferula assa-foetida oleo-gum-resin. *Biocatalysis and Agricultural Biotechnology*, *14*, 300–304. doi:10.1016/j.bcab.2018.03.014

About the Contributors

Nitin Agrawal, M.Pharm, Ph.D (Jadavpur University, Govt. University), is accomplished teacher & researcher in the field of Pharmaceutical Sciences. He has more than twelve years of teaching as well as research experience. He authored more than 15 research articles in several national and international journals, one book chapter, delivered invited lecture at RIPANS, Mizoram. He also attended UGC Sponsored workshop and given presentation in more than 15 national & international conferences in India and abroad. He has completed his B. Pharm in 2005, M. Pharm in 2008 in Pharmacognosy & phytochemistry. He has awarded Ph.D from Jadavpur University, Kolkata in 2015. He got Junior Research Fellowship in DBT funded project. Presently working as Head of the Department, Faculty of Pharmacy, Raja Balwant Singh Engineering Technical Campus, Bichpuri, Agra.

Aarif Ali is working in the department of the Clinical biochemistry University of Kashmir India as a full-time Ph.D. Scholar. He has joined the department in the year 2017. He is currently working on bovine subclinical mastitis under the guidance of Dr. Showkat Ahmad Ganie, Asst. Prof. in the Department of the Clinical Biochemistry University of Kashmir. He has completed M.sc in Clinical Biochemistry in 2014, from the Department of Clinical Biochemistry Kashmir University. He has done his M.Sc. project on 'Impact of some biochemical parameters and genetic polymorphism of SLC-30A8 in the risk of type-2 diabetes mellitus'. He also has worked on the project 'Genetic susceptibility to mastitis in cows reared in temperate regions of Kashmir' as a junior research fellow He has attended 8 th JK Science Congress at the University of Kashmir. International seminar on Accu-Pressure at the University of Kashmir. Expert Lecture on Stem Cell Therapy for Brain Tumors by Dr. Khalid Shah, Faculty at Harvard Medical School, Boston. He has attended several conferences national as well as international. He has 10 research publications along with 3 book chapters.

Akanksha Awasthi worked for the past six years as Assistant Professor in Vivek Group of Colleges, Bijnor Presently employed as Senior Assistant Professor in Pharmacology BBDNIIT, Lucknow, UP.

Basharat Ahmed Bhat works in the department of Bioresources as a Ph.D. scholar. He has joined the department in 2018. He is working on the "plant molecular biology and cancer biology" under the guidance of Dr. Manzoor Ahmed Mir, senior assistant professor in the depoart5ment of bioresources Kashmir University Srinagar. He has completed his M.sc in Bioresources in 2014, from the same department. He has done his MSc project on 'study on genetic diversity of some medicinal plants using RFLP markers'. He has completed his MPhil in 2017 from Baba Ghulam Shah Badshah University, Rajouri Jammu & Kashmir (BGSBU) On the topic 'Assessment of genetic diversity in parthenium hysterochorus an invasive plant species of ISSR/AFLP marker. He has also done his B.Ed. in the year 2016, from the ADVANCED Institute of education Cluster University Srinagar Kashmir. He has published two books on immunology and more than ten book chapters at international level.

Arghya Chakravorty, is continuing his Ph.D at Vellore Institute of Technology - Vellore, India. Earlier he was Adjacent Research Associate at Research & Development Section, SANCHARAN, 4289/2003 (A Socio Cultural Organization - Registered under Societies Registration Act 1860), Agartala – 799002, India and Post Graduate Teacher, Dept. of Biological Science, Brilliant Stars School, Tripura – 799114, India. He is also life member & Tripura State Chapter President as well as founder of "Foundation for Health & Environmental Research. Earlier he was Joint Secretory of "Society of Pharmaceutical & Educational Research". Recently he has started research career after completion of M.Sc in Microbiology from Hemwati Nandan Bahuguna Garhwal (Central) University, Uttrakhand, India; Verified Certification in Biothics: The Law, Medicine, and Ethics of Reproductive Technologies and Genetics from Harvard University, USA, under supervision of Prof. I. Glenn Cohen; Verified Certification in Customer Relationship Management from Indian Institute of Management – Banglore, India, under supervision of Prof. G Shainesh. She had received Appreciation Letter for the best performance in Academic and Research while working as Guest Lecturer in Doon (P.G) Paramedical College & Hospital, Dehradun for the session July 2017 to June 2018. He is also trained from Supercomputing Facility for Computational Biology and Bioinformatics, Indian Institute of Technology Delhi; School of Medical Science & Technology, IIT Kharagpur respectively. He has received Best Poster Award in " 1st International Conference on Current Research in Effective Methodology of Pharmaceutical and Life Sciences on 14th October 2017", jointly organized by Department of The Army, United States of America & National Forum of Pharmacy Students. Except this he has attended and participated in several Workshops/ Conferences/ Seminars at National and International levels. Till now he is an active member at Society of Pharmaceutical Education and Research and State President of Urrtakhand at National Forum of Pharmacy Student, an active reviewer of Journal of Emerging Technologies and Innovative Research. He has been successfully filled one utility and one design patent at India under The Patent Act, 1970 (39 of 1970) & The Patents Rules, 2003. Right now he is editing a book on "Nano-Biotechnology" with Prof. Amar P. Garg from CRC Press, Taylor & Francis Group, USA. His research interest is enzymology, antimicrobial resistance, Nano-biotechnology and public health. He was PI of two public health projects on topic of community medicine & those were presented at international conference RECYCLE 2020, conducted by Indian Institute of Technology – Guwahati.

Tashi Choedon is a Junior Professional at National Centre of Excellence and Advanced Research on Diets (NCEARD), Lady Irwin College, Nutritionist and Freelancer, New Delhi.

M. K. Dhanya is presently working as Assistant Professor (Plant Pathology) at Cardamom Research Station, Kerala Agricultural University, Pampadumpara, Idukki, Kerala. During the past 5 years, various research projects on crop protection aspects of spices were carried out and developed suitable management practices (including bio-agents and green labeled fungicides) against major diseases of cardamom and black pepper. Research on the correlation between weather parameters and pest and disease development in cardamom and black pepper was completed in the past years. Compatibility studies of various bio-agents including entomo pathogens with commonly used insecticides and fungicides in cardamom were also done. Worked on the effect of organic amendments on soil health and plants defense mechanism.

Studies on the effect of Mycorrhiza and PPFM on drought tolerance in black pepper was carried out. Study on the defense mechanisms in black pepper plants having disease tolerance against Colletotrichum infection was completed. Working on projects for identifying molecular markers for cardamom and black pepper. .Holding the position of major advisor as well as advisory committee member of masters' and PhD students' of Plant Pathology and Agricultural Entomology from College of Agriculture, Vellayani and Vellanikkara , Kerala Agricultural University. Guiding the dissertation works of B.Sc and M.Sc students from other Universities of Kerala. Identifying field problems and suggesting suitable remedies to the farmers of the district. Handling classes to farmers, traders, pesticide dealers and extension functionaries of the district in various plant protection aspects.

Gajra Garg is a keen learner and active researcher in the field of molecular biology with a specialisation in SCAR marker development for few crops of economic importance. The author had started her career as a Research associate in gov funded project, with an experience of almost 4 years of teaching at a private university.

Ashokkumar Kaliyaperumal is presently working as Assistant Professor in Plant Breeding and Genetics from Kerala Agricultural University, Cardamom Research Station, Pampadumpara, Idukki, Kerala, India. He has completed his graduation from Agricultural College and Research Institute, Killikulam, Tamil Nadu and his post-graduation and doctoral studies was Plant Breeding and Plant biotechnology, respectively from Tamil Nadu Agricultural University, Coimbatore, Tamil Nadu, India. He has completed his Post-Doctoral Research Fellow (2010-2014) from Department of Plant sciences, University of Saskatchewan, Saskatoon, Canada. He worked Assistant Professor (Plant Breeding/ Biotechnology) from School of Agriculture, PRIST Deemed University, Thanjavur, Tamil Nadu, India. He published about 50 scientific articles in international journals like Czech Journal of Genetics and Plant Breeding, Crop science, Food composition and analysis, Natural product research and Materials letters. He published 4 books in reputed publishers. He also published about 52 popular articles in Tamil and English in monthly science magazines. He obtained six awards from conference participation and his outstanding contributions in Agricultural research.

Nimisha Mathews is currently working as an Assistant Professor (Horticulture), Cardamom Research Station, Pampadumpara, Idukki, Kerala.

Isha Mishra took her Post Graduation in Pharmacy (Pharmaceutical Chemistry) from Teerthanker Mahaveer University, Moradabad and pursuing Ph.D. in Pharmacy from IFTM University, Moradabad. She has a good teaching and research experience in the field of Pharmacy. She has written two books and published over 17 articles including research and reviews in National and International Journals of repute. At present, she is working in Institute of Pharmaceutical Research, GLA University, Mathura, U. P.

Muthusamy Murugan studied MSc (Horticulture), PhD in Agro-Ecology and Bio-security. He worked tropical major spices crops such as Cardamom, Black pepper, Chilli and minor spices crops. The year 2014 onward working as a Professor and Head, CRS Pampadumpara. Currently directing all the research activities in Cardamom Research Station, Kerala Agricultural University, Pampadumpara, Idukki, Kerala.

Abhishek Nalluri is a doctoral researcher working on development of materials and relevant technologies for fuel cells applications. Acquired working knowledge on composites, water purification, surface and environmental engineering for various customised applications. Holder of prestigious Chinese government scholarship and nominated for best international researcher. Filed few Patent applications and publications.

Anima Nanda holds the post of Director - IQACat Sathyabama Institute of Science and Technology (Deemed to be University), Chennai, India. She was also the Dean for the School of Bio & Chemical Engineering hascredited with Ph. D. degrees in Microbiology from Berhampur University, Odisha. Dr. Nanda is a renowned professor heading four departments like, Department of Biomedical Engineering, Department of Biotechnology, Department of Bioinformatics and Department of Chemical Engineering with specialized in Microbial Nanotechnology. Her laboratory studies on the role of bacteria and fungi in human health by using nanotechnology to have a better control over broad spectrum antibiotics. Her publications proved the novel bio-nanomaterials synthesized in her lab by using various fungi and bacteria isolated from various sources have a targeted therapy against human pathogenic and broad spectrum antibiotic resistant bacteria in Septicemia (MRSA and MRSE), Multi Drug Resistant Tuberculosis (MDR Tb) and Extra Drug Resistant Tuberculosis (XDR Tb). In addition to this Dr. Nanda has been heavily involved in promoting microbial nanotechnology as the cornerstone in the field of biology in India. Currently she has two ongoing Govt. of India sponsored projects worth of 2 crore and two are in process. She has research tie up with reputed institutions in National and international level. She has worked with several eminent personalities of the world at various places. Apart from this she has more than 158 publications in high impacted national and international journals along with publications in international and national conferences. To her credit she has produced 11 Ph. D. students and 7 are continuing. She has delivered more than 73 lecturers as an invited speaker in national and international level. To her credit, Dr. Nanda has four patents on staircase climbing wheel chair for physically challenged person, biomimetic hand for amputee, mobile kit for stammering person and automated sensor alert for driver in drowsy condition. She has honored with Fellow of Natural Resources and Conservation and Fellow of Indian Aerobiological Society and also received twice best teacher award, gold medalist, best project award, chaired number of technical sessions and life member of varied societies including American Nano Society and Indian Nanomedicine and a reviewer of nature scientific journal.

Surya Raj is currently working in Cardamom Research Station as a Research Associate.

Sunita Rao is working in the field of nanotechnology and its association with the phytoremediation technology, Having teaching experience of almost 5 years in an agriculture university along with various private universities. Many students have been mentored by the author for the dissertation of masters and graduation courses.

Gulzar Ahmed Rather works in the department of biomedical engineering Sathyabama University Rajiv Gandhi Salai, Chennai Tamil Nadu, 600119 India as a full-time Ph.D. Scholar. He has registered the department in the year 2017. He is working on nanobiotechnology under the guidance of Dr. Anima Nanda Dean and Prof.in the department of Biomedical Engineering. He has completed his M.sc in Biochemistry in 2014, from the department of Biochemistry Kashmir University. He has done the project on 'Level of evaluation of knowledge, attitude, and behavior of people about Alternative Medicine, .He has got more than two years of teaching experience as a biology lecturer, from 2014-2016.He has attended the 8th JK Science Congress at the University of Kashmir. International seminar on Accu-Pressure at the University of Kashmir. Expert Lecture on Stem Cell Therapy for Brain Tumors by Dr. Khalid Shah, Faculty at Harvard Medical School, Boston. Attend Five days First National workshop on techniques in biotechnology (NWTBT-17) Which was organized by the Department of Biotechnology, School of Bio and chemical engineering Sathyabama University(18th to 22nd, 2017. Attended three days National workshop on Animal cell line techniques (NACL-2017) 22nd to 24th August 2017. He has received the best paper award in a ' International conference on Bioengineering on health and environment-2018. He has attended and published papers in the 6th International Conference on Nanotechnology for the better living 7-11 April 2019 jointly organized by the National Institute of Technology (NIT) Srinagar and Indian institute of technology(IIT) Kharagpur. Besides doing Ph.D. he is also teaching students' biochemistry at B.tech level in the Department of Biomedical Engineering, from time to time he also attended ISRO exam duties as an invigilator.

Thiravidamani Sathyan is pursuing Ph. D. (Agrl. Entomology) at the department of Agrl. Entomology, CPPS, TNAU, Coimbatore, Tamil Nadu. His research area is "Studies on the native isolates of Bt against the maize fall armyworm, Spodoptera frugiperda (J.E. Smith). He has published about 16 research articles (national and international), 9 book chapters, 18 research abstracts in several conferences and seminars, 20 popular articles, 9 leaflets and also edited a book. He has participated in several national and international conferences, seminars, symposium and workshops. More ever, he was the recipient of an award " M.A. Peer Mohamed Nazeer Memorial Award- 2014 " and was instrumental in the release of two promising small cardamom varieties KAU-PV3 and KAU-PV5 during 2018. He has guided four M.Sc. students and conducted few trainings for farmers and scientists. He is one among the life member of Agricultural Scientific Tamil Society (SciTSA), New Delhi and acted as a Co-PI in a plan project of KAU. His passion is uplifting farmers through minimising plant protection costs.

Priyanka Singh is Ph.D. in Food technology from Centre of Food Technology, University of Allahabad. She has earned B. Tech. in Agricultural Engineering M. Tech in Food Technology from SHUATS, Allahabad and PGDBM in Marketing Management. She has been awarded UGC- JRF and SRF in Home science and ASRB-NET in Food Technology. She has 7 years of experience of microbiological testing in food analysis and research laboratory (NABL Accredited) and 8 years of teaching experience at graduate and post graduate level. She has published 15 Research and Review papers in international journals.

Sonia Singh, M.Pharm Pharmacognosy (KLE's College of Pharmacy, Belgaum , Karnataka). She is an accomplished teacher as well as researcher in the field of Natural herbs. She has almost completed 12 years of teaching as well as research experience in GLA University, Mathura. She authored more than 15 research articles in several national and international journals. She has attended various workshops and national conferences. Presently, she is appointed as Assistant Professor in GLA University, Mathura, Uttar Pradesh, India.

Zoomi Singh is a nutritionist and experienced researcher in the field of Nutrition in Allahabad, with a demonstrated history of working in the Dietetics department at super-specialty hospitals. Currently pursuing Ph.D. in Nutritional Sciences from Centre of Food Technology, University of Allahabad, Prayagraj (From May 2016). Skilled in Diabetes and Weight Management, Health Promotion, Nutritional Counseling, Clinical Nutrition, and Medical Nutrition Therapy. Strong research professional with a Masters Degree in Nutritional Sciences from Centre of Food Technology, University of Allahabad and previously worked as a dietician in the hospital setting for 3-4 years. "Excellent Dietician" and "Academic Excellence" award holder, Life Member of Nutrition Society of India (LM No. 2018-0178). Also working as a Team Manager in Saksham Society- NGO, Jaipur. Pubshiled one book, 9 book chapters, and research papers, presented papers in various National and International Conferences and Seminars.

Urvashi Srivastava is a Research Scholar in the Center of Food Technology, University of Allahabad Prayagraj.

Vandana Verma is currently pursuing a PhD in Food Technology from Centre of Food Technology, IPS, University of Allahabad. She participated in a 3-month project entitled "Development of Ready to Serve (RTS) Beverages of Soymilk Blended With Strawberry Pulp" from Defence Food Research Laboratory (DFRL), Mysore. She participated in a four-week online course on AGMOOCS entitled "Functional Foods: Concept, Technology and Health Benefits" (November 2018) and an eight-week online course on "Fundamentals of Agriculture Extension" (May 2019). She has published 1 book (Development of RTS Soymilk Beverages Blended with Strawberry Pulp) and 1 paper (Optimization Process for the Development of Soymilk-Based Strawberry RTS Beverages) in the UGC listed journal, Plant Archives. She has also written 2 book chapters in the books "Food Technology from Health to Wealth & Future Challenges" and "Research Trends in Food Technology and Nutrition." She has participated in 2 national seminars, 2 international seminars, 2 national workshops and also presented in 2 poster presentations and one oral presentation.

Index

I

M

N

P

S

T

U

W

Z

www.ingramcontent.com/pod-product-compliance
Lightning Source LLC
LaVergne TN
LVHW080536300926
849162LV00007B/1617